Principles and Practice of
Pharmacology for Anaesthetists

This book is dedicated to our wives

Principles and Practice of Pharmacology for Anaesthetists

T.N. Calvey, BSc, MD, PhD (Liverpool), FRCA
Honorary Senior Research Fellow
Department of Anaesthesia
University of Liverpool
Formerly Honorary Consultant, Whiston Hospital

N.E. Williams, MB, ChB (Liverpool), FFARCS (England)
Formerly Consultant Anaesthetist, Whiston Hospital, and
Part-time Lecturer in Clinical Pharmacology
University of Liverpool

FIFTH EDITION

FOREWORD BY

Jackson Rees, MB, ChB, FFARCS
Formerly Honorary Director of Studies (Paediatric Anaesthesia) and
Clinical Lecturer, Department of Anaesthesia
University of Liverpool

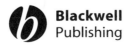

Blackwell
Publishing

First published 1981
Second edition 1991
Third edition 1997
Fourth edition 2001
Fifth edition 2008

1   2008

Library of Congress Cataloging-in-Publication Data

Calvey, T. N.
Principles and practice of pharmacology for anaesthetists / T. N. Calvey, N. E. Williams; foreword by Jackson Rees – 5th ed.
p. ; cm.
Includes bibliographical references and index.
ISBN 978-1-4051-5727-8 (alk. paper)
1. Anesthetics.   2.Pharmacology.   I. Williams, N. E. (Norton Elwy)   II. Title.
[DNLM: 1. Anesthetics–pharmacology. QV 81 C167p 2007]
RD82.C34 2007
615.1024617–dc22   2007006002

ISBN: 978-1-4051-5727-8

A catalogue record for this title is available from the British Library

Set in 9.25/11.5 Minion by Aptara Inc., New Delhi, India
Printed and bound in Singapore by Fabulous Printers Pte Ltd

Commissioning Editor: Martin Sugden
Editorial Assistant: Jamie Hartmann-Boyce
Development Editor: Adam Gilbert and Laura Murphy
Production Controller: Debbie Wyer

For further information on Blackwell Publishing, visit our website:
http://www.blackwellpublishing.com

The publisher's policy is to use permanent paper from mills that operate a sustainable forestry policy, and which has been manufactured from pulp processed using acid-free and elementary chlorine-free practices. Furthermore, the publisher ensures that the text paper and cover board used have met acceptable environmental accreditation standards.

Contents

Foreword to the First Edition

A book with a title such as this might be thought merely to present an account of the drugs used in anaesthesia. In this case, the authors have achieved much more. They have presented their subject in such a way as to give the reader an insight, which will make him not only a more competent anaesthetist, but one who will derive more satisfaction from his work by a more acute perception of the nuances of drug administration.

The authors demonstrate their awareness of the unique nature of anaesthesia amongst the disciplines of medicine. This uniqueness arises from the necessity of the anaesthetist to induce in his patient a much more dramatic attenuation of a wide range of physiological mechanisms than colleagues in other disciplines seek to achieve. He must also produce these effects in such a way that their duration can be controlled and their termination may be acute. The anaesthetist may be called upon to do this on subjects already affected by diseases and drugs which may modify the effects of the drugs which he uses. To be well-equipped to meet these challenges he needs a knowledge of the factors influencing the response to and the elimination of drugs, and of the mechanisms of drug interaction. Such knowledge is much more relevant to anaesthesia than to most other fields of medicine. The authors of this book have striven successfully to meet the needs of anaesthetists for a better understanding of these basic mechanisms of pharmacology. This is illustrated by the fact that one-third of the work is devoted to these principles. This should relieve the teacher of the frustration of having students who seem always to produce answers on the effects of drugs, but respond to the question 'Why?' with a stony silence.

Those sections of the book which deal with specific drugs show the same emphasis on mechanisms of action, thus giving life to a subject whose presentation is so often dull. The trainee who reads this book early in his career will acquire not only a great deal of invaluable information, but also an attitude and approach to the problems of his daily activity which will enhance the well-being of his patients and his own satisfaction in his work.

Jackson Rees

Preface

In this edition we have again attempted to provide a comprehensive scientific basis and a readable account of the principles of pharmacology, as well as some practical guidance in the use of drugs that is relevant to clinical anaesthesia. All the chapters have been thoroughly revised and updated with these concepts in mind, and an additional Chapter on Adverse Drug Reactions (Chapter 6) has been added, without increasing the overall size of the book. We hope that it will be of value to FRCA examination candidates, but also of interest to all anaesthetists.

In general, the book only deals with drugs that are currently available in Great Britain, so there is little mention of previously common but now discarded agents such as droperidol, trimetaphan, methohexitone or en-flurane. The structures of many commonly used agents have been included with their sites of isomerism, when appropriate, as we believe that these are generally more useful and informative than their chemical names. As in previous editions, recommended International Non-proprietary Names (rINNs) have been generally used for generic agents, although preference has been given to the current nomenclature for adrenaline and noradrenaline. As in previous editions, a comprehensive glossary covering the abbreviations and acronyms has been included to aid the reader.

Both authors are indebted to their wives for their help and forbearance during the preparation of the manuscript.

1 Drug Absorption, Distribution and Elimination

Drugs can be defined as agents that modify normal biological responses and thus produce pharmacological effects. These are frequently dependent on the transfer of drugs across one or more cellular membranes, whose structure and physicochemical properties govern the rate and extent of drug transfer.

Cellular membranes are usually about 10 nm wide and consist of a bimolecular layer of phospholipid and protein (Fig. 1.1). The lipid layer is relatively fluid, and individual phospholipid molecules can move laterally within the membrane. Extrinsic (peripheral) proteins are present on the external or internal aspect of the membrane. In contrast, intrinsic (integral) proteins traverse the entire width of the cell membrane and may form an annulus surrounding small pores or ion channels approximately 0.5 nm in diameter (Fig. 1.1). Both intrinsic and extrinsic proteins can act as enzymes or receptors and may mediate the active transport of drugs.

Approximately 5–10% of the cell membrane consists of carbohydrates, mainly glycolipids or glycoproteins. They are believed to be responsible for the immunological characteristics of cells and play an important part in molecular recognition. Many cell membranes also contain inorganic ions (e.g. Ca^{2+}).

Lipid cell membranes are excellent electrical insulators. Consequently, there may be differences in electrical potential across cellular membranes, which can facilitate or impede the passive transport of charged molecules through ion channels.

Transfer of drugs across cell membranes

In general, drugs may cross cell membranes by
- Passive diffusion
- Carrier transport

Passive diffusion

In most cases, drugs cross cell membranes by passive diffusion down a concentration gradient due to random molecular movements produced by thermal energy. The rate of drug transfer is directly proportional to the difference in concentration, and to the solubility of drugs in membranes, which is extremely variable. Highly polar substances (e.g. quaternary amines) are insoluble in membrane lipids and are unable to penetrate cellular membranes. In contrast, drugs with a high lipid solubility (e.g. diazepam, fentanyl) readily dissolve in membrane phospholipids and rapidly diffuse across cellular membranes. Other less lipid-soluble drugs (e.g. morphine) diffuse more slowly and their onset of action is often delayed.

Molecular size is a less important factor in the passive diffusion of drugs. Some low molecular weight compounds may diffuse through ion channels, or penetrate small intercellular or paracellular channels (particularly in 'leaky' epithelial membranes). In contrast, molecules larger than 100–200 Da are usually unable to cross cell membranes. The permeability of vascular endothelium is greater than other tissues, and most ionized compounds can readily cross capillary membranes.

Most drugs are weak acids or weak bases and are thus present in physiological conditions in both an ionized and a non-ionized form. Their ionization or dissociation can be represented by the equations:

$$AH \rightleftarrows A^- + H^+ \quad \text{(for acids)}$$
$$BH^+ \rightleftarrows B + H^+ \quad \text{(for bases)}$$

Weak acids and bases are predominantly present as the species AH and BH^+ in acidic conditions, but as A^- and B in alkaline conditions. The non-ionized forms AH and B are lipid soluble and can readily diffuse across cell membranes, while the ionized forms A^- and BH^+ are effectively impermeable. As the proportion of the drug that is present in the non-ionized form is dependent on pH, differences

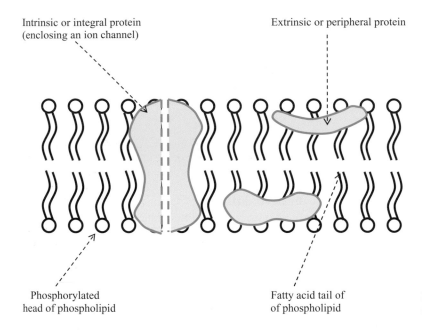

Intrinsic or integral protein (enclosing an ion channel)

Extrinsic or peripheral protein

Phosphorylated head of phospholipid

Fatty acid tail of of phospholipid

Fig. 1.1 The phospholipid and protein structure of a typical cell membrane.

in H^+ concentration across cellular membranes can provide a diffusion gradient for the passive transfer of the non-ionized form.

Consider a weak acidic drug that dissociates in the manner:

$$AH \rightleftharpoons A^- + H^+$$

From the Henderson–Hasselbalch equation, it can be shown that

$$pK_a - pH \rightleftharpoons \log \frac{[AH]}{[A^-]},$$

where [AH] and [A$^-$] are the concentrations of non-ionized and ionized forms and pK_a (the negative logarithm of the dissociation constant) is the pH value at which [AH] = [A$^-$]. If the pK_a of the drug is 6, at pH 2 (e.g. in gastric fluid), almost 100% is present in the form AH (Fig. 1.2). This non-ionized form will rapidly diffuse into plasma (pH 7.4) where approximately 96% will be converted to A$^-$, providing a concentration gradient for the continued diffusion of AH. Subsequent transfer of the drug to other sites will also be dependent on the relative pH gradient. At pH 8, as in interstitial fluid or alkaline urine, the concentration of AH is less than at pH 7.4. A gradient is thus created for the passive diffusion of AH across renal tubular epithelium, followed by its subsequent ionization to A$^-$ and elimination from the body (Fig. 1.2). By con-

trast, at a urine pH of 7 or less, the concentration of AH is greater in urine than in plasma, and the excreted drug will tend to diffuse back into plasma.

In a similar manner, pH gradients govern the non-ionic diffusion of weak bases that associate with hydrogen ions. In these conditions,

$$B + H^+ \rightleftharpoons BH^+$$

From the Henderson–Hasselbalch equation, it can be shown that

$$pK_a - pH \rightleftharpoons \log \frac{[BH^+]}{[B]},$$

where [BH$^+$] and [B] are the concentrations of the ionized and the non-ionized forms and pK_a is the pH value at which [BH$^+$] = [B]. If the pK_a of the basic drug is 7, at pH 2 (e.g. in the stomach), almost 100% is present as the ionized form BH$^+$ (Fig. 1.3). At pH 5.5 (e.g. in the small intestine), only 3% is present as the non-ionized form B, and thus available to diffuse across the cell membrane. Although the effective pH gradient does not facilitate the non-ionic diffusion of weak bases from the small intestine (pH 5.5) to plasma (pH 7.4), the continuous perfusion of intestinal capillaries provides a small concentration gradient for their absorption.

By contrast, weak bases at pH 7.4 (e.g. in plasma) are mainly present as the non-ionized species B. In these

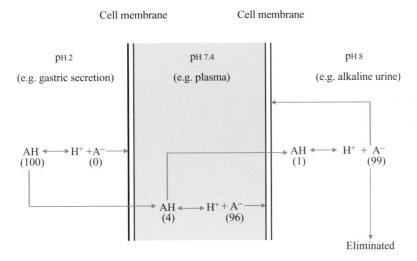

Fig. 1.2 Non-ionic diffusion of the weak acid AH ($pK_a = 6$). Only the non-ionized form AH can diffuse across cell membranes, and the diffusion gradient is dependent on pH differences between compartments or tissues. Numbers in parentheses correspond to the percentage of the drug present as AH and A^- at pH 2, 7.4 and 8.

conditions, there is a large concentration gradient that facilitates their diffusion into the stomach (pH 2) and into acid urine (pH 5). Following intravenous administration of fentanyl, the initial decline in plasma concentration may be followed by a secondary peak 30–40 minutes later. Fentanyl is a weak base which can diffuse from plasma (pH 7.4) to the stomach (pH 2), due to the large concentration gradient that is present, and its subsequent reabsorption from the small intestine is responsible for the secondary rise in the plasma concentration. Similarly, weak bases rapidly diffuse from plasma (pH 7.4) to urine (pH 5) as

the non-ionized species B, where they are converted to the ionic form BH^+ and rapidly eliminated (Fig. 1.3).

In theory, modification of urine pH can increase the proportion of weak acids ($pK_a = 3.0$–7.5) and weak bases ($pK_a = 7.5$–10.5) that are present in an ionized form in urine, and thus enhance their elimination in drug-induced poisoning. Although forced alkaline diuresis was once extensively used in drug overdosage, as with salicylates or phenobarbital, it has little or no place in current therapy. It is a potentially hazardous procedure that requires the infusion of relatively large amounts of fluid and the use of

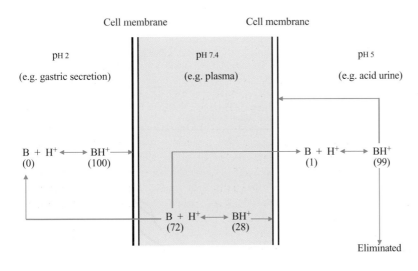

Fig. 1.3 Non-ionic diffusion of the weak base B ($pK_a = 7$). Only the non-ionized form B can diffuse across cell membranes, and the diffusion gradient is dependent on pH differences between compartments or tissues. Numbers in parentheses correspond to the percentage of the drug present as B and BH^+ at pH 2, 7.4 and 5.

loop diuretics or mannitol. In addition, pulmonary and cerebral oedema are possible complications, particularly in the elderly.

Carrier transport

Carrier transport can be divided into two main types:
- Facilitated diffusion
- Active transport

Facilitated diffusion

Facilitated diffusion is a form of carrier transport that does not require the expenditure of cellular energy. Many physiological substrates combine with specific sites on intrinsic proteins, resulting in conformational (allosteric) changes in protein structure. These changes facilitate the transcellular transport of many endogenous compounds. In these conditions, physiological substrates enter cells down a concentration gradient, but at a faster rate than anticipated from their lipid solubility or molecular size. Facilitated diffusion mediates the absorption of some simple sugars, steroids, amino acids and pyrimidines from the small intestine and their subsequent transfer across cell membranes.

Active transport

In contrast, active transport requires cellular or metabolic energy and can transfer drugs against a concentration gradient. In some instances, metabolic energy is directly produced from the hydrolysis of ATP (primary active transport). More commonly, metabolic energy is provided by the active transport of Na^+, or is dependent on the electrochemical gradient produced by the sodium pump, Na^+/K^+ ATPase (secondary active transport). It is generally considered that the drug or substrate initially combines with an intrinsic carrier protein (which may be an ion channel or Na^+/K^+ ATPase). The drug–protein complex is then transferred across the cell membrane, where the drug is released and the carrier protein returns to the opposite side of the membrane.

Active transport systems are saturable and specific and can be inhibited by other drugs (Chapter 4). They play a crucial role in the transfer of drugs across cell membranes at many sites, including the small intestine, the proximal renal tubule, the biliary canaliculus and the choroid plexus (Tables 1.1 and 1.2). A drug transport protein (P-glycoprotein) appears to play an important role as an efflux pump at many of these sites (i.e. it transports drugs from intracellular fluid across plasma membranes). Other

Table 1.1 Some acidic and basic drugs eliminated from plasma by active transport in the proximal renal tubule.

Acidic drugs	Basic drugs
Penicillins	Dopamine
Cephalosporins	Morphine
Salicylates	Neostigmine
Sulphonamides	Lidocaine
Thiazide diuretics	Quinidine
Furosemide	
Chlorpropamide	
Methotrexate	

active transport systems transfer physiological substrates across cell membranes. For example, at sympathetic nerve endings the transport of noradrenaline across the neuronal membrane (Uptake$_1$) is coupled to the active exclusion of Na^+ by the sodium pump.

Plasma concentration of drugs and their pharmacological effects

Although the plasma concentrations of drugs can usually be measured, it is often impossible to determine their effective concentration in tissues. In some instances, it may be possible to derive an approximate estimate of their concentration by pharmacokinetic techniques (Chapter 2). The principal factors that determine the plasma concentration of drugs are
- Absorption
- Distribution
- Metabolism
- Excretion

Table 1.2 Some acidic and basic drugs secreted from liver cells into biliary canaliculi.

Acidic drugs	Basic drugs
Amoxicillin	Vecuronium
Ampicillin	Pancuronium
Cefaloridine	Glycopyrronium
Sulphobromophthalein	Mepenzolate
Probenecid	
Rifampicin	

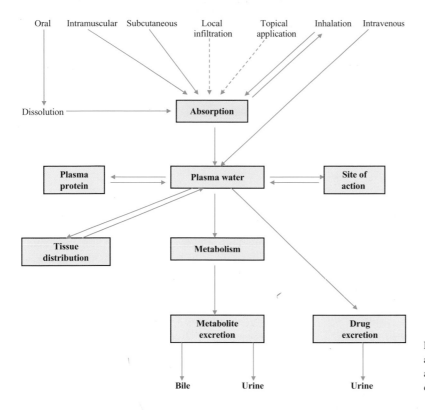

Fig. 1.4 The relation between drug absorption, distribution, metabolism and excretion, and the concentration of drugs at their site of action.

These factors also affect the concentration of drugs at their site of action (Fig. 1.4), and thus modify the magnitude and duration of their effects and the time course of drug action.

Drug administration

Drugs are most commonly administered orally, by subcutaneous, intramuscular, or intravenous injection, by local infiltration or by inhalation. Occasionally, drugs are given sublingually, rectally, or by application to other epithelial surfaces (e.g. the skin, nose or eye).

Oral administration

Oral administration is obviously most convenient and acceptable for the patient. Nevertheless, not all drugs can be taken orally. Some drugs are unstable in the acid medium of the stomach (e.g. benzylpenicillin, erythromycin), while others may irritate the gastric mucosa and cause nausea, vomiting or haemorrhage (e.g. salicylates, concentrated solutions of most salts). In recent years, these problems have been partially avoided by the use of enteric-coated tablets or slow-release preparations, which only dissolve in the upper small intestine.

When drugs are taken orally, there is usually a latent period of 30–120 minutes before they reach their maximum concentration in plasma. The presence of adequate drug concentrations in plasma is dependent on
• Drug dissolution
• Drug absorption
• The absence of significant first-pass effects in the gut wall or the liver

Drug dissolution
The dissolution of agents administered as tablets or capsules is essential before drug absorption can take place. Drug dissolution usually occurs in the stomach and may

be dependent on gastric acidity. Variations in the speed of dissolution and the rate and extent of gastric emptying can thus affect the amount of drug in solution in the upper part of the small intestine (where absorption mainly occurs).

Many pharmaceutical factors influence the dissolution of tablets and capsules, including particle size, chemical formulation, the inclusion of inert fillers and the outer coating of the tablet. In these circumstances, proprietary or generic preparations of the same drug may have different dissolution characteristics and thus produce a range of plasma concentrations after oral administration. At one time, differences in the potency of digoxin tablets suspected from clinical observations were eventually traced to variations in the dissolution of different preparations of the drug. Similarly, toxic effects were produced by diphenylhydantoin (phenytoin) tablets when an excipient (calcium sulphate) was replaced by lactose. In these conditions, dissolution was more rapid, resulting in faster and more extensive absorption, and higher blood levels of the drugs.

Sustained release preparations

Sustained release oral preparations usually consist of multi-lamellated erodable polymers and are designed to allow the slow continuous release of drugs. Other formulations may permit the release of fixed doses of a drug at regular intervals. Some preparations are osmotically active, or incorporate an ion-exchange resin that allows drugs to be released in solution at a defined ionic concentration and pH. Their use often results in greater convenience and safety, improves bioavailability and causes less variability in plasma concentrations. They may also reduce side effects, drug dosage, frequency of administration and cost.

Many drugs may be administered in this manner, including some opioid analgesics, NSAIDs, bronchodilators, antihypertensive drugs, antiarrhythmic agents and potassium salts.

Drug absorption

The absorption of drugs in the stomach and the small intestine is primarily dependent on their physicochemical properties, particularly their lipid solubility. Non-ionized compounds (e.g. ethyl alcohol) and low molecular weight substances (e.g. urea) readily cross cell membranes by passive diffusion and are easily and rapidly absorbed from the gut. Drugs that are weak acids (e.g. aspirin) are predominantly non-ionized and lipid-soluble in acidic conditions and partially diffuse into plasma from the stom-

ach. In contrast, basic drugs (e.g. propranolol, most benzodiazepines) are less ionized and more lipid-soluble in alkaline conditions and are preferentially absorbed from the duodenum (pH 5–6). Strong bases (e.g. quaternary amines) are always ionized in solution and are not significantly absorbed from the gut.

In practice, other factors influence the site of drug absorption. Mucosal surface area is more extensive in the upper small intestine than the stomach, and most drugs, whether acids or bases, are predominantly absorbed from the duodenum. Nevertheless, some non-ionized compounds and acidic drugs may be partially absorbed from the stomach and may produce a rapid increase in plasma concentration after oral administration.

Drugs that affect gastric motility

Compounds affecting gastric motility can modify drug dissolution, and influence the rate, but not the extent, of drug absorption. In particular, drugs that slow gastric emptying (e.g. atropine, morphine) decrease the rate of drug absorption. Other drug interactions, as between tetracyclines and iron, or colestyramine and digoxin, may affect the extent of drug absorption and thus modify systemic bioavailability. Drug absorption may be reduced in pathological conditions affecting the gastrointestinal tract, particularly in coeliac disease, Crohn's disease, obstructive jaundice, or after extensive resection of the small intestine.

Drug absorption and carrier transport

Although most drugs are absorbed from the stomach and small intestine by passive diffusion, occasionally absorption is dependent on carrier transport. Levodopa is absorbed by a carrier protein that normally transports amino acids, and fluorouracil is absorbed by the carrier that transports pyrimidine bases. In contrast, a carrier protein (P-glycoprotein) can transport many drugs from the intracellular environment to the intestinal lumen and actively opposes drug absorption. It is constitutively expressed on the luminal surface of most intestinal cells.

Subcutaneous and intramuscular administration

Some drugs do not produce adequate plasma concentrations or pharmacological effects after oral administration and are usually given subcutaneously or intramuscularly.

In particular, drugs broken down in the gut (e.g. ben-zylpenicillin, polypeptide hormones), are poorly or un-predictably absorbed (e.g. aminoglycosides), or drugs that have significant first-pass effects (e.g. opioid analgesics), are often given by these routes. Drugs are sometimes given by the intramuscular route when patients are intolerant of oral preparations (e.g. iron salts) or when patient compliance is known to be poor (e.g. in schizophrenia).

Absorption of drugs by subcutaneous or intramuscular administration is not usually dependent on the dissociation constant of the drug or its pH, but is often determined by regional blood flow. The onset of action of a drug given by intramuscular injection is usually more rapid and the duration of action shorter than when the subcutaneous route is used because of differences in the perfusion of muscle and subcutaneous tissues. The subcutaneous administration of relatively insoluble drugs or drug complexes is sometimes used to slow the rate of absorption and prolong the duration of action (e.g. with preparations of insulin or penicillin). In these conditions, the rate of dissolution of the drug from the complex and its subsequent absorption governs the duration of action.

Implantable subcutaneous preparations are sometimes used in hormone replacement therapy (e.g. estradiol and testosterone implants). Controlled release systems capable of an increased release rate on demand (by the external application of magnetic or ultrasonic fields, or the use of enzymes) are being developed.

Intravenous administration

Drugs are usually given intravenously when a rapid or an immediate onset of action is necessary. When given by this route, their effects are usually dependable and reproducible. This method of administration often permits the dose to be accurately related to its effects, and thus eliminates some of the problems associated with interindividual variability in drug response. Although most drugs can be safely given as a rapid intravenous bolus, in some instances (e.g. aminophylline) they must be given slowly to avoid the cardiac complications associated with high plasma concentrations. Irritant drugs must be given intravenously in order to avoid local tissue or vascular complications. Some drugs (e.g. diazepam) can cause local complications such as superficial thrombophlebitis after intravenous administration. It is uncertain if this is related to the pH of the injected solution. When drugs that release histamine from mast cells are given intravenously

(e.g. vancomycin, morphine) local or generalized vasodilatation and oedema ('flare and weal') in the surrounding tissues may be observed.

Mini-infusion pumps and syringe drivers

The development of mini-infusion pumps for intermittent intravenous drug delivery is particularly valuable in pain relief. Some of these devices incorporate electronic pumps to provide 'on-demand' bolus release of the drug according to the patient's needs. Alternatively, the use of gravity methods and balloon reservoir devices provide accurate mechanical control of drug administration. Battery-operated syringe drivers for the continuous administration of opioid analgesics are particularly valuable in the domiciliary management of patients with intractable pain associated with malignant disease.

Targeted drug delivery

Some delivery systems have been designed to selectively target drugs to their desired site of action, thus avoiding excessive toxicity and rapid inactivation. For instance, microparticulate carrier systems (e.g. liposomes, red cells, microspherical beads) have been occasionally used in the treatment of infectious and neoplastic diseases. Similarly, drugs conjugated with antibodies are sometimes used in the management of malignant disease. In these conditions, the more extensive use of 'pro-drugs' often leads to greater target specificity.

Other routes of drug administration

Transmucosal administration

Drugs are frequently applied to mucous membranes at various sites, including the conjunctiva, nose, larynx and the mucosal surfaces of the genitourinary tract, to produce topical effects. Antibiotics, steroids and local anaesthetic agents are commonly used for this purpose. Systemic absorption readily occurs due to the high vascularity of mucous areas, and local anaesthetics may produce toxic effects.

Alternatively, drugs may be administered to mucosal areas in order to provide a more rapid onset of systemic action and to avoid first-pass metabolism. The buccal route (i.e. the positioning of tablets between the teeth and the gum) may be used for the administration of glyceryl trinitrate, hyoscine and prochlorperazine. Similarly, oral transmucosal administration of opioid analgesics using drug impregnated 'lollipops' has been employed in the management of postoperative pain.

Nasal administration

Certain hypothalamic and pituitary polypeptides that are destroyed in the gut are given by nasal administration. A number of other drugs, including opioid analgesics, steroids, histamine antagonists, propranolol and vitamin B_{12}, can also be given by this route. These drugs may be partly absorbed from vascular lymphoid tissue on the nasal mucosa. Other evidence suggests that some drugs are rapidly absorbed from the nasal mucosa to the CSF and the cerebral circulation, since the submucous space of the nose is in direct contact with the subarachnoid space adjacent to the olfactory lobes. After nasal administration, the concentration of some drugs in the CSF may be significantly higher than in plasma.

Transdermal administration

Most drugs are poorly absorbed through intact skin. The stratum corneum is the main barrier to the diffusion of drugs, and its lipid lamellar bilayers prevent the penetration of polar compounds. Nevertheless, some extremely potent drugs with a high lipid solubility (e.g. glyceryl trinitrate, hyoscine) are absorbed transdermally and can produce systemic effects when applied to the skin. In these conditions, the stratum corneum may act as a reservoir for lipid-soluble drugs for several days after administration is stopped. The absorption of drugs from the skin may be influenced by the vehicle used for administration and can be increased by the use of various penetration enhancers (e.g. dimethyl sulfoxide).

Local anaesthetic preparations (EMLA, tetracaine gel) are frequently used to produce analgesia prior to venepuncture. An occlusive dressing and a relatively long contact time (30–45 min) are required to produce effective analgesia.

Infiltration techniques

Local anaesthetics are commonly infiltrated into the skin or mucous membranes when it is important to confine their action to a region or an area of the body; they are often combined with vasoconstrictors in order to restrict their absorption and prolong the duration of drug action. Alternatively, they may be injected at various sites on nerves and nerve plexuses to produce conduction anaesthesia. Local anaesthetics, analgesics and occasionally antibiotics may also be given by intrathecal injection.

Inhalation

The uptake and distribution of inhalational anaesthetic agents is dependent on their transfer from alveoli to pulmonary capillaries. Many factors, which include the inspired concentration, adequacy of pulmonary ventilation, lipid solubility and blood–gas partition coefficient of individual agents determine the rate of transfer (Chapter 8).

Corticosteroids and some bronchodilators are given to produce a local action on respiratory bronchioles and to avoid systemic effects. Particle size may influence their distribution to the site of action. In general, particles with a diameter greater than 10 μm are deposited in the upper respiratory tract. Particles with a diameter of 2–10 μm are deposited in bronchioles, while those with a diameter less that 2 μm reach the alveoli.

Drug distribution

After administration and absorption, drugs are initially present in plasma and may be partly bound to plasma proteins. They may subsequently gain access to interstitial fluid and intracellular water, depending on their physicochemical properties (in particular, their lipid solubility and ionic dissociation). Consequently, they may be rapidly distributed in other tissues and organs. When distribution is complete their concentration in plasma water and extracellular fluid is approximately equal.

The distribution of drugs in the body is extremely variable (Table 1.3). It may be assessed by preclinical studies in experimental animals or by pharmacokinetic methods. Some drugs are extensively protein-bound and are predominantly present in plasma. Similarly, ionized compounds cannot readily penetrate most cell membranes and are largely distributed in extracellular fluid. Consequently, these drugs usually have a low apparent volume of distribution. In contrast, lipid-soluble drugs with a relatively low molecular weight are widely distributed in tissues. For instance, ethyl alcohol, urea and some sulphonamides are evenly distributed throughout body water. These drugs usually have a volume of distribution similar to total body water. Other drugs penetrate cells and are extensively bound to tissue proteins, or are sequestered in fat. In these conditions, the volume of distribution is characteristically greater than total body water.

Following intravenous administration, some drugs are initially sequestered by well-perfused tissues, but are subsequently redistributed to other organs as the plasma

Table 1.3 The volumes of physiological compartments and the main sites of distribution of some common drugs.

Compartment	Volume (mL kg^{-1})	Drug (V: mL kg^{-1})
Plasma	50–80	Heparin (60) Tolbutamide (100) Warfarin (140)
Extracellular fluid	150–250	Acetylsalicylic acid (150) Atracurium (160) Chlorothiazide (200) Sulphamethoxazole (210) Mivacurium (210) Vecuronium (230)
Total body water Total body water + cell and tissue binding	500–700 >700	Ethyl alcohol (500) Bupivacaine (1000) Lidocaine (1300) Prilocaine (2700) Thiopental (2300) Morphine (3000) Pethidine (4400) Digoxin (8500)

Values for the distribution volume (V) of the drugs are shown in parentheses.

concentration declines. Approximately 25% of thiopental is initially taken up by the brain due to its high lipid solubility and the extensive blood supply of the CNS. As the plasma concentration falls, thiopental is progressively taken up by less well-perfused tissues which have a higher affinity for the drug. In consequence, intravenous thiopental is rapidly redistributed from brain to muscle and finally to subcutaneous fat. Redistribution is mainly responsible for its short duration of action, and its final elimination from the body may be delayed for 24 hours.

Some drugs tend to be localized in certain tissues or organs, for example, iodine is concentrated in the thyroid gland and tetracyclines in developing teeth and bone. The concentration of drugs in these tissues may be much greater than in plasma. Drugs that are widely distributed in tissues and concentrated in cells may have an extremely large volume of distribution, which is usually greater than total body water (e.g. phenothiazines, tricyclic antidepressants).

Blood–brain barrier
Structure

Many drugs are widely distributed in most tissues, but do not readily enter the CNS. In cerebral capillaries, endothelial cells have overlapping 'tight' junctions restricting passive diffusion. The surrounding capillary basement membrane is closely applied to the peripheral processes of astrocytes, which play an important part in neuronal nutrition (Fig. 1.5). To pass from capillary blood to the brain, most drugs have to cross the endothelium, the basement membrane and the peripheral processes of astrocytes by simple diffusion or filtration. Some drugs cannot readily cross these restrictive barriers, which are collectively referred to as the 'blood–brain barrier'.

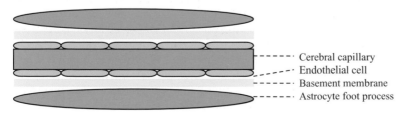

Cerebral capillary
Endothelial cell
Basement membrane
Astrocyte foot process

Fig. 1.5 Diagrammatic representation of the blood–brain barrier, showing the endothelial cells with tight junctions, the basement membrane and the foot processes of astrocytes.

Enzymatic blood–brain barrier

In addition to this structural barrier, there is also a metabolic or enzymatic blood–brain barrier, which is mainly associated with the peripheral processes of astrocytes. Many potentially neurotoxic agents (e.g. free fatty acids, ammonia) can readily cross the capillary endothelium, but are metabolized before they reach the CNS. Monoamine oxidase and cholinesterases are also present in capillary endothelium, and some neurotransmitters may be metabolized as they cross the blood–brain barrier. In addition, capillary endothelial cells express a transport protein (P-glycoprotein), which actively extrudes many drugs, including most opioids, from the CNS.

Consequently, the blood–brain barrier is not simply a passive and immutable structural barrier, but a dynamic membrane interface between the blood and the brain. Both its structure and function are dependent on trophic factors secreted by astrocytes. It develops during the first trimester of foetal life, but is immature at birth, when it is often less restrictive to drugs and endogenous substances than in adult life.

Drug permeability

Certain metabolic substrates and hormones, such as glucose, insulin, L-amino acids, L-thyroxine and transferrin, normally cross the blood–brain barrier by endocytosis or carrier transport. In addition, many low molecular weight, lipid-soluble drugs (e.g. general anaesthetics, local anaesthetics, opioid analgesics) can cross the barrier and enter the CNS, although their access may be restricted by P-glycoprotein. In contrast, when drugs are highly protein-bound (e.g. tolbutamide, warfarin), only the unbound fraction can readily diffuse from blood to the CNS, so that the concentration of these drugs in the brain may be 1–2% of the total plasma level. Drugs that are highly ionized (e.g. quaternary amines) cannot cross the blood–brain barrier, and muscle relaxants do not enter or affect the brain. Similarly, dyes that are protein-bound (e.g. Evans blue) and drugs with a large molecular weight (e.g. ciclosporin, erythromycin) do not readily cross the blood–brain barrier. Some drugs (e.g. benzylpenicillin) cannot penetrate the barrier or enter the brain unless its permeability is increased by inflammation (e.g. in bacterial meningitis). The normal impermeability of the blood–brain barrier can be modified by pathological changes, which include inflammation, oedema and acute and chronic hypertension.

Physiological deficiency

In some parts of the brain, principally the area postrema, the median eminence, the pineal gland and the choroid plexus, the blood–brain barrier is deficient or absent. In these areas, the diffusion of drugs and the exchange of endogenous substrates is not restricted. For example, in the choroid plexus drugs may freely diffuse from capillary blood to CSF across the relatively permeable choroidal epithelium. Similarly, the ependyma lining the cerebral ventricles does not appear to restrict the diffusion of most drugs. Neuropeptides and certain ionized compounds (e.g. benzylpenicillin, probenecid) may be actively secreted in the opposite direction, i.e. from cerebral ventricles into capillary blood.

Placental transfer
Structure and function

During late pregnancy, structural changes occur in the placenta, involving the gradual disappearance of the cytotrophoblast and the loss of chorionic connective tissue from placental villi. At term, maternal and foetal blood compartments are separated by a single layer of chorion (the syncytiotrophoblast) in continuous contact with the endothelial cells of foetal capillaries. Consequently, the placental barrier consists of a vasculosyncytial membrane, and from a functional point of view behaves like a typical lipid membrane. Most low molecular weight, lipid-soluble drugs are readily transferred across the placenta, and their rate of removal from maternal blood is dependent on placental blood flow, the area available for diffusion and the magnitude of the effective diffusion gradient. In contrast, large molecular weight or polar molecules cannot readily cross the vasculosyncytial membrane. Almost all drugs that cross the blood–brain barrier and affect the CNS can also cross the placenta, and their elimination by foetal tissues may be difficult and prolonged.

Drugs and the foetus

Some drugs that readily cross the placenta are known to produce foetal abnormalities if taken in pregnancy (Table 1.4). Many other drugs can readily diffuse from maternal plasma to the foetus and may cause complications when used in late pregnancy. These include inhalational anaesthetics, intravenous agents, local anaesthetics and many analgesics such as morphine and pethidine. Similarly, some β-adrenoceptor antagonists (e.g. propranolol) can cross the placenta and may cause foetal bradycardia and hypoglycaemia. When diazepam is used in late pregnancy as in the treatment of preeclampsia and eclampsia, it readily crosses the placenta, but is not effectively metabolized by the foetus. Several of its active metabolites (including both desmethyldiazepam and oxazepam)

Table 1.4 Drugs that may cause foetal damage or malformation (teratogenic effects) if taken during pregnancy.

Drug	Effect on foetus
Methotrexate	Hydrocephalus; neural tube defects
Tretinoin	Hydrocephalus
Phenytoin	Cleft lip and palate; cardiac defects
Sodium valproate	Neural tube defects
Oestrogens	Vaginal adenosis; testicular atrophy
Aminoglycosides	Cochlear and vestibular damage
Tetracyclines	Dental pigmentation; enamel hypoplasia
Carbimazole	Goitre; hypothyroidism
Propylthiouracil	Goitre; hypothyroidism
Warfarin	Nasal hypoplasia; epiphyseal calcification

accumulate in foetal tissues and can cause neonatal hypotonia and hypothermia. By contrast, ionized compounds (e.g. muscle relaxants) cannot readily cross the placenta.

Protein binding

Plasma protein binding plays an essential role in the transport and distribution of drugs. Most drugs are relatively lipid-soluble, but are only poorly soluble in plasma water. Consequently, binding to plasma proteins is essential for their transport in plasma.

Most drugs are reversibly bound to plasma proteins, according to the reaction:

unbound drug + protein $\rightleftarrows$ drug − protein complex

During perfusion, the unbound drug diffuses into tissues, and as its concentration in plasma falls, protein-bound drug rapidly dissociates. Consequently, a continuous concentration gradient is present for the diffusion of drugs from plasma to tissues.

Binding by albumin and globulins
Albumin usually plays the most important role in the binding of drugs. It has a number of distinct binding sites with a variable affinity for drugs, and mainly binds neutral or acidic compounds, including salicylates, indometacin, tolbutamide, carbenoxolone and oral anticoagulants. Some basic drugs and physiological substrates

such as bilirubin, fatty acids and tryptophan are also bound by albumin.

Globulins bind many basic drugs (e.g. bupivacaine, opioid analgesics). These drugs are mainly bound by β-globulins or by α_1-acid glycoprotein. Plasma globulins also play an important part in the binding of minerals, vitamins and hormones. Hydrocortisone (cortisol) is mainly transported in plasma by a specific globulin (transcortin) for which it has a high affinity.

Some drugs (e.g. pancuronium) are bound by both globulins and albumin. Indeed, the resistance to muscle relaxants that often occurs in liver disease may be due to their increased binding by plasma globulins.

Extent of plasma protein binding
The extent of plasma protein binding of drugs ranges from 0% to almost 100%, even among closely related drugs (Table 1.5). Thus, the binding of local anaesthetics to α_1-acid glycoprotein ranges from 6% (procaine) to 95% (bupivacaine). In some instances (diazepam, phenytoin, warfarin) unbound, pharmacologically active concentrations are only 1–5% of total plasma levels. The concentration of drugs in salivary secretions and CSF often reflects the level of the unbound drug in plasma. Alternatively, the concentration of the unbound drug can be determined by various *in vitro* techniques, such as equilibrium dialysis or ultrafiltration.

Table 1.5 Plasma protein binding of some common anaesthetic drugs.

Drug	Plasma protein binding (%)
Prilocaine	55
Lidocaine	65
Tetracaine	75
Ropivacaine	94
Bupivacaine	95
Morphine	30
Pethidine	64
Fentanyl	80
Alfentanil	90
Atracurium	<20
Vecuronium	<20
Pancuronium	30
Thiopental	80
Etomidate	75
Propofol	97
Diazepam	97

Drug competition and displacement

Drugs and endogenous substrates that are extensively bound to proteins may compete for (and be displaced from) their binding sites. In most instances, binding of drugs at clinical concentrations only occupies a small proportion of the available binding sites and does not approach saturation. Consequently, competition between drugs resulting in clinically significant displacement from plasma protein binding is extremely rare (Chapter 4).

Protein binding and drug elimination

The hepatic clearance of many drugs is limited by liver blood flow and is not restricted by plasma protein binding (which is a rapidly reversible process). Drug dissociation from binding to plasma proteins probably occurs within microseconds or milliseconds. By contrast, the hepatic perfusion time may be several seconds or more. Thus, extensive protein binding only decreases hepatic clearance when the ability of the liver to extract, metabolize or excrete the drug is low. Similarly, protein binding is unlikely to restrict the renal elimination of drugs, either by the glomerulus or the renal tubule. Only the unbound drug is secreted by the proximal tubule, but the resultant decrease in its plasma concentration leads to the immediate dissociation of protein-bound drug in order to maintain equilibrium. Indeed, a number of protein-bound drugs are completely cleared in a single passage through the kidney (e.g. benzylpenicillin).

Protein binding in pathological conditions

Binding to plasma proteins is modified in pathological conditions associated with hypoalbuminaemia, as in hepatic cirrhosis, nephrosis, trauma or burns. In these conditions, the concentration of the unbound drug tends to increase and may result in toxic effects (e.g. with phenytoin or prednisolone). Significant changes are particularly likely when high doses of drugs are used, or when drugs are given intravenously. In these conditions, binding to albumin and other plasma proteins may be saturated, causing a disproportionate increase in the concentration of the unbound drug. Tissues and organs that are well perfused (e.g. brain, heart, abdominal viscera) may receive a higher proportion of the dose, predisposing them to potential toxic effects. Similar effects may occur in elderly patients and in subjects with renal impairment, possibly due to alterations in the affinity of drugs for albumin. The plasma concentration of α_1-acid glycoprotein can also be modified by a number of pathological conditions including myocardial infarction, rheumatoid arthritis, Crohn's disease, renal failure and malignant disease, as well as operative surgery. In these conditions, the binding of basic drugs (e.g. propranolol, chlorpromazine) is increased, and the concentration of the free, unbound drug is reduced.

Drug metabolism

Most drugs are eliminated by drug metabolism, which mainly occurs in the liver. Nevertheless, certain drugs are partly or completely broken down by other tissues. Some esters that are used in anaesthesia are hydrolysed by plasma cholinesterase (e.g. suxamethonium, mivacurium) or red cell acetylcholinesterase (e.g. esmolol, remifentanil). In addition, drugs may be partly or completely metabolized by the gut (e.g. morphine, chlorpromazine), the kidney (e.g. midazolam, dopamine) or the lung (e.g. angiotensin I, prilocaine).

Nevertheless, the liver is mainly responsible for the breakdown of drugs. Hepatic metabolism decreases the concentration of the active drug in plasma, and thus promotes its removal from the site of action. This mainly involves the enzymatic conversion of lipid-soluble nonpolar drugs into water-soluble polar compounds, which can be filtered by the renal glomerulus or secreted into urine or bile.

Metabolism usually reduces the biological activity of drugs, and most metabolites have less inherent activity than their parent compounds. In addition, their ability to penetrate to receptor sites is limited because of their poor lipid solubility. Nevertheless, some drugs are relatively inactive when administered, and require metabolism to produce or enhance their pharmacological effects (Table 1.6). Other drugs may be metabolized to compounds

Table 1.6 Drugs that require metabolism to produce their pharmacological effects.

Drug	Active metabolite
Prontosil red	Sulphanilamide
Chloral hydrate	Trichlorethanol
Cyclophosphamide	Phosphoramide mustard
Cortisone	Hydrocortisone
Prednisone	Prednisolone
Methyldopa	Methylnoradrenaline
Proguanil	Cycloguanil
Enalapril	Enalaprilat

Table 1.7 Phase 1 reactions resulting in drug oxidation, reduction and hydrolysis.

Reaction	Site	Enzyme	Example
Oxidation	Hepatic endoplasmic reticulum	Cytochrome P450	Thiopental → pentobarbital
	Mitochondria	Monoamine oxidase	Dopamine → dihydroxyphenylacetaldehyde
	Hepatic cell cytoplasm	Alcohol dehydrogenase	Alcohol → acetaldehyde
Reduction	Hepatic endoplasmic reticulum	Cytochrome P450	Halothane → chlorotrifluoroethane
	Hepatic cell cytoplasm	Alcohol dehydrogenase	Chloral hydrate → trichlorethanol
Hydrolysis	Hepatic endoplasmic reticulum	Carboxyesterase	Pethidine → pethidinic acid
	Plasma	Cholinesterase	Suxamethonium → succinate + choline
	Erythrocyte	Acetylcholinesterase	Remifentanil → carboxylated derivatives
	Neuromuscular junction	Acetylcholinesterase	Acetylcholine → acetate + choline
	Hepatic cell cytoplasm	Amidase	Lidocaine → 2,6-xylidine + diethylglycine

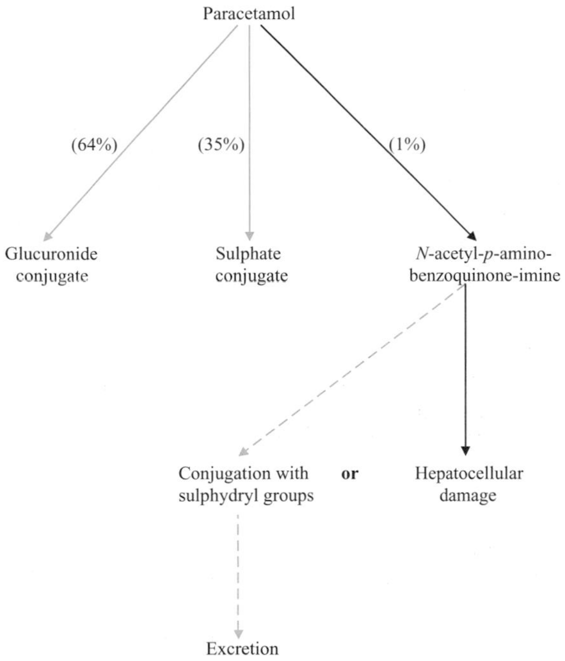

Fig. 1.6 The metabolism of paracetamol to the toxic metabolite *N*-acetyl-*p*-amino-benzoquinone-imine.

with a different spectrum of pharmacological activity (e.g. pethidine, atracurium). Certain antibiotics (e.g. ampicillin, chloramphenicol) may be administered orally as esters. In this form, they are better absorbed than their parent drugs and are subsequently hydrolysed to active derivatives.

Occasionally, drug metabolism results in the formation of compounds with toxic effects. Paracetamol, for example, is partially converted to *N*-acetyl-*p*-amino-benzoquinone-imine, and if this metabolite is not rapidly conjugated, it alkylates macromolecules in liver cells, resulting in necrosis (Fig. 1.6). Similarly, one of the metabolites of halothane (trifluoroacetyl chloride) is covalently bound by lysine residues in liver proteins, resulting in hepatocellular damage. The breakdown of halothane to reactive intermediate metabolites plays an important role in halothane hepatitis.

The enzymic changes carried out by the liver during drug metabolism are divided into two types. Phase 1 reactions (non-synthetic or functionalization reactions) usually result in drug oxidation, reduction or hydrolysis (Table 1.7). Phase 2 reactions (synthetic or conjugation reactions) involve combination of phase 1 reaction products (or unchanged drugs) with other groups, including glucuronide, sulphate, acetate or glycine radicals. Both phase 1 and phase 2 reactions increase the water solubility of drugs and promote their elimination from the body.

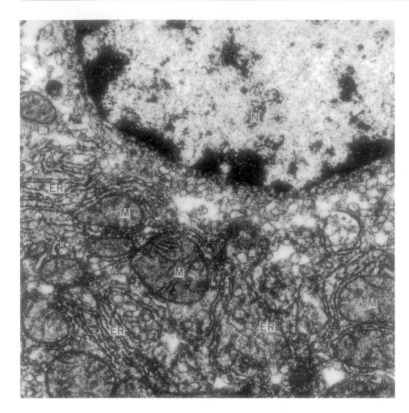

Fig. 1.7 Electron micrography of part of a mouse liver cell, showing mitochondria (M), endoplasmic reticulum (ER) and the nuclear membrane enclosing the nucleus (N) (×30,000).

Some drugs (e.g. sodium salicylate) are almost entirely metabolized by phase 2 reactions.

Phase 1 reactions

Most phase 1 reactions and glucuronide conjugation are carried out by the smooth endoplasmic reticulum or the microsomes (Fig. 1.7). Most drug oxidation and reduction, and some hydrolysis, is carried out by a non-specific microsomal enzyme system (cytochrome P450 or the 'mixed function oxidase system'). Cytochrome P450 consists of many distinct but genetically related forms of a superfamily of haem proteins. Their name is derived from their ability, in the reduced state, to combine with carbon monoxide and form a complex that maximally absorbs light at a wavelength of 450 nm.

Cytochrome P450

Drug oxidation by cytochrome P450 depends on the flavoprotein NADPH-CYP reductase, the electron donor NADPH and molecular oxygen (as well as cytochrome b_5 and NADPH-cytochrome b_5 reductase). The reaction in-volves a complex enzymatic cycle (Fig. 1.8), which results in the breakdown of molecular oxygen. A single oxygen atom (from O_2) is released as H_2O and the other is transferred to the substrate (D), according to the equation:

$$DH + O_2 + NADPH + H^+ \rightarrow DOH + H_2O + NADP^+$$

Cytochrome P450 enzymes may also mediate the reductive metabolism of certain drugs, such as halothane (Table 1.7). This is dependent on the ability of drugs to directly accept electrons from the reduced cytochrome P450 drug complex (Fig. 1.8) and is enhanced by hypoxia.

Isoforms of cytochrome P450

Different forms of human cytochrome P450 are classified by the similarity in their amino acid sequences into gene families and gene subfamilies. The members of each gene family (CYP 1, CYP 2 etc.) have a common amino acid sequence of 40% or more, while members of each subfamily (CYP 1A, CYP 1B etc.) have a sequence similarity of more than 55%. At the present time, 17 different gene families have been identified, and at least six of these

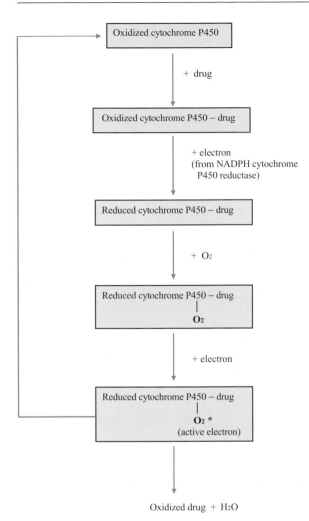

Fig. 1.8 The mixed-function oxidase system (cytochrome P450).

families (CYP 7, CYP 11, CYP 17, CYP 19, CYP 21 and CYP 27) appear to be solely concerned with the synthesis of steroids, bile acids and cholesterol, and play no part in drug metabolism. The CYP 1, CYP 2 and CYP 3 families account for more than 75% of hepatic cytochrome P450, and seven distinct isoforms (CYP 1A2, CYP 2C8, CYP 2C9, CYP 2C19, CYP 2D6, CYP 2E1, CYP 3A4) are responsible for most phase 1 reactions in man (Table 1.8). The individual isoforms have different but overlapping substrate specificities, metabolize drugs at different rates, and also differ in their susceptibility to enzyme induction and inhibition. Their expression in different organs is extremely variable, and some of them (e.g. CYP 2D6) are subject to genetic polymorphism.

The isoform CYP 2E1 is specifically responsible for defluorination and degradation of many common fluorinated inhalational agents. The rate of anaesthetic defluorination, as assessed by fluoride production, occurs in the order sevoflurane > enflurane > isoflurane > desflurane. Enzyme induction with ethanol or phenobarbital increases the rate of defluorination. CYP 2E1 may also be induced by fasting, obesity, diabetes, isoniazid, ketones and isopropyl alcohol (Table 1.8). In some cases, it may produce activation of some carcinogens.

Cytochrome P450 isoenzymes have also been identified at many extrahepatic sites. Cerebral isoenzymes are considered to play an important role in the regulation of certain steroids that control mood and sleep patterns.

Other phase 1 reactions

Although most drug oxidation and reduction is dependent on isoforms of cytochrome P450, some endogenous compounds (e.g. dopamine, tyramine) are metabolized by monoamine oxidase, which is predominantly present in mitochondria. Similarly, ethyl alcohol is oxidized and chloral hydrate is reduced by alcohol dehydrogenase, which is present in the cytoplasm of liver cells (Table 1.7).

Most esters and amides are primarily metabolized by hydrolysis. Drug breakdown may be dependent on certain microsomal enzyme systems (e.g. the carboxylesterases, which hydrolyse diamorphine to 6-monoacetylmorphine, and pethidine to pethidinic acid). Alternatively, it may occur in plasma (e.g. the hydrolysis of suxamethonium by butyrylcholinesterase), in erythrocytes (the hydrolysis of esmolol and remifentanil by acetylcholinesterase), or at the neuromuscular junction (e.g. the hydrolysis of acetylcholine). Many amides (e.g. lidocaine, prilocaine) are broken down in the liver by amidases.

Phase 2 reactions

Phase 2 reactions (synthetic reactions) involve the conjugation of other chemical groups with the oxidized, reduced or hydrolysed products of phase 1 reactions. Some relatively polar drugs may only be metabolized by phase 2 reactions. The metabolic changes that occur during phase 2 reactions usually involve the addition of glucuronide, sulphate, acetate, glycine or methyl groups to the products of phase 1 reactions. The most important of these reactions is glucuronide conjugation.

Table 1.8 The main forms of cytochrome P450 involved in hepatic drug metabolism in humans.

Enzyme isoform	Typical substrates	Inhibitors	Biological properties
CYP 1A2	Caffeine Clomipramine Imipramine Lisophylline Oestrogens Ondansetron Phenacetin Ropivacaine Theophylline R-warfarin	Benzoflavone Cimetidine Fluvoxamine Furafylline	13% of total hepatic cytochrome P450 Only present in liver Induced by phenobarbital, phenytoin, omeprazole, cigarette smoke Polycyclic aromatic hydrocarbons Cruciferous vegetables Marked interindividual variation in expression (40-fold)
CYP 2C8	Carbamazepine Diazepam Pioglitazone Paclitaxel Rosiglitazone Taxol Zopiclone	Cimetidine	4% of total hepatic cytochrome P450 Narrow substrate specificity Inducible by phenobarbital and rifampicin
CYP 2C9	Diclofenac Fluoxetine Ibuprofen Losartan Omeprazole Phenytoin S-warfarin	Fluconazole Fluvastatin Sulfaphenazole Sulfinpyrazone Trimethoprim	17% of total hepatic cytochrome P450 Individual variation in expression in human liver, due to genetic variants with low activity Unaffected by enzyme inducing agents
CYP 2C19	Citalopram Diazepam Imipramine S-mephenytoin Omeprazole Proguanil	Sulfaphenazole	3% of total hepatic cytochrome P450 Subject to genetic polymorphism A mutation is inherited as an autosomal recessive trait
CYP 2D6	β-blockers Codeine Dextromethorphan Flecainide Morphine Fluphenazine	Cimetidine Haloperidol Methadone Quinidine SSRIs	2–5% of total hepatic cytochrome P450 Metabolizes 25% of all drugs Subject to genetic polymorphism (debrisoquine/sparteine polymorphism); presents as autosomal recessive trait Catalyses many O-demethylation reactions
CYP 2E1	Desflurane Ethanol Enflurane Isoflurane Isoniazid Sevoflurane	Diallylsulphide Diethylcarbamate Disulfiram 4-methylpyrazole	6% of total cytochrome P450 Induced by fasting, obesity, ethanol, isoniazid and benzene Metabolizes small molecular weight halogenated compounds
CYP 3A4	Alfentanil Cortisol Ciclosporin Erythromycin Lidocaine Midazolam Nifedipine Testosterone	Cimetidine Ketoconazole Gestodene Grapefruit juice Propofol Troleandomycin	30–60% of total hepatic cytochrome P450 Metabolizes 50% of all drugs Catalyses many N-demethylated reactions Induced by barbiturates, rifampicin, phenytoin, glucocorticoids, St John's Wort

Table 1.9 Drugs that induce and inhibit cytochrome P450.

Inducers of cytochrome P450	Inhibitors of cytochrome P450
Barbiturates	Imidazoles (cimetidine, etomidate,
Phenytoin	ketoconazole, omeprazole)
Carbamazepine	Macrolide antibiotics (erythromycin, clarithromycin)
Rifampicin	Antidepressants
Griseofulvin	HIV protease inhibitors
Alcohol (chronic consumption)	Ciclosporin
Polycyclic hydrocarbons (tobacco	Amiodarone
smoke, grilled meat)	Gestodene
	Grapefruit juice

Glucuronide conjugation

The conjugation of drugs to glucuronides is mainly dependent on enzyme systems in the hepatic endoplasmic reticulum. The microsomal enzyme glucuronyl transferase catalyses the transfer of glucuronide residues from UDP-glucuronide to unconjugated compounds. This process is responsible for the conjugation of endogenous compounds (e.g. bilirubin, thyroxine) as well as many drugs (e.g. morphine, steroid hormones). Glucuronide conjugation usually results in the formation of acidic drug metabolites with a low pK_a (i.e. relatively strong acids) and consequently increases their water solubility.

Other conjugation reactions

Sulphate conjugation may occur in the gut wall or in the cytoplasm of the liver cell. The enzymes involved are normally concerned with the synthesis of sulphated polysaccharides (e.g. heparin). Sulphate conjugation may be the final step in the metabolism of chloramphenicol, isoprenaline, noradrenaline, paracetamol and certain steroids.

Drug acetylation may take place in several tissues (e.g. spleen, lung, liver). In the liver, Kupffer cells rather than hepatocytes may be responsible for conjugation, which involves the transfer of acetyl groups from coenzyme A to the unconjugated drug. The rate and extent of acetylation in man are under genetic control. Isoniazid, many sulphonamides, hydralazine and phenelzine are partly metabolized by acetylation.

Glycine conjugation occurs in the cytoplasm of liver cells. Bromosulphonphthalein and several other drugs are partly eliminated in bile as glycine conjugates.

Methylation is mediated by enzymes that are present in the cytoplasm of many tissues, and plays an important part in the metabolism of catecholamines by the enzyme catechol-0-methyltransferase.

Induction and inhibition of cytochrome P450

Induction

Several drugs selectively increase the activity of cytochrome P450, including phenytoin, carbamazepine and rifampicin (Table 1.9). Enzyme induction usually occurs within several days and increases liver weight, microsomal protein content and biliary secretion. Chronic alcohol consumption, brussels sprouts, and polycyclic hydrocarbons in tobacco and grilled meats, also increase the activity of certain isoforms. Polycyclic hydrocarbons mainly induce CYP 1A2, while barbiturates and phenytoin affect CYP 1A2 and CYP 3A4. Rifampicin is a potent inducer of CYP 2D6 and CYP 3A4, while ethyl alcohol induces CYP 2E1. Enzyme induction usually increases the activity of glucuronyl transferase, and thus enhances drug conjugation. In some instances, drugs may induce their own metabolism (autoinduction).

Induction of cytochrome P450 may have secondary effects on other enzyme systems. Hepatic enzyme induction decreases intracellular haem, reducing its inhibitory effects on porphyrin synthesis, and this may be significant in acute porphyria.

Inhibition

Many imidazole derivatives (e.g. omeprazole, etomidate) combine with the ferric (Fe^{3+}) form of haem, resulting in reversible non-competitive inhibition of CYP 3A4 and various other isoforms. Quinidine is a competitive inhibitor of CYP 2D6 (although it is not metabolized by this isoform). In addition, some synthetic corticosteroids (e.g. gestodene) are oxidized by CYP 3A4 and combine with it covalently ('suicide inhibition'). Furafylline affects CYP 1A2 in a similar manner. Many other drugs also inhibit some cytochrome P450 isoforms, particularly CYP 3A4 (Table 1.9). Enzyme inhibition may increase plasma concentrations of other concurrently used drugs, resulting in drug interactions (Chapters 4 and 5).

First-pass metabolism

After oral administration, some drugs are extensively metabolized by the gut wall (e.g. chlorpromazine, dopamine) or by the liver (e.g. lidocaine, pethidine) before they enter the systemic circulation ('presystemic' or 'first-pass metabolism'). In these conditions, oral administration may not produce adequate plasma concentrations in the systemic circulation and may result in an impaired response to drugs. First-pass metabolism by the liver is relatively common with drugs that have a high hepatic extraction ratio (i.e. when the concentration in the hepatic vein is less than 50% of that in the portal vein). In these conditions, clearance is primarily dependent on liver blood flow rather than the activity of drug-metabolizing enzymes, and drugs that reduce hepatic blood flow (e.g. propranolol) may influence the magnitude of the first-pass effect. Drugs are sometimes given by sublingual or rectal administration in order to avoid first-pass metabolism in the liver.

Individual differences in drug metabolism

When some drugs are administered in the same dose to different patients, plasma concentrations may vary over a 10-fold range. The phenomenon is sometimes due to interindividual differences in drug metabolism, which is an important cause of the variability in response to drugs (Chapter 5). Most of the available evidence suggests that the rate and the pattern of drug metabolism are mainly controlled by genetic factors, including sex, race and ethnicity. Some metabolic pathways are subject to genetic polymorphism (e.g. drug acetylation, ester hydrolysis). For example, individuals who are deficient in CYP 2D6 (Table 1.8) may have an impaired analgesic response to codeine, since they convert little or none of the drug to morphine.

Environmental factors, including diet, cigarette smoking, alcohol consumption and exposure to insecticides, are probably of lesser importance. However, interindividual differences in plasma concentrations and variable responses are sometimes related to drug interactions (Chapter 4), particularly with agents that induce or inhibit hepatic enzyme systems. Interactions with enzyme inducers or inhibitors are commoner with low extraction, extensively protein-bound drugs whose clearance is dependent on metabolism rather than hepatic blood flow. High extraction drugs whose clearance is dependent on hepatic blood flow are unlikely to be involved in significant metabolic reactions.

Drug metabolism may be related to age, and the hepatic metabolism of many drugs is modified in childhood and in the elderly. Neonates have impaired drug metabolizing systems, and some isoforms of cytochrome P450 and glucuronyl transferase may be relatively immature. In the elderly, drug metabolism is also modified, although altered environmental influences may be of more importance.

Pathological changes

Pathological changes may affect the metabolism and clearance of drugs in an unpredictable manner. In severe hepatic disease (e.g. cirrhosis or hepatitis), the elimination of drugs that are primarily metabolized may be impaired. The reduction in clearance may result in drug cumulation, and the urinary elimination of metabolites may be decreased. Liver disease may also enhance and prolong the effects of drugs that are metabolized by plasma cholinesterase. Any decrease in cardiac output (e.g. due to heart block, myocardial infarction or hypertension) may reduce the elimination of drugs whose clearance is dependent on hepatic blood flow. Renal disease usually has little or no effect on drug metabolism, although polar metabolites may accumulate in plasma and produce toxic effects. Thus, norpethidine (a demethylated metabolite of pethidine) is normally eliminated in urine, but in renal failure its excretion is impaired, and may sometimes cause cerebral excitation and convulsions.

Hepatic, renal and cardiac diseases are important factors affecting the variable response to drugs (Chapter 5).

Drug excretion

Almost all drugs and their metabolites are eventually eliminated from the body in urine or in bile. Small amounts of some drugs are excreted in saliva and in milk.

The molecular weight of drugs and their metabolites plays an important part in determining their route of

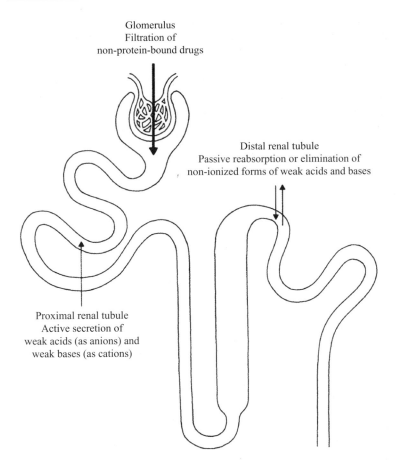

Glomerulus
Filtration of
non-protein-bound drugs

Distal renal tubule
Passive reabsorption or elimination of
non-ionized forms of weak acids and bases

Proximal renal tubule
Active secretion of
weak acids (as anions) and
weak bases (as cations)

Fig. 1.9 The renal elimination of drugs by glomerular filtration, proximal tubular secretion and distal tubular reabsorption or excretion. In the distal renal tubule, weak acids and weak bases may be reabsorbed or excreted into urine, depending on their pK_a values and the pH gradient between plasma and urine.

elimination. Most low molecular weight compounds and their metabolites are excreted in urine. By contrast, drugs with a higher molecular weight (above 400–500 Da in man) are preferentially eliminated in bile. Thus, biliary secretion plays an important part in the elimination of some muscle relaxants, many steroid conjugates and certain antibacterial drugs (Table 1.2).

The renal elimination of drugs is dependent on three separate processes that take place at different sites in the nephron (Fig. 1.9). These are
• Glomerular filtration
• Proximal tubular secretion
• Distal tubular diffusion

Glomerular filtration

Glomerular filtration is partly responsible for the elimination of poorly lipid-soluble drugs and drug metabolites in urine. Only the free or unbound fraction in plasma

water is available for filtration by the renal glomerulus. Nevertheless, since glomerular perfusion time is probably much longer than the dissociation time from the rapidly reversible binding to plasma proteins, significant amounts of protein-bound drugs may be filtered by the glomerulus.

Proximal tubular secretion

The active secretion of drugs by the proximal renal tubule may lead to their rapid elimination from the body. Proximal tubular secretion is an example of carrier transport, requires the expenditure of cellular energy, and may take place against a concentration gradient. A wide number of drugs and drug metabolites are partly eliminated by this process (Table 1.1). Acidic and basic drugs are secreted by two separate and distinct transport systems. These are located in related sites in renal tubule cells, and both have a requirement for cellular energy. Acidic drugs may compete with each other for tubular secretion, and basic drugs may interfere with the elimination of other bases or cations. Acids do not usually compete with or affect the secretion of bases. Occasionally, the competitive inhibition of the tubular transport of acids or bases is of practical significance (e.g. the inhibition of penicillin secretion by probenecid, or the reduction of urate transport by thiazide diuretics).

During tubular secretion, only the unbound drug is transferred from plasma to tubular cells. Nevertheless, protein or red cell binding does not apparently restrict tubular secretion, and some drugs that are significantly bound to plasma proteins (e.g. phenol red, some penicillins) are completely cleared by the kidney in a single circulation. As discussed above, this probably reflects the rapid dissociation from plasma protein in relation to the time required for renal tubular perfusion.

Distal tubular diffusion

In the distal renal tubule, non-ionic diffusion is partly responsible for the reabsorption and elimination of acids and bases. In this region of the nephron, there is a considerable H^+ gradient between plasma and acid urine. Most acidic drugs are preferentially excreted in alkaline urine, where they are present as non-diffusible anions. In acid urine, they are usually present as non-ionized molecules that can readily diffuse back into plasma. In these conditions, they are slowly eliminated from the body and their half-lives may be prolonged. For instance, the weak acid probenecid is actively secreted in the proximal renal tubule as an anion, i.e. R-COO$^-$. In acidic conditions (e.g. in the distal renal tubule), it is partially present in the non-ionized form R-COOH and is extensively reabsorbed. In consequence, its elimination from the body is relatively slow and its half-life is approximately 6–12 hours.

By contrast, basic drugs (e.g. secondary and tertiary amines) are preferentially excreted in acid urine (Fig. 1.3). In these conditions they can readily diffuse from plasma to urine where they are trapped as cations. This provides a gradient for the diffusion of the non-ionized drug from plasma to urine. Many basic drugs are highly lipid-soluble and extensively bound to plasma proteins and may not be significantly eliminated by glomerular filtration or by tubular secretion. Diffusion of the non-ionized fraction from the relatively alkaline plasma to acid urine (Fig. 1.3) may be the only method responsible for the elimination of these drugs. At one time, the effects of changes in urine pH on the elimination of weak acids and bases were sometimes utilized in the treatment of drug overdosage.

Biliary excretion

The biliary excretion of drugs and drug metabolites is usually less important than their renal elimination. Nevertheless, almost all drugs or their metabolites can be identified in bile after oral or parenteral administration (although only trace amounts of many compounds may be detected). Biliary excretion is usually the major route of elimination of compounds with a molecular weight of more than 400–500 Da.

Ionized or partly ionized drugs and their metabolites are usually eliminated from liver cells by active transport. High molecular weight anions (including glucuronide and sulphate conjugates) and cations (including quaternary amines) are actively transferred from hepatocytes to the biliary canaliculus by separate transport systems, which are dependent on Na^+/K^+ ATPase. Biliary secretion is relatively non-specific, saturable and can be competitively or non-competitively inhibited by other drugs. Thus, anions compete with each other for canalicular transport, while basic drugs interfere with the elimination of other bases or cations. In many respects, the biliary secretion of anions and cations is similar to their active transport in the proximal renal tubule, and accounts for the high concentrations of certain drugs in bile (in some instances, more than 100 times their plasma level).

The phenomenon is sometimes of practical significance. The visualization of contrast media during radiological examination of the biliary tract is dependent on their active secretion and concentration in bile. Similarly, the high concentrations of ampicillin and rifampicin that are eliminated in bile may account for their effectiveness in enteric infections. Many muscle relaxants are also present in high concentrations in bile. Monoquaternary compounds (e.g. vecuronium) are more extensively eliminated than their bisquaternary analogues (pancuronium), and this may partly account for the differences in their duration of action.

Enterohepatic circulation

Many compounds that are eliminated in bile as glucuronide conjugates are hydrolysed in the small intestine by bacterial flora that secrete the enzyme glucuronidase. After hydrolysis the unchanged drug is reabsorbed, metabolized and re-excreted as a glucuronide conjugate (Fig. 1.10). This 'enterohepatic circulation' of drugs may occur many times before compounds are finally eliminated from the body and is often associated with a substantial first-pass effect and a prolonged plasma half-life.

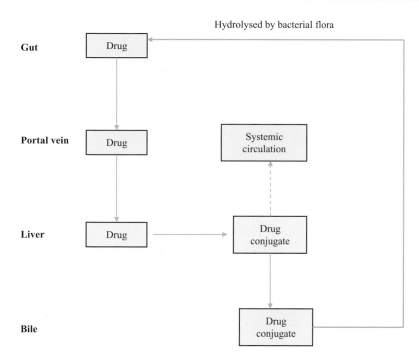

Fig. 1.10 The enterohepatic circulation of drugs. Only small amounts of the absorbed drug and its conjugates escape recirculation and enter the systemic circulation.

Many oestrogens have an extensive enterohepatic circulation. During broad-spectrum antibiotic therapy, oestrogen conjugates may not be hydrolysed in the small intestine, and their elimination in the gut is enhanced. This phenomenon may sometimes be responsible for the failure of oral contraception in these patients.

The trace amounts of many drugs that are eliminated unchanged in bile are probably directly transferred from hepatic arterial blood to intrahepatic bile ducts via the peribiliary plexus. The transference of drugs may be modified by the hormone secretin, which also increases bile flow by its action at this site.

Excretion in saliva and milk

Small amounts of most drugs are excreted unchanged in saliva and in milk. The elimination of drugs by these routes is usually dependent on simple physical principles. Non-protein bound, lipid-soluble, small molecular weight drugs can readily diffuse into saliva and milk, where their levels may be similar to the plasma concentration. As the pH of saliva and milk is slightly acid compared with plasma, the concentration of weak acids will be reduced (although weak bases may be slightly concentrated). Some ions (e.g. chloride, iodide) may be actively secreted into saliva and milk. Nevertheless, drug excretion by these routes is usually of little quantitative significance. Occasionally, the elimination of trace amounts of certain drugs in milk (e.g. many opioid analgesics and most hypnotic and tranquillising drugs) may make breast-feeding inadvisable when patients are on continual therapy. Muscle relaxants and their antagonists are not significantly eliminated in saliva or in milk.

Suggested reading

Bates, I.P. (1985) Permeability of the blood–brain barrier. *Trends in Pharmacological Sciences* **6**, 447–450.

Birkett, D.J., Mackenzie, P.I., Veronese, M.E. & Miners, J.O. (1993) *In vitro* approaches can predict human drug metabolism. *Trends in Pharmacological Sciences* **14**, 292–294.

Calvey, T.N. (2001) Enzymes. *Anaesthesia and Intensive Care Medicine* **2**, 322–323.

Calvey, T.N. (2005) Enzyme inducers and inhibitors: addition, subtraction and synergism. *Anaesthesia and Intensive Care Medicine* **6**, 139–140.

Chang, G.W.M. & Kam, P.C.A. (1999) The physiological and pharmacological roles of cytochrome P450 isoenzymes. *Anaesthesia* **54**, 42–50.

Cholerton, S., Daly, A.K. & Idle, J.R. (1992) The role of individual human cytochromes P450 in drug metabolism and clinical response. *Trends in Pharmacological Sciences* **13**, 434–439.

Fehrenbach, A. (1987) Drugs in breast milk. *British Journal of Pharmaceutical Practice* **9**, 288–290.

George, C.F. (1981) Drug metabolism by the gastro-intestinal mucosa. *Clinical Pharmacokinetics* **6**, 259–274.

Gonzalez, F.J. (1992) Human cytochromes P450: problems and prospects. *Trends in Pharmacological Sciences* **13**, 346–352.

Guengerich, F.P. (1989) Characterization of human microsomal cytochrome P-450 enzymes. *Annual Review of Pharmacology and Toxicology* **29**, 241–264.

Iohom, G., Fitzgerald, D. & Cunningham, A.J. (2004) Principles of pharmacogenetics – implications for the anaesthetist. *British Journal of Anaesthesia* **93**, 440–450.

Kharasch, E.D. & Thummel, K.E. (1993) Identification of cytochrome P450 2E1 as the predominant enzyme catalysing human liver microsomal defluorination of sevoflurane, isoflurane and methoxyflurane. *Anesthesiology* **79**, 795–807.

Krishna, D.R. & Klotz, U. (1994) Extrahepatic metabolism of drugs in humans. *Clinical Pharmacokinetics* **26**, 144–160.

Lieber, C.S. (1997) Cytochrome P-450 2E1: its physiological and pathological role. *Physiological Reviews* **77**, 517–544.

Lin, J.H & Lu, A.Y. (2001) Interindividual variability in inhibition and induction of cytochrome P450 enzymes. *Annual Review of Pharmacology and Toxicology* **41**, 535–567.

Okey, A.B. (1990) Enzyme induction in the cytochrome P-450 system. *Pharmacology and Therapeutics* **45**, 241–298.

Pardridge, W.M. (1988) Recent advances in blood–brain barrier transport. *Annual Review of Pharmacology and Toxicology* **28**, 25–39.

Pleuvry, B.J. (2002) Body compartments and drug distribution. *Anaesthesia and Intensive Care Medicine* **3**, 256–260.

Pleuvry, B.J. (2005) Factors affecting drug absorption and distribution. *Anaesthesia and Intensive Care Medicine* **6**, 135–138.

Routledge, P.A. (1986) The plasma protein binding of basic drugs. *British Journal of Clinical Pharmacology* **22**, 499–506.

Schinkel, A.H. (1997) The physiological function of drug-transporting P-glycoproteins. *Seminars in Cancer Biology* **3**, 161–170.

Somogyi, A. (1996) Renal transport of drugs: specificity and molecular mechanisms. *Clinical and Experimental Pharmacology and Physiology* **23**, 986–989.

Spatzeneger, M. & Jaeger, W. (1995) Clinical importance of hepatic cytochrome P450 in drug metabolism. *Drug Metabolism Reviews* **27**, 397–417.

Stoughton, R.B. (1989) Percutaneous absorption of drugs. *Annual Review of Pharmacology and Toxicology* **29**, 55–69.

Tamai, I. & Tsuji, A. (2000) Transporter-mediated permeation of drugs across the blood–brain barrier. *Journal of Pharmaceutical Sciences* **89**, 1371–1388.

Tanaka, E. (1999) Update: genetic polymorphism of drug metabolizing enzymes in humans. *Journal of Clinical Pharmacy and Therapeutics* **24**, 323–329.

Tucker, G.T. (1979) Drug metabolism. *British Journal of Anaesthesia* **51**, 603–618.

Tucker, G.T. (1994) Clinical implications of genetic polymorphism in drug metabolism. *Journal of Pharmacy and Pharmacology* **46**, 417–424.

Wood, M. (1997) Drug distribution: less passive, more active? *Anesthesiology* **87**, 1274–1276.

Zhang, Y. & Benet, L.Z. (2001) The gut as a barrier to drug absorption: combined role of cytochrome P450 3A and P-glycoprotein. *Clinical Pharmacokinetics* **40**, 159–168.

2 Pharmacokinetics

Pharmacokinetics was originally defined as the quantitative study and mathematical analysis of drug and drug metabolite levels in the body. More recently, the term has been generally applied to the processes of drug absorption, distribution, metabolism and excretion, and to their description in numerical terms. Pharmacokinetics is sometimes described as 'what the body does to drugs'.

Since 1960, many sensitive analytical techniques, including high performance liquid chromatography, mass spectrometry and radioimmunoassay, have been used to measure the concentration of many drugs and their metabolites in plasma and urine. Changes in drug concentration in relation to time have been assessed and used to derive pharmacokinetic constants that describe the behaviour of drugs in the body. These constants can be used to determine the loading dose and the rate of infusion required to maintain steady-state concentrations in plasma, and to predict the rate and extent of drug cumulation. They can also be used to predict the modification of drug dosage required in renal and hepatic disease, and to determine the possible effects of other agents and pathological conditions on drug disposition.

The two most important pharmacokinetic constants are
- Volume of distribution (V)
- Clearance (CL)

The volume of distribution represents the apparent volume available in the body for the distribution of the drug, while the clearance reflects the ability of the body to eliminate the drug.

These constants are related to the terminal or 'elimination' half-life of the drug, which is defined as the time required for the plasma concentration to decrease by 50% during the terminal phase of decline, by the expression:

$$t_{\frac{1}{2}} \propto \frac{V}{CL} = k \times \frac{V}{CL}$$

where k is a constant ($\ln 2 = 0.693$). Consequently, the terminal half-life is a hybrid constant, which depends on the primary pharmacokinetic constants V and CL. A prolonged terminal half-life may reflect an increased volume of distribution, a reduced clearance, or both these changes. Similarly, a shorter terminal half-life may represent a decreased volume of distribution, an increased clearance, or both phenomena. When the terminal half-lives of drugs are compared, differences between them do not necessarily reflect changes in drug elimination.

Volume of distribution

The volume of distribution represents the relation between the total amount of a drug in the body and its plasma concentration, and thus reflects the process of drug dispersal in the body. It is dependent on the partition coefficient of the drug, regional blood flow to tissues and the degree of plasma protein and tissue binding.

Although the volume of distribution is an apparent volume, and does not correspond to anatomical or physiological tissue compartments, it may be of some practical significance.

When measured by pharmacokinetic analysis, its value for various drugs in adults ranges from 50 to 21,000 mL kg^{-1} (Table 2.1). Drugs with a volume of distribution of 50–150 mL kg^{-1} are predominantly localized in plasma or are extensively bound by plasma proteins (e.g. heparin, warfarin). Drugs with a slightly higher distribution volume (150–250 mL kg^{-1}) are mainly present in extracellular fluid (e.g. muscle relaxants). Conversely, when the volume of distribution is greater than the presumed values for total body water (i.e. 500–700 mL kg^{-1}), there is extensive tissue distribution of drugs (although the specific sites of drug distribution cannot be determined or inferred). In these circumstances, the concentration in tissues may be higher than in plasma. The binding of drugs by tissue constituents is not uncommon, and drugs that are bound by tissues and have relatively high apparent volumes of distribution include fentanyl, digoxin, propofol,

Table 2.1 The volume of distribution of some common drugs in normal adult patients.

Drug	Volume of distribution (mL kg^{-1})	Volume of distribution (L 70 kg^{-1})
Heparin	58 (47–69)	4 (3–5)
Warfarin	140 (80–200)	10 (7–14)
Acetylsalicylic acid	150 (120–180)	11 (8–13)
Atracurium	160 (110–210)	11 (8–15)
Chlorothiazide	200 (120–280)	14 (8–20)
Vecuronium	230 (160–300)	16 (11–21)
Pancuronium	270 (200 340)	19 (14–24)
Ethanol	540 (490–590)	38 (34–41)
Alfentanil	800 (500–1100)	56 (35–77)
Lidocaine	900 (500–1300)	63 (35–91)
Bupivacaine	1050 (650–1450)	74 (46–102)
Prilocaine	2700 (2100–3300)	189 (147–231)
Morphine	3500 (2600–4400)	245 (182–308)
Pethidine	4000 (3100–4900)	280 (217–343)
Fentanyl	4000 (3600–4400)	280 (252–308)
Digoxin	5500 (4000–7000)	385 (280–490)
Propofol	8000 (4000–12,000)	560 (280–840)
Imipramine	18,000 (15,000–21,000)	1260 (1050–1470)
Chlorpromazine	21,000 (12,000–30,000)	1470 (840–2100)

The values shown are approximate and represent means and normal ranges (in parentheses).

most phenothiazines and most antidepressant drugs (Table 2.1).

The volume of distribution of drugs may be modified by age and physiological factors, since extracellular fluid volume is greater in infants and during pregnancy than in adults, and may also be affected by disease (e.g. renal and cardiac failure).

An appreciation of the total apparent volume of distribution of potentially toxic drugs may be relevant to the management of drug poisoning. Drugs with a large volume of distribution may take many hours or days to be entirely removed from the body. In contrast, drugs with a relatively small volume of distribution may be rapidly eliminated (as long as they are not significantly metabolized or extensively bound by plasma proteins).

Clearance

Clearance represents the volume of blood or plasma from which a drug would need to be completely removed in unit time in order to account for its elimination from the body. It is therefore a theoretical concept, since in practice drugs are incompletely removed from a rather larger volume of plasma. Clearance values are usually expressed as a volume cleared in unit time and are usually measured in mL min^{-1} or L h^{-1}.

Alternatively, clearance can be defined as the rate of drug elimination (in mg min^{-1}) per unit of blood or plasma concentration (in mg mL^{-1}), and

$$\text{plasma clearance (mL min}^{-1}\text{)}$$
$$= \frac{\text{rate of drug elimination (mg min}^{-1}\text{)}}{\text{plasma concentration (mg mL}^{-1}\text{)}}$$

Since plasma clearance is normally constant, the rate of drug elimination is directly proportional to plasma concentration.

Total body clearance is the sum of different ways of drug elimination that are carried out by various organs in the body:

$$CL = CL_R + CL_H + CL_X$$

where CL is total clearance, CL_R is renal clearance, CL_H is hepatic clearance and CL_X is clearance by other routes.

Renal clearance

In many instances, the renal clearance of drugs can be directly measured by classical methods,

i.e. renal clearance = rate of urine flow $(mL\ min^{-1})$

$$\times \frac{\text{urine concentration } (mg\ mL^{-1})}{\text{plasma concentration } (mg\ mL^{-1})}$$

Consequently, separate estimates may be obtained for renal clearance (CL_R) and extrarenal clearance (CL_{ER}), where $CL_{ER} = CL - CL_R$. These values may be useful in assessing the relative importance of renal and hepatic function in drug elimination. When the total body clearance of drugs is predominantly due to renal excretion (i.e. when $CL_R > 0.7\ CL$), drug cumulation may occur in renal failure or during renal transplantation. By contrast, when $CL_R < 0.3\ CL$, renal disease has little effect on drug elimination, and drug clearance is mainly dependent on metabolism or biliary excretion. Although these processes may be affected by liver disease, the effects of hepatic dysfunction on the clearance of drugs are usually less predictable.

Hepatic clearance

The clearance of most drugs from the body is dependent on the liver (either by hepatic metabolism and/or biliary excretion). In steady-state conditions, the removal of drugs by the liver can be expressed by the extraction ratio (ER). This can be defined as

$$ER = \frac{C_a - C_v}{C_a} = 1 - \frac{C_v}{C_a}$$

where C_a is the drug concentration in mixed portal venous and hepatic arterial blood, and C_v is the drug concentration in hepatic venous blood. The ER is an overall measure of the ability of the liver to remove drugs from the hepatic capillaries and reflects drug metabolism and biliary secretion.

The most generally accepted model of hepatic clearance assumes that the unbound concentration of drugs in hepatic venous blood and in liver cell water is equal. In these conditions, the elimination of drugs by the liver is dependent on

- Hepatic blood flow (Q)
- The proportion of unbound drug in blood (f)
- The rate of hepatic clearance $(CL_{intrinsic})$

Hepatic clearance represents the product of hepatic blood flow (Q) and the ER, i.e.

$$CL_H = Q \times ER$$

Hepatic clearance can also be expressed in terms of blood flow and 'intrinsic clearance' $(CL_{intrinsic})$, i.e.

$$CL_H = Q \times \frac{CL_{intrinsic} \times f}{Q + (CL_{intrinsic} \times f)}$$

$CL_{intrinsic}$ represents the rate at which liver water is cleared of drug (measured in $mL\ min^{-1}$) and f is the fraction of the drug unbound in blood. Intrinsic clearance is independent of blood flow and represents the maximum ability of the liver to irreversibly eliminate drugs by metabolism or biliary excretion. It has a unique value for different drugs and can be interpreted in terms of enzyme kinetics as the ratio V_{max}/K_m (page 37).

Low extraction drugs

When intrinsic clearance $(CL_{intrinsic})$ is relatively low compared to blood flow (Q), then

$$Q + (CL_{intrinsic} \times f) \approx Q$$

and

$$CL_H \approx CL_{intrinsic} \times f$$

In these circumstances, hepatic clearance depends only on intrinsic clearance and the fraction of the drug that is unbound in blood. This type of drug elimination ('capacity-limited' or 'restrictive elimination') is characteristic of the hepatic elimination of phenytoin, theophylline and warfarin, as well as most barbiturates and benzodiazepines. These drugs have a limited first-pass effect after oral administration and a low hepatic ER (i.e. <0.3). Their clearance is relatively low and is unaffected by alterations in liver blood flow, but is profoundly influenced by changes in hepatic enzyme activity. These changes may be induced by other drugs or environmental agents, as well as age, malnutrition or disease, which characteristically affect the hepatic clearance of these compounds. Consequently, drugs that induce cytochrome P450 (e.g. barbiturates, phenytoin, rifampicin) may increase the hepatic clearance of low extraction drugs, while drugs that inhibit this enzyme system (e.g. imidazoles, macrolide antibiotics) reduce the clearance of drugs that are poorly extracted by the liver.

Since $CL_H = (CL_{intrinsic} \times f)$, hepatic clearance is also dependent on the fraction of the unbound drug in blood and may be modified by plasma protein binding. Drugs that are only slightly bound (i.e. 20–30% or less) may be unaffected by changes in protein binding ('capacity-limited, binding-insensitive drugs'). On the other hand, the clearance and terminal half-life of extensively bound drugs will be modified by changes in protein binding ('capacity-limited, binding-sensitive drugs').

High extraction drugs

When intrinsic clearance ($CL_{intrinsic}$) is relatively large compared to blood flow, then

$$Q + (CL_{intrinsic} \times f) \approx CL_{intrinsic} \times f$$

and

$$CL_H \approx Q$$

In these conditions, hepatic clearance is relatively high (10–21 mL kg min^{-1} in adults) and is determined by liver blood flow ('flow-limited' or 'non-restrictive' elimination). The hepatic clearance of some opioid analgesics, local anaesthetics and propofol is flow-dependent (Table 2.2). The hepatic ER is usually high (i.e. 0.7 or more) and there is a substantial first-pass effect after oral administration. Their hepatic clearance may be modified by changes in liver blood flow, but is not influenced by alterations in hepatic enzyme activity or plasma protein binding.

Although this classification is useful, many drugs cannot be rigidly classified as low extraction or high extraction compounds. Their elimination may be partly dependent on intrinsic clearance (enzyme activity and/or biliary secretion) and partly on hepatic blood flow, depending on the conditions in which hepatic clearance is assessed. Nevertheless, these concepts provide a physiological approach to the hepatic clearance of drugs and illustrate the unpredictable relationship between plasma protein binding and drug elimination. When the hepatic clearance of drugs is dependent on intrinsic clearance (i.e. with low extraction drugs), significant protein binding may reduce the concentration of free drug and restrict its elimination. By

Table 2.2 The hepatic clearance of some common drugs in normal adult patients.

Drug	Hepatic clearance (mL min^{-1} kg^{-1})	Hepatic clearance (mL min^{-1} 70 kg^{-1})
Warfarin	0.05 (0.03–0.07)	3.5 (2.1–4.9)
Phenytoin	0.1 (0.07–0.13)	7 (4.9–9.1)
Diazepam	0.4 (0.3–0.5)	28 (21–35)
Theophylline	0.5 (0.3–0.7)	35 (21–49)
Temazepam	1.0 (0.7–1.3)	70 (49–91)
Chlorphenamine	1.7 (1.6–1.8)	119 (112–126)
Thiopental	2.9 (2.2–3.6)	203 (154–252)
Atracurium	6.2 (4.2–8.2)	434 (294–574)
Ketamine	6.6 (4.0–9.2)	462 (280–644)
Alfentanil	6.7 (4.3–9.1)	469 (301–637)
Fentanyl	13.0 (11.0–15.0)	910 (770–1050)
Lidocaine	17.0 (12.6–21.4)	1190 (882–1498)
Pethidine	17.0 (12.0–22.0)	1190 (840–1540)
Morphine	24.0 (14.0–34.0)	1680 (980–2380)
Propofol	28.1 (23.3–32.9)	1967 (1631–2303)

The values shown are approximate and represent means and normal ranges (in parentheses).

contrast, when clearance is dependent on hepatic blood flow, protein binding has little or no effect. Characteristically, the clearance of these drugs is relatively high and is dependent on and determined by liver blood flow (21 mL kg^{-1} min^{-1} in adults). The half-life may be modified by changes in liver blood flow, but is relatively insensitive to alterations in hepatic enzyme activity or plasma protein binding.

Measurement of clearance and volume of distribution

Clearance

Clearance is usually calculated from the equation:

$$CL = \frac{dose}{AUC}$$

where AUC is the area under the plasma concentration – time curve between $t = 0$ and $t = \infty$. The AUC can be estimated by the 'trapezoidal rule', which depends on the measurement and summation of the area of each trapezoid between successive sampling times and the corresponding plasma concentrations (Fig. 2.1). The area ('terminal area') between the plasma concentration and time of the

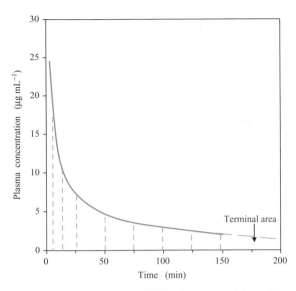

Fig. 2.1 Determination of the AUC by the trapezoidal rule. The area of each trapezoid between successive sampling times and the corresponding plasma concentrations is calculated, and the area between 0 and 150 minutes is derived by summation. The remaining terminal area between the plasma concentration and time of the final sample and $t = \infty$ is calculated from the slope of the terminal decline.

final sample and $t = \infty$ can be estimated from the slope of the terminal decline in plasma concentration.

Volume of distribution

The volume of distribution can be calculated from the product of the mean residence time (MRT) and the clearance, i.e., $V = \text{MRT} \times \text{CL}$. The MRT is the mean time that each drug molecule resides in the body; it can be determined from the relationship:

$$\text{MRT} = \frac{\text{AUMC}}{\text{AUC}}$$

where AUMC is the total area under the first moment of the plasma concentration – time curve (i.e. the area under the plasma concentration × time versus time curve, extrapolated to infinity).

Measurement of the volume of distribution and clearance by compartmental analysis

The volume of distribution and clearance of drugs can also be determined by compartmental analysis. A suitable

pharmacokinetic model is used to illustrate the distribution and elimination of the drug, and values for its volume of distribution and clearance are derived from the parameters of the model.

One-compartment open model

In the past, the pharmacokinetics of many drugs was described in terms of a simple, one-compartment open model (Fig. 2.2). The body is considered in a highly simplified manner as a single homogenous entity or

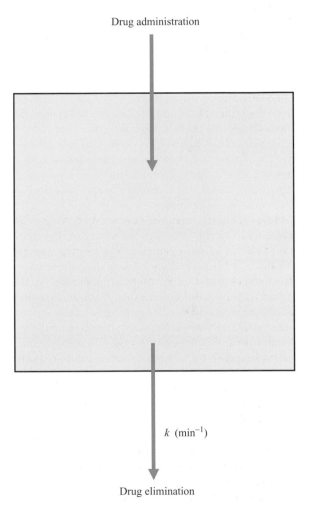

Fig. 2.2 A one-compartment open pharmacokinetic model. The constant k represents the elimination rate constant, measured in units of reciprocal time (e.g. min^{-1}). The concentration declines in a monoexponential manner, as expressed by the equation $C_t = C_0 e^{-kt}$.

compartment, and drugs are administered into and eliminated from this compartment. The rate of drug elimination (k) is assumed to be proportional to the amount of drug in the compartment at any time, while the concentration (C) decreases with time (t) in a monoexponential manner, as expressed by the equation $C_t = C_0 e^{-kt}$, where $e = 2.718$ (Appendix).

Although one-compartment models have the advantage of mathematical transparency and simplicity, they have considerable limitations, and are not consistent with the behaviour of most common drugs or anaesthetic agents.

Two-compartment open model

After intravenous injection, the concentration of most drugs in plasma rapidly declines due to their distribution. This decline is usually called the distribution or rapid disposition phase, and its rate and extent are mainly dependent on the physicochemical characteristics of the drug, particularly its molecular weight and lipid solubility. The distribution phase (or phases) is followed by a slower decline in plasma concentration (the terminal or elimination phase), which usually reflects its elimination by metabolism and excretion.

A typical biphasic decline occurs when a bolus dose of lidocaine (1 mg kg^{-1}) is given intravenously (Fig. 2.3). The initial fall in concentration due to drug distribution is followed by a slower decline due to drug elimination. When the logarithm of the plasma concentration of lidocaine is plotted against time, there is a linear relationship between the variables during the terminal elimination phase, and the decrease in plasma concentration can be resolved into two exponential components by extrapolation. In this procedure, the terminal decline in plasma concentration during the elimination or β-phase is extended to the ordinate (y-axis), which it intersects at point B. Subtraction of the extrapolated values from the initial data points gives a series of residual values which represent the initial (α) phase of exponential decline, and are defined by a regression line that intercepts the ordinate at A. Both α- and β-phases have characteristic slopes (α and β) and half-lives ($t_{1/2\alpha}$ and $t_{1/2\beta}$). The intercepts on the ordinate (A and B) represent the amount that each half-life contributes to the decrease in plasma concentration after intravenous lidocaine. Approximately 80% of the decrease in concentration occurs during the initial distribution phase.

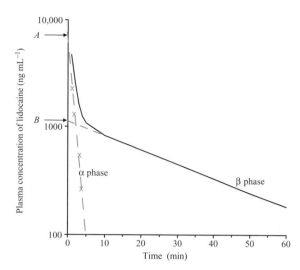

Fig. 2.3 Biexponential decline in the plasma concentration of lidocaine (1 mg kg^{-1}, i.v.). The abcissae (x-axis) shows the time in minutes, and the ordinate (y-axis) the plasma concentration of lidocaine (logarithmic scale). B represents the initial concentration of the slower β-phase of exponential decline, extrapolated to zero time. Extrapolated values on this line were subtracted from the initial data points to give a series of residual values ($\times$). The least squares regression line through these points corresponds to the rapid disposition α-phase, which intercepts the ordinate at A.

Numerical values for the slopes α and β can be derived from the equations:

$$\alpha = \frac{\ln 2}{t_{1/2\alpha}} \quad \text{and} \quad \beta = \frac{\ln 2}{t_{1/2\beta}}$$

and the plasma concentration (C_p) of lidocaine at time t is given by the expression representing the sum of the two exponential components, i.e.

$$C_p = Ae^{-\alpha t} + Be^{-\beta t}$$

where A and B are the intercepts on the ordinate, α and β are hybrid rate constants (i.e. they are dependent on other constants) and $e = 2.718$ (Appendix). Values for A, B, α and β can be derived by graphical methods, or more accurately determined by digital computer programs. In the case of lidocaine, the plasma concentration (C_p) at time t is given by the expression:

$$C_p = 8774e^{-0.895t} + 1147e^{-0.0309t}$$

where C_p is measured in ng mL^{-1} and t in minutes.

Lidocaine (1 mg kg^{-1}, i.v)

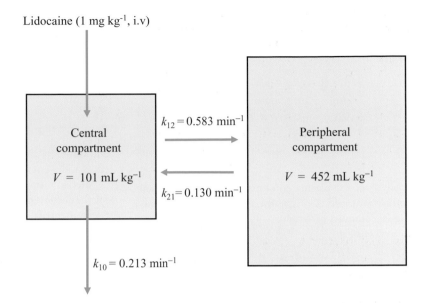

Fig. 2.4 A two-compartment open model for lidocaine disposition. The constants k_{12} and k_{21} govern drug transfer between the central and peripheral compartments. k_{10} is the elimination rate constant.

The biexponential decline in the plasma concentration of lidocaine can be interpreted in terms of a two-compartment open pharmacokinetic model (Fig. 2.4). The model consists of a relatively small central compartment, into which lidocaine is administered and from which it is eliminated, and a larger peripheral compartment. The rate of drug elimination is governed by the rate constant k_{10}, and reversible drug transfer between the two compartments is governed by the rate constants k_{12} and k_{21}. The central and the peripheral compartments have no direct physiological significance, and their parameters and constants are solely determined by the behaviour of lidocaine in the body.

The two-compartment model is essentially a theoretical concept which accounts for the observed biexponential decline in the plasma concentration of lidocaine. In the case of lidocaine (and most other drugs), the central compartment consists of extracellular fluid and some intracellular water of highly perfused organs. The peripheral compartment consists of less well-perfused tissues (e.g. most skeletal muscle, fat). During the distribution phase, the concentration of lidocaine in the central compartment falls rapidly as the drug is distributed to the peripheral compartment. After the occurrence of distribution equilibrium between the two compartments, removal of the drug is solely dependent on elimination, which is governed by the rate constant k_{10}.

Resolution of the model assumes that both distribution and elimination are first-order processes (i.e. that the rate

at which they occur is proportional to the amount of drug in each compartment). Differential equations can then be derived that express the rate of change of the amount of lidocaine in each compartment (dX_1/dt and dX_2/dt, where X_1 and X_2 are the amounts of drug in each compartment at time t). The solution of these differential equations for dX_1/dt and dX_2/dt, and the conversion of X_1 and X_2 to concentrations, gives expressions that relate the concentration of the drug in the central compartment and the peripheral compartment to the constants A, α, B and β, and to time.

In the case of the central compartment,

$$C_1 = Ae^{-\alpha t} + Be^{-\beta t}$$

This expression has an identical form to the equation that describes the biexponential decline in the plasma concentration of lidocaine after intravenous injection. Consequently, values for A, α, B and β can be derived from the measured plasma concentrations, and then used to derive other parameters of the two-compartment open model (e.g. the area under the plasma concentration – time curve (AUC), the clearance (CL), the volume of distribution (V), as well as the rate constants k_{12}, k_{10} and k_{21}), using the formulae:

$$\text{AUC} = \frac{A}{\alpha} + \frac{B}{\beta}$$

$$\text{CL} = \frac{\text{dose}}{\text{AUC}} = \frac{\text{dose}}{\frac{A}{\alpha} + \frac{B}{\beta}}$$

$$k_{21} = \frac{A\beta + B\alpha}{A + B}$$

$$k_{10} = \frac{\alpha\beta}{k_{21}}$$

$$k_{12} = \alpha + \beta - (k_{21} + k_{10})$$

$$V_{area} = \frac{dose}{\beta(AUC)} = \frac{dose}{\beta(A/\alpha + B/\beta)}$$

$$V_{ss} = \frac{dose}{A + B} \times \frac{k_{12} + k_{21}}{k_{21}}$$

Analysis of the plasma concentration of lidocaine after intravenous injection gave the following values, using a digital computer program:

$A = 8774$ ng mL^{-1}

$\alpha = 0.895$ min^{-1}

$t_{\frac{1}{2}\alpha} = 0.77$ min

$B = 1147$ ng mL^{-1}

$\beta = 0.0309$ min^{-1}

$t_{\frac{1}{2}\beta} = 22.4$ min

$AUC = 46692$ ng mL^{-1} min

$CL = 21.4$ mL min^{-1} kg^{-1}

$k_{21} = 0.130$ min^{-1}

$k_{10} = 0.213$ min^{-1}

$k_{12} = 0.583$ min^{-1}

$V_{area} = 693$ mL kg^{-1}

$V_{ss} = 553$ mL kg^{-1}

$V_1 = 101$ mL kg^{-1}

$V_2 = 452$ mL kg^{-1}

As shown above, two expressions for the volume of distribution (V_{area} and V_{ss}) can be calculated. V_{area} expresses the relation between the total amount of lidocaine in the body and its concentration in the central compartment during the terminal phase when distribution equilibrium has been established. V_{area} may overestimate the true volume of distribution when rapid drug elimination occurs and clearance is high. V_{ss} (the volume of distribution at steady state) is not dependent on the rate of drug elimination, and therefore usually provides the more accurate and reliable value. In the case of lidocaine, V_{area} (693 mL kg^{-1}) is greater than V_{ss} (553 mL kg^{-1}), although both values are similar to presumed values for total body water. The volume of the central compartment (101 mL kg^{-1}) is approximately twice the plasma volume, while the clearance of lidocaine is similar to liver blood flow (21 mL min^{-1} kg^{-1}).

Three-compartment models

Although the pharmacokinetics of many drugs is consistent with a two-compartment solution, models of greater complexity may provide a better interpretation of the experimental data. The decline in the plasma concentration of many opioids, as well as some muscle relaxants and intravenous anaesthetics, can often be resolved into three exponential components. Consequently, the plasma concentration C_p at time t is defined by the expression:

$$C_p = Ae^{-\alpha t} + Be^{-\beta t} + Ce^{-\gamma t},$$

and values for the intercepts (A, B and C) and the slopes (α, β and γ) of the three components can be obtained.

After an intravenous bolus dose (1 mg kg^{-1}) of propofol, the decline in plasma concentration is consistent with a triexponential decline. Its concentration rapidly decreases during the first 10 minutes, and then declines more slowly for approximately 4 hours (Fig. 2.5). Both these phases of drug distribution are due to the uptake of propofol by tissues and are followed by a slower decline in plasma concentration due to hepatic elimination (which is constrained by the slow return of propofol from peripheral tissues). When the logarithm of the plasma concentration of propofol is plotted against time, there is a linear relationship between the variables during the terminal elimination (γ) phase,

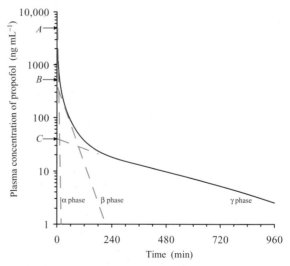

Fig. 2.5 Triexponential decline in the plasma concentration of propofol (1 mg kg^{-1}, i.v.). The abcissae (x-axis) shows the time in minutes, and the ordinate (y-axis) the plasma concentration of propofol (logarithmic scale). C is the initial concentration of the slowest γ-phase of exponential decline, extrapolated to zero time. A and B are the intercepts of the rapid α-distribution phase and the slower β-distribution phase of exponential decline.

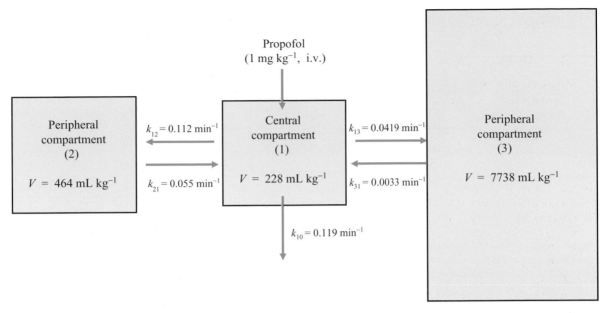

Fig. 2.6 A three-compartment open model for propofol disposition. Drug administration occurs into and elimination occurs from the central compartment. The constants k_{12}, k_{21}, k_{13} and k_{31} govern drug transfer between the central and the peripheral compartments. k_{10} is the elimination rate constant.

and the decrease in plasma concentration can be resolved into three exponential components by extrapolation. The three phases of exponential decline all have characteristic slopes ($\alpha = 0.301$ min^{-1}; $\beta = 0.0299$ min^{-1}; and $\gamma = 0.0024$ min^{-1}) and half-lives ($t_{1/2\alpha} = 2.3$ min; $t_{1/2\beta} = 23.2$ min; and $t_{1/2\gamma} = 289$ min). The intercepts on the ordinate (A, B and C) can be considered to represent the amount that each half-life contributes to the decrease in plasma concentration after the bolus dose of propofol. Almost all the decline in plasma concentration occurs during the α- and β-phases of drug distribution.

Since the number of compartments required to characterize drug behaviour is always equal to the number of phases of exponential decline, the decline in plasma concentration is interpreted in terms of a three-compartment model (Fig. 2.6). This consists of a relatively small central compartment, into which the drug is administered and from which it is eliminated, and two larger peripheral compartments that are both connected to the central compartment. One of the peripheral compartments is relatively small and well perfused, and reflects the initial fall in plasma concentration (α-phase), while the other peripheral compartment is larger and less well perfused, and is associated with the slower phase of distribution (β-phase). The rate of drug elimination is governed by

the rate constant k_{10}, and bidirectional (reversible) drug transfer between the central compartment and the peripheral compartments are governed by the rate constants k_{12} and k_{21} (compartment 2) and k_{13} and k_{31} (compartment 3).

Resolution of the three-compartment open model is essentially similar to the two-compartment model and depends on similar assumptions. Values for A, α, B, β, C and γ are derived from the pharmacokinetic analysis, and used to derive the parameters of the model, including the volume of distribution and the clearance. In some instances, the decrease in plasma concentration is best interpreted by a three-compartment model with elimination from one of the peripheral compartments (Fig. 2.7).

In practice, the distinction between two compartment and three compartment models may be relatively small, and the choice of model may be influenced by the accuracy of the analytical method used to measure drug concentration. Similarly, the timing of blood sampling may influence the choice of a pharmacokinetic model, since inappropriate sampling times may fail to identify the initial phase or the terminal phase of exponential decline. Consequently, technical, analytical and sampling factors may play an important part in determining the choice of pharmacokinetic model.

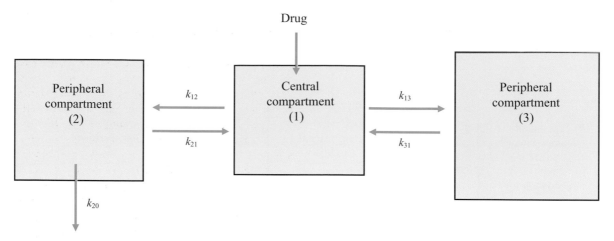

Fig. 2.7 A three-compartment open model. Drug administration occurs into the central compartment, but elimination occurs from a peripheral compartment. The constants k_{12}, k_{21}, k_{13} and k_{31} govern drug transfer between the central and the peripheral compartments. k_{20} is the elimination rate constant.

Physiological models

The distribution and elimination of some drugs, including thiopental, lidocaine and inhalational anaesthetics, have been described in terms of physiological perfusion models. These depend on the interpretation of drug distribution in terms of anatomical or physiological spaces, which have defined volumes, perfusion characteristics and partition coefficients that are specific for each drug. They are particularly useful in the modelling of drugs with effects that produce changes in physiological parameters (e.g. cardiac output, liver blood flow) and which can thus influence their own disposition.

In 1960, the disposition of thiopental was classically described by a physiological perfusion model, which illustrated the importance of redistribution in the termination of its action. The concentration of the drug in blood, skeletal muscle and subcutaneous fat at various times after its administration was shown to be consistent with a relatively simple model (consisting of a central blood pool and six tissue compartments). It was suggested that thiopental was primarily removed from the brain by lean body tissues (e.g. muscle) and that subcutaneous fat only played a subsidiary role. The model was subsequently refined by the inclusion of compartments representing drug metabolism, plasma protein binding and tissue binding. More recent models have predicted the occurrence of higher peak arterial concentrations in patients with a low cardiac output, and may account for the interindividual variability in

thiopental disposition in patients during induction of anaesthesia.

Physiological perfusion models have a number of distinct advantages. They can be used to predict drug concentrations at the site of action in tissues. Distribution and elimination can be precisely described, and they can also take account of local or general physiological changes during anaesthesia (e.g. alterations in cardiac output, regional blood flow and renal function). In some instances, they can accommodate intrasubject variability in drug disposition. Unfortunately, they depend on the detailed analysis of a significant amount of data, and the collection of appropriate tissue samples from anaesthetized patients may be undesirable or unethical.

Maintenance of constant plasma concentrations

Values for the volume of distribution and the clearance of drugs can be used in the design of individual dosage regimes when drugs are given by intravenous infusion. In these conditions, a loading dose and a continuous infusion can be used to produce accurate and constant plasma concentrations. The required loading dose (in $\mu g \, kg^{-1}$) is given by $C_p \times V$, and the rate of infusion (in $\mu g \, min^{-1} \, kg^{-1}$) by $C_p \times CL$, where C_p is the desired steady-state plasma concentration ($\mu g \, mL^{-1}$), V is the volume of distribution at steady state ($mL \, kg^{-1}$), and CL is the clearance

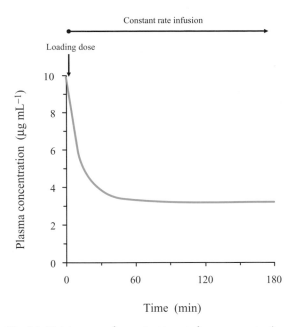

Fig. 2.8 Maintenance of a constant target plasma concentration (C_p) based on the equations: loading dose = $C_p \times V$; infusion rate = $C_p \times$ CL.

(mL min^{-1} kg^{-1}). When drugs are given intravenously for prolonged periods (e.g. opioid analgesics, induction agents) this method can be used to provide reproducible and constant plasma concentrations (Fig. 2.8). Unfortunately, it depends on accurate values for the volume of distribution and clearance of drugs, which may be subject to experimental error and considerable interindividual variability. In addition, the loading dose may result in transiently high plasma concentrations, and may therefore require modification, such as an initially rapid rate of infusion, rather than a loading dose.

More recently, the BET (bolus, elimination and transfer) method has been used to produce constant and reproducible plasma concentrations of drugs. This procedure is based on the use of an appropriate compartmental model. A bolus of drug sufficient to fill the central compartment to the required concentration is administered, followed by a continuous infusion at an exponentially declining rate to compensate for the disappearance of the drug from the central compartment and its transfer to one or more peripheral compartments. This method has been used with computer-controlled programmed infusion devices to deliver constant plasma concentrations of several anaesthetic agents (e.g. propofol, alfentanil), and to maintain them within the therapeutic range.

Target-controlled infusion systems

In recent years, target-controlled computer systems have been used to produce desirable plasma concentrations of drugs after intravenous infusion. In general, the parameters of three compartment models have been used as the input for pharmacokinetic simulation programs that control conventional intravenous infusion systems. Computer programs that can be used to control infusion systems for various drugs are generally available, and a variety of different algorithms can be used to regulate the infusion rate. Target-controlled infusion systems can alter the rate of infusion extremely rapidly (e.g. every 10 s) and thus rapidly achieve the target concentration. These systems rapidly achieve and maintain steady-state plasma concentrations, which can then be modified in a controlled manner according to the individual pharmacodynamic response.

Pharmacokinetic variability

Identical doses of drugs may result in wide differences in the plasma concentrations in different patients due to pharmacokinetic variability. These differences may be related to variability in the processes of absorption, distribution, metabolism and excretion (Chapter 1), or to physiological changes associated with age, obesity, gender or pregnancy. They may also be related to genetic variability or caused by interaction with other drugs (Chapter 4). Alternatively, they may be related to the effects of pathological changes on the clearance of drugs.

Hepatic disease

Hepatic disease may have relatively little effect on the pharmacokinetics of drugs, since the liver has a large reserve capacity and its metabolic functions may not be compromised until failure is extreme. In general, liver impairment will have the greatest effect on the elimination of drugs with a low intrinsic hepatic clearance (e.g. theophylline, diazepam, warfarin). The metabolic clearance of these drugs may be reduced in severe hepatic failure, resulting in a longer terminal half-life.

Renal disease

Chronic renal disease causes a reduction in creatinine clearance and the renal elimination of many drugs. In particular, the clearance of drugs that are almost entirely eliminated unchanged by the kidney (e.g. aminoglycoside antibiotics, digoxin) is reduced.

Renal failure may reduce the clearance and prolong the duration of action of some muscle relaxants. The action of gallamine and pancuronium is prolonged in renal failure, although the duration of action of other non-depolarizing agents is generally unaffected. These clinical findings are consistent with the effects of renal impairment on the clearance of these drugs.

Population pharmacokinetics

Population pharmacokinetic analysis attempts to take account of interindividual variability to derive constants and parameters that reflect drug disposition in the entire patient population. The use of summary statistics derived from individual pharmacokinetic studies is usually unreliable. A more acceptable method depends on the collection of a small number of individual blood samples from a large and varied population of patients. Analysis of the data can be used to assess intraindividual and interindividual variability, and attempts to relate the variation to patient characteristics, renal and hepatic function, and concurrently administered drugs. In 'non-linear mixed effects modelling', an attempt is made to integrate the inherent interindividual variability into a pharmacokinetic model by means of appropriate statistical parameters. Data from all individual patients are included, as well as a note of their identity. Population pharmacokinetic analysis usually depends on restricted individual data derived from a large number of subjects, as well as several assumptions (e.g. that the form of each individual plasma profile is identical to the population profile).

The differences between individual pharmacokinetic constants and the population value are then assessed in terms of measurable characteristics or 'fixed effects' (e.g. age, weight, creatinine clearance, hepatic clearance), while other unexplained sources of variability are described as 'random effects'. Population pharmacokinetics attempts to interpret as much variability as possible in terms of measurable characteristics or 'fixed effects'.

Duration of drug action

In some instances (e.g. organophosphorus compounds, phenoxybenzamine), the activity of drugs is dependent on their irreversible combination with enzymes or receptors. In these conditions, there is often no relationship between pharmacokinetic parameters and their duration of action. Their biological effects usually last for days or even weeks, long after their elimination from the body.

In most other conditions, the activity of drugs is dependent on the presence of an effective concentration at the site of action, which is in turn dependent on their plasma concentration. Consequently, if the plasma concentration is above the minimum effective level when drug distribution is complete, its subsequent rate of decline due to drug elimination may be a guide to the duration of action. In these circumstances, values for the terminal half-lives of drugs may be used as a guide to their length of action, particularly when drugs are administered orally.

Terminal half-life

The terminal half-life is usually defined as the time required for the plasma concentration to decrease by 50% during the terminal phase. Its value in agents that are commonly used in anaesthesia varies over an extremely wide range, from suxamethonium (3–5 min) to diazepam (24–48 h).

The terminal half-life is often closely related to the primary pharmacokinetic constants V and CL. In general terms,

$$t_{1/2} \propto \frac{V}{CL} = k \times \frac{V}{CL},$$

where k is a constant (ln 2; 0.693).

Consequently, the term is a hybrid constant, which depends on the values for V and CL. An increase in the terminal half-life of a drug may reflect an increased volume of distribution, a reduced clearance, or both these changes. A shorter half-life may represent a decrease in the volume of distribution, an increase in clearance, or both phenomena. Consequently, alterations in the terminal half-lives of drugs do not necessarily reflect changes in drug elimination.

When drugs are administered orally in identical doses at intervals that are equal to their terminal half-lives, there is a progressive rise in plasma concentration for approximately 4–5 half-lives until steady-state concentrations are reached (Fig. 2.9). The latent period before steady-state conditions occur can be avoided by the initial administration of a loading dose equal to twice the normal dose. Similarly, when drugs are given by continuous infusion, steady-state concentrations are reached after approximately 4–5 terminal half-lives. In general, drugs are best given at intervals that are approximately equal to their terminal

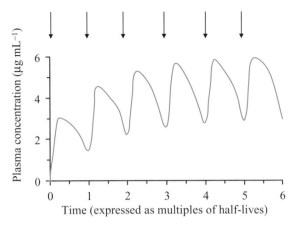

Fig. 2.9 The cumulation of drugs when they are administered (arrows) at intervals that are equal to their half-lives.

half-lives. In these conditions, there is often an acceptable compromise between the decline in drug concentrations after successive doses and the necessity for frequent drug administration in order to maintain an adequate plasma level.

In the case of some anaesthetic drugs (e.g. muscle relaxants), there is an approximate relationship between the terminal half-lives of individual drugs and the relative duration of action of conventional doses (Table 2.3). This relationship may not be present with other drugs (e.g. opioid analgesics), since they must cross the blood–brain barrier in order to produce their effects (Chapter 10).

Table 2.3 Plasma half-lives and approximate duration of action of conventional doses of some common muscle relaxants in adult patients with normal renal and hepatic function.

Drug	Plasma half-life (min)	Duration of action
Suxamethonium	3–5	Very short
Mivacurium*	2–8	Very short
Atracurium	18–22	Short
Cisatracurium	18–22	Short
Vecuronium	36–72	Short
Rocuronium	70–140	Intermediate
Gallamine	80–220	Intermediate
Pancuronium	110–150	Long

*Values for the two most active isomers (cis–trans mivacurium and trans–trans mivacurium).

Consequently morphine, which has a shorter terminal half-life than pethidine, has a longer duration of action. Similarly, when the effects of drugs are terminated by distribution or redistribution (e.g. intravenous barbiturates, benzodiazepines, some opioids) their duration of action is not predictably related to their terminal half-lives. After low doses of propofol ($1–2\ mg\ kg^{-1}$), the plasma concentration rapidly falls below the levels associated with anaesthesia due to its extensive tissue distribution (Fig. 2.5). In these conditions, the terminal half-life (4–11 h) is quite unrelated to its duration of action. Similar conclusions apply to fentanyl, alfentanil and thiopental, whose actions are normally terminated by their distribution in tissues.

Context-sensitive half-times

As explained above, the terminal half-lives of drugs may be an inaccurate indication of their disposition and duration of action after intravenous administration, since their concentrations may decline below effective levels during the initial phase or phases of drug distribution, i.e. before the terminal half-life becomes a dominant feature of the plasma concentration profile. In these conditions, the action of drugs is terminated by drug distribution, and 'context-sensitive half-times' provide a more accurate measurement of drug disposition and activity. The context-sensitive half-time can be defined as the time required for the plasma concentration to decrease by 50% at the end of a period of infusion designed to maintain a constant level. Even after prolonged periods of infusion, context-sensitive half-times are invariably less than their comparable terminal half-lives. Computer simulations suggest that the context-sensitive half-times of some drugs are independent of the duration of infusion. For instance, the half-time of remifentanil is 2–5 minutes for all infusion times of up to 8 hours. The context-sensitive half-times of some other drugs (for instance, alfentanil, midazolam, propofol) are moderately influenced by the duration of infusion, and the half-time of propofol increases 2–3 times (from 12 to 38 min) when the duration of infusion is increased from 1 to 8 hours (Table 2.4). Consequently, recovery from the effects of these drugs after short infusions is usually relatively rapid. In contrast, the context-sensitive half-time of fentanyl increases 10–12 times (from 24 to 280 min) when the infusion duration is increased from 1 to 8 hours, since significant amounts of the drug rapidly returns to plasma from peripheral tissues after the termination of prolonged infusions (Table 2.4).

Table 2.4 Context-sensitive half-times of some common anaesthetic agents.

Infusion duration (h)	Context-sensitive half-times (min)					
	Remifentanil	Alfentanil	Midazolam	Propofol	Thiopental	Fentanyl
1	2	36	34	12	78	24
2	2	53	45	16	100	50
3	3	55	60	18	120	108
4	3	56	63	25	138	175
5	3	57	67	30	157	218
6	3	58	70	32	167	250
7	3	59	72	35	172	268
8	4	60	75	38	180	280

These computer simulations suggest that the effects of fentanyl may last for at least several hours after prolonged infusions are stopped. By comparison, the residual effects of remifentanil, and to a lesser extent alfentanil, propofol and midazolam, are relatively transient, irrespective of the duration of infusion. The clinical usefulness of context-sensitive half-times has been questioned, since the decrease in plasma concentration required for recovery is not necessarily 50%. Nevertheless, they are a useful guide to the duration of action of drugs whose effects are normally terminated by distribution.

Although context-sensitive half-times are not pharmacokinetic constants and have no pharmacokinetic meaning, they provide a useful practical indication of the decline in plasma concentrations after infusions of a defined duration. In these conditions, they may also provide a guide to the likely duration of drug activity and the speed of recovery after infusions of different durations, and may therefore be of considerable value in the context of total intravenous anaesthesia.

More recently these ideas have been extended by the concept of 'relative decrement times', in which a pharmacodynamic model is integrated into the computer simulations of context-sensitive half-times.

Compartmental models and pharmacological effects

When drugs produce reversible effects at their site of action, there may be a close correlation between their plasma concentrations and their pharmacological effects. When the site of action is in the central compartment, there may be a relation between the amount of drug in the compartment and the observed response. Early studies suggested that the serum concentration of tubocurarine (and the amount of the drug in the central compartment) was closely correlated with its effects on neuromuscular transmission, suggesting that the action of the drug was in this compartment. More recently, it has been shown that a better interpretation of the pharmacokinetics and pharmacodynamics of muscle relaxants during onset and recovery is obtained when a separate 'effect compartment' is added to a pharmacokinetic model.

Drug hysteresis

When non-depolarizing muscle relaxants are infused, there is a latent period between the rise in their plasma concentration and the onset of neuromuscular blockade. When infusion ceases, the fall in plasma concentration occurs slightly earlier than the recovery in neuromuscular transmission. This phenomenon is known as anticlockwise hysteresis or temporal disequilibrium (Fig. 2.10). It has been shown to occur with many other drugs (e.g. intravenous anaesthetics, most opioid analgesics) and is usually attributed to slow drug–receptor kinetics or to the delayed access of drugs to their site of action ('the biophase').

Effect compartment

In the case of muscle relaxants, the occurrence of hysteresis or temporal disequilibrium has been rationalized by the addition of a separate 'effect compartment' (with distinct rate constants) to the central compartment of a pharmacokinetic model. The effect compartment is envisaged as a hypothetical and infinitely small compartment that has no significant effect on the kinetics of the pharmacokinetic model as a whole, but in which there is a hysteresis-free relationship between the plasma concentration and the pharmacological effect. At equilibrium,

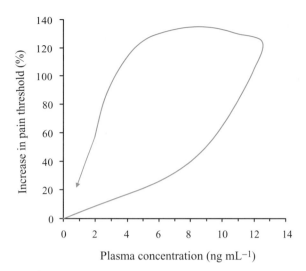

Fig. 2.10 An anticlockwise hysteresis loop, showing the relationship between the plasma concentration of an opioid and its analgesic effects.

there is no difference between the drug concentration in the central compartment and the effect compartment.

Saturation kinetics

When drug behaviour is analysed by pharmacokinetic models, it is usually assumed that distribution and elimination are first-order processes (i.e. that the rate of drug transfer from compartment to compartment is always proportional to drug concentration). This presumption is not necessarily correct. Many physiological processes concerned with drug distribution and elimination are dependent on carrier transport, and are potentially saturable, i.e. they have a maximum, finite, transport capacity. Similarly, many reactions concerned with drug metabolism are saturable, and proceed at a maximal and constant rate at high substrate concentrations. In these conditions, drug transport and metabolism occur at a high but constant rate that is independent of drug concentration. This type of kinetics is usually called saturation, zero-order or non-linear kinetics.

Michaelis–Menten enzyme kinetics

Metabolic reactions that are subject to saturation kinetics are consistent with Michaelis–Menten kinetics (Fig. 2.11). When saturation occurs, metabolism changes from the first-order process

$$dX/dt = -kX^1 = -kX$$

to a zero-order process

$$dX/dt = -kX^0 = -k$$

and is thus constant and independent of drug concentration.

These expressions can be derived from the Michaelis–Menten equation for enzyme kinetics as expressed in the form:

$$v = \frac{V_{\max}C_{\mathrm{p}}}{K_{\mathrm{m}} + C_{\mathrm{p}}}$$

where v is the rate of drug elimination, $V_{\max}$ is the maximum rate of drug elimination and C_{p} is the plasma concentration. K_{m} is an affinity constant (the Michaelis–Menten constant) which represents the affinity of the drug for the enzyme, carrier or transport system. It corresponds to the plasma concentration at which drug elimination is half its maximal rate (i.e. $v/V_{\max} = 0.5$). When the plasma concentration C_{p} is low (and $<K_{\mathrm{m}}$), then $v \approx (V_{\max}/K_{\mathrm{m}}) \times C_{\mathrm{p}}$.

Since $V_{\max}$ and K_{m} are both constants, $v \propto C_{\mathrm{p}}$, and the rate of drug elimination is directly proportional to the plasma concentration.

At higher plasma concentrations, C_{p} is greater than K_{m}, and $v \approx (V_{\max} \times C_{\mathrm{p}})/C_{\mathrm{p}}$, and $v \approx V_{\max}$. Thus, the rate of drug elimination becomes constant and approaches $V_{\max}$ at high concentrations, producing saturation kinetics (Fig. 2.11).

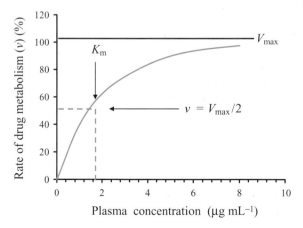

Fig. 2.11 Michaelis–Menten kinetics and drug metabolism. K_m corresponds to the plasma concentration at half the maximum rate of drug metabolism ($v = V_{\max}/2$). The rate of drug metabolism is linear (directly proportional to plasma concentration) below the K_m value. At higher concentrations the rate of drug metabolism becomes increasingly non-linear, and is constant when $v = V_{\max}$.

Clinical implications

In clinical practice saturation kinetics is relatively uncommon, since the capacity of carrier transport systems and metabolic reactions is normally much greater than effective drug concentrations. Nevertheless, in some instances, particularly with drugs that are predominantly eliminated by hepatic metabolism, saturation kinetics occurs *in vivo*. In these conditions, increases in drug dosage prolong the terminal half-life, and cause a disproportionate increase in steady-state plasma concentrations.

Saturation kinetics occurs during the metabolism of ethanol, salicylates and phenytoin due to the saturation of hepatic metabolic pathways. Ethyl alcohol is removed from plasma by alcohol dehydrogenase at the maximum rate of approximately 2 mmol $kg^{-1} h^{-1}$ (about 100 mg $kg^{-1} h^{-1}$) due to the limited availability of the cofactor NAD^+. Consequently, traces of alcohol can still be detected in blood for as long as 8 hours after the intake of 60 g or so (about 3 pints of beer). Saturation kinetics also occurs at subtherapeutic or therapeutic plasma concentrations of phenytoin (40–80 μmol L^{-1}), so that increments in dosage cause a disproportionate increase in plasma concentrations. A similar phenomenon occurs during the elimination of large or repeated doses of thiopental, so that the terminal half-life of the drug is increased and its pharmacological effects are prolonged due to saturation of hepatic metabolism.

Saturation kinetics may also occur in many patients after drug overdosage. It is uncertain whether this is due to saturation of hepatic metabolism, the toxic effects of drugs, or other factors. When drugs are eliminated by saturable processes, the subsequent decrease in plasma concentration is associated with reversion to linear, non-saturable kinetics. Consequently, the plasma half-life becomes progressively shorter during drug elimination, and the logarithm of the plasma concentration versus time curve is bell-shaped, rather than monoexponential or biexponential (Fig. 2.12).

The value and limitations of pharmacokinetic analysis

Pharmacokinetic models and constants have been widely used to design acceptable dosage regimes for the intravenous administration of anaesthetic agents. Automatic computer-controlled infusion pumps have been programmed with appropriate pharmacokinetic models and individual patient characteristics, and used to produce predetermined plasma concentrations of drugs ('target-controlled infusion'). More recently, 'feedback' devices

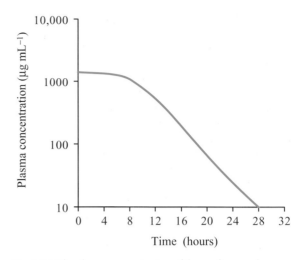

Fig. 2.12 The plasma concentration of drugs after overdosage. Initially drug metabolism is non-linear (saturation kinetics). As the plasma concentration falls, drug metabolism becomes linear (first-order) resulting in a shorter plasma half-life.

that monitor drug responses have been used to produce 'closed-loop' control of infusion systems. Nevertheless, there are a number of inherent problems involved in the consistent application of pharmacokinetic regimes in clinical practice.

In the first place, the pharmacokinetics of drugs whose distribution and elimination are consistent with a two- or three-compartment open model have been usually determined after intravenous administration, either with a bolus dose or a rapid infusion. In these conditions, the accurate determination of kinetic parameters is subject to a number of errors. The estimation of both the clearance (CL) and the volume of distribution (V) are critically dependent on the area under the plasma concentration–time curve between $t = 0$ and $t = \infty$ (AUC). In a two-compartment model, the AUC is determined from the relationship $A/\alpha + B/\beta$. Since A is usually large and α is relatively small, any errors in the determination of these constants may significantly affect the value of the AUC. After the intravenous injection of drugs, measurement of A and α may be extremely inaccurate since:

(1) They are dependent on derived rather than measured concentrations;

(2) They are usually determined from a relatively small number of data points;

(3) The plasma concentration of drugs is rapidly decreasing during the distribution phase, so that minor difficulties in the timing or removal of blood samples may

lead to considerable errors. Consequently, the pharmacokinetic parameters that are derived from the plasma concentration data may be relatively inaccurate and unreliable.

Values for the volume of distribution and clearance can be determined more accurately when drugs are administered by infusion. Pharmacokinetic constants applicable to a two- or three-compartment open model can then be derived from the postinfusion plasma concentration data by appropriate mathematical techniques. When drugs are given by continuous infusion, rapid distribution or redistribution may no longer occur (depending on the period of infusion), and the rapid decline in their plasma concentration during the α or fast disposition phase may be attenuated.

A further problem associated with the application of kinetic data to routine clinical practice is associated with the wide interindividual variability in both pharmacokinetics and pharmacodynamics. There is commonly a two or threefold variation in the plasma concentrations achieved by the same dosage regime in different patients. In addition, there is often a marked variability in interindividual pharmacodynamic responses to the same plasma concentration. The presence of pathological changes in cardiac, hepatic and renal function may be responsible for further interpatient variability. In these conditions, the application of highly variable pharmacokinetic and pharmacodynamic data, usually obtained in young and healthy volunteers, to surgical patients with compromised organ function is extremely questionable.

The value of pharmacokinetics depends on a reproducible and measurable relationship between the plasma concentration of drugs and their pharmacological effects. Pharmacokinetic analysis is of little practical use unless drug activity is a predictable function of plasma concentration. Unfortunately, the relationship between these levels and the biological effects of drugs may be unpredictable. In some instances, plasma concentrations do not reflect those at the biophase or site of action, and the relation between them is often complex. Some anaesthetic agents do not act in an entirely reversible manner (e.g. neostigmine). Others have active metabolites with similar effects to the parent drug (e.g. diazepam, thiopental), while some have an onset and duration of action unrelated to their pharmacokinetics (e.g. some opioids and local anaesthetics). In all of these instances, pharmacokinetic methods may be of little use in the accurate prediction of drug activity.

Finally, the use of many anaesthetic drugs as chiral or racemic mixtures (Chapter 3) may have pharmacokinetic implications. In most instances, their plasma concentrations have been determined by non-stereoselective methods. Since the proportion of stereoisomers in the original racemic mixture may rapidly change to an unknown ratio in the body, pharmacokinetic interpretation of the derived kinetic constants may be inaccurate and misleading. The generation of pharmacokinetic data on chiral drugs by methods that do not distinguish between the enantiomers has been rightly described as a waste of money on unscientific, sophisticated nonsense.

Bioavailability

When drugs are administered orally, the term bioavailability is often used to indicate the proportion of the dose that is present in the systemic circulation. Bioavailability can be defined as the rate and extent to which a drug is absorbed and becomes available at its site of action. The total amount of drug that is present in the systemic circulation is usually more important than its rate of absorption, and bioavailability is usually defined by reference to the area under the plasma concentration–time curve (AUC), which can be easily measured by the 'trapezoidal rule' (Fig. 2.1). After intravenous administration, drugs can be presumed to have a bioavailability of 100%; consequently, the bioavailability (%) of oral drugs can be defined as (see Fig. 2.13)

$$\frac{(\text{AUC}_{0-\infty} \text{ after oral administration})}{(\text{AUC}_{0-\infty} \text{ after intravenous administration})} \times 100$$

Alternatively, the absolute bioavailability of drugs can be measured from the total excretion of unchanged drug in urine after oral and intravenous administration.

High oral bioavailability

Some drugs have a high oral bioavailability (e.g. diazepam, warfarin). These compounds are relatively stable in gastrointestinal secretions, are well absorbed from the small intestine, have a low intrinsic hepatic clearance and first-pass effect, and are not significantly metabolized by the gut wall or the liver before they gain access to the systemic circulation.

Low oral bioavailability

Other drugs have a low oral bioavailability due to a number of factors. In the first place, some drugs are unstable or are broken down in the gastrointestinal tract (e.g. benzylpenicillin, many polypeptide hormones). Secondly, drugs may be poorly absorbed from the gut due to their low lipid

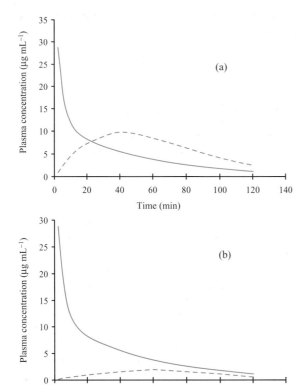

Fig. 2.13 Differences in the oral bioavailability of drugs. (a) High oral bioavailability; (b) low oral bioavailability. Plasma concentrations after intravenous administration (——); plasma concentrations after oral administration (- - -).

solubility or high molecular weight (e.g. neostigmine, glycopyrronium). Finally, high extraction drugs with a significant first-pass effect have a low systemic bioavailability due to their extensive metabolism by the gut and the liver (e.g. morphine, propranolol). First-pass metabolism reduces the amount of unchanged drug that enters the systemic circulation.

Differences in oral bioavailability

Differences in the oral bioavailability of drugs may be due to several causes. Numerous pharmaceutical factors can influence the dissolution of tablets and capsules. In these conditions, proprietary or generic preparations of the same drug may have different dissolution characteristics and thus produce a range of plasma concentrations after oral administration. These variations in drug dissolution mainly occur with relatively insoluble drugs that

are administered orally, and the subsequent differences in bioavailability may be clinically significant (page 6). Interindividual differences in hepatic blood flow and first-pass metabolism can also lead to variations in bioavailability. With 'flow-limited' hepatic clearance, any reduction in hepatic blood flow may lead to an increase in bioavailability. Drugs that induce or inhibit hepatic microsomal enzymes may also affect systemic bioavailability. For instance, cimetidine can increase the bioavailability of propranolol. Similarly, physiological changes (old age) and pathological factors (hepatic cirrhosis) can impair drug metabolism and increase bioavailability.

Plasma concentrations of lidocaine and propofol in Figs. 2.3 and 2.5 were not determined experimentally but were derived from published pharmacokinetic models. See Schnider *et al.* (1996); Marsh *et al.* (1991); Glen (2002).

Suggested reading

Benet, L.Z. & Galeazzi, R.L. (1979) Noncompartmental determination of the steady-state volume of distribution. *Journal of Pharmaceutical Sciences* **68**, 1071–1074.

Coetzee, J.F. (2005) Principles of intravenous drug infusion. *Anaesthesia and Intensive Care Medicine* **6**, 141–144.

Gibaldi, M. & Perrier, D. (1982) *Pharmacokinetics*, 2nd edn. New York: Marcel Dekker.

Glen, I. (2002) Pharmacokinetic analysis. *Anaesthesia and Intensive Care Medicine* **3**, 263–265.

Gupta, V.L. & Glass, P.S.A. (1998) Total intravenous anesthesia. In: Longnecker, D.E., Tinker, J.H. & Morgan, G.E. (eds.), *Principles and Practice of Anesthesiology*. St. Louis: Mosby, pp. 1260–1293.

Lin, J.H. & Lu, A.Y. (2001) Interindividual variability in inhibition and induction of cytochrome P450 enzymes. *Annual Review of Pharmacology and Toxicology* **41**, 535–567.

Marsh, B., White, M., Morton, N. & Kenny, G.N.C. (1991) Pharmacokinetic model driven infusion of propofol in children. *British Journal of Anaesthesia* **67**, 41–48.

Pleuvry, B. (2002) Pharmacodynamics: concentration–response relationships and hysteresis. *Anaesthesia and Intensive Care Medicine* **3**, 269–271.

Price, H.L., Kovnat, P.J., Safer, J.N., Conner, E.H. & Price, M.L. (1960) The uptake of thiopental by body tissues and its relation to the duration of narcosis. *Clinical Pharmacology and Therapeutics* **1**, 16–22.

Prys-Roberts, C. & Hug, C.C. (eds) (1984) *Pharmacokinetics of Anaesthesia*. Oxford: Blackwell Scientific Publications.

Riegelman, S., Loo, J.C.K. & Rowland, M. (1968) Shortcomings in pharmacokinetic analysis by conceiving the body to exhibit properties of a single compartment. *Journal of Pharmaceutical Sciences* **57**, 117–123.

Rowland, M. & Tozer, T.N. (1995) *Clinical Pharmacokinetics: Concepts and Applications*, 3rd edn. Baltimore: Williams & Wilkins.

Schnider, T.W., Gaeta, R., Brose, W., Minto, C.F., Gregg, K.M. & Schafer, S.L. (1996) Derivation and cross-validation of pharmacokinetic parameters for computer-controlled infusion of lidocaine in pain therapy. *Anesthesiology* **84**, 1043–1050.

Schuttler, J., Kloos, S., Schwilden, H. & Stoeckel, H. (1988) TIVA with propofol and alfentanil by computer assisted infusions. *Anaesthesia* **43**(Suppl), 2–7.

Shafer, S.L. & Varvel, J.R. (1991) Pharmacokinetics, pharmacodynamics, and rational opioid selection. *Anesthesiology* **74**, 53–63.

Stanski, D.R. & Watkins, W.D. (1982) *Drug Disposition in Anesthesia*. New York: Grune & Stratton.

Tozer, T.N. (1981) Concepts basic to pharmacokinetics. *Pharmacology and Therapeutics* **12**, 109–131.

Wilkinson, G.R. (1987) Clearance approaches in pharmacology. *Pharmacological Reviews* **39**, 1–47.

Wright, P.M.C. (1998) Population based pharmacokinetic analysis: why do we need it; what is it; and what has it told us about anaesthetics? *British Journal of Anaesthesia* **80**, 488–501.

Appendix

Exponential changes

Changes in the plasma concentration of drugs in relation to time can usually be expressed as mathematical equations containing one or more exponential terms. In the mathematical expression

$$10^3 = 1000$$

10^3 is an exponential term; the number 10 must be raised to the power or exponent of 3 in order to equal 1000. Equations of this type can be conveniently considered in terms of the common logarithms of numbers, which are defined as the power or exponent to which the base must be raised in order to give the number. Consequently, the logarithm of 1000 to base 10 is 3.

Since $10^a \times 10^b = 10^{a+b}$ and $10^a \div 10^b = 10^{a-b}$, the multiplication of numbers can be carried out by summating their logarithms, and the division of numbers by subtracting their logarithms, followed by an antilogarithmic transformation. Logarithms to base 10 ($\log_{10}$) are most commonly used for this purpose.

Natural or Napierian logarithms ($\log_e$ or $\ln$) are similar to common logarithms, but use the mathematical constant e (2.718) as their base. In numerical terms, e can be expressed as the limiting sum of an infinitely convergent series:

$$e = 1 + 1 + \frac{1}{2.1} + \frac{1}{3.2.1} + \frac{1}{4.3.2.1} \text{etc.}$$

and

$$e^x = 1 + x + \frac{x^2}{2.1} + \frac{x^3}{3.2.1} + \frac{x^4}{4.3.2.1} \text{etc.}$$

convergent for all finite values of x. Alternatively, e can be considered as an irrational number which can be expressed as the sum of a series:

$$e = \left(1 + \frac{1}{n}\right)^n \ (n \to \infty)$$

which can be expressed as the sum of a series:

The importance of the constant e is related to the mathematical interpretation of exponential changes, in which the rate of change in a variable is proportional to its magnitude. Exponential changes can be expressed mathematically in terms of natural logarithms. Many processes concerned with the absorption, distribution and elimination of drugs result in exponential changes in drug concentration in relation to time. In these exponential changes, the increase or decrease in the concentration of a drug is directly proportional to its magnitude, and in mathematical terms,

$$\pm \frac{dX}{dt} \propto X$$

$$\pm \frac{dX}{dt} = kX$$

where dX/dt is the rate of increase or decrease of the variable X during an infinitesimal moment of time t, k is a constant and X is the value of the variable at time t.

On integration of this expression between $t = 0$ and $t = \infty$

$$X = X_0 e^{kt} \text{(for exponential growth)}$$

$$X = X_0 e^{-kt} \text{(for exponential disappearance)}$$

where X is the value of X at any time t, X_0 is the initial value of X at zero time, e is the base of natural logarithms (2.718) and k is a constant.

In these conditions, X can be described as an exponential function of time.

Consider the equation for exponential disappearance

$$X = X_0 e^{-kt}$$

On taking natural logarithms,

$$\ln X = \ln X_0 - kt$$

and

$$\ln\left(\frac{X}{X_o}\right) = -kt$$

Consequently, $k = -\ln(X/X_0)/t$; in this equation k can be considered as a rate constant, and represents the proportional change in X in unit time. Alternatively, the rate of exponential change can be represented as the half-time (half-life) or as a time constant. Since

$$k = \frac{-\ln(X/X_o)}{t}$$

$$t = \frac{\ln(X/X_o)}{-k}$$

If $(X/X_0) = 1/2$, t represents the time for X to decline to half its original value, and

$$t = \frac{\ln(1/2)}{-k}$$

$$= \frac{\ln 2}{k}$$

$$= \frac{0.693}{k}$$

In these conditions, t represents the half-time (half-life) of the exponential change. Alternatively, if t represents the time required for X to decline to $1/e$ (37%) of its original value, and

$$\frac{X}{X_o} = \frac{1}{2.718} = \frac{1}{e}$$

$$t = \frac{\ln(1/e)}{-k}$$

$$= \frac{\ln(e^{-1})}{-k}$$

$$= \frac{-\ln e}{-k}$$

$$= \frac{1}{k}$$

In these conditions, t represents the time constant of the exponential change and is the reciprocal of the rate constant k.

3 Drug Action

The effects of drugs in humans usually depend on the modification of cellular function by agents with a relatively simple chemical structure. In some cases, including inhalational agents, local anaesthetics and non-depolarizing muscle relaxants, there is a reasonably close relationship between their chemical structure or physicochemical properties and their biological effects. In other instances, drugs that are closely related chemically (such as promazine and promethazine, which are structural isomers) have quite different pharmacological actions.

Dose–response relationships

Pharmacological effects are usually related to drug dosage by means of dose–response curves (Fig. 3.1). Although the plasma concentration of most drugs can be accurately measured, the relation between these values and their concentration at the site of action in the 'biophase' is often unclear or unknown. In some instances, it may be possible to obtain an approximation of their concentration from appropriate pharmacokinetic models (Chapter 2). Nevertheless, it is often difficult to study the relationship between drug doses or concentrations and pharmacological responses in *in vivo* conditions, and any observed correlation between them may be subject to significant inaccuracy.

Until 50 years ago, the observation and analysis of the effects of drugs was predominantly dependent on isolated tissue preparations, such as the frog rectus abdominis muscle, the rat phrenic nerve–diaphragm preparation and the guinea pig ileum. In these isolated preparations, a defined concentration of a drug can be added to a tissue bath, and the response obtained can be directly measured by appropriate techniques. Many of the effects of drugs that produce observable and measurable responses ('agonists') were originally assessed in these experimental conditions. In recent years, other techniques have been more widely used, such as the direct measurement of cellular or subcellular responses to drugs in *in vitro* conditions

or tissue culture. Human tissues removed during surgical operations have been used for similar purposes, either as isolated preparations or in tissue culture.

Dose–response curves

In both *in vivo* and *in vitro* conditions, the relationship between drug dosage and biological response is usually represented by a dose–response (or concentration–effect) curve. In most experimental situations, this curve has a hyperbolic shape (Fig. 3.1). Incremental increases in dosage progressively amplify the response obtained. As the dose is further increased, the proportional response diminishes, and eventually a maximum effect (E_{max}) is obtained which cannot be exceeded irrespective of the dose. Dose–response curves can be used to estimate E_{max} and the drug concentration required to produce 50% of the maximal response (EC_{50}). Differences between the EC_{50} values of drugs are frequently used to compare their potencies (i.e. the dose required to produce a given effect).

Log dose–response curves

Dose–response relationships are more commonly expressed semi-logarithmically, and in these conditions, the hyperbolic curve usually becomes sigmoid or S-shaped (Fig. 3.2). This transformation has a number of advantages. In particular, it is linear for most of its course (between approximately 20 and 80% of E_{max}), and it permits the simultaneous comparison and assessment of drugs with large differences in potency. In general, drugs that have a similar mechanism of action tend to have parallel log dose–response curves. Highly potent agents that produce responses at relatively low dose levels have a log dose–response curve which is displaced to the left, i.e. towards the *y*-axis. By contrast, drugs of lower potency have a log dose–response curve that is displaced to the right. Many drug antagonists displace agonist log dose–response curves to the right, without affecting the slope or the maximum response, and the extent of the parallel displacement can be used to measure antagonist affinity (page 60).

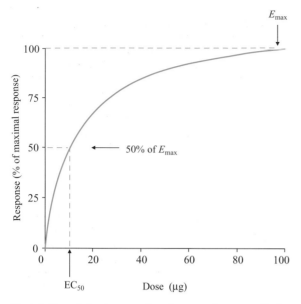

Fig. 3.1 The relation between drug dosage and response. Both axes are plotted on a linear scale, resulting in a hyperbolic curve. E_{max} represents the maximum response; EC_{50} is the dose required to produce 50% of the maximum response.

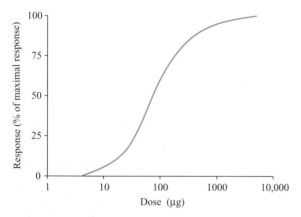

Fig. 3.2 A typical log dose–response curve (——), which is linear for most of its length (between 20 and 80% of the maximum response).

Atypical dose–response curves

Although most dose–response relationships are hyperbolic, and give rise to sigmoid log dose–response curves (Fig. 3.2), other types of concentration–effect relationship are not uncommon. Dose–response curves for agonists at nicotinic, glutamate and GABA receptors are

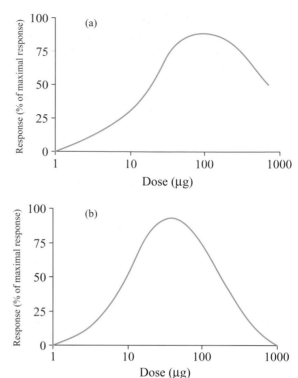

Fig. 3.3 Examples of atypical log dose–response relationships: (a) biphasic log dose–response curve; (b) bell-shaped log dose–response curve.

frequently sigmoidal. In some experimental situations, log dose–response curves are biphasic (e.g. the effects of noradrenaline and adrenaline on the rabbit heart) or even bell-shaped (e.g. the effects of histamine on vascular smooth muscle in the guinea pig pulmonary artery, Fig. 3.3). In some instances, drug concentrations at the site of action in the biophase may be much less than those bathing tissue preparations due to enzymic hydrolysis, tissue uptake or the presence of diffusion barriers.

Dose–response relationships in humans

In intact animals or in humans, the relation between drug dosage and response is often complicated by homeostatic reflexes and other factors, particularly plasma protein binding and the presence of active metabolites. Consequently, the plasma concentrations of drugs, or their presumed concentrations at their site of action, are usually related to their pharmacological effects. In these conditions, the slope of the plasma concentration–response curve may indicate the potential safety margin of a drug. When relatively steep plasma concentration–response relationships are present (e.g. fentanyl), toxic effects may be produced by relatively small incremental increases in dosage. By contrast, when more gradual plasma concentration–response relationships are present (e.g. diazepam), incremental increases in dosage are usually less hazardous.

Graded and quantal responses

Dose–response curves represent a graded or changeable response to incremental doses of drugs in different *in vivo* or *in vitro* conditions, rather than an all or none ('discontinuous' or 'quantal') response. At one time, quantal responses were widely used to measure the median effective dose (ED_{50}) and the median lethal dose (LD_{50}) of drugs in experimental conditions. The 'therapeutic index' was defined as the ratio of these values (i.e. LD_{50}/ED_{50}), in an attempt to reflect the relationship between the toxicity and effectiveness of drugs. In recent years, the limitations of this approach have been widely recognized and the use of these methods has greatly declined.

The basis of drug action

In some instances, the effects of drugs are solely dependent on their chemical or physical properties. Simple antacids act by neutralizing gastric acid, and are not significantly absorbed, although large doses may produce minor changes in systemic pH and acid–base status. Similarly, most acids and bases produce alterations in systemic and urinary pH due to the addition or removal of H^+ from body fluids.

The effects of chelating agents (Table 3.1) are also due to their chemical properties. Chelating agents usually produce their effects by combining with metallic ions, forming water-soluble complexes which are subsequently removed from the body. Consequently, they are often used in the treatment of heavy metal poisoning and certain other conditions.

The action of other drugs may be related to their physical properties. Both inhalational agents and local anaesthetics were formerly believed to act by producing non-specific physical changes in the lipid components of neuronal membranes, which subsequently produced secondary effects on ionic permeability and transport. Recent evidence suggests that both groups of drugs affect neuronal function in a more specific manner (Chapters 8 and 9).

Table 3.1 Chelating agents in current clinical use.

Chelating agent	Ions or elements chelated	Clinical use
Penicillamine	Lead	Heavy metal poisoning
	Mercury	Rheumatoid disease
	Copper	Wilson's disease
	Zinc	Cystinuria
Dimercaprol	Lead	Heavy metal poisoning
	Mercury	
	Arsenic	
	Gold	
Sodium calcium edetate	Lead	Heavy metal poisoning
Dicobalt edetate	Cyanide	Cyanide poisoning
Desferrioxamine	Iron	Iron poisoning
		Iron overload
	Aluminium	Aluminium overload

In most other circumstances, drugs produce their pharmacological effects by acting on protein targets, which may be

- Enzymes
- Receptors
- Ion channels
- Transport proteins

Enzymes

Many drugs produce their effects by inhibiting enzymes concerned with normal biochemical or metabolic processes (Table 3.2) and are often chemically related to the natural substrates that are metabolized by the enzyme. For example, allopurinol, a xanthine oxidase inhibitor, is a close chemical analogue of xanthine and hypoxanthine, which are normally converted by xanthine oxidase to uric acid.

Reversible enzyme inhibition

Most drugs that affect enzymes are reversible inhibitors, and compete with natural substrates for enzymes (e.g. edrophonium, enoximone, allopurinol). Their effects usually depend on the formation of a reversible enzyme-inhibitor complex, according to the equation:

$$\text{enzyme} + \text{inhibitor} \rightleftharpoons \text{enzyme} - \text{inhibitor complex}$$

Table 3.2 Common drugs whose effects are partly or totally due to enzyme inhibition.

Drug(s)	Inhibited enzyme
Acetazolamide	Carbonic anhydrase
Acetylsalicylic acid; NSAIDs	Cyclooxygenase
Aciclovir	Thymidine kinase
Allopurinol	Xanthine oxidase
Aminophylline; enoximone	Phosphodiesterase
Benserazide	Dopa decarboxylase
Benzylpenicillin	Bacterial wall transpeptidase
Chlorophenylalanine	Tryptophan hydrolase
Cytarabine	DNA polymerase
Disulfiram	Aldehyde dehydrogenase
Edrophonium; neostigmine; pyridostigmine	Acetylcholinesterase
Enalapril; lisinopril	Angiotensin converting enzyme
Methotrexate; trimethoprim	Dihydrofolate reductase
Methyldopa	Dopa decarboxylase
Moclobemide; phenelzine; selegiline	Monoamine oxidase
Sulphamethoxazole	Folate synthetase
Zidovudine	Reverse transcriptase

In some instances, enzyme inhibition is dependent on the formation of drug metabolites.

Formation of the enzyme–inhibitor complex is usually dependent on reversible, unstable chemical bonds (e.g. electrostatic bonds). Consequently, enzyme inhibition is often evanescent, and probably reflects the presence of drugs or their active metabolites in the immediate environment of the enzyme. As reversible enzyme inhibitors are eliminated from the body, their plasma concentration falls and inhibition decreases.

Neostigmine and related drugs are usually classified as reversible inhibitors of acetylcholinesterase and cholinesterase. These drugs initially combine reversibly with both enzymes, but subsequent inhibition is mainly dependent on carbamylation of the esteratic site, and involves the formation of a covalent chemical bond. This bond is slowly hydrolysed ($t_{1/2} = 36$ min), and the enzyme is gradually regenerated, although the drugs are hydrolysed (Chapter 10).

Irreversible enzyme inhibition

Irreversible enzyme inhibition depends on the formation of a stable chemical complex between the inhibitor and the enzyme. In these conditions, regeneration of the inhibited enzyme is usually impossible, and the enzyme must be resynthesized before its function is restored. Drugs that act by irreversible enzyme inhibition include organophosphorus insecticides, methotrexate and most monoamine oxidase inhibitors. These drugs have an extremely long duration of action and may produce effects for days or weeks after they are eliminated from the body. Aspirin has similar effects on platelet cyclooxygenase (COX-1), and irreversibly acetylates the enzyme for the duration of the platelet lifespan (approximately 7–9 days).

False metabolites

In some instances, drugs are converted by enzyme systems to metabolites that interfere with normal cellular function. Methyldopa is converted by sympathetic neurons to methyldopamine and methylnoradrenaline, and these metabolites replace noradrenaline in central and peripheral sympathetic nerve endings. Similarly, fluorouracil is metabolized to a false nucleotide intermediate, which cannot be converted to thymidylate by the enzyme thymidylate synthetase. Consequently, DNA synthesis is inhibited, resulting in cytotoxic effects.

Receptors

Most drugs produce their effects by combining with macromolecular sites in cells known as drug receptors. These sites are usually glycoproteins, and most of them were originally developed to enable cells to respond to endogenous hormones or neurotransmitters. Consequently, many of them have an important role in intercellular transmission, and form an integral part of the physiological mechanisms that are involved in signal transduction.

History

The concept of receptors was introduced at the end of the nineteenth century by J.N. Langley, in order to account for the highly specific actions of certain drugs on physiological systems, such as the effects of pilocarpine and atropine on salivary secretion, and the action of nicotine and curare on neuromuscular transmission. The German physician Paul Ehrlich also played an important part in the development of the concept of chemoreceptors in tissues. Ehrlich was clearly influenced by the work of Langley, and by his own studies on cross-resistance in antitrypanosomal drugs. The mathematical and quantitative aspects of drug–receptor reactions and drug responses were subsequently developed by A.J. Clark and J.H. Gaddum.

In subsequent work between 1930 and 1960, the nature and properties of drug receptors were mainly inferred from 'structure–activity' relationships. In these studies, an attempt was made to investigate the nature of drug–receptor interaction from the response of isolated tissues to a series of drugs with related chemical structures, as typified by the response of smooth muscle preparations to a series of choline esters. At this time, it was widely recognized that this was a relatively indirect approach to the study of the structure and properties of receptors.

Isolation and purification of receptors

Since 1965, it has been possible to isolate receptors from tissues and to study their properties in *in vitro* conditions, and their structure, function and organization can be determined by molecular biological techniques. Most receptors can now be complexed with radiolabelled ligands. For instance, the acetylcholine receptor at the neuromuscular junction is irreversibly bound by the radioiodinated α-toxins of certain snakes, such as α-bungarotoxin from the Taiwan banded krait and α-cobra toxin from the cobra. Intact receptors in cellular membranes can be solubilized by non-ionic detergents, radiolabelled and subsequently purified by affinity chromatography or related techniques, so that their amino acid sequences can be established. The corresponding base sequence of the messenger RNA (mRNA) can then be deduced and complementary DNA (cDNA) obtained by conventional cloning methods, using recombinant DNA technology. Subsequently, mRNA is generated by transcription of cDNA and injected into cultured cell lines *in vitro* ('transfection'), resulting in the expression of receptors by the cultured cells ('expression cloning').

In some instances, receptors expressed in stable cultured cell lines have been reconstituted with their transcription systems, and their molecular mechanisms have been studied. Similarly, receptor variants and subtypes have been cloned from cDNA libraries and expressed in cultured cells. Some receptor subtypes appear to have no known physiological functions, and in some instances 'orphan receptors' (receptors with no known endogenous ligands) have been identified. More recent techniques of expression cloning have been developed that do not depend on the isolation or purification of receptor proteins.

Receptor distribution

Radiolabelled compounds with a high affinity for specific receptors (radioligands) have also been widely used to study receptor distribution and heterogeneity. The distribution of nicotinic acetylcholine receptors in the brain has been studied, and muscarinic receptors in the heart, the small intestine, sympathetic ganglia and the brain have also been identified by various radiolabelled ligands (e.g. ^{3}H-pirenzepine). Similarly, dopamine receptors at various sites in the CNS have been identified by radiolabelled dopamine antagonists (e.g. ^{3}H-haloperidol). Both α- and ß-adrenoceptors can be specifically labelled and identified by different radioligands, which may be agonists (^{3}H-hydroxybenzylisoprenaline) or antagonists (^{125}I-iodocyanopindolol). Adrenoceptors are widely distributed in the body, and in some instances (α_2-receptors in platelets, ß$_2$-receptors in vascular smooth muscle) their presence is not associated with a nerve supply.

Receptor density

Changes in adrenoceptor density may be produced by endogenous hormones or drugs, or may be associated with various pathological conditions (e.g. bronchial asthma, congestive cardiac failure, thyrotoxicosis). In general, high catecholamine concentrations reduce the number and density of adrenoceptors ('down-regulation'). This phenomenon is partly due to the sequestration ('internalization') of receptors within cells, although receptor affinity may also be modified. In contrast, any fall in circulating epinephrine and norepinephrine, produced by drugs or by sympathetic denervation, increases the number of receptors ('up-regulation'). Similar changes in receptor density are probably produced by most neurotransmitters that act at synapses and neuroeffector junctions.

In some situations, 'up-regulation' of receptors may be partly responsible for the phenomenon of supersensitivity, defined as an excessive but essentially normal response to an agonist. After peripheral denervation or damage to skeletal muscle, the response to acetylcholine and other depolarizing agents is increased due to up-regulation of nicotinic receptors on the postsynaptic membrane (Chapter 10). Sympathetic denervation by surgical or pharmacological methods also increases peripheral responses to catecholamines. In these circumstances, the increased response is mainly related to impairment of the neuronal uptake of norepinephrine. Any increase in the number of adrenoceptors due to up-regulation probably plays a less important part.

Receptor sensitivity and specificity

Most receptors are extremely sensitive to their naturally occurring endogenous agonists, and only small concentrations are required to produce a significant response. Consequently, considerable amplification or enhancement of the initial stimulus may be required to produce a significant effect. In many instances, amplification is produced by regulatory G-proteins. Many receptor systems also show considerable specificity and selectivity, and characteristically respond to a limited range of agonists with a defined chemical structure, which are often closely related to their naturally occurring neurotransmitters or hormones. Many receptors also have a finite capacity, and the binding of endogenous agonists is often competitive and saturable ('high affinity, low capacity binding').

Cellular localization

Most drug receptors are present on the external surface of cells and are associated with the limiting cytoplasmic membrane. Important exceptions are receptors for steroid hormones, which are present in the cytoplasm or the nuclear membrane of certain cells (target cells). Steroid hormones are bound by specific receptor proteins. Their activation modifies messenger RNA, and thus indirectly affects ribosomal protein synthesis.

Receptor activation

Receptor activation depends on two essential attributes of an agonist, affinity and efficacy. Affinity is the tendency of an agonist to combine with a receptor, while efficacy refers to the tendency of the agonist–receptor complex to induce a pharmacological response.

The reversible combination of an agonist with the receptor ('receptor occupancy') is the primary event that initiates a sequence of biophysical and biochemical reactions, such as ion transport, enzyme activation and protein synthesis, resulting in a pharmacological response (Fig. 3.4). Four main biophysical or biochemical changes appear to mediate a wide range of different responses to endogenous neurotransmitters, hormones and drugs:

• Direct changes in ion channel permeability
• Increased or decreased synthesis of intracellular metabolites
• Enhanced tyrosine kinase activity (autophosphorylation)
• Modification of DNA transcription

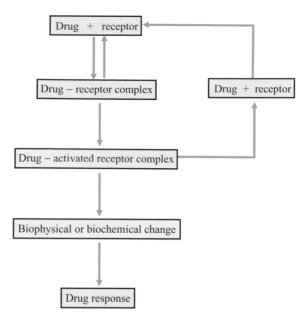

Fig. 3.4 General sequence of reactions involved in the combination of a drug with a receptor and the generation of a biological response. The drug combines reversibly with the receptor, causing its activation and resulting in biophysical or biochemical changes that mediate the biological response. The drug–receptor complex then dissociates resulting in the regeneration of the drug and the receptor.

Direct changes in ion channel permeability

In some instances, receptor activation directly affects ion channels in synaptic membranes, resulting in a selective or non-selective increase in ionic permeability. In these conditions, the receptor contains an intrinsic ion channel which is part of the same molecular complex. Receptor activation is usually evanescent, and causes an immediate increase in ionic permeability, which only lasts for several milliseconds.

Acetylcholine receptors at the neuromuscular junction

The acetylcholine receptor at the neuromuscular junction is the classical example of a receptor with an intrinsic ion channel (Chapter 10). The acetylcholine receptor is an integral membrane protein with a molecular weight of approximately 250 kDa. In adult man, it consists of

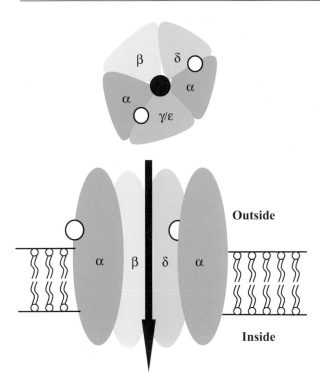

Outside

Inside

Fig. 3.5 Diagrammatic representation of the nicotinic receptor at the neuromuscular junction. The receptor consists of five subunits (α, α, β, γ or ε, and δ) surrounding the central transmembrane ion channel. It has two binding sites for acetylcholine (at the α–γ/ε and α–δ interfaces). (a) View of the receptor from above; (b) vertical cross-section of the receptor in the muscle cell membrane. acetylcholine-binding sites ($\circ$); ion channel ($\downarrow$).

five subunits (α, α, β, ε, δ), which cross the postsynaptic membrane and surround an ion channel (Fig. 3.5).[1] The α-subunits have a molecular weight of approximately 40 kDa, and each contains an acetylcholine-binding site at the interface with a different subunit (ε or δ). The phospholipid composition of the surrounding membrane may influence the combination of the α-subunits with acetylcholine and their subsequent conformational changes resulting in receptor activation.

When an action potential reaches the motor nerve terminal, acetylcholine is released and diffuses across the synaptic cleft. Combination of acetylcholine with both its receptor sites on the α-subunits results in conformational

changes that open the ion channel. Ion channel opening is an extremely rapid 'all or none' event that lasts for 1–2 milliseconds, and results in the transfer of approximately 10,000 ions (Na^+, K^+ or Ca^{2+}) during each millisecond that the channel is open. These ionic changes result in multiple single channel currents, which summate to produce an endplate current. If the localized endplate potential reaches a critical amplitude (a depolarization of approximately 10–15 mV), a muscle action potential is propagated along the muscle fibre.

Other nicotinic acetylcholine receptors

All nicotinic acetylcholine receptors have the same basic structure and consist of five subunits with an intrinsic ion channel. Nevertheless, many different molecular varieties of α- and β-subunits have been identified. Nicotinic receptors at presynaptic, ganglionic and CNS sites have a different molecular constitution, and most ganglionic receptors only contain α- and β-subunits.

Some receptors for other neurotransmitters have a similar molecular structure and are directly coupled to selective or non-selective ion channels. In these conditions, receptor activation results in channel opening and a rapid increase in permeability to one or more ions (Table 3.3).

Increased or decreased synthesis of intracellular metabolites

Receptor activation often modifies the activity of specific membrane-bound enzymes, resulting in an increased or

Table 3.3 Neurotransmitter receptors that contain an intrinsic ion channel (ionotropic receptors).

Receptor type	Ionic selectivity
Acetylcholine (nicotinic receptors)	Na^+, K^+, Ca^{2+}
GABA$_A$	Cl^-
Glutamate	
NMDA* receptors	Na^+, K^+, Ca^{2+}
AMPA† receptors	Na^+, K^+, Ca^{2+}
Kainate receptors	Na^+, K^+, Ca^{2+}
Glycine	Cl^-
5-HT$_3$	Na^+, K^+, Ca^{2+}

*NMDA, *N*-methyl-D-aspartate.
†AMPA, α-amino-3-hydroxy-5-methyl-4-isoxazole proprionic acid.

[1] In the foetus, the ε-subunit is replaced by the γ-subunit, which has different electrical and biophysical properties.

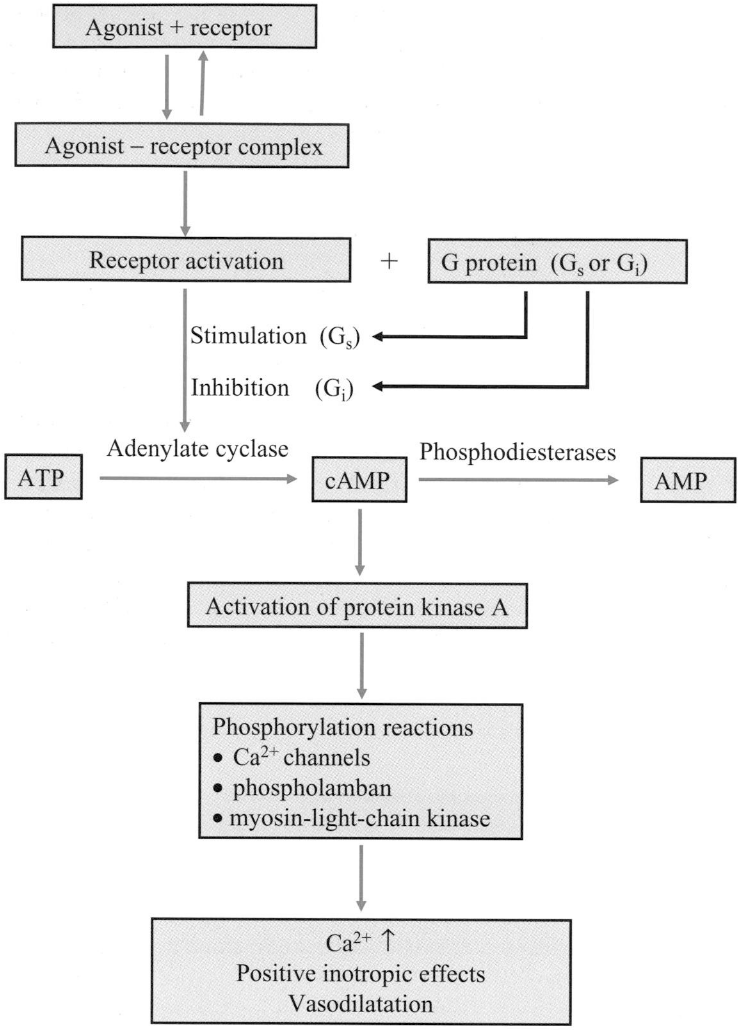

Fig. 3.6 Receptor activation and the formation of cAMP from ATP by adenylate cyclase. After receptor activation, GTP-binding proteins stimulate or inhibit adenylate cyclase. cAMP is formed and subsequently converted to AMP by phosphodiesterases.

decreased concentration of intracellular metabolites. Consequently, these mediators form a link between receptor activation and drug responses and are usually referred to as intermediate or second messengers.

The most important intermediate messengers are
• Cyclic adenosine monophosphate (cAMP)
• Inositol phosphates and diacylglycerol (IP and DAG)
• Cyclic guanosine monophosphate (cGMP)

Cyclic adenosine monophosphate

Cyclic adenosine monophosphate (cAMP) is synthesized from adenosine triphosphate (ATP) by the enzyme adenylate cyclase (Fig. 3.6). Many drugs and hormones which combine with receptors in cell membranes can affect the activity of adenylate cyclase, and thus modify the synthesis of cAMP. All these receptor systems are indirectly coupled to adenylate cyclase by regulatory G-proteins. All G-protein coupled receptors ('metabotropic receptors') have a similar molecular structure, consisting of a single long polypeptide chain with seven transmembrane regions ('domains').

Regulatory G-proteins

There are numerous different types of regulatory G-proteins. The effects of many drugs and endogenous compounds are mediated by receptors coupled to G_s, a

Table 3.4 Receptors with effector pathways that are dependent on activation of G_s, stimulation of adenylate cyclase, and the increased synthesis of cAMP.

ACTH receptors
Adenosine A_2-receptors
Adrenergic β-receptors (β_1, β_2 and β_3)
Dopamine D_1- and D_5-receptors
Glucagon receptors
Histamine H_2-receptors
5-Hydroxytryptamine 5-HT$_4$, 5-HT$_6$ and 5-HT$_7$ receptors
Vasopressin V_2-receptors

stimulatory G-protein, and adenylate cyclase. Consequently, receptor activation results in increased enzyme activity and enhanced synthesis of cAMP. All the ß-adrenergic effects of catecholamines are mediated by an increase in cAMP, and its significance was first recognized by Sutherland and Rall during their studies of the effects of adrenaline on glycogenolysis in isolated liver cells. More

recently, it has been recognized that increases in intracellular cAMP mediate effects at many other receptor sites (Table 3.4). In contrast, if the regulatory protein is G_i, receptor agonists inhibit the enzyme and decrease the synthesis of cAMP (Fig. 3.6).

Structure and function of G-proteins

Regulatory G-proteins consist of three different subunits, α, β and γ. In the inactive state, the α-subunit is bound by GDP. Receptor activation results in dissociation of the β–γ units and the binding of GTP by the α-units (i.e. GTP/GDP exchange), resulting in varying forms of an α–GTP complex which is then transferred to adenylate cyclase (Fig. 3.7). After enzyme stimulation (G_s) or inhibition (G_i), the α–GTP complex is rapidly hydrolysed to GDP and then recombines with the β–γ units to reform the inactive G-protein (α–GDP – β–γ), which can then be reactivated by another agonist–receptor complex. Since G_s and G_i can be repeatedly activated by a single drug–receptor complex, G-proteins can produce considerable

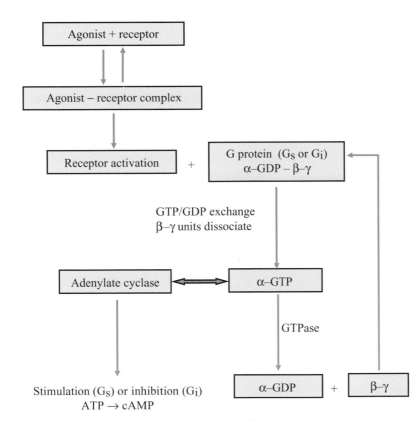

Fig. 3.7 The role of regulatory G proteins in the stimulation (by G_s) or inhibition (by G_i) of adenylate cyclase. The regulatory proteins G_s and G_i consist of three subunits, α, β and γ. In the inactive state, the α-subunit is bound to GDP. Receptor activation results in the binding of G_s or G_i by the receptor, followed by GTP/GDP exchange (GDP dissociates from the α-subunits and is replaced by GTP); the β–γ subunits also dissociate. The α–GTP complex then combines with adenylate cyclase, producing activation (G_s) or inhibition (G_i) of the enzyme. The α–GTP complex is rapidly broken down to α–GDP, which then recombines with the β–γ subunits to reform the inactive G protein. GDP, guanosine diphosphate; GTP, guanosine triphosphate.

amplification of the biological stimulus, and many drugs whose action is mediated by cAMP are extremely potent agents. The β–γ subunits may also have an important role in intracellular signalling.

G-proteins and bacterial endotoxins

Regulatory G-proteins are affected by some bacterial exotoxins. Cholera toxin causes persistent excitation of G_s by ADP-ribosylation of its α-subunit, resulting in the continuous activation of adenylate cyclase and accumulation of cAMP. Most of the symptoms and signs of cholera are due to the effects of the toxin on intestinal epithelium. In a similar manner, pertussis toxin produces ADP-ribosylation of the α-subunit of G_i and G_o, inhibiting the synthesis of cyclic AMP.

G-proteins in other systems

G-proteins play an important role in many other cellular systems. Some receptor systems cause activation of the third main type of regulatory G protein (G_q) which mediates the activation of phospholipase C and the breakdown of phosphoinositides (page 53). In some systems, G-proteins (G_i or G_o) directly control the gating of ion channels. The β–γ units probably mediate K^+ channel opening in α_2, M_2, M_4 and opioid receptors, resulting in hyperpolarization and inhibitory effects (Chapters 11 and 13).

Inhibition of adenylate cyclase

The effects of some drugs and hormones are dependent on the activation of receptors that are coupled to the regulatory protein G_i, resulting in inhibition of adenylate cyclase and decreased synthesis of cAMP. The effects of opioids at μ-, κ- and δ-receptors, and the action of noradrenaline on α_2-receptors are partly dependent on this mechanism. In addition, some of the effects of acetylcholine, adenosine, dopamine, glutamate and somatostatin are dependent on the attenuation of adenylate cyclase activity and the decreased synthesis of cAMP (Table 3.5).

In some instances, opposing or complementary physiological responses may be dependent on the activation and inhibition of adenylate cyclase, as shown by the effects of sympathetic and vagal tone on heart rate and cardiac contractility. An increase in cardiac sympathetic tone causes ß$_1$-receptor activation, resulting in enhanced synthesis of cAMP. In contrast, increased vagal tone activates myocardial muscarinic M_2-receptors, reducing cAMP.

Table 3.5 Receptors with effector pathways that are dependent on activation of G_i, inhibition of adenylate cyclase and the decreased synthesis of cAMP.

Adenosine A_1- and A_3-receptors
Adrenergic α_2-receptors
Dopamine D_2-, D_3- and D_4-receptors
Glutamate $mGlu_2$, $mGlu_3$, $mGlu_4$, $mGlu_6$, $mGlu_7$ and $mGlu_8$
$GABA_B$ receptors
5-Hydroxytryptamine $5-HT_1$ receptors
Muscarinic M_2- and M_4-receptors
Opioid receptors (μ, δ, κ and N/OFQ)

Effects and metabolism of cyclic AMP

Intracellular cAMP is rapidly bound by the regulatory (R) units of protein kinase A (PKA). The free catalytic (C) units of PKA are then activated, resulting in extensive protein phosphorylation, including the phosphorylation of voltage-dependent calcium channels, phospholamban (a regulatory protein in the sarcoplasmic reticulum) and myosin light chain kinase (Fig. 3.6). Consequently, Ca^{2+} mobilization in the heart is increased and vasodilatation occurs. In addition, activation of PKA increases lipolysis, glycogenolysis and protein synthesis.

After stimulation of adenylate cyclase by G_s, increased intracellular concentrations of cAMP rapidly return to their resting level, due to their metabolism by phosphodiesterase (PDE) enzymes, which convert cAMP to AMP (Fig. 3.6). The related cyclic nucleotide cGMP is also converted to GMP by phosphodiesterase. At least seven different families of PDE isoenzymes are present in mammalian cells, with different specificities, tissue distributions, and sensitivity to enzyme inhibition by drugs (Table 3.6). PDE III, and to a lesser extent, PDE IV play an important part in the hydrolysis of cAMP.

Phosphodiesterase inhibitors

When PDE enzymes are inhibited, the effects of cAMP may be prolonged, producing similar effects to the activation of receptors linked to G_s, i.e. an increase in intracellular cAMP. Several drugs primarily act by the reversible inhibition of one or more forms of the enzyme. Many methylxanthines (e.g. aminophylline, caffeine) non-selectively inhibit PDE isoenzymes in many tissues, producing positive inotropic effects on the heart, vasodilatation, relaxant effects on bronchial smooth muscle, inhibition of platelet aggregation and lipolysis.

Table 3.6 The primary substrates, tissue distribution and selective inhibitors of phosphodiesterase isoenzymes.

Isoenzyme family	Primary substrate	Tissue distribution	Selective inhibitors
I	cAMP	Brain Heart Liver Kidney	Vinpocetine
II	cGMP	Heart Adrenal cortex	
III	cAMP	Heart Blood vessels Bronchi Platelets	Pimobendan Milrinone Inamrinone Enoximone Peroximone
IV	cAMP	Brain Heart Bronchi Macrophages	Rolipram Cilomilast Roflumilast
V	cGMP	Platelets Penis	Dipyridamole Zaprinast Sildenafil Tadalafil Vardenafil
VI	cGMP	Retina	

In contrast, other drugs with a structural relationship to the natural substrate cAMP (e.g. enoximone, peroximone) selectively inhibit PDE III, which is predominantly present in the heart and vascular smooth muscle (Table 3.6). Consequently, their effects are mainly restricted to the cardiovascular system, and these agents are primarily used for their positive inotropic effects. Similarly, selective inhibitors of PDE IV have bronchodilator and anti-inflammatory effects, while inhibitors of PDE V are inhibitors of platelet aggregation or enhance penile erection.

Inositol phosphates and diacylglycerol

The mobilization of Ca^{2+} in many tissues is associated with the increased hydrolysis and turnover of the inositol phosphates ('phosphoinositides'), a minor group of membrane phospholipids. The occupation of receptor sites by agonists activates the enzyme phospholipase C, which hydrolyses the membrane phospholipid PIP_2 (phosphatidylinositol 4,5-bisphosphate) to IP_3 (inositol 1,4,5-trisphosphate) and DAG (diacylglycerol) (Fig. 3.8). Receptor occupation is not directly linked to the activa-tion of phospholipase C, but is mediated by a regulatory G protein (G_q), which behaves in an identical way to the regulatory proteins G_s and G_i in the cAMP-adenylate cyclase system. The activation of phospholipase C, in a similar manner to the activation of adenylate cyclase, is dependent on the formation of an α-subunit–GTP complex (Fig. 3.7). Both products of the hydrolysis of PIP_2 (IP_3 and DAG) are intracellular messengers. IP_3 is subsequently converted intracellularly to an inositol tetraphosphate (IP_4) whose role is uncertain, but may be involved in Ca^{2+} mobilization.

Inositol trisphosphate

Inositol trisphosphate (IP_3) combines with intracellular receptors in the endoplasmic reticulum, resulting in the opening of Ca^{2+} channels in the reticular membrane, with a subsequent increase in cytoplasmic Ca^{2+}, which is normally low (about 10^{-7} M, 100 nmol L^{-1}). Subsequently, free intracellular Ca^{2+} is bound by the regulatory protein troponins in cardiac and skeletal muscle, and calmodulin in most other tissues. Combination of Ca^{2+} with troponin C in cardiac and skeletal muscle plays an essential role in muscle contraction, allowing interaction to occur between myosin and actin filaments (Chapter 10). In other tissues, combination of Ca^{2+} with calmodulin causes conformational changes in the protein, exposing sites, which can interact with a wide variety of effectors, particularly protein kinases such as myosin light chain kinase and phosphorylase kinase. Consequently, the Ca^{2+}-calmodulin complex mediates a wide range of responses, including protein synthesis, changes in ionic permeability, glandular secretion and smooth muscle contraction (Fig. 3.8). The action of many hormones and neurotransmitters depends on receptor mechanisms that are mediated by the activation of PLC and the hydrolysis of PIP_2 to IP_3 (Table 3.7).

Diacylglycerol

DAG activates the enzyme protein kinase C, which binds Ca^{2+} and is then translocated to the plasma membrane where it mediates the phosphorylation of a wide variety of membrane proteins (e.g. enzymes, receptors, ion channels). Protein kinase C is also activated by phorbol esters (carcinogenic compounds produced by certain plants). DAG can be degraded by phospholipase A_2 to arachidonic acid, which is subsequently metabolized to prostaglandins and leukotrienes (Chapter 11). The phosphokinases A and C play a central role in the effector responses to receptor activation.

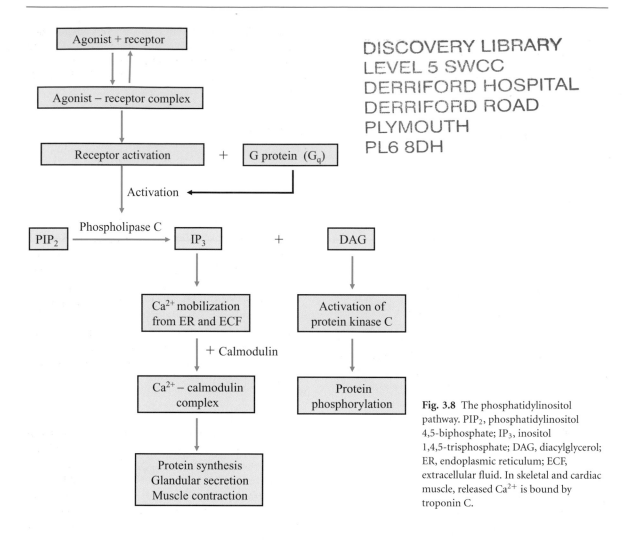

Fig. 3.8 The phosphatidylinositol pathway. PIP_2, phosphatidylinositol 4,5-biphosphate; IP_3, inositol 1,4,5-trisphosphate; DAG, diacylglycerol; ER, endoplasmic reticulum; ECF, extracellular fluid. In skeletal and cardiac muscle, released Ca^{2+} is bound by troponin C.

In practice, it is believed that activation of a single receptor or receptor subtype can be mediated by multiple G proteins, or by different subunits of a single G protein, that are concerned with several intermediate messengers. In addition, cAMP can increase intracellular Ca^{2+}, and modify responses to Ca^{2+}, and phosphorylation of many enzymes and proteins by protein kinases often results in a significant increase in their Ca^{2+} sensitivity. Indeed, Ca^{2+} are generally considered to be the universal messenger in mediating the response of cells to receptor activation and are responsible for the regulation of many forms of cellular activity.

Cyclic guanosine monophosphate

The cyclic nucleotide cGMP has a limited role as an intermediate messenger and mediates the effects of some hormones and neurotransmitters, although it is much less important than cAMP. It is synthesized from GTP by the enzyme guanylate cyclase, which exists in two distinct forms and cellular locations:

- Membrane-bound guanylate cyclase
- Cytoplasmic (soluble) guanylate cyclase

Membrane-bound guanylate cyclase

Occasionally, receptor systems in cell membranes possess inherent guanylate cyclase activity, increasing the synthesis of cGMP from GTP. In these conditions, the activation of guanylate cyclase is not dependent on G proteins, but appears to be due to the 'autophosphorylation' of tyrosine residues in the enzyme. For instance, the effects of natriuretic peptides on renal and vascular smooth muscle cells are mediated by receptors with inherent guanylate

Table 3.7 Receptors with effector pathways that are dependent on activation of G_q and phospholipase C, resulting in the formation of inositol 1,4,5-trisphosphate (IP_3).

Adrenergic α_1-receptors
Angiotensin AT_1-receptors
Endothelin receptors
Glutamate $mGlu_1$- and $mGlu_5$-receptors
Histamine H_1-receptors
5-Hydroxytryptamine 5-HT_2 receptors
Muscarinic M_1-, M_3- and M_5-receptors
Vasopressin V_1-receptors

cyclase activity, so that receptor activation increases the intracellular synthesis of cGMP.

Cytoplasmic (soluble) guanylate cyclase

Cytoplasmic (soluble) guanylate cyclase is a different form of enzyme that increases the intracellular formation of cGMP from GTP. The subsequent activation of cGMP-dependent protein kinases results in the phosphorylation of membrane proteins and ion channels, decreased Ca^{2+} entry in vascular smooth muscle and vasodilatation. K^+ channels are also activated by cGMP, resulting in hyperpolarization. Soluble guanylate cyclase contains a haem group, which binds nitric oxide (NO), and many of the effects of NO on neurons and blood vessels are indirectly mediated by the enzyme.

Metabolism of cGMP

The metabolism of cGMP is dependent on one or more of the phosphodiesterase family of enzymes, and some isoforms (PDE II, III and V) have a high affinity for cGMP (Table 3.6). Inhibition of PDE V by dipyridamole prevents platelet adhesion. In contrast, inhibition by sildenafil prolongs and enhances penile erection due to its dependence on the local synthesis of cGMP by soluble guanylate cyclase. Occasionally, high doses of these drugs cause visual disturbances in sensitive individuals due to their non-specific effects on PDE VI.

Nitric oxide

Although NO is not an intracellular messenger produced by receptor activation, many of its effects are mediated by soluble guanylate cyclase and cGMP.

The physiological role of NO was first elucidated during studies of 'endothelium-derived relaxing factor' (EDRF), which showed that acetylcholine-induced relaxation of blood vessels was dependent on a factor derived from vascular endothelium. It was subsequently shown that the activity of EDRF was dependent on the formation and release of NO by endothelial cells, and that EDRF and NO were identical.

Synthesis of NO

In most cells, NO is synthesized from L-arginine by nitric oxide synthase (NOS), which exists in three distinct isoforms:
- Neuronal (nNOS)
- Endothelial (eNOS)
- Inducible (iNOS)

All three enzyme isoforms are haem proteins with molecular similarities to cytochrome P450, and have binding sites for arginine, Ca^{2+}-calmodulin and flavine nucleotides. Both neuronal and endothelial NOS are Ca^{2+}-dependent, 'constitutive' enzymes that are present in normal physiological conditions. In contrast, inducible NOS is a Ca^{2+}-independent and 'non-constitutive' isoform that is synthesized in inflammatory cells by pathological changes. Its activity is normally approximately 1000 times greater than either nNOS or eNOS.

Neuronal NOS

Neuronal NOS is responsible for the synthesis of NO in most peripheral and central neurons. In the peripheral nervous system, NO is synthesized by non-adrenergic, non-cholinergic (NANC) neurons in the adventitial wall of blood vessels, and regulates the control of smooth muscle function in many organs and tissues (e.g. stomach, small intestine, uterus). In the penis, the release of NO from NANC nerves activates guanylate cyclase and increases the synthesis of cGMP, causing relaxation of the corpus cavernosum and erection. In the CNS, NO synthesis is enhanced by the increase in intracellular Ca^{2+} and calmodulin binding that are produced by activation of NMDA glutamate receptors. NO subsequently diffuses into adjacent cells, activates guanylate cyclase and increases synthesis of cGMP. It may also be involved in retrograde neurotransmission and regulate synaptic plasticity.

Endothelial NOS

Endothelial NOS is present in vascular endothelium and certain other tissues, including myocardial cells, osteoblasts and platelets, and is responsible for the synthesis of NO at these sites. NO then diffuses from the endothelium to vascular smooth muscle cells, where it activates

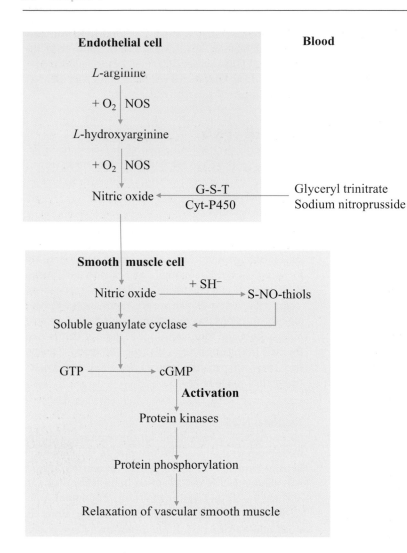

Fig. 3.9 The synthesis, release and action of nitric oxide in vascular smooth muscle. NOS, nitric oxide synthase; G-S-T, glutathione S-transferase; Cyt-P450, cytochrome P450; SH, sulphydryl groups; S-NO-thiols, S-nitrosothiols.

soluble (cytoplasmic) guanylate cyclase, increasing cGMP synthesis and activating cGMP-dependent protein kinases (Fig. 3.9). These changes cause phosphorylation of membrane proteins, a decrease in Ca^{2+} entry and relaxation of vascular smooth muscle. NO also reacts with intracellular SH^- groups in amino acids and proteins, and the S-nitrosothiol compounds formed are potent vasodilators. In physiological conditions, acetylcholine, bradykinin and the shear stress of blood flow increase the synthesis of NO by endothelial cells and cause cGMP-dependent relaxation of vascular smooth muscle. In addition, NO may act in conjunction with prostacyclin as an inhibitor of platelet aggregation and adhesion, and has negative inotropic effects. Its continuous synthesis and release by endothe-

lial cells plays an important functional role in the control of peripheral resistance and vascular smooth muscle tone.

Receptor activation is occasionally mediated by NO synthesis and release. The activation of muscarinic M_3-receptors in blood vessels increases endothelial NO synthesis; subsequently NO diffuses into smooth muscle cells and increases the formation of cGMP, producing vasodilatation.

Inducible NOS
Inducible NOS is a Ca^{2+}-independent, non-constitutive enzyme that can be induced in most immune and

inflammatory cells, as well as in endothelial cells and microglia. Its synthesis is induced by bacterial liposaccharides and endotoxins, interferon γ, tumour necrosis factor α, interleukin 1ß and other cytokines. In pyrexia, the synthesis and expression of iNOS frequently increases nitrate excretion, and similar changes commonly occur in bacterial sepsis and endotoxaemia. Synthesis of NO by inflammatory cells is a major cause of delayed hypotension in shock, and its formation and conversion to peroxynitrite is an important factor in the cytotoxicity induced by activated macrophages.

The induction of iNOS is inhibited by many glucocorticoids and is mainly responsible for the anti-inflammatory effects of these drugs (Chapter 17).

Therapeutic applications

Certain vasodilator drugs, including glyceryl trinitrate (GTN) and sodium nitroprusside (SNP) are metabolized to NO and thus produce relaxation of vascular smooth muscle. Both GTN and SNP are highly lipid-soluble drugs, and readily diffuse from blood vessels to vascular endothelium and smooth muscle cells. They are then metabolized to NO and nitrosothiols by glutathione-S-transferases and cytochrome P450 enzymes, resulting in activation of soluble guanylate cyclase, increased synthesis of cGMP and vasodilatation (Fig. 3.9).

Low concentrations of inhaled NO (30–50 ppm) produce pulmonary vasodilatation, and have been used in pulmonary hypertension and the adult respiratory distress syndrome (ARDS), with encouraging results. In the circulation, NO is rapidly inactivated by haem and reversibly bound by globin. Consequently, it has a circulatory half-life of approximately 5–7 seconds and does not significantly affect the systemic circulation.

Enhanced tyrosine kinase activity (autophosphorylation)

Extracellular activation of membrane receptors may cause the association of adjacent paired receptors, resulting in the intracellular phosphorylation of their own tyrosine residues ('autophosphorylation'). Insulin receptors consist of two extracellular α-units and two intracellular β-units, which are linked by S–S bonds, forming a β–α–α–β tetrameric molecule. The binding of insulin by the two α-units results in enhanced tyrosine kinase activity in the β-units, and the subsequent phosphorylation of amino acid residues in other intracellular proteins.

Similar receptors mediate cellular responses to many cytokines and interleukins, as well as natriuretic peptides and related transmitters. Thus natriuretic peptide receptors have catalytic functions, with inherent guanylate cyclase activity on their intracellular aspects.

Modification of DNA transcription

Steroid hormones and their synthetic analogues produce their effects by combining with nuclear receptors and indirectly affecting protein synthesis. Steroid receptors are usually discrete nuclear proteins that are widely expressed, although their density in different cells is extremely variable. All steroid hormones are highly lipid-soluble and diffuse across cellular membranes where they are bound by steroid receptors, usually in the cytoplasm or the nuclear membrane. The binding of steroids by the receptor protein results in the activation of adjacent amino acid residues that normally bind DNA, usually known as 'zinc fingers'. The activation of these high-affinity DNA binding sites results in their association with specific sequences in DNA ('steroid regulatory or hormone response elements') and the induction or repression of adjacent genes that control protein synthesis. The binding of receptors by different steroid hormones, i.e. corticosteroids, oestrogens, or progestogens, results in the activation of distinct DNA sequences, and thus produces an entirely different pattern of protein synthesis. Irrespective of the hormonal stimulus, gene transcription is either repressed or induced, resulting in rapid changes in RNA polymerase activity, mRNA and ribosomal protein synthesis. Nevertheless, the physiological effects of steroid hormones are often delayed for several hours.

The anti-inflammatory effects of glucocorticoids are mainly due to their combination with intracellular steroid receptors, and the subsequent modification of DNA and RNA synthesis (Chapter 17).

Ion channels and transport proteins

In addition to their effects on enzymes (page 45) and receptors (page 46), drugs may also directly act on ion channels and transport proteins. In particular, drugs may affect Na^+, K^+ or Ca^{2+} channels. Local anaesthetics produce blockade of voltage-sensitive Na^+ channels in excitable membranes (Chapter 9), and oral hypoglycaemic agents block K_{ATP} channels in pancreatic β-cells, resulting in depolarization and insulin secretion (Chapter 17). Diazoxide and thiazide diuretics open K^+ channels in vascular smooth muscle, producing hyperpolarization, vasodilatation and a reduction in blood pressure (Chapter 14), while some antianginal drugs produce similar effects in myocardial cells (nicorandil, Chapter 15). Finally, calcium channel blockers affect L-type Ca^{2+} channels in the heart or vascular smooth muscle (Chapters 14 and 15).

Analysis of drug–receptor reactions

Occupation theory

The classical analysis of drug responses in terms of the combination of agonists with receptors ('occupation theory') was introduced by A.J. Clark in the 1930s. It depends on the assumption that each drug molecule combines with a receptor in a reversible manner, forming a drug–receptor complex. In these conditions, it can be shown that the fraction of receptors occupied by the drug is equal to

$$\frac{[D]}{K_d + [D]}$$

where $[D]$ is the concentration of free (unbound) drug and K_d is the equilibrium dissociation constant of the drug–receptor complex at equilibrium (Appendix I).

If the total number of receptors remains constant, this expression can be represented graphically as a rectangular hyperbola. As the concentration of the drug is increased, the fraction of receptors that are occupied rises progressively and approaches an asymptote (with almost 100% receptor occupation) at high drug concentrations (Fig. 3.10). If drug concentration is plotted on a logarithmic axis, a characteristic sigmoid curve is obtained from which the numerical value of K_d can be derived. If it is assumed that the pharmacological response is proportional to the fraction of receptors occupied by the drug ('fractional occupancy') the relationship between the log dose and the effect will also be represented by a sigmoid curve. As previously noted, this type of relationship is often observed (Fig. 3.1), and the log dose–response curve has a characteristic sigmoid shape (Fig. 3.2). Until the 1950s, these classical concepts ('occupation theory') were generally accepted, and it was considered that the pharmacological responses of tissues to drugs were directly and linearly related to the proportion of receptors occupied by the agonist.

Spare receptors (receptor reserve)

In 1956, Stephenson identified certain apparent anomalies in occupation theory and suggested a number of im-

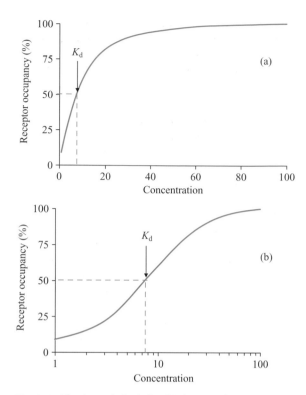

Fig. 3.10 The theoretical relationship between drug concentration and the fraction of receptors occupied by the drug. It is assumed that each agonist molecule combines with the receptor in a non-cooperative manner. K_d represents the equilibrium dissociation constant of the drug–receptor complex at equilibrium, i.e. the concentration required to occupy 50% of the receptor sites at equilibrium. In (a) concentration is plotted on a linear scale; in (b) concentration is plotted on a logarithmic scale.

portant modifications. It was proposed that maximal responses to agonists could be produced by the occupation of a small proportion of receptors and that 'spare receptors' were present at many sites. The presence of a receptor reserve generally ensures that maximal pharmacological effects can be produced by relatively low concentrations of drugs or endogenous transmitters. It is now generally considered that spare receptors are present in smooth muscle, but are rather less common in most other situations.

Nevertheless, it is accepted that a receptor reserve is present on the postsynaptic membrane at the neuromuscular junction, and that occupation of only 25% of the receptors by acetylcholine may be required to produce a maximal contractile response to indirect stimulation. Similarly, a fractional occupancy of only 50% may be required to produce a sustained tetanic response. Consequently, neuromuscular blockade by non-depolarizing agents may be dependent on the occupation of more than 50% of postsynaptic receptors before any effects on function are observed.

Efficacy and intrinsic efficacy

Stephenson also proposed that drug responses were not directly proportional to the fraction of receptors occupied by the agonist, as predicted by occupation theory. Consequently, two different drugs could produce equal responses, although they occupied different proportions of the receptor population. This property of agonists was defined as their efficacy or strength, and drugs that could only produce a half-maximal response were considered to have an efficacy of unity (on a scale between 0 and a number greater than 1). Subsequently, the definition of efficacy has been broadened, and the concept of intrinsic efficacy has been developed. Intrinsic efficacy has been used to explain differences in the potency and efficacy of agonists in different tissues, even though they are acting on the same receptor.

Positive cooperativity

It is now widely recognized that the classical occupation theory is an outdated and simplistic approach to drug action, and that many pharmacological effects are complex and non-linear functions of receptor occupation. In many instances, the relation between concentration and response is sigmoidal (S-shaped) rather than hyperbolic as predicted by occupation theory.

For example, when drugs act at nicotinic, glutamate or GABA receptors, log dose–response curves are frequently sigmoidal, and their shape is believed to reflect the presence of multiple agonist binding sites on a single macromolecular complex. The binding of a drug molecule by a single receptor site often produces conformational (allosteric) changes and alters the affinity of the remaining receptor sites for additional drug molecules. Consequently, the affinity of the remaining receptor sites for agonist molecules may be increased or decreased. This concept ('cooperativity') was originally advanced by Monod, Wyman and Changeux in the mid-1960s in order to explain the allosteric properties of enzymes. Certain protein molecules (e.g. haemoglobin) are known to combine with their substrates (oxygen) in this manner, and the combination of haemoglobin with a molecule of oxygen affects its affinity for additional molecules of oxygen. Other substances (e.g. 2,3-diphospho-glycerate, nitric ox-

ide, carbon monoxide) may also bind to haemoglobin at different sites and significantly decrease its affinity for oxygen.

Neuromuscular junction

A comparable phenomenon probably occurs at the neuromuscular junction. When the effects of acetylcholine or other agonists on nicotinic cholinergic receptors at the neuromuscular junction are studied, the relationship between drug concentration and response is usually sigmoid. This is consistent with the presence of two agonist binding sites on each receptor macromolecule, which are present on the α–γ and α–δ subunit interfaces of the nicotinic receptor (Chapter 10). Binding of acetylcholine at one site increases its affinity for the other agonist binding site, although simultaneous occupation of both sites is essential for channel opening.

In other experimental situations, log dose–response curves are biphasic or even bell-shaped (Fig. 3.3). Both biphasic and bell-shaped log dose–response curves may be due to agonists acting on two opposing receptor populations that mediate different effects (e.g. activation and inhibition of vascular smooth muscle). Complex dose–response curves of this type can usually be unmasked by selective antagonists.

Drug antagonism

Drug antagonists characteristically prevent or decrease pharmacological responses to agonists. In general, drug antagonism can be divided into three types:
- Reversible competitive antagonism
- Irreversible competitive antagonism
- Non-competitive antagonism

In both reversible and irreversible competitive antagonism, agonists compete for and combine with the same binding site as antagonists. In contrast, non-competitive antagonism does not depend on competition for the same binding sites on receptors.

Reversible competitive antagonism

The ability of drugs to combine with receptors ('affinity') is determined by simple intermolecular forces and is distinct from the capacity to produce receptor activation ('intrinsic activity'). Intrinsic activity and efficacy are similar concepts, although intrinsic activity is usually measured on a scale between 0 and 1.

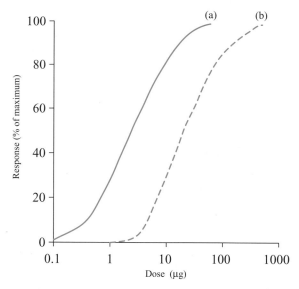

Fig. 3.11 The effect of reversible competitive antagonists on the log dose–response curve. (a) In the absence of an antagonist; (b) in the presence of an antagonist. The log dose–response curve is displaced to the right in a parallel manner. The slope of the curve and the maximum response is unaffected.

Since agonists combine with receptors and induce pharmacological responses, they possess both receptor affinity and intrinsic activity. In contrast, reversible competitive antagonists combine reversibly with receptors but do not induce pharmacological responses, i.e. they possess receptor affinity but no intrinsic activity. Consequently, they do not cause receptor activation or induce the biochemical and biophysical changes that result in drug responses. Most reversible competitive antagonists can be completely displaced from receptors by a sufficiently high concentration of any agonist that acts at the same site. They typically displace the log dose–response curve to the right in a parallel manner, so that the slope and the maximum response obtained are unaffected (Fig. 3.11).

The Schild equation

A number of reversible competitive antagonists are commonly used in anaesthetic practice (Table 3.8). Their potency can be compared by their dose ratios, i.e. the ratio or factor by which the dose of the agonist must be raised to produce an equivalent response in the presence of the antagonist. It can be shown that

$$\text{dose ratio} - 1 = \frac{[A]}{K_{d(A)}} \text{ (the Schild equation)}$$

Table 3.8 Reversible competitive antagonists that are used in anaesthetic practice.

Drug	Endogenous neurotransmitter antagonized
Atropine Glycopyrronium Hyoscine	Acetylcholine (muscarinic sites)
Atracurium Cisatracurium Pancuronium Rocuronium Vecuronium	Acetylcholine (nicotinic sites at the motor endplate)
Atenolol Esmolol Propranolol	Adrenaline and noradrenaline (β-effects)
Prochlorperazine Domperidone Metoclopramide	Dopamine
Chlorphenamine Promethazine Alimemazine	Histamine (H$_1$-effects)
Cimetidine Ranitidine	Histamine (H$_2$-effects)
Ondansetron Granisetron Tropisetron Dolasetron	5-Hydroxytryptamine (at 5-HT$_3$ receptors)
Naloxone Naltrexone	Endorphins
Flumazenil	? Endogenous benzodiazepines

where $[A]$ is the molar concentration of the antagonist and $K_{d(A)}$ is the equilibrium dissociation constant of the antagonist–receptor complex. It is comparable with the equilibrium dissociation constant of the drug–receptor complex (K_d), and its reciprocal in numerical terms (the affinity constant) reflects the affinity with which antagonists bind to receptors. When the log (dose ratio − 1) is plotted against log $[A]$, $K_{d(A)}$ can be easily derived from the intercept on the x-axis.

pA$_2$ values

The relationship between log $[A]$ and log (dose ratio − 1) can be used to compare the potency of competitive antagonists, using their pA$_2$ values. The pA$_2$ value represents the negative logarithm of the molar dose of antagonist required to produce a dose ratio of 2. In these conditions, $K_{d(A)} = [A]$, and pA$_2 = -\log K_{d(A)}$. Determination of

Table 3.9 The pA$_2$ values of reversible competitive antagonists of acetylcholine at muscarinic receptors.

Drug	pA$_2$ value
Hyoscine	9.5
Glycopyrronium	9.5
Atropine	9.0
Promethazine	7.7
Chlorpromazine	7.5
Amitriptyline	6.7
Pethidine	5.8
Sotalol	5.1
Propranolol	5.0
Imipramine	3.4

Drugs with the highest pA$_2$ values are the most potent antagonists of acetylcholine. Potencies are expressed on a logarithmic scale; thus atropine is 10,000 times more potent than propranolol as an antagonist of acetylcholine.

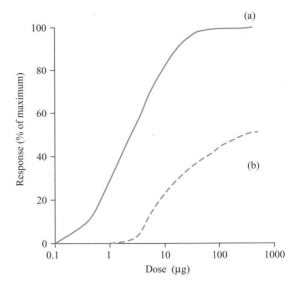

Fig. 3.12 The effect of irreversible competitive antagonists on the log dose–response curve. (a) In the absence of an antagonist; (b) in the presence of an antagonist. The log dose–response curve is displaced to the right in a non-parallel manner by the antagonist (i.e. its slope is decreased), and the maximum response is reduced.

the pA$_2$ values of drugs is a convenient way of comparing the potency of a series of reversible competitive antagonists, with the most potent compounds having the highest pA$_2$ values (Table 3.9). These values are entirely independent of the characteristics and the relative potency of the agonist, as long as the different antagonists compete with the agonist for the same receptor population.

Irreversible competitive antagonism

Irreversible competitive antagonists compete with agonists, but only slowly dissociate from receptor sites, so that the total number of receptors available for combination with agonists is reduced. This type of antagonism is usually due to the formation of stable chemical bonds between the antagonist and the receptor, or to disorientation and distortion of the receptor molecule. Irreversible antagonists characteristically decrease the slope of the log dose–response curve (i.e. there is a non-parallel displacement of the curve to the right) and also decrease the maximal response produced by the agonist (Fig. 3.12), since they decrease the number of receptors available to combine with the agonist. They often have a long duration of action, and their effects are usually unrelated to their pharmacokinetics or their plasma concentration.

Characteristic examples of irreversible antagonism are the effects of phenoxybenzamine on α-adrenoceptors, and the action of α-bungarotoxin on acetylcholine receptors at the neuromuscular junction.

Despite these differences, the precise distinction between reversible and irreversible antagonism is not always clear. Many tissues contain a receptor reserve that allows a maximum response to be obtained at a relatively low receptor occupancy. In these conditions, an irreversible decrease in the total number of receptor sites may not initially reduce the maximal response, and may displace the log dose–response curve to the right in a parallel manner. Irreversible antagonists may therefore produce initial effects that are consistent with reversible antagonism. Higher concentrations, and prolonged exposure, may be required to produce unequivocal features of irreversible antagonism. In other instances, irreversible antagonism may be preceded by a reversible phase.

Non-competitive antagonism

Other types of drug antagonism do not depend on competition between agonists and antagonists for the same receptor binding sites. Non-competitive antagonism may be due to

- Conformational changes in receptors
- Direct combination between agonists and antagonists
- Physiological (functional) antagonism
- Pharmacokinetic antagonism

Conformational changes in receptors

In some instances, non-competitive antagonism is due to conformational (allosteric) changes in receptors, in which antagonists reduce the affinity of receptors for agonists. For instance, the tachycardia commonly induced by gallamine is partly due to a reduction in the affinity of cardiac muscarinic receptors for acetylcholine.

Direct chemical combination between agonists and antagonists

Non-competitive antagonism may be dependent on direct chemical combination between agonists and antagonists, so that the effects of agonists are prevented or diminished. For instance, the effects of some metallic ions can be neutralized by various chelating agents (Table 3.1), and this type of chemical antagonism is widely used in the management of heavy metal poisoning. Similarly, the anticoagulant effects of heparin are antagonized by protamine due to the neutralization of the acidic sulphate groups in heparin by the basic arginine residues in protamine.

Physiological or functional antagonism

In physiological or functional antagonism, drugs acting on two independent receptor systems that normally mediate opposing responses are used simultaneously to antagonize their respective actions. Thus, histamine causes contraction of bronchial smooth muscle, while adrenaline causes relaxation. Consequently, adrenaline is a physiological or functional antagonist of histamine, since it can oppose or negate its bronchoconstrictor effects. In some instances, this type of antagonism occurs in physiological conditions and is responsible for the opposite effects of sympathetic and parasympathetic tone in effector systems.

Pharmacokinetic antagonism

Pharmacokinetic interactions may reduce the plasma concentration and activity of other drugs by affecting their absorption, distribution, metabolism or excretion (Chapter 4).

Agonists, partial agonists and inverse agonists

Agonists have two distinct characteristics:
- Receptor affinity (the capacity to combine with receptors)
- Intrinsic activity or efficacy (the ability to cause receptor activation)

Full or complete agonists have both receptor affinity and maximal intrinsic activity (unity), and thus produce the maximal response of which the system is capable. Reversible competitive antagonists also have receptor affinity (as reflected by their pA_2 values; Table 3.9) and compete with agonists for receptors. Nevertheless, they have no inherent intrinsic activity and therefore do not produce pharmacological effects.

Partial agonists

Partial agonists are drugs with variable receptor affinity and some intrinsic activity, which is greater than that of competitive antagonists (zero) but less than that of full agonists (unity). Consequently, partial agonists can produce either agonist or antagonist effects, depending on the circumstances in which they are used (Fig. 3.13). In low doses or concentrations, they usually produce agonist effects; in the presence of small concentrations of a full agonist, additive effects are observed. When the response to the full agonist equals the maximum response to the partial agonist, the latter has no apparent action. When high concentrations of the full agonist are present, the partial agonist acts as a competitive antagonist and reduces the response to the agonist.

Partial agonist activity is dependent on receptor expression, receptor density and the efficiency of effector systems, which may vary in different tissues. Consequently, drugs that are partial agonists in one tissue or system may be full agonists or antagonists in another.

Drugs with partial agonist activity

At least two groups of drugs have some partial agonist activity that may be of clinical significance in man:
- β-Adrenoceptor antagonists
- Opioid analgesics

Many β-adrenoceptor antagonists possess some partial agonist activity ('intrinsic sympathomimetic activity') and may produce sympathomimetic effects (Table 13.5). These actions may be of some importance when ß-adrenoceptor antagonists are used in the management of patients with borderline congestive cardiac failure. Nevertheless, in patients with high sympathetic tone and enhanced noradrenaline release, all β-adrenoceptor antagonists tend to reduce cardiac output and may result in clinical deterioration.

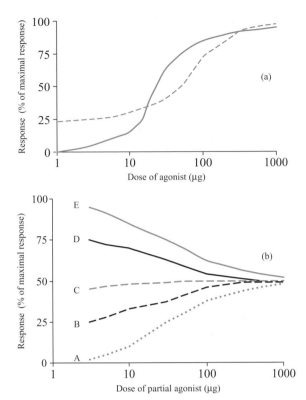

Fig. 3.13 (a) Dose–response relationship for a full agonist in the presence of a constant concentration of a partial agonist. Solid line (_____), response to full agonist alone; broken line (_ _ _), response to full agonist in presence of a partial agonist. At low concentrations of the full agonist, the partial agonist increases the response, due to their combined intrinsic activities. At higher concentrations of the full agonist, the response is reduced, since the partial agonist (intrinsic activity <1) competes with the full agonist (intrinsic activity = 1) for receptor occupancy. At extremely high concentrations, the partial agonist is completely displaced from receptors, so the maximal responses are identical. (b) Dose–response relationship for a partial agonist in the presence of increasing concentrations of a full agonist (represented by the curves A–E). At lower concentrations of the full agonist (A and B) the partial agonist has additive effects, due to their combined intrinsic activities; at higher concentrations of the full agonist (D and E) the partial agonist has antagonist effects, since it competes with the full agonist for receptor occupancy. When the response to the full agonist equals the maximal response to the partial agonist alone (C), little or no effect is observed.

Table 3.10 Opioid analgesics with partial agonist activity at μ- or κ-receptors.

| | Partial agonist activity at opioid receptors | |
Drug	μ-Receptors	κ-Receptors
Nalorphine		+
Pentazocine		++
Cyclazocine		++
Butorphanol		+++
Nalbuphine		++
Buprenorphine	++	

Some synthetic opioid analgesics are partial agonists at some opioid receptors (Table 3.10). In consequence, they may show agonist or antagonist activity, depending on the circumstances in which they are used. The analgesic effects of full agonists (e.g. morphine, pethidine) may be partially antagonized by partial agonists (e.g. buprenorphine, pentazocine).

Inverse agonists

In normal conditions, most receptor systems are quiescent unless activated by agonists. Nevertheless, in some conditions receptor systems show spontaneous basal or 'constitutive' activity and activate effector systems without being bound by agonists. Constitutive activation appears to be relatively common when receptor populations are overexpressed and may be related to physiological or pathological changes in the number of receptors.

Inverse agonists inhibit the spontaneous constitutive activation of receptor systems and may therefore produce opposite effects to agonists or act as competitive antagonists. In general, they are best considered as agents with receptor affinity and negative intrinsic activity. Inverse agonists can compete with full agonists, partial agonists and competitive antagonists for receptors depending on their relative affinity for receptors.

Drugs that are inverse agonists typically produce pharmacological effects that are opposite to those of full agonists. For example, some simple methyl, ethyl and propyl esters of the ß-carbolines (ß-CCM, ß-CCE and ß-CCP) are competitive antagonists of most benzodiazepines and antagonize the anticonvulsant, anxiolytic and sedative effects of these drugs. When given alone, ß-CCM and ß-CCE commonly produce excitatory or convulsant effects due to their inverse agonist activity. A similar phenomenon may occur with the benzodiazepine antagonist flumazenil, which occasionally acts as an inverse agonist by causing anxiety or precipitating convulsions in susceptible patients (Chapter 12). These effects are believed to be due to inverse agonist activity.

Similarly, the over expression of β-receptors can result in the activation of adenylate cyclase and the synthesis of cAMP without the binding of β-receptors by agonists. In these conditions, β-adrenoceptor antagonists with inverse agonist activity may decrease resting heart rate in cardiac failure and be more useful in the control of some tachyarrhythmias.

Desensitization

Desensitization can be defined as a decrease in cellular sensitivity or responsiveness due to the continuous or repeated exposure to agonists. It is usually observed in *in vitro* conditions (e.g. in isolated tissues or cultured cells).

Acute desensitization

Acute desensitization usually occurs rapidly and is readily reversible. In experimental conditions, it was originally observed when nicotinic agonists were applied to the motor endplate at the neuromuscular junction. In man, it is sometimes produced by large or repeated doses of suxamethonium, although this phenomenon is more commonly referred to as tachyphylaxis or rapid tolerance (Chapter 5).

This type of acute desensitization is sometimes explained by the conversion of the receptor to an inactivated and desensitized form. Although the receptor can still bind agonists, it cannot open the ion channel or cause depolarization at the motor endplate. Many agonists and some antagonists may have a preferential affinity for the desensitized receptor.

Acute desensitization also occurs with β-adrenoceptors. Although they are able to bind agonists, desensitized β-adrenergic receptors cannot activate G-proteins or adenylate cyclase. These changes are believed to be related to the phosphorylation of specific amino acid residues in the receptor.

Chronic desensitization

Chronic desensitization usually develops more slowly and is not easily reversible. It is often associated with the loss or sequestration of receptors from effector cells by

- Endocytosis ('internalization')
- Irreversible conformational changes
- Receptor degradation
- Receptor 'down-regulation'

Chronic increases in hormonal or transmitter release may cause receptor 'down-regulation', and may occur at both cholinergic and adrenergic synapses. Receptor 'down-regulation' occurs when receptors are exposed to excess concentrations of agonists, as when bronchial smooth muscle cells are exposed to sympathomimetic amines with ß2 effects.

Chronic desensitization due to receptor loss may also occur in pathological conditions associated with autoimmune processes (e.g. myasthenia gravis).

Suggested reading

Berridge, M. (1997) Elementary and global aspects of calcium signalling. *Journal of Physiology* **499**, 291–306.

Carafoli, E. (2002) Calcium signaling: a tale for all seasons. *Proceedings of the National Academy of Sciences USA* **99**, 1115–1122.

Changeux, J.-P., Giraudat, J. & Dennis, M. (1987) The nicotinic acetylcholine receptor; molecular architecture of a ligand-regulated ion channel. *Trends in Pharmacological Sciences* **8**, 459–465.

De Ligt, R.A.F., Kourounakis, A.P. & Ijzerman, A.P. (2000) Inverse agonism at G protein-coupled receptors: pathophysiological significance and implications for drug discovery. *British Journal of Pharmacology* **130**, 1–12.

Fergusson, S.S.G. (2001) Evolving concepts in G protein-coupled receptor endocytosis: the role in receptor desensitization and signaling. *Pharmacological Reviews* **53**, 1–24.

Gilman, A.G. (1987) G proteins: transducers of receptor-generated signals. *Annual Review of Biochemistry* **56**, 615–649.

Kenakin, T. (1997) *Pharmacologic Analysis of Drug–Receptor Interactions*, 3rd edn. New York: Lipincott-Raven.

Monod, J., Wyman, J. & Changeux, J.-P. (1965) On the nature of allosteric transitions: a plausible model. *Journal of Molecular Biology* **12**, 88–118.

Palmer, R.M.J., Ferrige, A.G. & Moncada, S. (1987) Nitric oxide accounts for the biological activity of endothelium-derived relaxing factor. *Nature* **327**, 524–526.

Pleuvry, B.J. (2004) Receptors, agonists and antagonists. *Anaesthesia and Intensive Care Medicine* **5**, 350–352.

Prince, R.J. (2004) Ion channels. *Anaesthesia and Intensive Care Medicine* **5**, 348–349.

Quinn, A.C., Petros, A.J. & Vallance, P. (1995) Nitric oxide: an endogenous gas. *British Journal of Anaesthesia* **74**, 443–451.

Rang, H.P., Dale, M.M., Ritter, J.M. & Moore, P.K. (2003) *Pharmacology*, 5th edn. Edinburgh: Churchill-Livingstone.

Schwinn, D.A. (1993) Adrenoceptors as models for G protein-coupled receptors: structure, function and regulation. *British Journal of Anaesthesia* **71**, 77–85.

Stephenson, R.P. (1956) A modification of receptor theory. *British Journal of Pharmacology* **11**, 379–393.

Sutherland, E.W. & Rall, T.W. (1960) The relation of adenosine-3′,5′-phosphate and phosphorylase to the actions of catecholamines and other hormones. *Pharmacological Reviews* **12**, 265–299.

Zaugg, M. & Schaub M.C. (2004) Cellular mechanisms in sympatho-modulation of the heart. *British Journal of Anaesthesia* **93**, 34–52.

Appendix I

Kinetic analysis of drug–receptor reactions

The classical analysis of drug responses depends on the assumption that each drug molecule combines with a receptor in a reversible manner, forming a drug–receptor complex, i.e.

$$D + R \underset{k_2}{\overset{k_1}{\rightleftharpoons}} DR$$

where D is the number of free (unbound) drug molecules, R is the number of free receptors, DR is the number of occupied receptor sites, k_1 the association rate constant and k_2 the dissociation rate constant. At equilibrium, the rates of association and dissociation are equal; if D, R and DR are expressed as molar concentrations (i.e. $[D]$, $[R]$ and $[DR]$), then

$$k_1[D][R] = k_2[DR]$$

and

$$\frac{k_2}{k_1} = \frac{[D][R]}{[DR]} = K_d$$

where K_d is the equilibrium dissociation constant and reflects the affinity with which drugs bind to receptors. When K_d is high, there is a low affinity for drug receptors, and when K_d is low, there is high receptor affinity. In numerical terms, K_d represents the concentration of the drug required to occupy half the receptor sites at equilibrium.

If R_t is the total number of receptors,

$$[R_t] = [R] + [DR]$$

and

$$[R] = [R_t] - [DR]$$

thus

$$K_d = \frac{[D][R]}{[DR]} = \frac{[D]([R_t] - [DR])}{[DR]}$$

and

$$[D]([R_t] - [DR]) = K_d[DR]$$

thus

$$[D][R_t] - [D][DR] = K_d[DR]$$

and

$$[D][R_t] = K_d[DR] + [D][DR]$$
$$= [DR](K_d + [D])$$

consequently

$$\frac{[DR]}{[R_t]} = \frac{[D]}{K_d + [D]}$$

and

$$f = \frac{[D]}{K_d + [D]}$$

since the fraction of receptors occupied (f) is given by

$$f = \frac{[DR]}{[R_t]}$$

This equation (the Langmuir or Hill–Langmuir equation) was originally derived by A.V. Hill in 1909. A similar relationship was used by Langmuir to characterize the absorption of gases to metal surfaces.

Appendix II

Drug isomerism

Isomers can be defined as two or more different drugs with identical numbers of atoms; consequently, they have the same chemical composition, molecular formula and molecular weight. They are difficult to define in terms of their physical, chemical or biological properties, since these may be almost identical or quite different, depending on the type of isomerism that is involved.

There are two main types of isomerism:
• Structural isomerism
• Stereoisomerism

Structural isomerism

Structural isomers have the same molecular formula but different chemical structures because their atoms are not arranged in the same manner. Isoflurane and enflurane are a well-known example of structural isomerism. Both drugs have the same molecular formula ($C_3 H_2 Cl F_5 O$), but individual atoms are not arranged in the same manner in relation to the common carbon atom structure of the two agents.

The actions of structural isomers may be relatively similar (e.g. isoflurane and enflurane), or their actions and uses may be quite different (e.g. promethazine and promazine). Structural isomers do not usually present problems of identification, since they are easily recognized as entirely different drugs, with distinctive names.

Tautomerism

In tautomerism or dynamic isomerism, two unstable structural isomers are present in equilibrium.

One isomer can be reversibly and rapidly converted to the other by physical changes (e.g. pH changes). In alkaline solution (pH 10.5), sodium thiopental is ionized and water-soluble. On injection into plasma (pH 7.4), the drug becomes non-ionized and undergoes tautomerism, thus increasing its lipid-solubility (Chapter 7).

Stereoisomerism

Stereoisomers are two or more different substances with the same molecular formula and chemical structure, but a different configuration, i.e. their atoms or chemical groups occupy different positions in space, and thus differ in their spatial arrangements. Stereoisomers can be classified into two main groups:

• Enantiomers
• Diastereomers

Enantiomers

Enantiomers (literally, substances of opposite shape) are pairs of stereoisomers that are non-superimposable mirror-images of each other. This type of stereoisomerism is dependent on the presence of a chiral centre in the molecular structure of certain drugs, which is usually a single carbon atom with four different substituent atoms or groups. Drugs with this type of structure (chiral drugs) have a mirror-image that cannot be superimposed on their original configuration, and they therefore exist as R (rectus) and S (sinistra) isomers. These two forms are distinguished by the orientation of different substituents around the chiral centre. Enantiomers are also optically active and can rotate polarized light to the right (the (+) or (d) form) or the left (the (−) or (l) form). Individual isomers are

therefore referred to as R(+), S(−), R(−) or S(+) isomers. Equal mixtures of the two forms (racemic mixtures), with the prefixes (±) or (dl), have no optical activity.

Diastereomers

Diastereomers are pairs of stereoisomers that are not enantiomers (i.e. not mirror images). Diastereomers characteristically have different physical and chemical properties. For example, they do not have the same melting point or solubility, and they do not take part in chemical reactions in the same manner. Some of the stereoisomers of atracurium, mivacurium and tramadol are diastereomers.

Differences between stereoisomers

In terms of stereoisomerism, anaesthetic agents can be divided into four main groups (Table 3.11).

• Achiral drugs
• Drugs administered as single stereoisomers
• Drugs administered as mixtures of two stereoisomers
• Drugs administered as mixtures of more than two stereoisomers

There may be differences in the pharmacodynamic activity and pharmacokinetic properties of individual isomers. Although R and S isomers have the same structure, they have a different configuration, i.e. their substituent groups occupy different positions in space. Consequently, the two enantiomers may form different three-dimensional relationships in the asymmetric environment of receptors and enzymes, which are almost entirely composed of L-amino acids with stereoselective properties. In these conditions, there may be differences between the R and S enantiomers, since their relationship with specific receptor sites and enzymes may not be identical.

There are often differences in the potency of individual enantiomers, for example, S(+)-isoflurane is slightly more potent than its R(−) enantiomer, while S(+)-ketamine is 3–4 times more potent than R(−)-ketamine. Occasionally, one stereoisomer is almost inactive, and l-atropine, l-noradrenaline and l-adrenaline are approximately 50–100 times more potent than their d-enantiomers. When differences in potency are present, they are often expressed by the stereo-specific index (eudismic ratio), which represents the relation between the activity of the more active isomer (the eutomer) and its less active antipode (the distomer). Stereo-specific indices of 100 or more are not uncommon and may be due to differences in either the affinity or the intrinsic activity of individual enantiomers.

Table 3.11 Some achiral and chiral drugs that are commonly used in anaesthetic practice.

| Achiral | Chiral | | |
	One isomer	Two isomers	More than two isomers
Propofol	Etomidate	Thiopental	Mivacurium
Nitrous oxide	Ropivacaine	Ketamine	Atracurium
Tetracaine	Levobupivacaine	Halothane	
Lidocaine	Cisatracurium	Isoflurane	
Fentanyl	Pancuronium	Desflurane	
Alfentanil	Vecuronium	Prilocaine	
Remifentanil	Morphine	Bupivacaine	
Pethidine	Hyoscine	Atropine	
Neostigmine		Tramadol	
Edrophonium		Dobutamine	
Dopamine		Glycopyrronium	

Although some chiral drugs are administered as single isomers, most of them are used as equal, racemic mixtures of two enantiomers.

There may also be important differences in the type of pharmacological activity produced by the enantiomers. Thus, one isomer may be an agonist, while its enantiomer is a partial agonist or competitive antagonist.

There are also differences in the metabolism and pharmacokinetics of individual stereoisomers, and one enantiomer may be more rapidly metabolized than its antipode. R(+)-propranolol, R(−)-prilocaine and S(+)-ketamine are more rapidly metabolized than their enantiomers, and have a greater intrinsic hepatic clearance. Paradoxically, the metabolism of S(+)-ketamine is inhibited by R(−)-ketamine, and this may account for the relatively prolonged action of the racemic mixture. Some inactive enantiomers undergo unidirectional metabolic conversion ('inversion') to their antipodes. R(−)-ibuprofen and R(−)-ketoprofen are converted to their active S(+)-enantiomers in the intestine and the liver, which are 100–160 times more potent than their R(−)-enantiomers. Both S(+)-ibuprofen and S(+)-ketoprofen are now used clinically as single isomer preparations (dexibuprofen and dexketoprofen).

Differences in the metabolism and disposition of the R and S enantiomers of many chiral drugs may affect their pharmacokinetics, and individual drug enantiomers may have different half-lives, clearances and volumes of distribution (Chapter 2).

Practical considerations

Many anaesthetic agents are normally administered as chiral mixtures of two stereoisomers or more complex isomeric mixtures. In many instances, there are differences in the pharmacodynamic properties and pharmacokinetic behaviour of the individual isomers (e.g. ketamine, bupivacaine and atracurium). Occasionally, the enantiomers of chiral drugs have different but complementary actions, and both stereoisomers make an important contribution to the overall pharmacological profile of the drug (e.g. tramadol, dobutamine). The use of these drugs as chiral mixtures is clearly essential.

In other instances, the use of stereoisomeric mixtures has been widely accepted, although it appears to have few practical advantages. Recent progress in chemical technology has greatly simplified the separation and preparation of individual stereoisomers by asymmetric chemical synthesis, or by chiral inversion of one enantiomer. In addition, drug regulatory authorities in many countries have encouraged the introduction of new drugs as single stereoisomers. Consequently, since 1990 most new drugs have been introduced as single enantiomers, and in some instances previously available mixtures have been reintroduced as single stereoisomers (e.g. atracurium, bupivacaine). In the future, it seems likely that this trend will continue.

4 Drug Interaction

Drug interaction is the modification of the effects of one drug by another. Many of these reactions are clinically unimportant, while others form an integral part of medical or anaesthetic practice. A familiar example is the use of neostigmine to antagonize the effects of non-depolarizing neuromuscular blocking agents and the concomitant use of atropine to prevent the muscarinic effects of the anticholinesterase drug. However, a minority of interactions are hazardous or potentially fatal, and it is therefore important for the anaesthetist to be aware of their possible occurrence. Interactions may occur between drugs that are administered concurrently during anaesthesia; alternatively, reactions may be associated with prescribed drugs or self-medication. It is thus essential for a full drug history to be available prior to the administration of anaesthesia. Nevertheless, the assessment of drug interactions in humans must be undertaken with a sense of balance. Reports of adverse effects based on single case histories or circumstantial and anecdotal evidence are of little value, particularly when the mechanisms involved are obscure.

The incidence of adverse drug reactions and presumably of interactions increases with the number of drugs a patient receives. One hospital study showed that the rate was 7% in those taking 6–10 drugs and 40% in those taking 16–20 drugs. Comparable figures for anaesthetic practice, where the patient may receive as many as 10 drugs as part of the anaesthetic regimen, are unknown. However, most of the interactions that occur in anaesthesia are well known and are usually predictable from an appreciation of the pharmacology of the drugs concerned.

Nomenclature

Drug interactions are often described in terms of four phenomena:
- Summation
- Antagonism
- Potentiation
- Synergism

Summation

Summation is defined as the additive effects produced when two or more drugs with similar actions are given simultaneously. For example, when two different inhalational agents are used concurrently (e.g. nitrous oxide and isoflurane), their potencies and effects are usually additive (Chapter 8). Similarly, when drugs with anticholinergic properties are used simultaneously (e.g. atropine and amitriptyline), they produce additive effects on salivary secretion. Since their effects are solely due to the summation of their separate activities, they are not a true example of drug interaction.

Antagonism

Antagonism is the attenuation or prevention of pharmacological responses to agonists by other drugs (Chapter 3). In most instances, it is due to reversible competitive antagonism, such as between naloxone and opioid analgesics, or propranolol and β-adrenoceptor agonists. Occasionally, it is irreversible (e.g. phenoxybenzamine and noradrenaline) and is due to the failure of the antagonist to dissociate from the receptor site. Alternatively, antagonism may be due to pharmacokinetic factors such as reduced drug absorption or enzyme induction, or to the formation of complexes between drugs, as occurs between heparin and protamine, or heavy metals and chelating agents.

Potentiation

Potentiation is usually defined as the enhancement of the effects of one drug by another when the two drugs have dissimilar pharmacological activities (e.g. midazolam and erythromycin, or digoxin and thiazide diuretics). The mechanisms involved in potentiation are usually pharmacokinetic (e.g. enzyme inhibition), or involve changes in acid–base and electrolyte balance.

Synergism

Synergism refers to the supra-additive effects of two drugs with similar pharmacological properties and closely related sites of action, which produce an effect in combination which is greater than anticipated from summation, as shown by the hypnotic effects of benzodiazepines and concomitantly administered intravenous induction agents. Synergism may also occur between vecuronium and atracurium at the neuromuscular junction, and has been attributed to the different affinities of drugs with diverse molecular structures for binding sites on the two α-subunits of the acetylcholine receptor.

Isoboles

Synergism is often defined and interpreted by isoboles, i.e. graphs showing equi-effective combinations of drugs. Isoboles were first used approximately 120 years ago to illustrate the antagonism between physostigmine and atropine. Each axis on the graph corresponds to the dosage of a drug, whose individual values for a given effect (e.g. hypnosis) have previously been determined by probit analysis of the dose–response relationship. The median effective dose (ED_{50}) of each agent is plotted on the coordinates of the graph, which are then joined by a straight line between the axes. When equi-effective combinations of two drugs approximate to this line, the effects of drugs are merely additive. However, when equi-effective combinations lie below this line, the interaction is considered to be synergic. In contrast, when the corresponding reference points to the equi-effective combination of the two drugs lies above the line, it is considered that drug antagonism is present (Fig. 4.1).

Limitations of isoboles

In the past, the analysis of interactions between drugs by the use of isoboles has been viewed with considerable circumspection. The method has been regarded as rather empirical and appears to take little account of any differences in the dose–response relationships of the two drugs. Nevertheless, current evidence suggests that isoboles can be used to distinguish between additive and synergic effects when the drugs concerned act at, or are bound by, the same receptor or enzyme site. However, combinations of drugs that act at different sites cannot be analysed by isoboles, since agents with purely additive effects may give rise to isoboles that are incorrectly attributed to synergism. Nevertheless, they are a convenient method of demonstrating the coexistent effects of two drugs so that the lowest dose combination necessary to produce the desired effect can be defined.

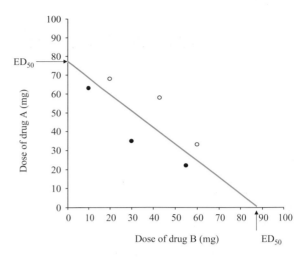

Fig. 4.1 Diagrammatic illustration of an isobole. The two axes show the median effective doses (ED50) for two drugs (A and B) that are required to produce a specific pharmacological effect (e.g. loss of response to command, onset of neuromuscular blockade). The ED_{50} values are joined by a straight line between the axes. When equi-effective combinations of the two drugs approximate to this line, their effects are considered to be additive. However, when equi-effective combinations fall below this line, their effects are considered to reflect synergism (●); if they fall above the line (○), they are considered to reflect drug antagonism.

Mechanisms of drug interactions

In this chapter, a general account is given of the pharmacological mechanisms that are usually responsible for drug interactions in humans. Reactions with specific groups of drugs that are commonly used in anaesthetic practice are then considered in more detail.

The mechanism of drug interactions may be considered in three groups:
• Pharmaceutical interactions
• Pharmacokinetic interactions
• Pharmacodynamic interactions

Pharmaceutical interactions

Pharmaceutical interactions are due to chemical or physical reactions that occur *in vitro*. These interactions may be responsible for the loss of activity of drugs, or for their aggregation or precipitation in solution, which occasionally has serious consequences.

Chemical
Chemical deterioration or decomposition
Most drugs, including anaesthetic agents, must be stored before use and in many instances may undergo deterioration or decomposition. When stored in a powder or solid form, decomposition tends to occur more slowly. The addition of water or a mixing agent may accelerate the rate of decomposition of certain drugs (e.g. thiopental), particularly when more concentrated solutions are formed, or when dextrose or saline is used as a solvent. Other drugs (e.g. most catecholamines) are decomposed by light, or are sensitive to changes in temperature (e.g. suxamethonium).

Drug precipitation
Mixing of solutions with different pH values may result in drug precipitation. For example, thiopental is invariably used as a sodium salt and is only ionized and water-soluble in alkaline conditions (pH 10–11). Conversely, many other drugs including local anaesthetics, analgesics and most sympathetic amines are weak bases that can only exist in aqueous solutions as acid salts (sulphates or hydrochlorides) at a pH of 4–5. Mixing these dissimilar solutions in the same syringe or in an infusion set usually causes precipitation of free acid and base. The addition of drugs such as suxamethonium to a solution of thiopental results in rapid alkaline hydrolysis and thus inactivation of the muscle relaxant. Similarly, the addition of calcium salts to infusion lines containing bicarbonate solutions will result in significant precipitation of insoluble calcium carbonate, and the addition of drugs or electrolytes to fat emulsions (e.g. intralipid) or concentrated solutions (e.g. 20% mannitol) may result in the aggregation or precipitation of the mixture.

Direct chemical combination or degradation
Direct chemical combination may also produce drug interaction *in vitro*. A classical example was the use of the inhalational anaesthetic trichlorethylene in anaesthetic circuits incorporating soda lime, leading to the production of the potentially neurotoxic vapour dichloracetylene. More recently, it has been recognized that carbon monoxide may be produced in circle systems when isoflurane or desflurane is administered in the presence of warm and dry soda lime, and may cause significant levels of carboxyhaemoglobin in anaesthetized patients. Sevoflurane may also undergo some decomposition when used with warm soda lime in low flow anaesthesia systems, and sig-

nificant amounts of a potentially nephrotoxic vinyl ether ('Compound A') may be produced.

Similarly, when penicillin derivatives are added to infusion fluids containing amino acids, drug–protein complexes are formed that can induce the formation of cytophilic antibodies (IgE). These reactions may result in the development of Type I hypersensitivity reactions.

Racemization
Racemization (epimerization) may also occur in solution, and involves a change in the steric configuration of molecules. A change in the pH of catecholamine solutions may convert (l)-adrenaline to (d)-adrenaline, with an almost total loss of potency.

Physical
Solvent system polarity
Solvent system polarity (the solubility of a drug or drug solvent in aqueous solution) may be important when relatively insoluble agents such as diazepam or propofol are present in organic solvents and are subsequently added to aqueous solutions. In these conditions, precipitation may occur, and its extent will depend on the relative volume and concentration of both drug and aqueous solution.

Interactions with glass or plastic
Drugs may also interact with the administration sets through which they are given. Some drugs may have the tendency to adhere to the surface of their containers, as may occur with insulin in glass or plastic syringes (adsorption). Similarly, nitroglycerine and other lipophilic drugs may be bound by different types of plastic.

Other physical phenomena which may occur include 'salting out', when electrolytes are added to supersaturated solutions such as mannitol, and 'emulsion cracking', when calcium salts are added to fat emulsions.

Prevention of pharmaceutical interactions
Pharmaceutical interactions are often predictable and are not usually an important cause of complications in anaesthetic practice. Their occurrence can be minimized by a number of simple precautions. If possible, only one drug should be added to each unit of a crystalloid solution. No additives should be incorporated in infusions of blood, blood products, lipid emulsions, amino acid preparations or hypertonic fluids. The addition of drugs to acid or alkaline solutions should be avoided. Solutions must be thoroughly mixed before administration and this is

particularly important when potassium salts are added to intravenous fluids. Solutions containing additives are preferably prepared in the pharmacy and should be clearly labelled. When additives are used in the wards or theatre, the manufacturers' data sheet or a table of drug incompatibilities should be consulted. A pharmacist or drug information centre can usually resolve any problems.

Pharmacokinetic interactions

Pharmacokinetic interactions occur in the body and are due to an alteration in the disposition of one drug by another. In these circumstances, the concentration of a drug at its site of action may be modified. These interactions are usually classified by their effects on the processes of

- Dissolution or absorption
- Distribution
- Metabolism
- Elimination

Dissolution or absorption
Gastric pH and motility

Drug dissolution usually takes place in the stomach, and the solubility of some drugs (e.g. tetracyclines) is critically dependent on acid conditions. In these circumstances, drugs affecting gastric pH (e.g. antacids, H_2-receptor antagonists) will influence the degree of absorption. Most drugs are absorbed in the more alkaline medium of the small intestine. Agents that affect the speed of gastric emptying will alter the rate of delivery of other drugs to their site of absorption and consequently influence their uptake. Metoclopramide stimulates gastric emptying and increases the rate of uptake of many drugs administered by mouth. In contrast, opioid analgesics and antimuscarinic agents that slow gastric emptying have the converse effect. When drugs affect gastric motility, the total amount of orally administered drugs absorbed usually remains unaltered. However, the bioavailability of digoxin is reduced by metoclopramide and increased by propantheline. Conversely, the absorption of levodopa is reduced in the presence of antimuscarinic drugs, presumably because of an increased time of exposure to metabolism by the intestinal mucosa.

Intestinal absorption

Drug interactions in the small intestine may decrease absorption when chelates or other insoluble complexes are formed. Thus, the absorption of tetracyclines is reduced by the simultaneous administration of calcium, magnesium or iron salts, and the resin colestyramine may decrease the absorption of many other drugs including warfarin, digoxin and thyroxine.

Subcutaneous and intramuscular absorption

The absorption of drugs administered by subcutaneous or intramuscular injection is determined by the aqueous solubility of the drug at tissue sites, the extent of local metabolism and peripheral blood flow. Drugs prepared in organic solvents (e.g. diazepam, phenytoin) may precipitate in tissues, and this may account for any decrease in bioavailability compared to that after oral administration. Sympathomimetic amines and β-adrenoceptor antagonists can significantly modify skin and muscle blood flow. If extensive metabolism of the parenterally administered drug occurs at tissue sites, bioavailability may be affected.

Distribution
Inhalational agents

The uptake and distribution of inhalational agents is significantly influenced by minute ventilation and cardiac output. The rate of rise of alveolar concentration, which is correlated with the induction of anaesthesia, is largely determined by ventilation. Consequently, respiratory depressants may slow the rate of onset of anaesthesia. Conversely, drugs that reduce cardiac output increase the rate of rise of alveolar concentration and the rate of induction may be increased (Chapter 8).

Displacement from protein binding

After administration and absorption, drugs are present in plasma in simple solution or bound to carrier proteins or erythrocytes. They are subsequently transported to organs and tissues by the vascular system.

The transport of drugs in the circulation usually involves their binding by plasma proteins. Acidic drugs are usually bound by albumin, and basic drugs are bound by other plasma protein constituents such as lipoproteins, α_1-acid glycoprotein and γ-globulin. In most instances binding sites are relatively non-specific and are subject to competition by a wide variety of drugs.

Nevertheless, it is doubtful whether displacement from plasma proteins alone is an important factor in drug interactions in humans. Any enhanced effects are likely to be small and transient, since the increase in the concentration of unbound drug in plasma is usually counterbalanced by increased renal and hepatic clearance. A new steady state is thus established, with the total amount of drug in plasma reduced but the unbound fraction unchanged, and drug distribution to the site of action is unaffected. Basic drugs have a wide availability of binding sites and plasma levels of α_1-acid glycoprotein may be considerably elevated following surgery and in many disease processes.

Significant interactions may occur between acidic drugs with a low volume of distribution which are predominantly present in plasma, and where the ratio between the effective and toxic dose is small (e.g. anticoagulants). Drugs that displace warfarin from plasma proteins (e.g. phenylbutazone, some sulphonamides) may enhance its therapeutic effects and produce toxic side effects. However, drugs that lead to clinical interactions with warfarin may also affect its metabolism, presumably by competing at enzymatic sites, where protein configuration may be important.

Interactions may occur between drugs that are extensively bound by tissue proteins. The antimalarial drugs mepacrine and pamaquin are both bound by hepatic proteins and may displace each other into extracellular fluid. It is unclear whether this phenomenon is responsible for clinically significant drug interactions in humans.

Metabolism

Drug interactions affecting metabolism mainly occur in the liver, although drug metabolism can also occur in the intestinal mucosa, plasma and lung parenchyma, and may be due to interference with a number of different physiological or biochemical processes.

First-pass metabolism

After oral administration, some drugs are extensively metabolized by the liver before they gain access to the systemic circulation. First-pass metabolism may be an important cause of the diminished response to certain drugs when given orally, as occurs with most opioid analgesics. In the case of drugs with a high extraction ratio that are extensively cleared by the liver, the magnitude of the first-pass effect is dependent on liver blood flow. Drugs that modify hepatic perfusion may affect the proportion of the oral dose that enters the systemic circulation. Thus, the oral bioavailability of some opioid analgesics may be increased by drugs that reduce liver blood flow (e.g. propranolol, inhalational anaesthetics). Cimetidine, which is also a potent inhibitor of liver enzymes, enhances the systemic bioavailability of propranolol by a reduction in hepatic blood flow.

Enzyme induction

Drug interaction in the liver may be due to effects on enzymes that are responsible for drug metabolism. The activity of cytochrome P450 and other microsomal enzymes can be enhanced by certain drugs (Table 4.1), and the rate and extent of drug metabolism may be increased. Chronic alcohol consumption and polycyclic hydrocarbons in tobacco and grilled meats may also induce certain isoforms of cytochrome P450. Polycyclic hydrocarbons mainly induce CYP 1A1 and CYP 1A2, while barbiturates and phenytoin mainly affect CYP 1A2 and CYP 3A4. Rifampicin is a potent inducer of CYP 2D6 and CYP 3A4, while ethyl alcohol induces CYP 2E1. Most enzyme-inducing agents also increase liver weight, microsomal protein content and the rate of biliary secretion. Enzyme induction usually increases glucuronyl transferase activity and thus enhances drug conjugation. In some instances, drugs may induce their own metabolism (autoinduction). Induction of cytochrome P450 may have secondary effects on other enzyme systems. For example, enzyme induction usually decreases intracellular haem, reducing its inhibitory effects on porphyrin synthesis, which may be significant in acute porphyria.

Enzyme induction is a common and important cause of drug interactions and normally takes place over several days. The rate of metabolism of the inducing agent itself, as well as other drugs, may be increased with a subsequent reduction in concentration and pharmacological effects. Conversely, withdrawal of the inducing drug will allow the serum concentration and the plasma half-life to increase, and toxicity may result if the dose is not adjusted. This is exemplified by the interaction between barbiturates and warfarin anticoagulants. Barbiturates are potent enzyme-inducing agents, and can alter the rate of metabolism of other drugs within 2 days of administration, with increasing effects over several weeks. It is unclear whether

Table 4.1 Agents that induce hepatic cytochrome P450.

- Barbiturates
- Phenytoin
- Carbamazepine
- Rifampicin
- Griseofulvin
- Ethyl alcohol (chronic consumption)
- Polycyclic hydrocarbons (tobacco smoke, grilled meat)
- Insecticides
- Corticosteroids
- St. John's Wort (a popular herbal medicine)

the repeated use of thiopental as an induction agent can lead to clinically significant enzyme induction.

Some hepatic enzyme systems that are concerned with drug metabolism are unaffected by enzyme induction (e.g. monoamine oxidase).

Inhalational anaesthesia and enzyme induction

Many inhalational anaesthetics produce complex effects on cytochrome P450 and other microsomal enzyme systems. Most fluorinated agents appear to be metabolized by the isoform CYP 2E1 (Chapter 1), which is induced by ethyl alcohol and variably affected by inhalational anaesthetics. Anaesthesia with inhalational agents may possibly cause induction, inhibition or have biphasic effects on CYP 2E1 and related enzyme systems. In addition, the metabolic response to surgery may profoundly affect hepatic drug metabolism.

Enzyme inhibition

Other agents may inhibit many microsomal enzyme systems and thus prevent or delay the metabolism of other drugs. Isoforms of cytochrome P450 and other hepatic enzymes concerned with drug metabolism may be inhibited in a competitive or a non-competitive manner by many drugs (Table 4.2). Enzyme inhibition may increase plasma concentrations of other concurrently used drugs, resulting in drug interactions.

Competitive inhibition may result when two drugs are in competition for the same metabolic pathway (e.g. tolbutamide and sulphonamides). Other drugs (e.g. quinidine) are competitive inhibitors of CYP 2D6, but are not substrates of this enzyme isoform.

Table 4.2 Agents that inhibit hepatic cytochrome P450.

- Imidazoles (ketoconazole, itraconazole, omeprazole, cimetidine, etomidate)
- Macrolide antibiotics (erythromycin, clarithromycin)
- Antidepressants
- HIV protease inhibitors
- Ciclosporin
- Amiodarone
- Gestodene
- Allopurinol
- Quinidine
- Disulfiram
- Grapefruit juice

Non-competitive inhibition may also occur and some imidazole compounds can form a complex with the ferric form of haem in CYP 3A4 and certain other isoforms (e.g. CYP1A2, CYP2C8, CYP 2D6). Other irreversible inhibitors (e.g. gestodene, diethylcarbamate) are oxidized by CYP 3A4 and then form a covalent bond resulting in enzyme destruction ('suicide inhibition').

Some compounds are not metabolized by hepatic enzymes but are broken down by cholinesterases in plasma (e.g. suxamethonium, mivacurium). Drugs that inhibit cholinesterase (e.g. edrophonium, neostigmine) or inhibit its synthesis (e.g. cyclophosphamide) may prolong the effect of suxamethonium and mivacurium.

Elimination

Drugs are principally eliminated from the body by the liver, the kidneys, the lungs or the gut. Drug interactions are possible when any of these routes are involved.

Hepatic elimination

Drug interactions affecting hepatic elimination may be due to competition for biliary excretion. Both anions (e.g. ampicillin) and cations (e.g. vecuronium) are concentrated and excreted in bile by transport processes that require cellular enzymes (e.g. Na^+/K^+-ATPase). These systems are usually saturable, and other anions and cations may compete with and reduce their transport and elimination. This interaction is rarely of practical significance.

Other drugs (e.g. morphine, oestrogens) are excreted in the bile as water-soluble conjugates (glucuronides or sulphates). Some of these conjugates are metabolized to their parent compounds by the gut flora and subsequently reabsorbed (enterohepatic recirculation). When bacterial flora are inhibited by antibiotics this recycling will not occur, and this may explain the occasional failure of oral contraception when used with oral penicillins or tetracyclines.

Renal elimination

Compounds that alter urine pH may influence the rate and the extent of elimination of other drugs. The duration of action and the proportion of the dose metabolized by the liver may also be modified. In general, drugs that are weak acids or weak bases may be present in solution in both ionized and non-ionized forms and the relative proportions of the two forms are dependent on pH. In alkaline urine, significant amounts of some weak acids are ionized. In these conditions, they cannot readily diffuse back into

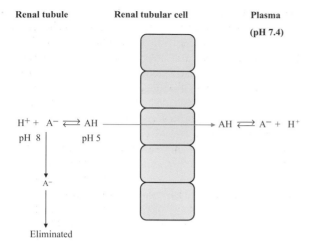

Renal tubule   Renal tubular cell   Plasma (pH 7.4)

$$H^+ + A^- \rightleftharpoons AH$$

pH 8   pH 5

$$AH \rightleftharpoons A^- + H^+$$

A^-

Eliminated

Fig. 4.2 Elimination of weak acids in alkaline and acidic urine. Weak acids are present in the renal tubule in an ionized and a non-ionized form (A^- and AH). Only AH can diffuse across tubular cell membranes ($\rightarrow$). At pH 8, most of the drug in the renal tubule is present as A^- and is eliminated in urine ($\downarrow$). At pH 5, more of the drug is present in the non-ionized form (AH), which can diffuse back across the renal tubule ($\rightarrow$) and is eliminated to a lesser extent. Similar factors apply to the elimination of weak bases.

plasma across the renal tubule, and are therefore eliminated in urine (Fig. 4.2). By contrast, in neutral or acidic urine a higher proportion of the drug is non-ionized, so that diffusion back into plasma is facilitated and excretion is reduced.

On the other hand, weak bases (e.g. tricyclic antidepressants, opioid analgesics) are more highly ionized in acidic urine and their elimination is enhanced. In contrast, the presence of an alkaline urine promotes the reabsorption of basic drugs in the renal tubule.

At one time, these principles were used in the treatment of drug overdosage. Although modification of the pH of urine may lead to other interactions, these are not usually of clinical significance.

Drug interactions involving renal function are sometimes related to competition for active transport. Both acid and basic drugs and their metabolites are partially eliminated from plasma by secretion in the proximal renal tubule. This process is competitive and may be subject to interference by other drugs. Benzylpenicillin is a weak acid that is actively secreted by the proximal renal tubule. Consequently, it has a relatively short half-life (30–40 min), which can be prolonged by other drugs that compete with it for active transport (e.g. probenecid, NSAIDs, most di-

uretics). The elimination of endogenous substances can also be inhibited by drugs. Many thiazide diuretics compete with urates for tubular secretion in the proximal renal tubule. In these conditions, the plasma urate concentration may be increased and acute gout can be precipitated.

Pulmonary elimination

The rate of removal of inhalational anaesthetic agents is principally determined by minute ventilation and cardiac output. Drugs that affect either of these factors (e.g. respiratory depressants and some antiarrhythmic drugs) can reduce the rate of elimination and thus prolong the effects of volatile and gaseous agents.

Gastrointestinal elimination

Some highly basic and lipid-soluble drugs (e.g. pethidine, fentanyl) may diffuse from plasma into the stomach, and subsequent reabsorption from the small intestine may result in a secondary peak effect. This gastroenteric recirculation process may be modified by drugs, which either influence splanchnic blood flow or produce changes in gastric pH.

Pharmacodynamic interactions

Interactions at receptor sites

Pharmacodynamic interactions occur at the site of action of drugs, and many are related to additive, synergistic or antagonistic effects at receptor sites. Such interactions are frequently beneficial, for example the use of protamine to reverse the anticoagulant effects of heparin, or the use of β-adrenergic antagonists to reverse adrenaline-induced tachycardia. Alternatively, adverse interactions can occur; for instance, chlorpromazine and related drugs block α-adrenoceptors and may therefore enhance the hypotensive effect of other drugs. Some pharmacodynamic interactions are related to the additive or synergistic effects of drugs on the CNS (e.g. ethyl alcohol and benzodiazepines) the autonomic nervous system (e.g. atropine and tricyclic antidepressants) or the cardiovascular system (e.g. β-adrenoceptor antagonists and calcium channel blockers). Many examples of competitive and noncompetitive antagonism (Chapter 3) can be classified as pharmacodynamic interactions. In addition, a number of important interactions are related to interference with the active transport of drugs to their site of action, such as the potentiation of the effects of noradrenaline by tricyclic antidepressant drugs.

Other pharmacodynamic interactions

Not all pharmacodynamic interactions are related to additive, synergistic or antagonistic effects at receptor sites. Disturbances of fluid and electrolyte balance play a role in some interactions. Thiazides and loop diuretics reduce serum K^+ and thus increase the sensitivity of Na^+/K^+-ATPase to inhibition by digoxin, resulting in enhanced Na^+/Ca^{2+} exchange, raised cardiac contractility and improved atrioventricular conduction. Similarly, the toxicity of lithium salts can be enhanced by Na^+ depletion produced by thiazide diuretics, since Na^+ and Li^+ are treated in a similar manner by the body.

Drug interactions in anaesthetic practice

Drug interactions in anaesthetic practice may occur between pre-existing drug therapy and general or local anaesthetic agents, muscle relaxants, analgesics and drugs used for premedication. Interactions may also occur between anaesthetic agents and their adjuvants.

In some instances, the pharmacological basis of drug interaction is unknown or obscure. From the anaesthetist's point of view, it is often more important to be aware of the more common established interactions that may be encountered or anticipated.

Interactions with general anaesthetic agents

Interactions may occur with both intravenous and inhalational agents. *In vitro* drug interactions can occur when solutions of lower pH are added to solutions of thiopental (pH 10–11). These *in vitro* interactions are well known and are easily avoided. Other interactions with general anaesthetics may occur *in vivo* and may involve:
- Other respiratory depressants
- Antiarrhythmic and antianginal agents
- Sympathomimetic amines
- Antihypertensive agents
- Drugs that modify electrolyte balance
- Muscle relaxants
- Enzyme-inducing agents
- Enzyme-inhibiting agents
- Nephrotoxic agents

Other respiratory depressants

Drugs with a significant respiratory depressant effect can modify the uptake, distribution and elimination of inhalational anaesthetic agents. However, once anaesthesia is established, all drugs that depress CNS activity are considered to have summative effects. The minimum alveolar concentration (MAC) value of many fluorinated agents, which reflects their potency in steady-state conditions, is reduced by about 30% when diazepam is also administered. Similar effects have been shown or may be predicted when opioid analgesics, hypnotics, tranquillisers, antidepressants and certain antihypertensive agents (e.g. clonidine) have been used. Nitrous oxide will accelerate the uptake of other inhalational agents by the 'concentration' and 'second gas' effects relating to its high diffusing capacity, but in steady-state conditions, the MAC values of different inhalational agents are additive (Chapter 8).

Conversely, the concomitant use of CNS stimulants (e.g. theophylline) may increase anaesthetic requirements and MAC values.

Antiarrhythmic and antianginal agents

Organic nitrates, β-adrenoceptor antagonists and calcium channel-blocking agents are commonly used in the management of angina, and the last two groups of drugs are also effective as antihypertensive and antiarrhythmic agents. Treatment with these drugs should always be continued until the immediate preoperative period as the risks of rebound phenomena, such as worsening of angina symptoms and the reappearance of arrhythmias far outweigh those due to drug interactions which may occur during anaesthesia. The percutaneous administration of glyceryl trinitrate in the management of angina is sometimes continued during anaesthesia, although the theoretical risk of potentiation of systemic hypotension or reflex tachycardia must be borne in mind.

β-Adrenoceptor antagonists and calcium channel-blocking agents

Bradycardia is frequently encountered during anaesthesia in patients receiving β-adrenoceptor antagonists. Severe bradyarrhythmias may result in hypotension and has been observed following the absorption of timolol eye drops. Pharmacokinetic parameters may be of some importance, as inhalational agents and propranolol can both reduce liver blood flow.

Many volatile anaesthetic agents have significant calcium channel-blocking activity or interfere with the mobilization of intracellular Ca^{2+}, although significant problems with therapeutic doses of calcium antagonists are unlikely. However, additive or synergistic effects may occur, and their combined effects on cardiac output and peripheral vascular tone is more likely to lead to intraoperative hypotension. In addition, certain calcium channel-blocking agents, especially verapamil and diltiazem, can produce some degree of heart block, which may be enhanced by inhalational anaesthesia.

Combined treatment with both β-adrenoceptor antagonists and calcium channel-blocking agents requires special vigilance during anaesthesia. β-Adrenoceptor antagonists will depress the reflex responses associated with some calcium channel blockers (e.g. nifedipine) and augment their effects by reducing Ca^{2+} channel availability, an effect which may be due to reduced intracellular synthesis of cAMP. In addition, the reduction in cardiac output associated with β-adrenoceptor antagonists and some calcium channel-blocking agents may also modify the pharmacokinetic behaviour of inhalational agents and effectively increase their potency by secondary reflex mechanisms which facilitate cerebral blood flow. Similarly, the effects of inhalational agents on hepatic perfusion and intrinsic clearance may increase plasma levels of antiarrhythmic agents.

Amiodarone

The antiarrhythmic agent amiodarone may cause a significant increase in bradyarrhythmias, complete heart block and pacemaker dependence in patients undergoing cardiac surgery and receiving various anaesthetic regimes. This may reflect the additive effect of anaesthetic drugs when used with antiarrhythmic agents with a long elimination half-life.

Sympathomimetic amines

Sympathomimetic amines with β-adrenergic activity may precipitate dangerous or fatal tachyarrhythmias during inhalational anaesthesia. Factors that can lead to an increase in endogenous production of adrenaline (e.g. hypoxia, hypercarbia, reflex stimulation) may increase the risk. Similar problems are encountered when cocaine, which inhibits the reuptake of noradrenaline, is used to promote mucosal surface anaesthesia and vasoconstriction in ENT surgery. Dysrhythmias are less common with the fluorinated ethers in common use than with halothane (Table 4.3).

Interactions with sympathomimetic amines are mainly encountered when these drugs are administered during anaesthesia. Indirectly acting sympathomimetic

Table 4.3 Doses of submucosal adrenaline required to induce ventricular extrasystoles in the presence of inhalational agents (median effective dose at 1.25 MAC).

Inhalational agent	Dose
Halothane	2.1 μg kg^{-1}
Isoflurane	6.7 μg kg^{-1}
Enflurane	10.9 μg kg^{-1}
Sevoflurane	≈7 μg kg^{-1}
Desflurane	≈7 μg kg^{-1}

amines (e.g. ephedrine, metaraminol) and related drugs (e.g. theophylline) may have a greater propensity to induce arrhythmogenic effects than directly acting catecholamines.

Ketamine produces central stimulation of sympathetic activity, resulting in raised catecholamine levels. Both tachyarrhythmias and the development of seizures have been reported with the concurrent use of theophylline, which has similar central and peripheral actions.

Cardiovascular effects have also been reported during anaesthesia associated with the prior administration of levodopa. These interactions appear to be dose related since large doses tend to produce tachyarrhythmias and vasoconstriction, presumably due to its metabolite dopamine. With smaller doses, vasodilatation usually predominates.

Arrhythmias induced by sympathomimetic amines during inhalational anaesthesia can usually be prevented or controlled by β-adrenoceptor antagonists.

Antihypertensive agents

During general anaesthesia, hypotensive responses may be induced by a number of drug interactions. Most of these reactions are due to the additive effects of drugs that affect arterial pressure. For instance, thiopental and sevoflurane tend to lower blood pressure and may interact with α- or β-adrenoceptor antagonists or with other drugs that can produce vasodilatation (e.g. chlorpromazine, morphine). These actions are predictable and may be desirable in normotensive patients during anaesthesia.

In hypertensive patients on drug therapy, severe hypotension may occur during general anaesthesia, or postural hypotension may be seen on recovery. Induction agents are particularly liable to induce such responses in treated hypertensive patients. Thiopental reduces cardiac output and often decreases blood pressure in both hypertensive and normotensive subjects. Similarly, inhalational agents, via negative inotropic or chronotropic effects or by a reduction in peripheral resistance, may lead to falls in systemic pressure that are exaggerated in hypertensive subjects. Treated hypertensive patients carry a greater risk of perioperative hypotension than normotensive subjects. However, if attention is given to circulating volume requirements and appropriate modification of the dosage of anaesthetic agents is made, drug interaction should not be a major problem.

Nevertheless, severe and unexpected hypotension has been observed during anaesthesia for patients receiving angiotensin-converting enzyme (ACE) inhibitors. This may reflect the failure of the normally protective renin–angiotensin–aldosterone system associated with decreased renal perfusion during general anaesthesia. It has been suggested that an intravenous infusion should be commenced for all patients who are receiving ACE inhibitors prior to induction of anaesthesia.

Drugs that modify electrolyte balance

Drugs affecting electrolyte balance may also contribute to the occurrence of cardiac arrhythmias during inhalational anaesthesia. Drugs that lower serum K^+ (most diuretics, corticosteroids, insulin) may induce supraventricular or ventricular ectopic beats during inhalational anaesthesia, particularly in patients who are digitalized. Conversely, drugs that induce hyperkalaemia (e.g. suxamethonium, potassium-sparing diuretics) tend to impair cardiac conduction and may cause sinoatrial block. Agents that lower serum Ca^{2+} (e.g. calcitonin, blood transfusions) depress cardiac contractility and may predispose to cardiac arrhythmias. Additional factors unrelated to drug administration may also be involved (e.g. reflex stimulation).

Muscle relaxants

Volatile anaesthetic agents increase the neuromuscular block induced by non-depolarizing muscle relaxants (page 79). They may also induce dual block when patients are concomitantly receiving repeated doses of suxamethonium (page 180).

Enzyme-inducing agents

Thiopental and other agents used in anaesthesia can potentially induce the activity of drug-metabolizing enzymes. It is therefore possible that the plasma concentration and effects of other drugs concurrently used (e.g. anticoagulants, anticonvulsants) could be reduced. However, underlying disease and associated trauma may have a depressant effect on drug metabolism and lead to higher plasma concentrations of drugs administered in the postoperative period.

Inhalational anaesthetics produce complex effects on cytochrome P450 and other microsomal enzyme systems. Most fluorinated agents are metabolized by the isoform CYP 2E1, which is induced by ethyl alcohol and variably affected by fluorinated agents. Anaesthesia with inhalational anaesthetics may cause induction, inhibition or have a biphasic effect on CYP 2E1 and related enzyme systems. In addition, the metabolic response to surgery may profoundly affect hepatic drug metabolism.

Enzyme-inhibiting agents

In clinical concentrations, propofol has a modest inhibitory effect on some isoforms of cytochrome P450, particularly CYP 1A1, CYP 2A1 and CYP 2B1. Experimental and clinical studies suggest that propofol may potentially alter the metabolism of fentanyl and alfentanil. In addition, imidazole derivatives (including etomidate) can inhibit drug hydroxylation by CYP 3A4 and other isoforms (Chapter 7).

Nephrotoxic agents

After administration of sevoflurane, there is a limited increase in the urinary excretion of fluoride ions. In addition, sevoflurane can interact with soda lime to form a potentially nephrotoxic vinyl ether ('compound A'). Although there is no clinical evidence that sevoflurane or isoflurane can produce renal damage, this possibility should be recognized when other nephrotoxic agents (e.g. aminoglycoside antibiotics) are used concurrently.

Interactions with local anaesthetic agents

Although local anaesthetics are extensively used in current practice, undesirable or adverse drug reactions are uncommon. Nevertheless, interactions involving local anaesthetic solutions are a potential risk when they are administered to patients receiving certain other drugs. Preparations of local anaesthetics often contain vasoconstrictors, which delay absorption and usually produce a beneficial drug interaction by increasing the duration of anaesthesia. Interactions with other drugs can occur with either the vasoconstrictor or the local anaesthetic agent. Other constituents of local anaesthetic solutions (reducing agents, preservatives, fungicides) have not been incriminated in drug interactions. Nevertheless, the addition of hyaluronidase to local anaesthetic solutions may significantly enhance tissue penetration and reduce the duration of blockade.

In the past, noradrenaline was occasionally used as a vasoconstrictor in local anaesthetic solutions. Injected noradrenaline, as well as the endogenous hormone, is predominantly removed from tissues and synapses by active transport into sympathetic nerve terminals (Uptake$_1$). This mechanism can be blocked by most tricyclic agents and their derivatives, which compete with noradrenaline for Uptake$_1$. Consequently, the pressor response to noradrenaline is significantly potentiated by these agents, and the effects of adrenaline may also be increased. Infusion or injection of noradrenaline, adrenaline or other α-adrenoceptor agonists such as phenylephrine to patients on tricyclic drugs may cause a marked rise in blood pressure, which can precipitate subarachnoid haemorrhage. There is some evidence that pancuronium may also sensitize tissues to noradrenaline by a similar mechanism.

The potential hazards of adrenaline and noradrenaline in patients receiving tricyclic antidepressants are well known. Nevertheless, current opinion suggests that provided adrenaline is used in local anaesthetic solutions, and proper attention is given to dosage and technique, clinically significant drug interactions will not occur. It should be recognized that tricyclic agents themselves may induce complex side effects on the cardiovascular system including postural hypotension, tachycardia, delayed AV conduction and T wave prolongation.

In general, local anaesthetic solutions can interact with:
• Muscle relaxants and their antagonists
• Sulphonamides
• Other drugs (e.g. clonidine, ketamine)

Muscle relaxants and their antagonists

Local anaesthetics can enhance the effects of both depolarizing and non-depolarizing muscle relaxants on neuromuscular transmission. High concentrations of esters (e.g. procaine) can compete with suxamethonium for cholinesterase, prevent its hydrolysis, and enhance depolarizing block. Conversely, the effects of local anaesthetic esters may be prolonged by drugs that inhibit cholinesterase (e.g. neostigmine, cytotoxic drugs).

Many local anaesthetics can also augment non-depolarizing block, although their mechanism of action is uncertain. Local anaesthetics decrease acetylcholine release from the nerve terminal and stabilize the postsynaptic receptor and the muscle cell membrane. These effects can clearly contribute to and enhance non-depolarizing blockade.

Sulphonamides

The antibacterial effects of sulphonamides are dependent on the antagonism of para-aminobenzoate, which is essential for nucleic acid synthesis in certain organisms. Drugs that release para-aminobenzoate in tissues, such as procaine and related esters, can overcome this antagonism and prevent the bacteriostatic effects of sulphonamides. Instances of this interaction have only rarely been reported and its significance is now mainly of historical interest. Nevertheless, local anaesthetic preparations containing procaine or amethocaine should be avoided for patients with infections that are being concurrently treated with sulphonamides or sulphonamide combinations (e.g. co-trimoxazole).

Other drugs

Clinical reports and experimental studies suggest that the cardiovascular toxicity of local anaesthetic amides is increased in the presence of calcium channel blockers (e.g. verapamil, nifedipine), and additive effects on myocardial contraction and conduction are likely. The administration of either clonidine or ketamine with local anaesthetic agents can increase the duration of extradural (and spinal) blockade, and both pharmacokinetic and pharmacodynamic factors may be involved. Conversely, a significant failure rate of spinal anaesthesia using bupivacaine has been reported in those patients with either a high alcohol intake, long-term treatment with non-steroidal anti-inflammatory drugs (e.g. indometacin) or both. The mechanism of such apparent drug antagonism is obscure.

Interactions with muscle relaxants and their antagonists

The intensity and duration of action of muscle relaxants can be affected by many other drugs. Interactions of this type may be associated with prescribed or self-administered oral therapy, with parenteral or locally applied preparations, or with agents concurrently used in the course of anaesthesia.

Interactions with muscle relaxants and their antagonists may occur with:
• General anaesthetics
• Local anaesthetics
• Drugs that affect cytochrome P450

- Drugs that affect electrolyte balance
- Drugs that modify acid–base balance
- Antibiotics
- Cholinesterase inhibitors
- Other drugs

General anaesthetics
Non-depolarizing relaxants

Most inhalational agents will affect both the pharmacodynamic activity and the kinetic behaviour of non-depolarizing neuromuscular blocking agents. The increase and prolongation of myoneural blockade is dependent on the nature and concentration of the anaesthetic agent. Isoflurane, sevoflurane and desflurane generally produce a greater effect than halothane at equivalent MAC values. The mechanism of skeletal muscle relaxation is not entirely clear, but may be due to central actions, presynaptic effects or to an altered sensitivity of the postsynaptic receptor or the muscle cell membrane. Alternatively, the variable potencies of individual inhalational agents may reflect different effects on presynaptic Ca^{2+} influx at the neuromuscular junction.

Volatile anaesthetics may also affect the kinetic disposition of muscle relaxants. When gradually increasing concentrations of fluorinated agents are administered neuromuscular junction sensitivity increases, but the rate of equilibration between the plasma concentration of the relaxant and the onset of paralysis will decrease. This reflects decreased perfusion to the neuromuscular junction, resulting in a reduction in the rate of drug delivery.

There is no evidence that intravenous induction agents in common use interact with non-depolarizing agents.

Suxamethonium

The duration of action of a single dose of suxamethonium is not usually affected by intravenous or inhalational anaesthesia. Nevertheless, if volatile agents are used concurrently, the transition from phase I (depolarizing) to phase II (non-depolarizing) blockade may occur at a lower total dosage of suxamethonium when repeated doses are given. Isoflurane may accelerate the onset of phase II blockade and potentiate its intensity. The mechanisms involved in this interaction are not entirely clear, but may involve translocation of Ca^{2+} at pre- and postsynaptic sites.

The muscarinic effects of suxamethonium may be enhanced by propofol, possibly due to its absence of any central vagolytic activity.

Local anaesthetics

Most local anaesthetic agents enhance the effects of non-depolarizing agents on neuromuscular transmission. Many other drugs have local anaesthetic or membrane-stabilizing properties and can also augment non-depolarizing blockade, including phenothiazines, tricyclic antidepressants, antihistamines, quinidine and some barbiturates. It is unclear whether these effects are due to presynaptic or postsynaptic actions on neuromuscular transmission.

In addition, local anaesthetic esters may compete with suxamethonium for cholinesterase and prolong depolarization blockade.

Drugs that affect cytochrome P450

Drugs that affect cytochrome P450 may modify the elimination of muscle relaxants that partly or predominantly depend on hepatic metabolism (pancuronium, rocuronium, vecuronium). Drugs that induce cytochrome P450 (Table 4.1) may reduce their effects and duration of action, in spite of their membrane-stabilizing effects. Conversely, drugs that inhibit cytochrome P450 or reduce hepatic perfusion (Table 4.2) may have the opposite effect.

Drugs that affect electrolyte balance

Electrolytes or drugs that modify electrolyte balance or mobilization, in particular those affecting Mg^{2+}, Ca^{2+} and K^+, may profoundly influence neuromuscular transmission.

Magnesium ions

Magnesium ions prevent Ca^{2+} entry into the presynaptic nerve terminal, thus decreasing acetylcholine release and reducing the amplitude of the endplate potential. Consequently, non-depolarizing blockade is augmented and depolarization blockade may be antagonized.

Calcium ions and calcium channel-blocking agents

Calcium ions play an important part in the presynaptic release of acetylcholine and in subsequent muscle contraction (i.e. in excitation–contraction coupling). Consequently Ca^{2+} salts and drugs that raise Ca^{2+} concentrations (e.g. parathormone) may increase acetylcholine release and enhance excitation–contraction coupling.

Conversely, drugs that decrease Ca^{2+} concentrations or interfere with Ca^{2+} transport and intracellular mobilization may decrease acetylcholine release and prolong neuromuscular blockade. In the presence of Ca^{2+} channel blockers, prolonged effects of vecuronium and atracurium have been reported. The problem is likely to be enhanced by volatile anaesthetic agents, particularly by isoflurane.

Potassium ions

Drugs that increase plasma K^+ (e.g. spironolactone, triamterene) decrease the resting membrane potential of muscle and may augment depolarization blockade. In contrast, drugs that induce hypokalaemia (corticosteroids, β-adrenoceptor agonists, insulin) increase the resting potential and may enhance the effects of non-depolarizing agents. Changes in plasma K^+ may also modify transmitter release. In the presence of hypokalaemia the dosage of non-depolarizing agents should usually be reduced. Conversely, the dose of suxamethonium may need to be increased.

Disturbances in electrolyte balance, particularly K^+, may also be a factor in possible interactions between corticosteroids and muscle relaxants. In these conditions, both potentiation and antagonism have been described.

Drugs that modify acid–base balance

Neuromuscular blockade can be modified by changes in acid–base balance. In particular, both respiratory acidosis and metabolic alkalosis appear to enhance and prolong non-depolarizing blockade. Any drug which induces respiratory acidosis (e.g. opioid analgesics, barbiturates) or metabolic alkalosis (e.g. thiazide diuretics, antacids) may therefore enhance the response to non-depolarizing agents. The effect of other alterations in acid–base balance on neuromuscular blockade is less clear.

Any increased response to muscle relaxants in the presence of respiratory acidosis and metabolic alkalosis is probably due to changes in intracellular pH and K^+ balance. During hypokalaemia, the resting membrane potential of excitable tissues is increased, resulting in an enhanced response to non-depolarizing agents.

In vitro studies suggest that changes in acid–base balance may also affect the ionization of certain muscle relaxants in *in vivo* conditions (e.g. vecuronium, rocuronium). In addition, both cisatracurium and atracurium have pH-dependent physicochemical properties, and extreme changes in acid–base balance in the physiological range may affect their duration of action.

Antibiotics

Some antibiotics can induce neuromuscular blockade and may enhance the effects of non-depolarizing agents. Occasionally, suxamethonium blockade is also enhanced. This phenomenon was first observed when antibiotic sprays containing streptomycin or neomycin were applied to the peritoneum after abdominal surgery. In these conditions, hypoventilation may supervene postoperatively due to the local effects of the antibiotic on neurotransmission in the diaphragm. Similar interactions after the systemic administration of antibiotics are relatively rare, and usually involve the aminoglycosides, colistin, clindamycin or tetracyclines. In these circumstances, neuromuscular block is probably dependent on several factors that may vary with different antibiotics.

Neuromuscular blockade induced or complicated by aminoglycosides is variably affected by anticholinesterase drugs and is more commonly antagonized by calcium salts (e.g. calcium gluconate 2–3 mg kg^{-1} min^{-1} for 5 min). The neuromuscular blockade induced by such antibiotics may be due to competition for calcium-binding sites in the nerve terminal or the pre-junctional membrane. In the case of tetracyclines, localized chelation of Ca^{2+} may be involved. By contrast, neuromuscular blockade which is induced by colistin or clindamycin is usually unaffected by anticholinesterases and calcium salts. These interactions are usually managed by controlled ventilation until normal neuromuscular function is restored, although the experimental agent 4-aminopyridine is sometimes effective. Enhancement of neuromuscular blockade usually occurs when non-depolarizing agents are administered to patients on antibiotics, although similar effects may be induced when antibacterial drugs are given to patients with myasthenia gravis.

Cholinesterase inhibitors

Many drugs inhibit or compete for plasma cholinesterase and may thus affect the enzymatic hydrolysis of suxamethonium and mivacurium, including:

- Edrophonium, neostigmine and pyridostigmine
- Organophosphorus insecticides (e.g. malathion)
- Tetrahydroaminacrine and hexafluorenium
- Local anaesthetic esters (cocaine, procaine and tetracaine)
- Other agents

Clinically significant interactions are particularly likely in heterozygous subjects with inherited variants in cholinesterase (Chapter 6).

Edrophonium, neostigmine and pyridostigmine

These quaternary amines primarily inhibit acetylcholinesterase and are used to antagonize non-depolarizing blockade. They also inhibit plasma cholinesterase and can therefore decrease the metabolism and prolong the duration of action of suxamethonium and mivacurium.

Tetrahydroaminacrine and hexafluorenium

In the past, tetrahydraminacrine and hexafluorenium were deliberately used to inhibit plasma cholinesterase and prolong the action of suxamethonium. Similar drugs that are used in the symptomatic treatment of Alzheimer's disease (e.g. donepezil, galantamine, rivastigmine) also inhibit acetylcholinesterase and cholinesterase.

Local anaesthetic esters

Although local anaesthetic esters decrease the metabolism of suxamethonium and mivacurium, clinically significant interactions are extremely rare.

Other agents

Pancuronium is a moderately potent inhibitor of plasma cholinesterase and may prolong the action of drugs that are normally metabolized by the enzyme.

Bambuterol is an inactive carbamate ester which is converted to an active β_2-agonist (terbutaline) by cholinesterase, and the residual carbamate groups can selectively inhibit the enzyme.

Metoclopramide, aprotinin and cimetidine are weak inhibitors of plasma cholinesterase.

Cyclophosphamide, and possibly thiotepa, may inhibit the synthesis of cholinesterase and prolong the duration of action of suxamethonium.

Certain immunosuppressants (e.g. azathioprine, ciclosporin) can antagonize the effects of some non-depolarizing agents. The mechanisms are obscure but in the case of the ciclosporin–pancuronium interaction, the Cremophor used as a vehicle for ciclosporin has been implicated. There are occasional reports of prolongation of neuromuscular blockade with the concurrent use of a number of other drugs, including benzodiazepines, lithium carbonate, H_1-antagonists and chloroquine.

Interactions with opioid analgesics

Opioid analgesics are extensively used in anaesthesia, and drug interactions with other agents are of particular concern to the anaesthetist. In current practice, fentanyl, alfentanil and remifentanil are most frequently used to provide intraoperative analgesia, while morphine is most commonly used postoperatively. In most cases drug interactions with opioids are readily predictable from the pharmacological effects of these agents. Drug interactions may occur with:

- Other central depressants
- Opioid antagonists and partial agonists
- Drugs that affect cytochrome P450
- Drugs given orally
- Monoamine oxidase inhibitors

Other central depressants
General anaesthetics

Effective analgesic doses of opioids tend to cause sedation and invariably produce some respiratory depression. Their depressant effects may be enhanced by both intravenous and inhalational anaesthetic agents. Respiratory depression induced by opioids can decrease the rate of removal of general anaesthetics given by inhalational techniques and thus prolong their effects.

Phenothiazines

Many phenothiazines augment the analgesic, sedative, respiratory depressant and hypotensive effects of opioids. The mechanisms associated with this interaction are complex and may involve summation or synergism at receptor sites. Other factors, including the pharmacological effects of drug metabolites and changes in hepatic blood flow, may also be important.

Benzodiazepines and tricyclic antidepressants

Benzodiazepines can enhance the sedative effects of opioid analgesics, and this combination may lead to problems in elderly patients or those with respiratory disease. Tricyclic antidepressants may also enhance the effects of opioid analgesics, possibly due to both the increased bioavailability of morphine and an intrinsic analgesic effect of the antidepressant agent.

Opioid antagonists and partial agonists

The effects of opioid analgesics can be modified by drugs that compete for opioid receptors in the CNS. Both naloxone and naltrexone are pure antagonists with no agonist activity, and competitively antagonize the effects of opioid analgesics. By contrast, other antagonists (e.g. pentazocine) also possess some agonist activity. These drugs (partial agonists) antagonize some of the effects of other opioid analgesics, but also produce central effects (e.g. dysphoria, analgesia, respiratory depression) due to their intrinsic activity at different opioid receptors. Interactions between pure and partial agonists are complex and dose related and may depend upon the timing of drug administration. They may present clinically as:

(i) Enhancement of respiratory depression if the two drugs are given simultaneously;

(ii) Decreased analgesic efficacy of the pure agonist after prior administration of the partial agonist;

(iii) The development of opioid withdrawal symptoms if the partial agonist is administered subsequently.

Analgesia and respiratory depression induced by buprenorphine, a partial agonist with no antagonistic activity, is not usually reversed by naloxone. This may reflect the slow dissociation of buprenorphine from opioid receptors.

Drugs that affect cytochrome P450
Enzyme induction

Drugs with significant enzyme-inducing properties (Table 4.1) may reduce the plasma concentration and effects of methadone and enhance withdrawal symptoms due to an increase in hepatic metabolism. Similarly, carbamazepine may decrease the plasma concentration of tramadol and reduce its analgesic efficacy. The concurrent use of oral contraceptives significantly increases the clearance of morphine, suggesting that the oestrogen component can significantly enhance glucuronyl transferase activity.

Enzyme inhibition

Most opioid analgesics are extensively metabolized in the liver by certain isoforms of cytochrome P450, particularly CYP 2D6 and CYP 3A4. Inhibitors of these enzymes (Table 4.2) can increase the plasma concentration and effects of fentanyl and alfentanil.

Drugs given orally

Most opioid analgesics delay the oral absorption of many other drugs by decreasing gastric motility and slowing down the rate of gastric emptying. Conversely, the rate and extent of absorption of oral morphine can be enhanced by drugs that increase gastric motility (e.g. metoclopramide). The urinary elimination of some analgesics (e.g. pethidine, fentanyl) is increased by drugs that induce acidosis. Since these opioids are extensively metabolized, their enhanced elimination in acid urine is of little value in the treatment of drug overdosage, although it is sometimes of value in the detection of drug dependence. The excretion of methadone is also increased in acid urine.

Nausea and vomiting are common side effects of many opioid analgesics which are modified by antiemetic drugs (e.g. chlorpromazine, ondansetron). Antagonism of dopamine receptors in the chemoreceptor trigger zone in the area postrema, and of 5-HT$_3$ receptors at central and peripheral sites, may be responsible for the decrease in opioid-induced nausea and vomiting.

Monoamine oxidase inhibitors

Pethidine is an opioid analgesic of low potency and a short duration of action, which is not commonly used in current anaesthetic practice. Dangerous interactions may occur between pethidine and monoamine oxidase inhibitors (MAOIs), which primarily interfere with the mitochondrial metabolism of monoamines (e.g. tyramine, dopamine), and have effects that can persist for 2–3 weeks after administration is stopped. Two types of reaction have been reported. Excitatory signs and symptoms, including agitation, mental confusion, headache, rigidity, hyperreflexia, hyperpyrexia and convulsions are probably due to an increase in intraneuronal and intrasynaptic 5-HT ('the serotonin syndrome'). Inhibitory effects, including respiratory depression, circulatory collapse and coma may be due to inhibition of hepatic microsomal enzyme systems by MAO inhibitors and accumulation of pethidine and its metabolites in the body. The serotonin syndrome may also occur when pethidine is given to patients on selegiline (a selective inhibitor of type B MAO), or moclobemide (a reversible inhibitor of type A MAO). It has been suggested that the syndrome may be due to inhibition of serotonin reuptake by central neurons, and is best treated with 5-HT$_{2A}$ antagonists, such as oral cyproheptadine or intravenous chlorpromazine.

Although similar interactions have occasionally been reported with some other opioids, they appear to be relatively uncommon. Nevertheless, the use of methadone, dextromethorphan, dextropropoxyphene and tramadol should probably be avoided in patients on MAO inhibitors. Morphine, codeine, oxycodone and buprenorphine do not interact with MAO inhibitors to cause serotonin toxicity, although dose titration may be necessary to avoid depressant side effects. Fentanyl, alfentanil and remifentanil also appear to be relatively safe.

Interactions with non-opioid analgesics

Non-steroidal anti-inflammatory drugs (NSAIDs) are frequently used to provide postoperative analgesia and are one of the commonest groups of drugs involved in drug interactions in general medical practice. Aspirin and related compounds have been particularly associated with clinically significant drug interactions. In most instances, these interactions have only been reported with chronic administration of large and repeated doses of these drugs, and the possible effect of single doses or restricted use is difficult to evaluate. Nevertheless, important interactions may occur with:

- Oral anticoagulants
- Antihypertensive drugs
- Uricosuric agents
- Paracetamol and co-proxamol

Oral anticoagulants

Aspirin and other NSAIDs can predispose to or induce haemorrhage in patients on anticoagulants (particularly warfarin). Although warfarin is strongly bound to plasma albumin (98–99%), this drug interaction is not related to the displacement from plasma protein binding. Aspirin and similar drugs may cause bleeding due to gastric mucosal damage and inhibit platelet aggregation by acetylation of platelet COX-1 in the hepatic portal circulation. In large doses, aspirin also reduces the synthesis of prothrombin. However, NSAIDs may predispose to or induce haemorrhage in patients on warfarin due to a pharmacodynamic rather than pharmacokinetic interaction. The use of standard doses of aspirin should be avoided in patients receiving warfarin, although low-dose aspirin (up to 75 mg daily) appears to be relatively safe. The parenteral use of diclofenac and ketorolac is also contraindicated in the presence of anticoagulants, including both warfarin and low-dose heparin.

Antihypertensive drugs

Prostacyclin (PGI_2) and possibly other vasodilator prostaglandins (e.g. PGD_2, PGE_2) produce important effects on the renal circulation, causing vasodilatation, renin release and promoting Na^+ excretion by inhibiting its reabsorption in the proximal renal tubule. Synthesis of prostacyclin (PGI_2) is mainly dependent on COX-2, and NSAIDs that inhibit this enzyme (e.g. indometacin, piroxicam, diclofenac) inhibit the renal excretion of Na^+, causing salt and water retention and increasing blood pressure. They may also impair or antagonize the effects of other drugs used in the treatment of hypertension and heart failure (e.g. diuretics, ACE inhibitors, β-adrenoceptor antagonists). Aspirin and most other related drugs have been less commonly implicated. Nevertheless, refractory hypertension or oedema may develop during treatment with NSAIDs and appropriate adjustment of the dosage of antihypertensive drugs may be necessary. This interaction may be implicated in some cases of postoperative hypertension.

Uricosuric drugs

Aspirin and other salicylates produce dose-dependent effects on tubular secretion in the kidney. Aspirin can decrease the urinary elimination of urates and may antagonize the effects of uricosuric agents (e.g. probenecid, sulfinpyrazone), which are concurrently administered. Salicylates may also interfere with the removal of other drugs that rely on active transport processes in the proximal tubule (e.g. methotrexate) and can potentiate their effects.

Paracetamol and co-proxamol

Drug interactions involving paracetamol appear to be extremely uncommon, although its absorption may be modified by colestyramine and its metabolism may be increased in the presence of anticonvulsants and oral contraceptives. However, a number of compound preparations containing paracetamol may also include codeine (co-codamol), dihydrocodeine (co-dydramol) or dextropropoxyphene (co-proxamol). Dextropropoxyphene poisoning is not infrequently associated with excessive consumption of alcohol and may be complicated by respiratory depression and heart failure. Dextropropoxyphene may also prolong and enhance the effects of oral anticoagulants, and interactions with the antimuscarinic compound orphenadrine have also been reported.

Interactions with drugs used for premedication and sedation

Drugs which induce sleep (hypnotics) or which relieve anxiety (tranquillisers) are closely related and are frequently prescribed in general medical practice. Benzodiazepines are commonly administered in the preoperative period. Diazepam is often used for premedication to allay anxiety prior to surgery, and temazepam may be prescribed as a hypnotic on the night before operation. In addition, intravenous benzodiazepines (e.g. diazepam, midazolam) are used to induce sedation during endoscopy and minor surgical procedures. Other drugs with sedative or antimuscarinic properties (e.g. antihistamine

compounds, atropine) may also be used for premedication. Significant drug interactions can occur with:
- Other central depressants
- Drugs that affect cytochrome P450
- Phenothiazines and butyrophenones
- Other drugs

Other central depressants

Doses of tranquillisers or sedatives that relieve anxiety and tension may induce drowsiness and cause loss of concentration in susceptible subjects. These drugs should not be given to ambulant patients without warning them of the possible hazards of their administration, particularly in relation to driving. Furthermore, all tranquillisers and sedatives may interact with other agents that have depressant effects on the CNS. Their effects may also be enhanced during the concurrent administration of antidepressant drugs, although authentic reports of this interaction are rare. The effects of drugs that induce respiratory depression may also be magnified. In contrast, aminophylline and caffeine can antagonize the CNS effects induced by benzodiazepines.

Drugs that affect cytochrome P450
Enzyme induction

Some drugs that induce hepatic enzymes (Table 4.1) can increase the rate of metabolism of most benzodiazepines, including diazepam and midazolam, and reduce the magnitude and duration of their effects. Conversely, both diazepam and chlordiazepoxide may inhibit the metabolism of phenytoin and increase its toxicity.

Enzyme inhibition

Drugs that inhibit cytochrome P450 (Table 4.2) can retard and decrease the metabolism of benzodiazepines. For example, the H_2-receptor antagonist cimetidine and other imidazoles (e.g. ketoconazole, omeprazole) bind to some isoforms of cytochrome P450, inhibit the metabolism of diazepam and related compounds, and may increase their sedative effects. Similarly, in patients on erythromycin the plasma concentration of midazolam is markedly increased and prolonged hypnosis and amnesia may occur due to inhibitory effects on the isoform CYP 3A4. Diltiazem and verapamil may have similar effects on the disposition of midazolam, since they are also competitive substrates for the isoform CYP 3A4. The sedative effects of diazepam may also be increased by other drugs that reduce its clearance (e.g. isoniazid, probenecid).

Phenothiazines and butyrophenones

Phenothiazines and butyrophenones are sometimes used during anaesthesia, mainly for their antiemetic effects. These drugs have central antidopaminergic properties which may be inhibited in patients on levodopa. On the other hand, the mutual antagonism between these drugs and levodopa may result in the exacerbation of extrapyramidal disorders. Metoclopramide is an antagonist at dopamine receptors at both peripheral and central sites. It may also increase the bioavailability of levodopa by its effects on gut motility and the resultant interaction is therefore unpredictable.

Phenothiazines potentiate the sedative and analgesic properties of drugs used in anaesthesia by their effects on central pathways, augment hypotensive responses to inhalational and neuromuscular blocking agents by α_1-adrenoceptor antagonism, and produce summation with anticholinergic drugs at muscarinic sites. When phenothiazines are given with α-adrenoceptor antagonists or tricyclic antidepressants, concentrations of both drugs are increased, with a resultant enhancement of their clinical effects. Mechanisms involving enzyme inhibition and/or effects on liver blood flow may be involved.

Other drug interactions

Drugs with significant antimuscarinic properties that are used for premedication (e.g. atropine, hyoscine) have a marked antisialagogue effect and may decrease the effect of other drugs which are given sublingually (e.g. glyceryl trinitrate, buprenorphine). Antimuscarinic drugs may also antagonize the effects of certain antiemetic agents (e.g. domperidone, metoclopramide) on the gut by opposing mechanisms on gastric emptying. When patients receive premedication with atropine, the risk of emergence delirium associated with ketamine is increased.

The prevention of adverse drug interactions

Although adverse drug interactions cannot be entirely prevented, their incidence may be minimized by an appreciation of their causation. In the first place, many interactions occur with prescribed or self-administered oral therapy and it is therefore important to take a drug history before the administration of any other agent. Second, the possibility of adverse interactions rises exponentially as the number of drugs administered is increased. Third, drug interactions are more likely when drug elimination is prolonged, as in hepatic or renal disease or in elderly patients. Finally, adverse interactions are more common with agents which have a relatively steep dose–response curve, or when there is little difference between the toxic and therapeutic doses of the drugs involved.

Suggested reading

Calvey, T.N. (1993) Synergy and isoboles. *British Journal of Anaesthesia* **70**, 246–247.

Gillman, P.K. (2005) Monoamine oxidase inhibitors, opioid analgesics and serotonin toxicity. *British Journal of Anaesthesia* **95**, 434–441.

Halsey, M.J. (1987) Drug interactions in anaesthesia. *British Journal of Anaesthesia* **59**, 112–123.

Johnston, R.R., Eger, E.I., II & Wilson, C. (1976) A comparative interaction of epinephrine with enflurane, isoflurane and halothane in man. *Anesthesia and Analgesia* **55**, 709–712.

Karalliedde, L. & Henry, J. (1998) *Handbook of Drug Interactions*. London: Arnold.

Oikkola, K.T., Aranko, K., Saarnivaara, L., *et al.* (1993) A potentially hazardous interaction between erythromycin and midazolam. *Clinical Pharmacology and Therapeutics* **53**, 298–305.

Pleuvry, B.J. (2005) Pharmacodynamic and pharmacokinetic drug interactions. *Anaesthesia and Intensive Care Medicine* **6**, 129–133.

Riley, B.B. (1970) Incompatibilities in intravenous solutions. *Journal of Hospital Pharmacy* **28**, 228–240.

Rolan, P.E. (1994) Plasma protein displacement interactions – why are they still regarded as clinically significant? *British Journal of Clinical Pharmacology* **37**, 125–128.

Soni, N. (1987) Mechanisms of drug interactions (Appendix III). In: Feldman, S., Scurr, C.F. & Paton, W. (eds.), *Drugs in Anaesthesia: Mechanisms of Action*. London: Edward Arnold, pp. 408–427.

Stockley, I.H. (2000) *Drug Interactions*, 5th edn. London: The Pharmaceutical Press.

Thummel, K.E. & Wilkinson, G.R. (1998) *In vitro* and *in vivo* drug interactions involving human CYP3A. *Annual Review of Pharmacology and Toxicology* **38**, 389–430.

Wood, M. (1991) Pharmacokinetic drug interactions in anaesthetic practice. *Clinical Pharmacokinetics* **21**, 285–307.

Variability in Drug Response

There is a wide variability in the response of different patients to identical doses of the same drug. Drugs do not always produce the same effect in all subjects and may not even produce identical responses when given to the same patient on different occasions. Consequently, dose–response curves obtained in man may only be directly applicable to individual subjects. Nevertheless, they are often used to illustrate the results obtained in a large sample derived from a relatively homogeneous population of subjects. In these conditions, a sigmoid log dose–response curve can be used to express the results, although it often disguises the high degree of interindividual variability (Fig. 5.1).

Variability in the response to drugs can be considered as part of the general phenomenon of inherent or intrinsic biological variability. Both physiological responses and pharmacological phenomena are subject to considerable interindividual variability. Although this variability can be expressed by the enumeration of individual results, this is usually unnecessary and impractical, since a large number of observations may be involved. More commonly, the distribution and variability of individual measurements (variables) is expressed in terms of two 'descriptive statistics':

These two statistics reflect

(1) The central tendency or midpoint of the data, expressed by the
   - Mode (the most commonly occurring value)
   - Median (the central or middle value that divides the results into two equal groups)
   - Mean (the arithmetic average)
(2) The variability or scatter of individual values, expressed by the
   - Frequency (how often each observation occurs)
   - Interquartile range (the middle 50% of values)
   - Standard deviation (the root mean square deviate)

The choice of the parameter or statistic that is used to express the central tendency and the scatter of a series of individual results depends on the 'level of measurement' of the data. In general, there are three 'levels of measurement' of biological data:
- Nominal
- Ordinal
- Continuous

Nominal measurements

Nominal or categorical measurements depend on the classification of data or subjects into groups that are solely dependent on their names or characteristics. Thus, patients can be classified as male or female, premedicated or unpremedicated, conscious or unconscious etc. In general, quantal ('all-or-none') measurements are also nominal. All measurements within a group are equivalent to each other, and there are no quantitative differences between individual members.

The central tendency of nominal measurements is usually expressed as the most frequently occurring value, or the mode; thus, in the numerical series, 1, 2, 3, 3, 5, 5, 5, 6, 7, 9, 9, the mode is 5. The distribution of nominal measurements is expressed by the frequency of their occurrence (Table 5.1).

Nominal measurements can be considered as the lowest level of description of data and are only used when measurements are obtained by unsophisticated techniques.

Ordinal measurements

Ordinal measurements (ranked data) depend on the ranking of the underlying data into a sequence or order that depends on their magnitude or relationship to each other. Individual data can usually be graded as lower (<) or greater (>) than other members of the series, although they cannot be given a precise quantitative value. At their best, ordinal or ranked data can be regarded as semi-quantitative. For instance, pain scores on a visual analogue scale (Fig. 5.2)

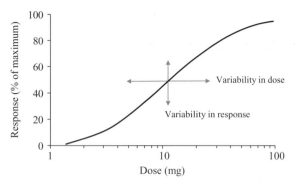

Fig. 5.1 Log dose–response curve showing the variability in dosage required to produce the same response (↔), and the variability in response produced by a single dose (↕) in a population of subjects.

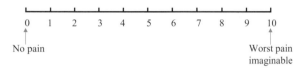

Fig. 5.2 A commonly used visual analogue scale for pain. The scale is a horizontal line which is 10 cm long. The origin of the line represents a score of 0 (i.e., no pain), while the end of the line corresponds to a score of 10 (the worst pain imaginable). The patient is asked to indicate the point on the line that corresponds best to their pain.

and Apgar scores are ordinal measurements, since they can be placed in an order in which their relationship to each other is defined (although their quantitative value is imprecise).

The central tendency of ordinal measurements is expressed as the median, or the middle value in a range of numbers (Table 5.1). Thus, in 11 patients with postoperative pain scores of 1, 2, 3, 3, 5, 5, 5, 6, 7, 9, 9, the

Table 5.1 Descriptive statistics used to describe the central tendency and variability of nominal, ordinal and continuous data.

Level of measurement	Descriptive statistic	
	Central tendency	Variability
Nominal	Mode	Frequency
Ordinal	Median	Interquartile range
Continuous	Mean	Standard deviation

median score is 5. The median is sometimes defined as the 50th percentile, since it divides the numerical observations or results into two equal halves, i.e. 50% of the observations are below the median while 50% are above. The distribution or variability of ordinal measurements can be expressed as the range (1–9), or more correctly as the interquartile range (3–7), which corresponds to the 25th–75th percentiles of the ranked values.

Pain scores are not accurate quantitative data, since their magnitude merely implies that a higher value represents more intense pain than a lower one. It is therefore incorrect to express pain scores as a mean and standard deviation (or standard error), since this implies that the scores have a defined numerical value. Ordinal measurements can be considered as an intermediate level of measurement for the expression and description of data.

Continuous measurements

Continuously variable measurements are quantitative data, and there is a precisely defined and measurable difference between the individual observations or values. Measurements of drug concentrations and responses, heart rate and blood pressure are continuously variable data, since they have a defined numerical value, and equal differences between individual values are comparable to each other. Continuously variable measurements are the highest level of description that can be used for biological and clinical data.

The central tendency of continuous measurements is expressed as the arithmetic mean or average ($\bar{x}$):

$$\text{mean } (\bar{x}) = \frac{\Sigma x \text{ (the sum of their individual values)}}{n \text{ (the number of results or observations)}}$$

The scatter of the individual observations about the mean (i.e. their distribution or variability) is usually described by the standard deviation (Table 5.1).

Standard deviation

The standard deviation ('root mean square deviate') is a commonly used indicator of scatter that is used for continuously variable data and is derived from the sum of the squares of the numerical differences ('deviate') between each individual value and the mean (i.e. $\Sigma[x_1 - \bar{x}]^2 + [x_2 - \bar{x}]^2 + [x_3 - \bar{x}]^2$ etc.). The 'mean deviate' from the mean is given by

$$\text{mean deviate} = \frac{\sum (x - \bar{x})}{n}$$

However, the numerator of this equation ($\Sigma(x - \overline{x})$) will clearly be zero when the (+) and (−) signs of individual results are taken into account, since the mean is defined as the value at which the summated positive and negative deviations are equal. This problem can be eliminated by squaring the deviations about the mean before their summation, and subsequently finding their mean value: this results in an expression for the mean square deviate (more commonly known as the variance):

$$\text{variance} = \frac{\Sigma (x - \overline{x})^2}{n}$$

The original units for the deviation about the mean can be restored by taking the square root of the variance, resulting in an expression for the root mean square deviate or standard deviation:

$$\text{standard deviation} = \sqrt{\left(\frac{\Sigma (x - \overline{x})^2}{n} \right)}$$

This expression can be used to estimate the standard deviation when n is >30. However, the standard deviation in continuously variable data is more usually based on a relatively small sample (i.e. < 30 values), which is only a small part of a much larger, unsampled population of results. In these conditions, it can be shown that a slight modification (Bessel's correction) gives a rather better estimate of the population standard deviation, using the expression:

$$\text{standard deviation} = \sqrt{\left(\frac{\Sigma (x - \overline{x})^2}{n - 1} \right)}$$

In practice, it is unnecessary to calculate each deviation from the mean (i.e. $[x_1 - \overline{x}]$, $[x_2 - \overline{x}]$, $[x_3 - \overline{x}]$ etc.), and to square and summate them, since it can be shown that $\Sigma (x - \overline{x})^2 = \Sigma x^2 - (\Sigma x)^2/n$. Consequently, the standard deviation of samples when $n < 30$ can be defined as

$$\text{standard deviation} = \sqrt{\left(\frac{\Sigma x^2 - (\Sigma x)^2/n}{n - 1} \right)}$$

Most electronic calculators that are designed for statistical use can automatically calculate the mean and the standard deviation, after the individual data values have been entered.

Variance

The variance ('mean square deviate') is the square of the standard deviation. It is defined (when $n < 30$) by the expression:

$$\text{variance} = \left(\frac{\Sigma x^2 - (\Sigma x)^2/n}{n - 1} \right)$$

The denominator of the variance ($n - 1$) defines the number of 'degrees of freedom'. It is one less than the number of observations or results, because only ($n - 1$) results are independent from each other, and the value of the nth result is determined by the values of the remainder.

Coefficient of variation

The variability or scatter of different observations cannot be compared by their standard deviations when the means are very dissimilar, or when they are calculated in different units. For example, in SI units, the weight of a group of 36 patients was 68.0 ± 20.4 kg (mean $\pm$ SD). When expressed in Imperial units, their weight was 150 ± 45 lb. The variability of the measurements must be identical, although their standard deviations are different. Clearly, the standard deviations of different groups cannot be compared unless their units of measurement are identical. This problem can be avoided by the use of the coefficient of variation, which expresses the standard deviation as a percentage of the mean:

$$\text{coefficient of variation (\%)} = \frac{\text{standard deviation}}{\text{mean}} \times 100$$

Since the standard deviation and the mean are measured in the same units, the coefficient of variation is independent of the units of measurement. In the above example, the coefficient of variation of body weight was 30%, whether measured in kg or lb.

Standard error of the mean

The mean ($\overline{x}$) and standard deviation (SD) of a small sample (e.g. $n < 30$) from a large population (e.g. $n > 1000$) are often used to provide an estimate of the population mean (μ) and the population standard deviation (σ). Clearly, different samples of the population may provide different estimates of μ and σ. The accuracy of the sample mean ($\overline{x}$) in comparison with the population mean (μ) can be estimated by the standard error of the mean (SEM):

$$\text{standard error of the mean} = \frac{\text{SD}}{\sqrt{n}}.$$

Clearly, the larger the size of the sample, the more accurate is the sample mean as an estimate of the population mean, and the smaller is the calculated value for the SEM.

Confidence limits

The SEM can also be used to predict the range within which the population mean will lie.

When $n > 30$, there is a 95% chance that the true population mean μ lies within 2 standard errors of the sample mean $\bar{x}$. In the example previously discussed, a group of 36 patients had a body weight of 68.0 ± 20.4 kg (mean $\pm$ SD); consequently:

$$\text{mean} \pm \text{SEM} = 68.0 \pm \frac{20.4}{\sqrt{36}}\,\text{kg} = 68.0 \pm 3.4\,\text{kg}$$

There is a probability of 95% that the true mean of the population lies within the range: mean $\pm$ 2 SEM (in the example above, this range is 61.2–74.8 kg). Approximately 95% of the sample means obtained by repeated sampling of the entire population will also lie within this range. Thus, the range from [mean $-$ (2 $\times$ SEM)] to [mean $+$ (2 $\times$ SEM)] represents the interval within which the true population mean is likely to lie, and is called the 95% confidence limits of the mean. By these methods, a small sample can be used to make inferences and predictions about the parent population from which the sample was obtained.

The SEM is sometimes incorrectly used to indicate the variability of individual values in the sample (possibly because it is always less than the standard deviation from which it is derived). However, the variability or scatter of individual values in a population sample should always be described by the standard deviation.

Frequency distribution curves

The variability of individual observations in a population sample can also be expressed as a histogram or a frequency distribution curve. For example, the variability in the dosage of a drug required to produce a specific pharmacological effect in 100 subjects can be expressed in this way (Fig. 5.3). Each shaded rectangle represents the additional number of patients responding to each 10 mg increment in dosage (e.g. 50–60 mg, 60–70 mg, 70–80 mg etc.). A frequency distribution curve can then be superimposed on the histogram and used to determine the probability of obtaining a response to a given dose in one subject. The data can also be plotted as a cumulative frequency distribution curve (Ogive) by calculating the proportion of patients that respond to a given dose, or to a dose below it (Fig. 5.4).

The normal distribution

The frequency distribution curve, shown in Fig. 5.3, is roughly symmetrical and bell-shaped and is an example

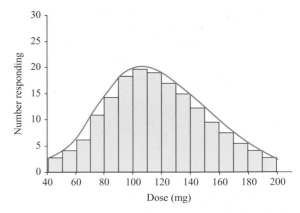

Fig. 5.3 Histogram showing the variability in dosage required to produce a specific effect. Each rectangle represents the number of patients that respond to each 10 mg increment in dosage. A frequency distribution curve (——) has been imposed on the histogram, showing that the data approximately corresponds to a normal or Gaussian distribution.

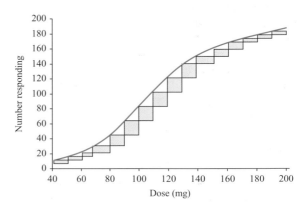

Fig. 5.4 A cumulative frequency distribution curve (——) or Ogive representing the summated results of Fig. 5.3.

of a common type of frequency distribution known as a normal or Gaussian[1] distribution. In many instances, the central tendency and variability of biological or clinical data is consistent with a normal distribution. The central tendency of a normal distribution is equal to the mean value, while the variability is expressed by the standard deviation (Fig. 5.5). Clearly, the shape and form of the Gaussian curve are not critical but are determined by the variability of the underlying data in relation to the mean. The curve is high and narrow when the coefficient of

---

[1] Johann Karl Friedrich Gauss (1777–1855).

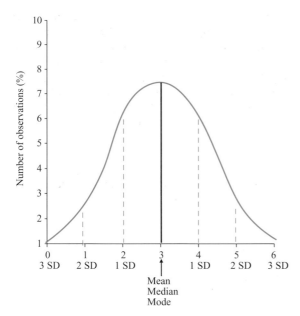

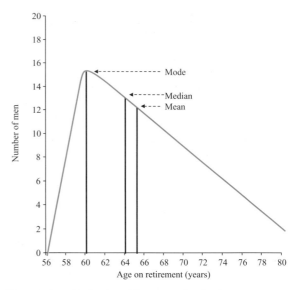

Fig. 5.5 A symmetrical frequency distribution curve in a large population which is consistent with a normal distribution. The mean, the median and the mode are all identical, and the variability is expressed by the standard deviation (SD). The mean ± 1 SD includes 67% of the results, the mean ± 2 SD includes 95% of the results and the mean ± 3 SD includes 99% of the results.

Fig. 5.6 A positively skewed frequency distribution curve showing the retirement age of a male population. In a positively skewed distribution, the mean is usually greater than the median or the mode.

variation is low, but small and wide when the coefficient of variation is high.

In a normal distribution, the mean (average value), the median (the central value that divides the sample into two equally sized groups) and the mode (the most commonly occurring value) are identical (Fig. 5.5). In addition, 67% of the values are within one standard deviation of the mean (i.e. mean ± 1 SD); 95% of the values are within two standard deviations of the mean (i.e. mean ± 2 SD); and 99% of the values are within three standard deviations of the mean (i.e. mean ± 3 SD). These statistics will also apply to a sample from a normally distributed population, as long as the sample size is sufficiently large ($n > 30$).

Skewed distributions

Biological or clinical observations may be positively or negatively skewed (Fig. 5.6). In a skewed distribution, the mean, median and mode are all different, and the median may be a better indication of the central tendency of the results. Similarly, the standard deviation may not be a reliable estimate of the variability of the underlying population.

Positively skewed data can usually be manipulated to conform to a normal distribution by a logarithmic transformation. In these conditions, parametric statistical tests designed for normally distributed data can be used on the transformed observations.

Tests of statistical significance

In general, tests of statistical significance are of two main types:
- Parametric tests
- Non-parametric tests

Parametric statistical tests

Most parametric statistical tests rely on the assumption that the variability of the two or more groups of results that are analysed are consistent with a normal distribution. Many of these tests are quite 'robust' and can be used for continuously variable data whose distribution is not grossly abnormal. They should not be used with ordinal or ranked data. Parametric statistical tests usually depend on the comparison of the mean values of two or more samples in relation to their variability. The most commonly used parametric tests (Table 5.2) are
- Student's *t* test (for paired and unpaired data)
- Analysis of variance (ANOVA, for paired and unpaired data)

Table 5.2 Commonly used tests of statistical significance.

Parametric tests	Non-parametric tests
Student's *t* test*	Mann–Whitney test
Analysis of variance (ANOVA)*	Wilcoxon signed rank test
	Wilcoxon ranked sum test
	Kruskal–Wallis test
	Friedman test

*These tests can be used for both paired and unpaired data.

Non-parametric statistical tests

Non-parametric tests (rank tests) do not make any assumptions about the distribution of the data or the population from which it is derived. They are most commonly used for comparing ordinal or ranked data (e.g. Apgar scores, pain scores), in which individual results or observations can be assigned a rank and arranged in order in relation to each other. Although they can also be used with parametric data, quantitative differences between their numerical values will be largely ignored or obscured.

Non-parametric tests of statistical significance include (Table 5.2):
• Mann–Whitney test
• Wilcoxon signed rank test
• Wilcoxon rank sum test
• Kruskal–Wallis test
• Friedman test

Hypothesis testing

Tests of statistical significance are widely used in hypothesis testing, in order to predict whether there are real differences between different groups or treatments, or whether these differences could have occurred by chance.

In general, there are three main steps in hypothesis testing:
(1) Form a null hypothesis, which assumes that there are no real differences observed between the groups or treatments, i.e. any differences observed are due to random variability.
(2) Calculate the probability that any differences observed are due to chance by the use of an appropriate statistical test.
(3) If the probability is more than 5% ($P > 0.05$) accept the null hypothesis and conclude that any differences between the groups are due to chance variations. On the other hand, if the probability is less than 5% ($P < 0.05$)

reject the null hypothesis and conclude that the differences between the groups are unlikely to be due to chance. In a small proportion of cases, the conclusions reached by hypothesis testing may be incorrect, resulting in Type I or Type II errors. In a Type I error, P is < 0.05, although there is no real difference between the populations or groups. In a Type II error, P is > 0.05, despite the presence of a real difference between the groups.

Physiological and social factors that affect the response to drugs

A number of physiological and social factors may affect the response to drugs (Table 5.3), including:
• Age
• Pregnancy
• Tobacco
• Alcohol

Childhood
Drug absorption

In the neonatal period, absorption of drugs is slower than in children or adults due to a longer gastric emptying time and an increase in intestinal transit time. Nevertheless, oral drugs may be more extensively absorbed due to their greater contact time with the intestinal mucosa. The gastric contents are less acidic, and some drugs such as benzylpenicillin and ampicillin will have greater overall oral absorption. Vasomotor instability observed in neonatal life may result in the unreliable absorption from tissue sites after subcutaneous or intramuscular administration.

Table 5.3 The principal causes of variability in drug responses.

Physiological and social	Pathological conditions	Other causes
Age	Liver disease	Idiosyncrasy
Pregnancy	Renal disease	Hypersensitivity
Tobacco	Respiratory diseases	Supersensitivity
Ethyl alcohol	Cardiac diseases	Tachyphylaxis
	Neurological diseases	Tolerance
	Endocrine diseases	

Drug distribution

The distribution of drugs is influenced by several factors including tissue mass, fat content, blood flow, membrane permeability and protein binding. Total body water as a percentage of body weight falls from 87% in the preterm baby to 73% at 3 months, and subsequently decreases to 55% in adult patients. Consequently, doses of water-soluble drugs that are calculated by scaling down adult doses in proportion to body weight can result in lower tissue concentrations in infants and neonates. However, drug distribution is also affected by the lower body fat content and by the increased permeability of the blood–brain barrier in the neonate, and lipid-soluble drugs may be relatively concentrated in the CNS. In addition, the decrease in plasma protein levels in the neonate leads to the increased availability of unbound drug, resulting in enhanced pharmacological activity and drug metabolism. Any change in plasma pH during neonatal life may influence the degree of drug ionization and thus affect the membrane permeability of both acidic and basic drugs.

Drug metabolism and renal elimination

The rate of drug metabolism depends on both the size of the liver and the activity of microsomal enzyme systems. In neonatal life, hepatic enzyme activity, particularly glucuronide conjugation, is initially immature and may not assume the adult pattern for several months. In older children, enzyme activity is similar to adults, although most drugs are metabolized at faster rates due to the relatively greater liver volume.

In the neonatal period, glomerular filtration rates are 20–40% of those in adults, and drugs removed from the body by this means (e.g. digoxin, aminoglycoside antibiotics) are eliminated relatively slowly. Glomerular filtration rates comparable to those in adults occur at about 4 months of age.

Practical implications

These physiological and kinetic differences have significant practical implications. In the neonate, dose regimes for water-soluble drugs should be related to surface area rather than body weight, in order to produce similar blood levels to those in adults. However, the increased volume of distribution and the decreased renal clearance results in a longer elimination half-life, and dose intervals should therefore be prolonged. In addition, the effects of drugs on the neonatal CNS may be enhanced after administration in labour (e.g. morphine, diazepam). This phenomenon may

be due to the increased fraction of non-protein-bound drug, delayed hepatic metabolism, the presence of active metabolites or greater permeability of the CNS due to immaturity of the blood–brain barrier.

For many years, it was considered that neonates were relatively resistant to suxamethonium but highly sensitive to non-depolarizing agents, particularly during the first 10 days of life. More recent studies with atracurium infusions indicate that dose requirements in the neonate in proportion to body weight do not differ greatly from those at other ages. Any variations in dose requirement may be related to lower body temperatures in the newborn, and the subsequent effect on drug distribution.

In older children, protein binding, hepatic microsomal enzyme activity, renal function and the permeability of the blood–brain barrier are similar to adults, and so differences in drug disposition are less likely. Nevertheless, drug dosage is best expressed in terms of surface area due to the proportional increase in body water during childhood. More frequent rates of administration, especially of less polar compounds, may be necessary due to the relative increase in liver blood flow. Differences in pharmacodynamic activity between children and adults may also be present, but are not easy to assess.

Maturity and old age

Elderly patients often respond differently to standard adult doses of drugs and are more likely to react adversely to drugs prescribed in hospital. Compliance with drug therapy may be unreliable due to failing memory, confusion and poor eyesight.

Pharmacokinetic changes

In contrast to the neonate, there is a reduction in the proportion of total body water and a relative increase in body fat. Although drug absorption is not appreciably modified, the volume of distribution of polar drugs is reduced and their plasma and tissue concentrations are effectively increased. Since plasma albumin levels tend to fall with age, the unbound fraction of certain drugs (e.g. phenytoin, tolbutamide) increases, thus enhancing their availability to cells and tissues.

At the age of 65, hepatic blood flow may be 45% less than normal values in younger adults, and experimental evidence suggests that the activity of microsomal enzyme systems declines to a similar extent. Consequently, the systemic bioavailability of drugs that are subject to low or high hepatic clearance is increased, with enhancement of their pharmacological effects. Similarly, glomerular filtration and tubular secretion decline with age, and the elderly patient is therefore at risk from drugs with a low therapeutic index (e.g. digoxin, gentamicin, lithium).

Anaesthetic implications

Enhanced effects of drugs used in anaesthesia should be anticipated in the elderly. Dose–response studies have shown that the requirements of thiopental diminish with increasing age. Pharmacokinetic factors, including plasma protein binding, lowered volume of distribution and increased accumulation in fat, as well as pharmacodynamic factors play their part in this phenomenon. Similarly, the unbound fraction of pethidine is four times higher than in the young, indicating that the dose of the drug should be reduced in the elderly.

Changes in receptor numbers or sensitivity may account for some alterations in drug responses, such as the increased analgesia in elderly patients who are given opioid analgesics for postoperative pain. Altered sensitivity to drug concentrations at receptor sites may also occur with nitrazepam, warfarin and some β-adrenoceptor antagonists.

The minimum alveolar concentration (MAC values) of all inhalation anaesthetics in steady-state conditions progressively declines with advancing age, and anaesthetic requirements are significantly depressed. Comparative data for intravenous induction agents can be superimposed on these results (Fig. 5.7). The decline in anaesthetic requirement may be due to pharmacodynamic factors that are based upon underlying anatomical, biochemical or functional changes associated with ageing.

Pregnancy
Physiological changes

Plasma volume and cardiac output are both increased during pregnancy (by 50% and 30% respectively), with maximum values achieved at 30–34 weeks gestation. The clearance of many drugs (e.g. phenytoin) may be enhanced in pregnancy due to increased cardiac output, and the subsequent increase in hepatic and renal blood flow. The increase in cardiac output, associated with the modest hyperventilation that normally occurs during pregnancy, enhances the rate of uptake and elimination of inhalational anaesthetic agents.

Pharmacokinetics in pregnancy

The absorption, distribution and elimination of drugs alter during pregnancy. Slower gastric emptying results in

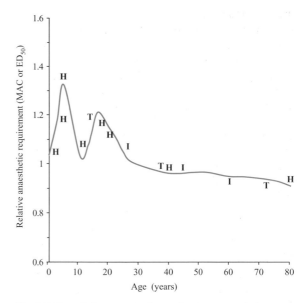

Fig. 5.7 The relative anaesthetic requirement expressed as a multiple of the minimum alveolar concentration (MAC) or median effective dose (ED_{50}) for various inhalational and intravenous anaesthetic agents. Requirements normalized for established values in young healthy adults. H, halothane, I, isoflurane, T, thiopental.

the increased uptake of drugs absorbed in the stomach (e.g. alcohol) and the delayed absorption of those that are principally absorbed in the upper gastrointestinal tract (e.g. aspirin, paracetamol). Drug absorption may be further delayed by the concurrent use of opioids. Disturbances of gut motility during pregnancy have been related to changes in the relative amounts of gastric acid and mucus secretion, and increased progesterone levels during pregnancy may cause relaxation of smooth muscle in many organs.

Changes in plasma protein binding also occur during pregnancy. The binding of many drugs (e.g. diazepam, propranolol, theophylline) to albumin and globulins is decreased, particularly during the last trimester. It has been suggested that exogenous substances in plasma may interfere with protein binding. Decreased plasma protein binding increases the volume of distribution of theophylline and prolongs its terminal half-life.

The pharmacokinetics of thiopental is modified in pregnant patients during Caesarean section. The volume of distribution is increased, although plasma protein binding and clearance are not markedly altered. Consequently, the elimination half-life of the drug is prolonged.

Enzymatic changes during pregnancy

Decreased sensitivity to insulin occurs in pregnancy and may be due to the placental lactogen insulinase that degrades the hormone. Other enzymes whose activity is increased in pregnancy include alkaline phosphatase and β-glucuronidase, which is secreted by the intestinal mucosa and hydrolyses glucuronide conjugates eliminated in bile. Consequently, the effects of some drugs may be potentiated in pregnancy due to their increased enterohepatic recirculation (e.g. analgesics, antibiotics). In addition, the placenta contains a wide range of enzymes that are concerned with the metabolism of neurotransmitters and other endogenous compounds.

Tobacco smoking

Tobacco smoking results in the induction of some isoforms of cytochrome P450 (particularly CYP 1A2). The rates of elimination of drugs that are metabolized by this enzymatic pathway are generally greater in smokers, although there is a considerable overlap. The metabolism of theophylline, imipramine and pentazocine is increased, although the breakdown of diazepam, pethidine and warfarin is not significantly affected.

Clinical studies suggest that smokers require more opioids to obtain relief from pain, are less sedated by benzodiazepines and may obtain reduced benefit from β-blockers and nifedipine in angina. Not all these differences arise from alterations in the rate of drug metabolism, although the exact mechanism is often unclear.

Ethyl alcohol (ethanol)

Chronic consumption of ethyl alcohol increases the metabolic capacity of the liver and induces some isoforms of cytochrome P450 (e.g. CYP 2E1). Pharmacodynamic tolerance also occurs, and higher blood concentrations are required to produce intoxication in alcohol-tolerant subjects than in normal individuals. Cross-resistance occurs between many sedative drugs (e.g. benzodiazepines) and alcohol due to both pharmacodynamic (CNS) tolerance and more rapid metabolism. The resistance to thiopental frequently encountered in chronic alcoholic patients is undoubtedly due to tolerance at a cellular level, as the duration of action of thiopental is determined by redistribution rather than by metabolism. Changes in GABA availability, as well as changes in the number and nature of $GABA_A$ receptors, may also play a part in this phenomenon.

Similar concepts may apply to the reported tolerance of chronic alcoholics to inhalational agents, although these do not take into account the state of agitation of patients who may be on the edge of withdrawal symptoms. Nevertheless, they are only relevant after prolonged prior exposure to alcohol has occurred. After the acute ingestion of alcohol, the administration of other CNS depressants may lead to supra-additive effects. The half-life of barbiturates may also be increased presumably due to competition with alcohol for microsomal enzymes.

Pathological conditions that affect the response to drugs

- Liver disease
- Renal disease
- Respiratory diseases
- Cardiac diseases
- Neurological diseases
- Endocrine diseases

Liver disease
Pharmacokinetic changes

Hepatic drug clearance may be affected by liver disease in several different ways. For instance, there may be alterations in hepatic blood flow, affecting both total flow and the degree of intrahepatic shunting, plasma protein binding and intrinsic clearance. The effects of liver disease on drug disposition are complex and vary according to the type and duration of liver pathology. They may also be associated with a reduction in renal blood flow.

Muscle relaxants

These changes can be illustrated by studies with pancuronium in different types of liver disease. Obstructive disorders lead to decreased clearance, presumably due to the decreased elimination of pancuronium and its metabolites in the bile, and a slower recovery from neuromuscular blockade. In contrast, in hepatic cirrhosis the increased volume of distribution, associated with changes in plasma protein binding, results in lower plasma concentrations and decreased uptake at receptor sites. The apparent 'resistance' to the effects of the drug is consistent with original observations on the response of patients with liver disease to tubocurarine.

Severe liver disease may also impair the production of cholinesterase. The metabolism of suxamethonium, mivacurium and local anaesthetic esters may be delayed, particularly if there is an associated genetic abnormality of the enzyme.

General anaesthetics

In chronic hepatic dysfunction the dose requirements of thiopental are decreased and its duration of action is prolonged. These effects are consistent with decreased plasma protein binding, resulting in an increase in the unbound fraction that crosses the blood–brain barrier, and a prolonged distribution half-life.

General anaesthesia also affects the hepatic clearance of other drugs due to alterations in cardiac output and redistribution of regional blood flow. Splanchnic perfusion is invariably decreased and the elimination of drugs with a high hepatic clearance (e.g. opioid analgesics, local anaesthetics, β-adrenoceptor antagonists) is reduced. The problem may be accentuated in the presence of preexisting liver disease.

Renal disease
Pharmacokinetic changes

In renal failure, responses to many drugs are enhanced and prolonged, with increased toxicity due to the retention of metabolites. In addition, the accumulation of organic acids may lead to metabolic acidosis, with significant effects on drug disposition and competition for active tubular transport.

Changes in protein binding also occur in renal failure. The plasma protein binding of acidic drugs is usually decreased in uraemic patients. Basic drugs show a more variable response, although there is an increase in the free fraction of some drugs (e.g. diazepam, morphine). Endogenous binding inhibitors can accumulate in renal failure and thus increase the unbound concentration of drugs in plasma.

Thiopental

The dosage requirements of thiopental are often reduced in renal failure. These changes may be due to an increase in the free fraction of the drug, altered permeability of the blood–brain barrier or abnormal cerebral metabolism.

Opioid analgesics

Renal clearance is partly responsible for the removal of opioid analgesics and their metabolites. Dose requirements are reduced in renal failure, and active metabolites (e.g. morphine-6-glucuronide, norpethidine) may accumulate. Fentanyl, alfentanil and remifentanil undergo rapid and extensive metabolism and their metabolites have little or no activity or toxicity. Consequently, in renal fail-

ure they may have considerable advantages compared with other opioid analgesics.

Muscle relaxants

Renal impairment may affect the elimination of some muscle relaxants (e.g. pancuronium) which is partly eliminated unchanged. Occasionally, resistance to the onset of neuromuscular blockade is observed clinically and may be related to altered drug distribution and changes in plasma protein binding. The elimination of atracurium and cisatracurium is unaffected by renal failure, since they are spontaneously degraded by Hofmann elimination. Similarly, vecuronium is unaffected by renal failure, since it is predominantly eliminated in bile. Variability in the response to suxamethonium in renal disease only occurs when there is associated hyperkalaemia.

Local anaesthetics

The duration of local anaesthetic blockade may be reduced in renal failure, possibly because drug removal from the site of action is facilitated by an associated increase in cardiac output.

Diazepam

The terminal half-life of diazepam is reduced in chronic renal failure from approximately 97 to 37 hours. In addition, the elimination of active metabolites is decreased and their sedative effects are prolonged. Protein binding is lower and the volume of distribution of the unbound drug is decreased. The clinical significance of these changes is unclear.

Respiratory disease

A variable response to several drugs used in anaesthesia (and in other situations) may occur in patients with chronic respiratory disorders.

Chronic obstructive airways disease

In chronic obstructive pulmonary disease (COPD), the respiratory centre may become insensitive to CO_2 and only respond to the hypoxic drive. Consequently, the respiratory depressant effects of opioid analgesics and induction agents may be exaggerated, and the administration of benzodiazepines in doses used for endoscopy may cause CO_2 narcosis. Similarly, the response to some muscle relaxants may be variable due to acid–base changes and electrolyte imbalance. The co-existence of bronchospasm may lead to further problems when drugs that release histamine (e.g.

morphine, atracurium) or constrict bronchial muscle (e.g. propranolol, neostigmine) are used.

Inhalational anaesthesia

Ventilation–perfusion abnormalities occur during inhalational anaesthesia and may be enhanced by pre-existing respiratory disease. The rate of induction of anaesthesia with poorly soluble agents (e.g. nitrous oxide, desflurane) may well be delayed, but is less affected when more soluble agents are used. When surgical anaesthesia is achieved, hypoventilation can be a problem if spontaneous ventilation is maintained. Exaggerated effects on respiratory function may occur, and the activity of the accessory muscles appears to be abolished at relatively light planes of anaesthesia.

Cardiac disease

Systemic disorders often present with one or more different clinicopathological patterns, such as congestive cardiac failure, fixed-output cardiac dysfunction, ischaemic heart disease, conduction defects and associated dysrhythmias and arterial hypertension. Consequently, there may be considerable differences in the response to drugs in patients with pre-existing cardiovascular disease.

General anaesthetics

Most general anaesthetic agents can induce depressant effects on different cardiovascular parameters, including myocardial contractility, systemic vascular resistance, coronary blood flow, baroreceptor reflex activity and circulating catecholamine levels, and these effects are undoubtedly enhanced when patients have a diminished cardiac reserve. The resultant clinical features may be extremely complex. In some cases anaesthetics may be extremely hazardous, for instance, in patients with constrictive pericarditis the myocardial depressant effects of thiopental can induce profound hypotension and pulmonary oedema. Similarly, isoflurane is a potent coronary vasodilator, but may induce maldistribution of myocardial blood flow in the presence of ischaemic heart disease (the 'steal' effect). Alternatively, beneficial effects may be achieved, as demonstrated by the reduction in cardiac work and systemic afterload which occurs when moderate concentrations of halothane are administered to patients with congestive cardiac failure.

Hypertension

In hypertensive patients, exaggerated changes in blood pressure may occur after the induction of anaesthesia. Although these effects are usually more pronounced when hypertension is untreated, no specific anaesthetic agent has been incriminated and the mechanism of this response remains unclear.

Arrhythmias

Pre-existing arrhythmias may be enhanced by drugs with significant cardiac muscarinic effects (e.g. suxamethonium), which can alter the autonomic balance in the myocardium.

Neurological disease
Myasthenia gravis

Patients with myasthenia gravis are extremely sensitive to non-depolarizing blockade, but are usually resistant to depolarizing agents. Both phenomena have been used as diagnostic tests in myasthenic patients. The differential effects of depolarizing and non-depolarizing drugs in myasthenia are due to the occupation and destruction of acetylcholine receptors at the motor endplate by immunoglobulin antibodies. In these conditions, the endplate potential induced by acetylcholine release is decreased, so that the effects of non-depolarizing agents are enhanced.

In myasthenia gravis, many different muscle groups may be affected to a variable extent, and the reaction to muscle relaxants is usually unpredictable. In general, neuromuscular blocking agents should be avoided in myasthenic patients undergoing major surgery including thymectomy, since they may induce prolonged postoperative paralysis. Nevertheless, low doses of vecuronium and atracurium have been successfully used to produce neuromuscular blockade in patients with myasthenia gravis who are undergoing surgical procedures. Suxamethonium has also been used, although large doses may be required to produce muscle relaxation, and elimination of the drug may be retarded by concurrent anticholinesterase therapy.

Eaton–Lambert syndrome

In the Eaton–Lambert (myasthenic) syndrome, there is a defect in the release of acetylcholine from the motor nerve terminal. Voluntary muscle weakness improves with exercise, and an increase in twitch amplitude is usually observed during tetanic stimulation. The condition may accompany various malignant diseases, particularly bronchial carcinoma. In general, there is a marked sensitivity to all muscle relaxants, with resistance to the effects of anticholinesterases.

Dystrophia myotonica

Dystrophia myotonica is an inherited disorder in which the primary defect is in the muscle fibre itself. The signs and symptoms include mental disturbances, cataracts, testicular atrophy, premature baldness and various endocrine disturbances. The underlying muscle dysfunction results in generalized muscular weakness, including those involved in respiration and deglutition, associated with prolonged contracture after stimulation. The latter is particularly noticeable by difficulty in releasing the grip after shaking hands. There is a high incidence of cardiomyopathy with abnormalities of cardiac conduction that are linked to the disorder, and these may reflect the underlying muscle pathology. After administration of suxamethonium, excessive quantities of K^+ may be released from abnormal muscle, producing prolonged and generalized myotonia and enhancing any existing dysrhythmia. In dystrophia myotonica, suxamethonium is absolutely contraindicated and the response to non-depolarizing neuromuscular blocking agents is unpredictable. Their duration of action may be normal or prolonged, and reduced doses should be used. Undue sensitivity to the effect of respiratory depressants (e.g. general anaesthetic agents, opioid analgesics) may also be anticipated, and the administration of volatile agents may induce cardiotoxic effects.

Other neurological disorders

In neurological diseases in which muscle wasting is a predominant feature, in particular motor neuron disease, long-standing spinal injuries, and the advanced stage of multiple sclerosis, there is often increased sensitivity to the effects of suxamethonium. Degeneration of the motor endplate is followed by receptor up-regulation outside its immediate vicinity, and the entire sarcolemma responds to acetylcholine and other agonists. The efflux of K^+ is greatly increased, and there is a possibility of dysrhythmias or cardiac arrest.

In some other neurological diseases such as muscular dystrophies, Friedreich's ataxia and Huntington's chorea, unpredictable responses to both depolarizing and non-depolarizing agents may occur. In Duchenne progressive muscular dystrophy, hazards associated with induction and recovery have been reported, which are likely to be due to the associated cardiomyopathy. The use of suxamethonium may lead to the development of hyperpyrexia.

In neurological disorders associated with autonomic disturbances, typified by diabetic autonomic neuropathy, acute polyneuritis and Shy–Drager syndrome, enhanced falls in arterial pressure may occur after the administration of most general anaesthetic agents or other drugs with significant cardiovascular effects due to the inadequacy of compensatory baroreceptor mechanisms.

Endocrine disease

Myxoedema

In myxoedematous patients, there may be an increased response to drugs acting on the CNS, including opioid analgesics and various general anaesthetic agents. Various factors, including a decreased efficiency of microsomal enzyme systems, alterations in drug distribution due to associated bradycardia or congestive cardiac failure, prolonged gastrointestinal transit and changes in body temperature may be involved.

Thyrotoxicosis

Thyrotoxicosis affects drug metabolism, and specific pharmacokinetic studies have shown some enhancement of microsomal drug oxidation. In hyperthyroidism, binding of both acidic and basic drugs to plasma proteins is decreased, and there may be evidence of sympathetic overactivity. A varying response to a number of drugs used during anaesthesia may therefore be anticipated.

Adrenal disease

Adrenocorticosteroids exert permissive effects on catecholamines. An exaggerated response to drugs that reduce systemic blood pressure may occur in patients with inadequate adrenal function, and replacement therapy should always be provided (Chapter 17).

In patients with a phaeochromocytoma, drugs that release histamine or induce dysrhythmias may induce exaggerated hypertensive responses or disorders of cardiac conduction. Similarly, patients with carcinoid tumours are also at risk of developing tachyarrhythmias and hypertension when drugs with histamine releasing activity are administered.

Pharmacological causes of variable responses to drugs

Other causes of differences or variability in drug responses include:

- Idiosyncrasy
- Hypersensitivity

- Supersensitivity
- Tachyphylaxis
- Tolerance

Both idiosyncrasy and hypersensitivity are considered in Chapter 6.

Drug supersensitivity

Receptor down-regulation

Receptors play an important part in the regulation of physiological and biochemical functions and are subject to regulatory and homeostatic control. The continual stimulation of receptors by agonists leads to a reduction in their numbers, density and activity ('down-regulation'). This is exemplified by the refractory response that may follow the administration of β-adrenoceptor agonists in the treatment of bronchial asthma and is associated with a reduction in the number of functioning β-adrenoceptors in bronchial smooth muscle. The phenomenon is partly due to the sequestration ('internalization') of receptors within cells, although receptor affinity may also be modified. Adrenergic receptor density is also modified in a number of other pathological conditions (e.g. congestive cardiac failure, thyrotoxicosis).

Receptor up-regulation

By contrast, any decrease in catecholamine production, either following drug therapy or sympathetic denervation, increases the synthesis and numbers of adrenoceptors ('up-regulation') and may also diminish the neuronal uptake of catecholamines. Similar changes in receptor density are probably produced by most neurotransmitters that act at synapses and neuroeffector junctions. In these conditions, there may be hyperreactivity or supersensitivity to the effects of drugs that act on these receptors. The phenomenon of 'up-regulation' may explain the rebound effects which result from the sudden withdrawal of certain antihypertensive drugs (e.g. β-adrenoceptor agonists, clonidine) following their long-term administration and may account for the production of tardive dyskinesia by phenothiazines and its potentiation by dopamine precursors. The increase in receptor numbers also plays an important part in the exaggerated response to vasopressor drugs in those patients receiving adrenergic neuron-blocking agents.

Up-regulation of receptors may be responsible for the significant hyperkalaemia occurring after administration of suxamethonium to patients with severe burns or spinal cord injuries. In these conditions, extrajunctional receptors develop on the surface of the muscle fibre outside the motor endplate, and the total number of acetylcholine receptors may increase 100 times. Consequently, the ionic changes associated with the depolarization of skeletal muscle by suxamethonium may produce significant hyperkalaemia, and in extreme cases, serum K^+ levels may be doubled.

Tachyphylaxis

Tachyphylaxis can be defined as a rapid decrease or a reduction in the response to identical doses of an agonist within a short period of time. It is sometimes used to refer to the phenomenon of acute receptor desensitization, or to the occurrence of rapid drug tolerance.

Suxamethonium

Tachyphylaxis sometimes develops after the repeated administration of suxamethonium and may precede the development of phase II ('dual') blockade. This may be related to the slow dissociation of suxamethonium from the cholinergic receptor, so that receptor occupancy remains high when a second dose of the drug is given.

Sympathomimetic amines

Tachyphylaxis is more commonly applied to the effects of drugs that act by releasing endogenous transmitters from cells or nerve endings. In these conditions, the response to repeated doses of the drug rapidly declines presumably due to transmitter exhaustion. Tachyphylaxis is classically observed after the administration of indirectly acting sympathomimetic amines (e.g. ephedrine, xylometazoline) but may also occur with drugs that release dopamine (e.g. amantidine, tetrabenazine). In anaesthetic practice, a form of tachyphylaxis commonly occurred when ganglion-blocking agents were infused to produce controlled hypotension during surgery.

Tolerance

Drug tolerance refers to the gradual decrease in the activity of drugs, which usually occurs over a period of days or weeks.

Opioid analgesics

Tolerance classically occurs with opioid analgesics and may be related to the down-regulation of opioid receptors. Experimental studies suggest that some tolerance to opioids can develop within several hours of their administration. A physiological negative feedback system may result in modification of the synthesis or release of enkephalins or endorphins, resulting in altered responsiveness of cells in the CNS. Alternatively, opioid tolerance may be related to up-regulation of glutamate transmission via NMDA receptors and increased production of nitric oxide in the CNS.

Organic nitrates

Tolerance to nitrates was first observed in munition workers exposed to nitroglycerine during the manufacture of gelignite. Similarly, tolerance may also develop to the haemodynamic and vasodilator effects of organic nitrates and sodium nitroprusside during their continuous administration. The use of intermittent regimes of drug therapy may avoid the gradual attenuation of their therapeutic effects, although it may also expose the patient to the further risk of anginal episodes during the nitrate-free period.

Organic nitrates readily penetrate vascular smooth muscle cells and are metabolized intracellularly to NO, which combines with sulphydryl groups (SH^-) to form active S-nitrosothiols. Tolerance may be due to the depletion of sulphydryl groups from vascular smooth muscle, thus preventing the formation of S-nitrosothiols. In some studies, the administration of sulphydryl donors such as N-acetylcysteine has been shown to delay or prevent tolerance to nitrates.

Barbiturates

Tolerance may also occur to the effects of barbiturates and possibly other centrally acting drugs. Increased drug metabolism due to the autoinduction of the CYP 1A2 isoform of cytochrome P450 may be partly responsible.

Suggested reading

Altman, D.G. (1991) *Practical Statistics for Medical Research*. London: Chapman & Hall.

Armitage, P. & Berry, G. (1987) *Statistical Methods in Medical Research*, 2nd edn. Oxford: Blackwell Scientific Publications.

Bulpitt, C.J. (1987) Confidence intervals. *Lancet* **i**, 494–497.

Christiensen, J.H. & Andreasen, F. (1978) Individual variation in the response to thiopental. *Acta Anaesthetica Scandinavica* **22**, 303–313.

Churchill-Davidson, H.C. & Wise, R.P. (1963) Neuromuscular transmission in the newborn infant. *Anesthesiology* **24**, 271–278.

Crooks, J., O'Malley, K. & Stevenson, I.H. (1976) Pharmacokinetics in the elderly. *Clinical Pharmacokinetics* **1**, 280–296.

Dundee, J.W. & Gray, T.C. (1953) Resistance to d-tubocurarine chloride in the presence of liver damage. *Lancet* **ii**, 16–17.

Duvaldestin, P., Agoston, S., Henzel, D., *et al.* (1978) Pancuronium pharmacokinetics in patients with liver cirrhosis. *British Journal of Anaesthesia* **50**, 1131–1136.

Friis-Hansen, B. (1961) Body water compartments in children. Changes during growth and related changes in body composition. *Pediatrics* **28**, 169–181.

Gardner, M.J. & Altman, D.G. (1989) *Statistics with Confidence*. London: British Medical Journal.

Greenblatt, D.J., Sellers, E.M. & Shader, R.I. (1982) Drug therapy: drug disposition in old age. *New England Journal of Medicine* **306**, 1081.

Keslin, I. (2002) Statistics. *Anaesthesia and Intensive Care Medicine* **3**, 428–433; and **4**, 203–205.

Kirkwood, B.R. (1980) *Essentials of Medical Statistics*. Oxford: Blackwell Scientific Publications.

Muravchick, S. (1986) Immediate and long-term nervous system effects of anaesthesia in elderly patients. *Clinics in Anesthesiology* **4**, 1035–1048.

Perucca, E. & Crema, A. (1982) Plasma protein binding of drugs in pregnancy. *Clinical Pharmacokinetics* **7**, 336–352.

Rylance, G. (1981) Drugs in children. *British Medical Journal* **282**, 50–51.

Smith, C.L. & Bush, G.H. (1985) Anaesthesia and progressive muscular dystrophy. *British Journal of Anaesthesia* **57**, 1113–1118.

Vestal, R.E. (1978) Drug use in the elderly: a review of problems and special considerations. *Drugs* **16**, 358–362.

Wilkinson, G.R. & Shenker, S. (1975) Drug disposition and liver disease. *Drug Metabolism Reviews* **4**, 139–175.

6 Adverse Drug Reactions

Adverse drug reactions are believed to be responsible for 3–5% of all admissions to hospital and occur in 10–20% of inpatients. They can present clinically in many different ways, ranging in severity from mild skin rashes to the production of malignant and teratogenic changes. In the UK, the Commission on Human Medicines is responsible for collecting reports of suspected or definitive adverse reactions to drugs through the Yellow Card scheme.

Classification

Adverse drug reactions can be classified into two groups:
- Type A ('augmented') reactions
- Type B ('bizarre') reactions

Type A reactions
Type A reactions are relatively common and are often related to the main pharmacological effects of drugs (Table 6.1). They are particularly likely to occur in drug toxicity, in the elderly or in patients with renal or hepatic impairment. They can be divided into two types:
(1) Primary reactions, which are due to an exaggeration of a normal or intended clinical response (e.g. insulin-induced hypoglycaemia).
(2) Secondary reactions ('side effects'), which are not directly related to the desired clinical effects of drugs (e.g. hypotension produced by subarachnoid anaesthesia).
Type A reactions are responsible for 80–90% of all adverse reactions to drugs. They usually have a prevalence of more than 1 in 1000 (0.1%) and are readily identified in preclinical and clinical trials. Individual patients often vary in their susceptibility to Type A reactions, which can be produced by varying doses of a given drug in different individuals. Nevertheless, almost all Type A reactions can occur in every patient who is given high doses of the drug. For example, many of the Type A reactions produced by morphine are invariably present with high dose regimes. In some instances (e.g. respiratory depression), individual

variation in patient response corresponds to a characteristic S-shaped (sigmoid) curve (Fig. 6.1).

Type B reactions
Type B reactions are usually unrelated to the main pharmacological effects of drugs and are often dose-independent, relatively uncommon and unpredictable. In general, their prevalence is less than 1 in 1000 (0.1%) and they may not be identified in clinical trials involving less than 10,000 patients. Although they are much less common than Type A reactions, they are a significant cause of serious adverse responses to drugs. In many patients, the aetiology of Type B reactions is obscure. In other instances, they are clearly related to two main factors:
- Genetic predisposition (idiosyncrasy)
- Drug hypersensitivity

Adverse reactions due to genetic predisposition

In anaesthetic practice, at least three important adverse reactions are idiosyncratic and directly related to genetic predisposition:
- Suxamethonium apnoea
- Malignant hyperthermia
- Hepatic porphyria
Other examples of idiosyncratic reactions are:
- Hereditary methaemoglobinaemia
- Hereditary resistance to warfarin
- Haemolytic anaemia (antimalarial drugs)
- Toxic reactions to certain drugs (isoniazid, hydralazine and phenelzine)
- Hypotensive responses (debrisoquine)
- Alcohol-induced facial flushing (chlorpropamide)

Suxamethonium apnoea
Suxamethonium normally has a short duration of action due to its rapid hydrolysis by plasma cholinesterase.

Table 6.1 Some common Type A adverse reactions to drugs.

Drug	Adverse reaction
Aspirin	Tinnitus
Chlorphenamine	Sedation
Digoxin	Heart block
Insulin	Hypoglycaemia
Morphine	Respiratory depression
Phenytoin	Ataxia
Salbutamol	Muscle tremor
Amitriptyline	Xerostomia
Warfarin	Haemorrhage

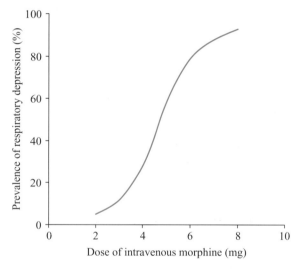

Fig. 6.1 Interindividual variation in response to intravenous morphine.

Certain genetic variants of the enzyme may decrease the rate of hydrolysis of suxamethonium and extend its duration of action, resulting in prolonged apnoea. Delayed metabolism may also predispose to tachyphylaxis and dual block.

Genetic variants

Genetic variants in plasma cholinesterase were originally investigated by enzymatic analysis and interpreted in terms of four allelomorphic genes identified at a single locus on chromosome 3q. These genes (*U, A, F* and *S*) encode the normal or usual enzyme (U), the atypical enzyme (A), the fluoride-resistant enzyme (F) and the absent or silent enzyme (S).

The atypical enzyme is the commonest genetic variant and was originally distinguished from the normal or wild-type enzyme by its resistance to inhibition by the local anaesthetic dibucaine (cinchocaine). The 'dibucaine number' was defined as the enzyme inhibition (%) produced by dibucaine (10^{-5} mol L^{-1}), using benzoylcholine as the substrate. Normal homozygotes (UU) have dibucaine numbers of 80, heterozygotes for the atypical enzyme (UA) have dibucaine numbers of 60, while homozygotes for the atypical enzyme (AA) have dibucaine numbers of 20. The four allelomorphic genes are consistent with 10 genotypes, and three of these genotypes (AA, AS and SS) are commonly associated with a prolonged response to conventional doses of suxamethonium (Table 6.2). Their total prevalence in Caucasian populations is about 1 in 1000 (0.1%).

DNA analysis

In recent years, this simple conceptual framework has been extended and rationalized by DNA analysis, and the complete amino acid sequence of human plasma cholinesterase and its main variants has been established by molecular genetic techniques. The atypical enzyme (AA) has a single point mutation at nucleotide 209 (GAT to GGT), which changes codon 70 from aspartate to glycine. At least 40 other naturally occurring mutations have been described. Some of these mutations only cause quantitative changes in enzyme activity (usually reductions), although their kinetic properties are relatively normal (variants H, J, K and S). They may be difficult to detect by standard activity and inhibition tests, since they are qualitatively similar to the normal enzyme. The silent cholinesterase phenotype (SS) is associated with at least 20 different structural alterations in DNA.

Other anaesthetic drugs

The duration of action of atracurium and mivacurium, but not esmolol and remifentanil, may also be prolonged by genetic variants in plasma cholinesterase. Although this often occurs with mivacurium, particularly when homozygotes (AA) or heterozygotes (UA) for the atypical enzyme are involved, it does not appear to be of clinical significance with other drugs.

Other genetic variants

A separate distinct chromosomal locus is associated with two further genetic variants ($E_{Cynthiana}$ and C_5), which may be responsible for increased cholinesterase activity.

Table 6.2 The classical genetic variants of human plasma cholinesterase.

Genotype	Approximate prevalence per 1000 population	Dibucaine number	Prolonged response to suxamethonium
UU	950	80	No
UA	40	60	Occasionally
UF	4	75	Occasionally
US	6	80	Occasionally
AA	<1	20	Yes
AF	<1	50	Occasionally
AS	<1	20	Yes
FF	<1	65	Occasionally
FS	<1	65	Occasionally
SS	<1		Yes

Malignant hyperthermia
Genetic basis
Malignant hyperthermia (malignant hyperpyrexia) is a rare but potentially fatal complication of anaesthesia and is usually inherited by autosomal dominant transmission. In about 60% of cases, the condition is linked to a mutation in the ryanodine gene (*RYR1*) on chromosome 19q (the long arm of chromosome 19). In some instances, mutations at other autosomal loci, particularly chromosomes 1q, 3q, 5q and 7q, are involved. *RYR1* normally encodes the ryanodine receptor in the sarcoplasmic reticulum, which is activated in response to depolarization of the T-tubules (and dihydropyridine receptors) in skeletal muscle. Ryanodine receptor activation results in Ca^{2+} release from the sarcoplasmic reticulum and initiates myosin–actin interaction and muscle contraction (Fig. 6.2).

Clinical effects
In malignant hyperthermia, exposure to 'triggering agents' (i.e. suxamethonium or fluorinated anaesthetics) results in excessive Ca^{2+} release from the sarcoplasmic reticulum, producing muscle rigidity and damage with release of K^+, myoglobin and creatine kinase into the circulation. Metabolic stimulation results in hypercapnia, hypoxaemia, tachycardia, metabolic and respiratory acidosis and hyperthermia.

Mortality
At one time, the mortality of malignant hyperthermia was relatively high (about 70%). In recent years, it has declined to 1–5%, mainly due to earlier recognition of the

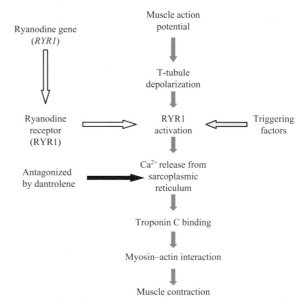

Fig. 6.2 Excitation–contraction coupling in skeletal muscle and the role of the ryanodine receptor (RYR1).

condition, improvements in monitoring and the use of dantrolene sodium (which uncouples ryanodine receptor activation from Ca^{2+} release).

Familial susceptibility
The familial susceptibility to malignant hyperthermia can be confirmed by muscle biopsy and *in vitro* contracture testing with various agents. In these conditions, there is

an abnormal contractile response to halothane and caffeine, with a greater increase in tension than in normal muscle. Similar effects are produced by ryanodine and chlorocresol. After the diagnosis has been established, genetic counselling and family screening by DNA analysis are essential.

Hepatic porphyria

Clinical presentation

In acute intermittent porphyria and variegate porphyria, acute attacks can be precipitated by certain drugs, particularly those that induce and increase the synthesis of hepatic cytochrome P450. Exacerbations of acute intermittent porphyria, with the increased synthesis of porphobilinogen and other porphyrins, are often associated with neuromuscular weakness and paralysis, progressive demyelination and neuropathy, neuropsychiatric disturbances and abdominal pain. The urine usually contains porphobilinogen and uroporphyrin and may turn red when allowed to stand in daylight for several hours. Similar phenomena, as well as cutaneous manifestations, usually occur in variegate porphyria. Nevertheless, other types of porphyria, such as erythropoietic porphyria and porphyria cutanea tarda, are not adversely affected by thiopental. Even in acute intermittent porphyria, barbiturates do not always induce an attack.

Porphyrin synthesis

In humans, the porphyrin derivative haem has an essential role as the prosthetic group of various haemoproteins, including haemoglobin, myoglobin, cytochrome oxidase and cytochrome P450. Its formation depends on the enzyme δ-aminolaevulinic acid synthetase (ALA synthetase), which catalyses the synthesis of δ-aminolaevulinic acid (ALA) and porphobilinogen from succinate and glycine (Fig. 6.3). Porphobilinogen is subsequently converted to hydroxymethylbiline, protoporphyrinogen, protoporphyrin and haem in the liver and in bone marrow. In physiological conditions, free haem causes feedback inhibition of the activity of ALA synthetase and thus normally controls porphyrin synthesis. In the acute porphyrias, notably acute intermittent porphyria and variegate porphyria, there is reduced activity of one or more synthetic enzymes in this pathway. Although haem synthesis may be decreased, and precursor porphyrins such as porphobilinogen and protoporphyrinogen can accumulate in tissues, many patients remain asymptomatic for prolonged periods.

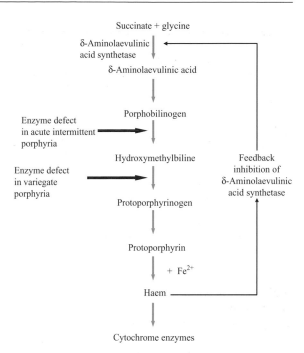

Fig. 6.3 The hepatic synthesis of haem and the cytochrome enzymes.

Enzyme induction

Drugs that induce cytochrome P450 (as well as some other drugs that are metabolized by the enzyme) increase the incorporation of haem into cytochrome P450. In these conditions, free haem is decreased, resulting in enhanced activation of ALA synthetase. The synthesis of porphyrin precursors is greatly increased and may cause acute attacks of the disease. Although all drugs that induce, affect or are metabolized by cytochrome P450 should be avoided, acute porphyria is particularly associated with certain agents (Table 6.3). The use of these drugs may lead to widespread demyelination of peripheral and central pathways, resulting in sensory changes and motor paralysis. Some haem derivatives (haematin, haem arginate) suppress the enhanced activity of ALA synthetase and have an important role in the treatment of acute attacks.

Hereditary methaemoglobinaemia

The local anaesthetic prilocaine often causes dose-related methaemoglobinaemia and cyanosis due to its oxidative metabolite o-toluidine. A number of other drugs (e.g. some nitrites and sulphonamides) can also oxidize haemoglobin (Fe^{2+}) to methaemoglobin (Fe^{3+}). In normal conditions, haemoglobin is readily regenerated from

Table 6.3 Drugs that are most commonly involved in acute porphyric reactions.

- Barbiturates
- Phenytoin
- Carbamazepine
- Rifampicin
- Ethyl alcohol
- Cephalosporins
- Benzodiazepines
- Sulphonamides
- Sulphonylureas
- Oral contraceptives
- Steroids

Many other agents are sometimes suspected or implicated.

methaemoglobin by the enzyme methaemoglobin reductase. When this enzyme is deficient or absent, persistent and long-lasting methaemoglobinaemia can be produced by these drugs. Haemoglobin can be readily regenerated by suitable reducing agents (ascorbic acid, methylene blue).

Hereditary resistance to warfarin

Hereditary resistance to warfarin and other oral anticoagulants can occur as an autosomal dominant trait in both man and in experimental animals. The most probable cause of the condition is an inherited abnormality in the hepatic enzyme diaphorase (epoxide reductase), which reduces its sensitivity to warfarin (and other coumarins). Diaphorase normally reduces inactive vitamin K epoxide to active vitamin K and is inhibited by warfarin and other coumarin anticoagulants. In addition, patients with a genetic deficiency in antithrombin III may be extremely resistant to warfarin.

Haemolytic anaemia with antimalarial and other drugs

In patients with an inherited deficiency in erythrocyte glucose-6-phosphate dehydrogenase (G6PD), haemolysis, haemolytic anaemia and jaundice may occur after exposure to certain drugs (e.g. dapsone, doxorubicin). This reaction may also occur after eating or inhaling the pollen of the bean *Vicia fava* (favism). Absence or deficiency of G6PD prevents the regeneration of NADPH, which normally maintains reduced glutathione in red cells and protects them from the effects of oxidative drugs.

Toxic reactions to some drugs in slow acetylators

The hepatic enzyme system that mediates acetylation reactions (*N*-acetyltransferase) shows genetic polymorphism. Consequently, there is a bimodal distribution in the plasma concentration of certain drugs that are metabolized by acetylation (e.g. isoniazid, hydralazine) and the toxic effects of these agents predominantly occur in patients who are slow acetylators of the parent drugs.

Miscellaneous idiosyncratic reactions

Other idiosyncratic or genetically determined disorders associated with drug administration include:

- Defective drug oxidation affecting CYP 2D6, causing excessive hypotension after normal oral dosage of debrisoquine.
- Increased intraocular pressure, which may occur after the chronic use of steroid eye drops.
- Intense facial vasodilatation induced by alcohol in patients on chlorpropamide.

Toxic reactions to gold, levamisole and procainamide have been related to specific HLA (human lymphocyte antigen) subtypes. Similarly, digoxin toxicity and thromboembolism induced by oral contraceptives have been associated with differences in ABO blood groups. Racial differences in drug responses may also occur, although they are not usually classified as idiosyncratic reactions.

Adverse reactions due to drug hypersensitivity

Hypersensitivity or allergic responses are abnormal reactions to drugs that are dependent on immunological factors and usually involve the formation of antibodies. Approximately 10% of adverse reactions to drugs are caused by drug hypersensitivity and its associated humoral responses. Most drugs are low molecular weight compounds, and many of them can act as haptens which can conjugate with tissue proteins to form relatively stable complexes. Hypersensitivity reactions to drugs can be divided into four main types, depending on the mechanism involved:

- Type I (immediate-type hypersensitivity)
- Type II (cytolytic reactions)
- Type III (immune complex-mediated responses)
- Type IV (delayed, cell-mediated responses)

Table 6.4 Pharmacological mediators commonly released during Type I hypersensitivity.

- Histamine
- Heparin
- Platelet-activating factor (PAF)
- Prostaglandins and leukotrienes
- Interleukins and cytokines

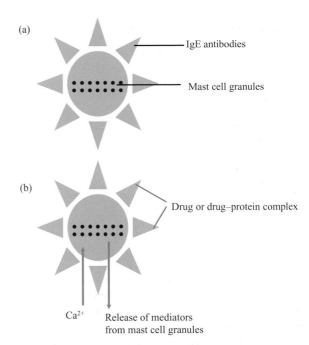

Fig. 6.4 The mechanism of Type I hypersensitivity. (a) Drugs combine covalently with proteins and induce the formation of IgE antibodies, which become attached to mast cells; (b) On subsequent exposure to the drug or drug–protein complex, cross-linking and Ca^{2+} entry occurs resulting in mast cell degranulation and the release of pharmacological mediators.

Type I hypersensitivity (immediate-type hypersensitivity)

Type I hypersensitivity is believed to be responsible for many of the severe adverse reactions associated with drugs, and other types of hypersensitivity are of lesser importance.

Immunological mechanism

In Type I hypersensitivity, drugs or their metabolites act as haptens which combine covalently with endogenous plasma or tissue proteins to form an antigenic drug–protein complex. Alternatively, foreign enzymes or proteins can act as antigens. The resultant antigen or antigenic complex induces the formation of IgE antibodies (by B lymphocytes and plasma cells), which become attached to mast cells in various tissues of the body, particularly the skin, bronchial and intestinal mucosa, vascular capillaries and basophil leucocytes. On subsequent exposure to the antigen, adjacent IgE molecules on mast cell membranes are bound by the hapten or antigen. Subsequently, Ca^{2+} enters mast cells, resulting in their degranulation and the release of pharmacological mediators (Table 6.4). Since adjacent IgE molecules are linked by the antigen or hapten (Fig. 6.4), Type I hypersensitivity is only commonly seen with drugs that form multivalent protein complexes, or are inherently divalent due to the presence of symmetrical molecular features (e.g. most muscle relaxants).

Sensitizing agents

Type I hypersensitivity reactions are not uncommon after administration of certain drugs or other agents. In general medical practice, Type I hypersensitivity responses are most frequently seen in atopic patients who are given penicillins or cephalosporins. These groups of antibiotics are structurally related and may show cross-sensitivity reactions in approximately 15% of patients. Their metabolites or degradation products (particularly penicillinoyl derivatives) are believed to be the main antigenic determinants.

Other agents that are less commonly implicated include:
- Aspirin and NSAIDS
- Radiological contrast media
- Foreign proteins (streptokinase, asparaginase, heparin, vaccines, blood products)
- Desensitization regimes
- Latex rubber
- Insect stings, reptile venom and snake venom
- Certain foods (fish, eggs, cow's milk, peanuts, tree nuts, sesame and pulses)

In anaesthetic practice, hypersensitivity responses are most frequently associated with
- Muscle relaxants
- Antibiotics
- Thiopental
- Latex rubber
- Chlorhexidine

As many as 60% of cases involve reactions with muscle relaxants, which appear to be commonest with suxamethonium, atracurium and rocuronium. At least 50% of these cases show cross-reactivity or cross-sensitivity with other neuromuscular blocking agents. A further 30% involve reactions to latex or chlorhexidine. Reactions to chlorhexidine occur when it is used to sterilize the skin, or during the insertion of central venous or epidural catheters.

Clinical features

The clinical features often depend on the provoking stimulus. Systemic allergens (e.g. drugs, insect stings and venom) usually cause hypotension, cardiovascular shock or bronchospasm. Ingestion of foods often results in facial, labial and laryngeal oedema, while skin contact causes urticaria.

Anaphylaxis

The term anaphylaxis is often used to describe hypersensitivity reactions that are associated with extreme hypotension and respiratory difficulty due to bronchospasm and/or laryngeal oedema.

Bronchospasm is often a feature of anaphylaxis, although it may occur independently. It is mainly due to the local formation and release of leukotrienes C_4, D_4, and E_4 ('cysteinyl-leukotrienes') from mast cells in the bronchial mucosa.

Anaphylactoid reactions

Histamine and similar vasoactive factors may be directly released from mast cells and basophils by many drugs and other agents. These non-immunological effects are often referred to as anaphylactoid reactions, since they may be difficult or impossible to distinguish clinically from the anaphylactic responses associated with Type I hypersensitivity.

Causative agents

Many agents can produce local or generalized histamine release from mast cells, including:
- Basic drugs (morphine, atracurium, suxamethonium, vancomycin)
- Solubilizing agents (Cremophor EL)
- Radiocontrast media (fluorescein, iopamidol, ioversol and iohexol)
- Intravenous dyes (methylene blue and isosulphan blue)
- Colloidal plasma expanders (dextrans, hydroxyethyl starch and gelatin)
- Polypeptides (polymyxin B, bradykinin, substance P and anaphylatoxins)

Local anaphylactoid reactions

Localized and transient anaphylactoid reactions are not uncommon in anaesthetic practice, particularly when high concentrations of drugs are rapidly injected into small blood vessels. They may occur more frequently when several different drugs are administered through small infusion needles. In these conditions physicochemical combination may result in the production of colloid aggregates, resulting in histamine release. Local anaphylactoid reactions are usually due to the disruption and degranulation of mast cells in the walls of blood vessels, and present clinically as vasodilation, local oedema or skin reactions.

The anaphylactoid responses induced by the solubilizing agent Cremophor EL and by large polysaccharide molecules (large molecular weight dextrans, hydroxyethyl starch, gelatin and possibly heparin) may depend on activation of the alternate complement pathway and the conversion of complement C3 to the anaphylatoxins C3a and C5a. These agents subsequently combine with receptors in mast cells causing the release of histamine and other vasoactive peptides.

Systemic anaphylactoid reactions

Severe systemic anaphylactoid reactions occasionally cause circulatory collapse or bronchospasm, and their treatment is identical to anaphylaxis. It may be difficult to detect patients who are susceptible to systemic anaphylactoid reactions, although individuals with a history of atopy (asthma, hay fever or eczema), or with a previous or family history of adverse responses are particularly vulnerable. Although some drugs appear to be relatively safe, at least two intravenous agents (propanidid and althesin) have been withdrawn because of their association with severe anaphylactoid reactions. Preoperative prophylaxis with both H_1- and H_2-receptor antagonists may confer some degree of protection in susceptible patients.

Plasma tryptase

Both anaphylactic and anaphylactoid reactions result in increases in plasma histamine and tryptase (a neutral protease released from the secretory granules in mast cells). Almost all the tryptase in the body is localized in mast cell granules, and the half-life of the enzyme in the circulation after mast cell degranulation is about 3 hours. Basal concentrations of tryptase range from 0.8 to 1.5 ng mL^{-1}, and increase to 10–15 ng mL^{-1} after anaphylactoid or mild anaphylactic reactions. Higher concentrations (20–25 ng mL^{-1}) usually occur in severe anaphylactic reactions. After mast cell degranulation, maximal concentrations of tryptase are usually present in plasma within 1 hour. If possible, samples of serum (about 5 mL) should be obtained for enzyme analysis as soon as possible, and at 1 hour and 6–24 hours after the reaction. Patients should subsequently be fully investigated and referred to an allergist for skin testing in order to identify the causative agent. The presence of antigen-specific IgE antibodies in serum can usually be identified and measured by a radioallergosorbent test (RAST).

After anaphylactic reactions, the basophil granule protein CD63 and the transmembrane protein CD203c are rapidly and specifically expressed by the plasma membrane. It is possible to test for these markers *in vitro*, using flow cytometry.

All suspected or proven anaphylactic reactions should be reported to the CSM on a 'Yellow Card' and patients should be advised to carry an anaesthetic hazard card or Medic-Alert bracelet.

Other adverse effects

Occasionally, other adverse effects of drugs resemble anaphylactic and anaphylactoid reactions.

For instance, salicylates and other NSAIDs may increase the conversion of arachidonic acid to various leukotrienes (particularly LTC_4 and LTD_4), which are important mediators of bronchoconstriction secondary to inflammation of the airways. Consequently, bronchospasm induced by aspirin or other NSAIDs may be related to the increased synthesis of leukotrienes, rather than to anaphylaxis or anaphylactoid reactions.

Type II hypersensitivity (cytolytic reactions)

In Type II hypersensitivity, drugs typically combine with proteins in erythrocyte, granulocyte or platelet cell membranes. The resultant antigenic complex induces the synthesis of IgG or IgM antibodies, which subsequently cross-react with antigenic sites in blood cell membranes (and complement), causing cellular lysis or agglutination.

Type II hypersensitivity reactions include
- Haemolytic anaemia (sulphonamides, methyldopa)
- Leucopenia or agranulocytosis (phenothiazines, carbimazole, clozapine)
- Thrombocytopenia (heparin, thiazides)
- Pancytopenia

Halothane hepatitis is probably a Type II hypersensitivity reaction. An oxidative metabolite of halothane (trifluoroacetyl chloride) is covalently bound by lysine residues in hepatic cell membrane proteins. In susceptible patients, the alkylated membrane protein acts as an antigen, resulting in the synthesis of antibodies, which cross-react with hepatocyte proteins, causing acute liver necrosis.

Type III hypersensitivity (immune complex-mediated responses)

In type III hypersensitivity, soluble antigens (e.g. bacterial toxins) react with circulating antibodies (IgG) forming precipitin complexes, which cause the fixation of complement. In normal conditions, precipitins are removed by the reticuloendothelial system, but when excess antigen is present, immune complexes are deposited in the vascular endothelium. Type III hypersensitivity reactions are responsible for serum sickness, a systemic generalized response that may ensue 7–14 days after drug administration. They may also be the basis for some of the pathological changes in acute glomerulonephritis, polyarteritis nodosa and rheumatoid arthritis.

Type IV hypersensitivity (delayed, cell-mediated responses)

In delayed hypersensitivity, antibody formation is not involved and the reaction solely results from the combination of antigens or haptens with T lymphocytes. The antigen or hapten is introduced by contact or injection, forms a complex with macrophages and then combines covalently with receptors on the lymphocyte membrane. This process results in lymphocyte mitosis and the local release of lymphokines (e.g. tumour necrosis factor α, interferon γ). A local inflammatory reaction usually occurs within 24–48 hours, resulting in erythema, induration, blistering and exfoliation, due to the accumulation of macrophages and lymphocytes at the site of injection.

Delayed hypersensitivity is responsible for the positive response to the Mantoux reaction and occurs in most forms of contact dermatitis, whether produced by metals or drugs. It is also a factor in many drug rashes, erythema multiforme (the Stevens–Johnson syndrome) and in the morbilliform rashes that are sometimes induced by ampicillin and amoxicillin in patients with glandular fever or chronic lymphatic leukaemia.

Hypersensitivity responses associated with anaesthesia

Hypersensitivity responses to anaesthetic drugs are not infrequent and can occasionally be life-threatening. In many instances, commonly used drugs such as thiopental or suxamethonium are involved, and colloid infusions may have been administered. It may be particularly difficult to detect patients who are at risk from such responses, although those with a history of atopy (asthma, hay fever or eczema) or with a previous or family history of adverse reactions must be considered as vulnerable. It has been suggested that some drugs are relatively safe (etomidate, vecuronium, fentanyl, local anaesthetic amides). Pretreatment with both H1- and H2-receptor antagonists (e.g. chlorphenamine and ranitidine) may confer some protection in susceptible patients.

Although 'halothane hepatitis' is an extremely rare hypersensitivity response, it is usually unpredictable and can only be prevented by avoiding the clinical use of the drug.

Not all the adverse responses to drugs in 'normal' individuals can be related to immunological mechanisms or to underlying genetic disorders. In some cases, adverse responses can be considered as an extension of the pharmacological effects of the agent, or may reflect intrinsic toxicity that is primarily dependent on the chemical properties of the drug or its metabolites. These Type A adverse effects are usually dose-dependent and can usually be reproduced in animals. Adverse responses of this type have become less frequent because of increased understanding of the structural features of drugs that contribute to their intrinsic toxicity. In addition, these toxic effects are frequently disclosed in preclinical and clinical trials.

Adverse reactions to drugs during foetal life

Drugs that are administered during pregnancy may cross the placental barrier and adversely affect the foetus. The placenta consists of a vascular syncytial membrane, with the functional properties of a typical lipid barrier. Lipid-soluble, low molecular weight drugs are readily transferred across the placental membrane, and their rate of removal from maternal blood is predominantly affected by

- Placental blood flow
- Diffusional area
- Concentration gradient

In practice, all lipid-soluble drugs that cross the blood–brain barrier also cross the placenta, and their elimination by foetal tissues may be prolonged. In contrast, polar (ionized) or large molecular weight compounds do not readily cross the placenta.

Anaesthetic agents

Inhalational anaesthetics, thiopental, propofol and most opioid analgesics can diffuse from maternal plasma to the foetus, and when used in labour may produce respiratory depression in the newborn. Similar effects may be produced by some sedative and hypnotic drugs. When diazepam is used in late pregnancy in pre-eclampsia and eclampsia, it readily crosses the placenta, but is only slowly metabolized by the foetus. Its active metabolites desmethyldiazepam and oxazepam accumulate in foetal tissues and can cause neonatal hypotonia and hypothermia.

Other drugs

Lipid-soluble β-adrenoceptor antagonists (propranolol, oxprenolol) can cross the placenta and may cause foetal bradycardia. In addition, foetal hypoglycaemia may be induced by insulin, oral hypoglycaemic agents or some β-adrenoceptor antagonists.

Teratogenic effects

More serious effects are produced by drugs taken during pregnancy that produce foetal damage or malformation (teratogenic changes). In early pregnancy (0–18 days), drugs that affect cell division (cytotoxic agents, folate antagonists) may affect formation of the blastocyst and cause foetal death. Nevertheless, foetal abnormalities are more commonly produced by drugs that are administered during organogenesis (2 weeks–2 months), including phenytoin and antithyroid drugs (Table 1.4). In some instances, the effects of drugs may be delayed for many years. When stilboestrol was used in late pregnancy, alteration in the maternal hormonal environment produced vaginal dysplasia and malignancy in female offspring after a latent period of 10–20 years.

Suggested reading

Axon, A.D. & Hunter, J.M. (2004) Anaphylaxis and anaesthesia – all clear now? *British Journal of Anaesthesia* **93**, 501–503.

Dean, G. (1971) *The Porphyrias: A Story of Inheritance and Environment*, 2nd edn. London: Pitman, pp. 1–118.

Ellis, F.R. & Halsall, P.J. (2002) Malignant hyperthermia. *Anaesthesia and Intensive Care Medicine* **3**, 222–225.

Ewan, P.W. (1998) Anaphylaxis. *British Medical Journal* **316**, 1442–1445.

Fisher, M. (1995) Treatment of acute anaphylaxis. *British Medical Journal* **311**, 731–733.

Iohom, G., Fitzgerald, D. & Cunningham, A.J. (2004) Principles of pharmacogenetics – implications for the anaesthetist. *British Journal of Anaesthesia* **93**, 440–450.

James, M.F.M. & Hift, R.M. (2000) Porphyrias. *British Journal of Anaesthesia* **85**, 143–153.

Jensen, F.S., Schwartz, M. & Viby-Mogensen, J. (1995) Identification of human plasma cholinesterase variants using molecular biological techniques. *Acta Anaesthesiologica Scandinavica* **39**, 142–149.

Kalow, W. (1993) Pharmacogenetics: its biological roots and the medical challenge. *Clinical Pharmacology and Therapeutics* **54**, 235–241.

Kroigaard, M., Garvey, L.H., Menne, T. & Husum, B. (2005) Allergic reactions in anaesthesia: are suspected causes confirmed on subsequent testing? *British Journal of Anaesthesia* **95**, 468–471.

La Du, B.N. (1995) Butyrylcholinesterase variants and the new methods of molecular biology. *Acta Anaesthesiologica Scandinavica* **39**, 139–141.

Laroche, D., Vergnaud, M.C., Sillard, B., *et al.* (1991) Biochemical markers of anaphylactoid reactions to drugs: comparison of plasma histamine and tryptase. *Anesthesiology* **75**, 945–949.

McIndoe, A. (2001) Recognition and management of anaphylactic and anaphylactoid reactions. *Anaesthesia and Intensive Care Medicine* **2**, 402–403.

Mertes, P. M. & Laxenaire, M.-C. (2002) Allergic reactions occurring during anaesthesia. *European Journal of Anaesthesiology* **19**, 240–262.

Mertes, P.M., Laxenaire, M.-C. & Alla, F. (2003) Anaphylactic and anaphylactoid reactions occurring during anesthesia in France in 1999–2000. *Anesthesiology* **99**, 536–545.

Neugut, A.I., Ghatak, A.T. & Miller, R.L. (2001) Anaphylaxis in the United States: an investigation into its epidemiology. *Archives of Internal Medicine* **161**, 15–21.

Plaud, B., Donati, F. & Debaene, B. (2002) Anaphylaxis during anaesthesia. *British Journal of Anaesthesia* **88**, 604–606.

Pleuvry, B.J. (2005) Pharmacokinetics: familial variation in drug response. *Anaesthesia and Intensive Care Medicine* **6**, 243–244.

Stewart, A.G. & Ewan, P.W. (1996) The incidence, aetiology and management of anaphylaxis presenting to an accident and emergency department. *Quarterly Journal of Medicine* **89**, 859–864.

7 Intravenous Anaesthetic Agents

History

Intravenous anaesthetic agents are usually defined as drugs that induce loss of consciousness in one arm–brain circulation time (normally 10–20 s), when given in an appropriate dosage. In the late nineteenth and early twentieth century many drugs were administered intravenously in an attempt to produce rapid unconsciousness. These included several opiates, chloral hydrate, bromethol, infusions of chloroform and ether, and various preparations of the available barbiturate derivatives. Unfortunately, problems with delayed onset, prolonged duration of anaesthesia and the toxic effects of individual drugs were common.

Barbiturates

A milestone in anaesthetic practice was achieved with the advent of the barbiturates, which had a rapid onset of hypnotic activity and an extremely short duration of action. Hexobarbital was first used in Germany in 1932 by Weese and Scharpff, and its rapid onset of action was responsible for its acceptance as an induction agent. It was soon superseded by thiopental, which was independently studied by Lundy and Waters in the USA. The potential hazards of thiopental (particularly when used alone in large doses) were not fully appreciated until the disaster at Pearl Harbour in 1941. In subsequent years, thiopental became widely accepted as an intravenous induction agent. However, many thiobarbiturates have essentially similar properties, and in some respects it is remarkable that the drug has stood the test of time.

Methohexital (an oxybarbiturate) was introduced in the UK in 1959, and until recently it was sometimes used as an induction agent. Although induction and recovery from anaesthesia and its elimination from the body were rapid, it had a number of significant disadvantages, including localized pain on injection, the occurrence of excitatory side effects and a tendency to induce tachycardia. Nevertheless, the drug was widely used in dental anaesthesia and in day-case surgery. Because of production difficulties, it is no longer generally available in the UK.

Steroids

In 1941, Hans Selye reported on the ability of certain steroids to produce reversible sleep in animals. The development of many of these drugs was precluded because of their hormonal effects, although several steroids have been used as anaesthetic agents. In the late 1950s, hydroxydione was introduced into anaesthetic practice; it had a marked hypnotic potency, but no hormonal activity. Because of the poor solubility of the drug, administration was dependent on its continuous infusion in a large volume of saline, and the onset of action was delayed. A polymerized and more concentrated preparation was subsequently produced, but unfortunately led to the frequent occurrence of thrombophlebitis and the use of hydroxydione was discontinued.

Althesin, a combination of the steroids alphaxolone and alphadolone, became available in 1972. Despite its many advantages, the occurrence of anaphylactic or anaphylactoid phenomena, particularly bronchospasm and severe hypotension, led to the withdrawal of the drug in 1984. These phenomena were probably related to the polyethoxylated castor oil (Cremophor EL), which was used with Althesin to increase the solubility of the steroid.

Minaxolone, a water-soluble steroid, was studied in clinical trials in 1979. Its use was associated with a significant incidence of excitatory effects. In addition, it was shown to induce neoplasia in experimental animals and development was subsequently discontinued.

Eltanolone (5β-pregnanolone) is a water-insoluble steroid which was reformulated as an emulsion and evaluated in clinical studies. Although induction was rapid and reliable and haemodynamic changes were minimal, it occasionally induced convulsions and had no advantages when compared with other induction agents.

Eugenol derivatives

Eugenol is chemically related to phenoxyacetic acid and is one of the main constituents of oil of cloves. The eugenol derivative propanidid was used as an occasional induction agent for approximately 20 years, but was withdrawn in 1983. Propanidid is an ester that is poorly soluble in water, and preparations of the drug also contained Cremophor EL, which occasionally produced bronchospasm and profound hypotension. In addition, propanidid caused various excitatory side effects.

Other agents in current clinical use

Phencyclidine was used in the 1950s as an induction agent, but was soon discarded because of severe psychotomimetic reactions. The related compound ketamine was introduced in 1970. Although it does not produce loss of consciousness in one arm–brain circulation time, it is usually classified as an induction agent. In spite of several disadvantages, the drug has a definite (though limited) role in anaesthetic practice.

Etomidate was introduced into clinical practice in 1974 and is an imidazole ester with hypnotic activity but little or no analgesic effects. Although the drug has a high margin of safety, it has several disadvantages that have restricted its use as an anaesthetic agent.

Propofol is a chemically inert phenolic derivative with anaesthetic properties. Its clinical use in a Cremophor EL formulation was first described in 1977. It was subsequently reformulated as an aqueous emulsion in 1985. Propofol has a rapid onset and symptom-free recovery and few adverse effects, which have undoubtedly contributed to its current popularity. It is widely used as an induction agent, particularly in day-case procedures, and for the maintenance of anaesthesia by infusion techniques.

Intravenous induction agents

All intravenous induction agents must be administered in aqueous solution, or as an oil or an emulsion that is readily miscible with plasma. In addition, they must be partially or entirely non-ionized and lipid-soluble in plasma at pH 7.4, in order to cross the blood–brain barrier and produce rapid loss of consciousness. These conflicting physicochemical requirements are resolved in various ways, either by the use of alkaline solutions, or by the administration of lipid-soluble drugs in water-miscible oils and emulsions. Consequently, bases, buffers or solubilizing agents are frequently added to solutions of anaesthetic agents.

In the UK, the following drugs are currently used as intravenous induction agents:

- Thiopental
- Propofol
- Etomidate
- Ketamine

Although benzodiazepines, opioids and neuroleptic agents are sometimes used to induce anaesthesia, they do not produce rapid loss of consciousness in therapeutic doses and are not usually considered to be intravenous induction agents.

Thiopental

Chemistry

Thiopental is 5-ethyl-5′-(1-methylbutyl)-2-thiobarbituric acid and is the sulphur analogue of pentobarbital. The sodium salt is a pale yellowish-white powder with a bitter taste and an alliaceous (garlic-like) odour. It readily dissolves in deionized water producing an alkaline solution due to its ionized sulphur atom (S^-), which has strongly basic properties and attracts H^+. In plasma the drug is predominantly present in an undissociated form (thiopental acid), which rapidly undergoes tautomerism (dynamic isomerism) into a structural isomer with high lipid-solubility (Fig. 7.1). Immediately after intravenous injection, crystal formation in plasma may occur due to the alteration in pH (from 10.5 to 7.4). However, this is of little importance since thiopental is rapidly diluted by the collateral venous return. The drug used clinically is a racemic mixture of two stereoisomers due to the presence of a single chiral carbon atom in the methylbutyl side chain.

Solutions of thiopental sodium (2.5%, w/v; pH 10.5) are commonly used to induce intravenous anaesthesia. Commercial preparations of the drug usually contain 6 parts of sodium carbonate to 100 parts of thiopental sodium by weight in nitrogen-filled ampoules. Sodium carbonate

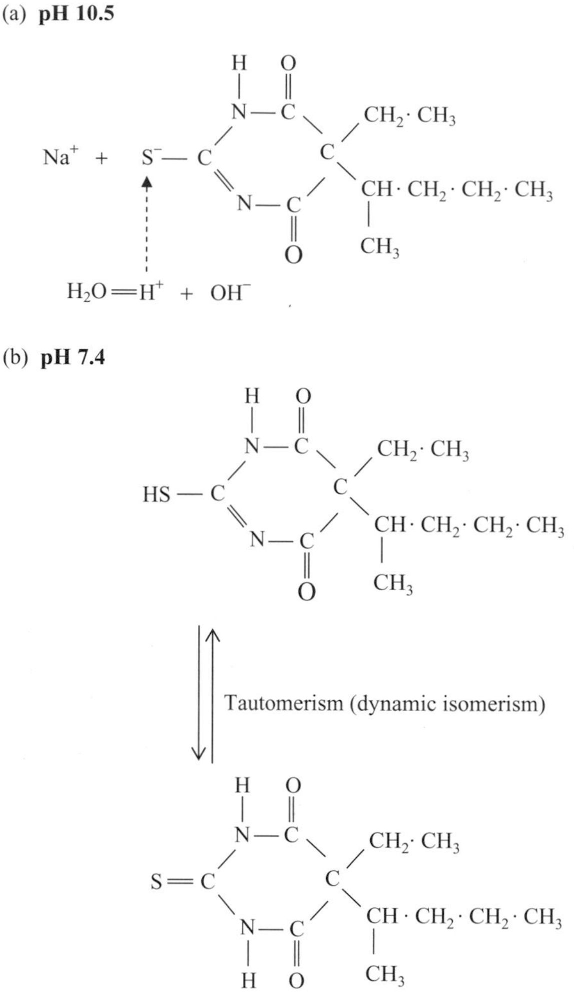

(a) **pH 10.5**

(b) **pH 7.4**

Tautomerism (dynamic isomerism)

Fig. 7.1 The ionization and tautomerism of thiopental sodium. (a) Thiopental sodium is soluble in water forming an alkaline solution due to its ionized sulphur atom (S^-) which has strong basic properties and attracts H^+; (b) In plasma (pH 7.4), the drug is initially present as undissociated, water-insoluble thiopental acid, which rapidly undergoes tautomerism (dynamic isomerism) into a highly lipid-soluble isomer.

produces free hydroxyl ions (OH^-) in solution and is added to prevent the precipitation of the insoluble free thiopental acid by H^+ derived from atmospheric CO_2 and carbonic acid. Solutions of thiopental sodium may remain stable at room temperature for up to 2 weeks (and for longer at 4°C), but should be immediately discarded if they become cloudy. They are not normally used more than 48 hours after preparation.

Because of their alkaline pH, 2.5% solutions of thiopental are usually bacteriostatic, but are incompatible with many basic drugs. In general, thiopental should not be mixed with oxidizing agents, acidic solutions, or drugs normally administered as sulphates, chlorides or hydrochlorides.

Mode of action

Although thiopental and other barbiturates may affect many receptors, it is generally accepted that their primary action is on $GABA_A$ receptors, which are widely distributed in the CNS. $GABA_A$ receptors are transmembrane proteins with five distinct subunits (usually $2\alpha:2\beta:1\gamma$), surrounding an intrinsic ion pore that is selectively permeable to chloride ions (Fig. 7.2). Since the subunits may be present in 3–6 different isoforms, $GABA_A$ receptors are a heterogenous group of related receptors rather than a single entity. Both the α- and β-subunits are believed to contribute to the GABA-binding site, which is closely related to the chloride channel. $GABA_A$ receptors are present as a macromolecular complex that includes specific binding sites for benzodiazepines, barbiturates and steroids, as well as some pro-convulsive drugs (e.g. picrotoxin).

GABA is the main inhibitory neurotransmitter in the brain and probably mediates presynaptic and postsynaptic inhibition at more than 50% of all synapses. It is normally synthesized from glutamate by the enzyme glutamate decarboxylase and is rapidly broken down by GABA transaminase (Fig. 7.3). In the presence of GABA, the ion channel in $GABA_A$ receptors allows chloride ions to diffuse into the neuron, resulting in hyperpolarization, decreased neuronal excitability and postsynaptic inhibition.

Thiopental and other barbiturates mainly act by increasing the duration of GABA-dependent chloride channel opening. This effect is partly mediated by the GABA-binding site, and partly by a distinct barbiturate binding site associated with the β-subunits and closely related to the ion channel (Fig. 7.2). Benzodiazepines affect $GABA_A$ receptors in a rather different manner, since they have a greater affinity for α- and γ-subunits of the GABA receptor, and increase the frequency of channel opening.

Most barbiturates appear to have little effect on anion-selective glycine channels that mediate neuronal inhibition, particularly in the spinal cord. In common with most other general anaesthetic agents, they may have some effect on transmitter-gated channels mediating neuronal activity and may modulate the effects of various excitatory neurotransmitters, including glutamate, acetylcholine, adenosine and 5-HT. Nevertheless, these effects

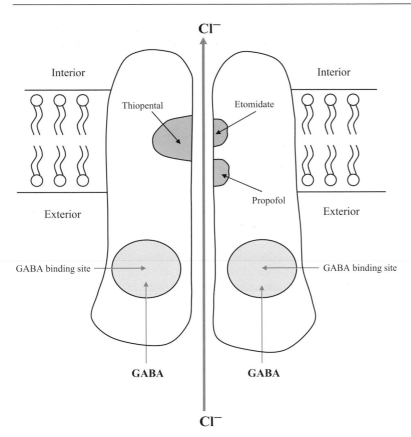

Fig. 7.2 The GABA$_A$ receptor contains an intrinsic ion channel that is selectively permeable to chloride ions. Thiopental, propofol and etomidate are believed to affect one or more modulatory sites that are distinct from the GABA binding site but closely related to the chloride channel.

do not appear to be germane to their mechanism of anaesthetic action.

Effects on the central nervous system

The effects of thiopental on the CNS are closely related to the dose and the rate of administration of the drug. After a normal induction dose (3–5 mg kg^{-1}), the rapid loss of consciousness is principally due to two factors. In the first place, brain tissue is extremely vascular and normally receives about 25% of the cardiac output. Secondly, thiopental is highly lipid-soluble at pH 7.4 due to its tautomerism (oil: water solubility coefficient = 500–700) and more than 90% of the drug in the cerebral capillaries immediately crosses the blood–brain barrier.

Consequently, the initial loss of consciousness during the induction of anaesthesia is usually smooth and rapid, and excitatory effects are rare (Table 7.1). The onset of sleep is often preceded by one or more deep breaths and may be associated with rapid eye movements and asso-

ciated EEG changes. Characteristically, the EEG shows a variable amplitude and high frequency pattern (predominantly at 20–30 Hz), which is usually replaced by slow wave activity as anaesthesia deepens. The high frequency response may be due to the selective depression of inhibitory neurons in the reticular formation, and probably accounts for the enhanced reflex response to surgical stimulation, increased vagal activity and laryngospasm, and hyperalgesia. These effects may be shown to occur when small doses of thiopental are administered, or are observed clinically during recovery from anaesthesia.

As anaesthesia deepens due to the increased cerebral uptake of thiopental, cortical responsiveness declines and EEG wave forms of low voltage become predominant. As the dose is increased, effects on the brainstem are produced. Respiratory depression is due to a direct action on the respiratory centre and its pontine connections, and the sensitivity to CO_2 is decreased in proportion to the depth of anaesthesia. Consequently, PaCO$_2$ increases, pH falls and apnoea may occur. In deep barbiturate anaesthesia,

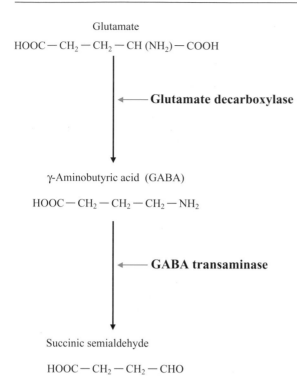

Glutamate

$$HOOC-CH_2-CH_2-CH(NH_2)-COOH$$

← **Glutamate decarboxylase**

γ-Aminobutyric acid (GABA)

$$HOOC-CH_2-CH_2-CH_2-NH_2$$

← **GABA transaminase**

Succinic semialdehyde

$$HOOC-CH_2-CH_2-CHO$$

Fig. 7.3 The synthesis of GABA from glutamate in the CNS. After its release from presynaptic nerve endings, the neurotransmitter is rapidly broken down to succinic semialdehyde by the enzyme GABA transaminase.

hypoxic drive mediated by aortic and carotid chemoreceptors may play an important part in the maintenance of respiration. In clinical practice, the respiratory effects of thiopental may be considerably modified by the degree of surgical stimulation and by the concomitant use of other central depressant drugs.

Thiopental and other barbiturates also decrease cerebral metabolism and reduce oxygen consumption. Cerebral blood flow, cerebral blood volume and CSF pressure fall during barbiturate anaesthesia due to the decreased production of CO_2. Consequently, thiopental has been used for cerebral resuscitation or to reduce raised intracranial pressure. These effects may be modified by any changes in systemic $PaCO_2$ produced by respiratory depression, which will tend to increase intracranial pressure.

Effects on the cardiovascular system

Normal induction doses cause a variable degree of hypotension in fit patients. Particular problems may occur in hypovolaemic states, patients with cardiovascular

disease or those who are concurrently receiving drugs that affect the sympathetic nervous system. In these conditions, the ability of the cardiovascular system to compensate for the haemodynamic effects of thiopental is impaired and dose requirements are reduced. The reduction in blood pressure is primarily due to decreased stroke volume and cardiac output, although there may be a compensatory reflex increase in systemic vascular resistance. High doses of thiopental directly depress cardiac contractility due to its local anaesthetic (membrane stabilizing) effects, and are hazardous in patients with a fixed cardiac output (Table 7.1).

During thiopental anaesthesia, there is a fall in glomerular filtration rate, renal plasma flow and electrolyte and water excretion. There may also be an increase in the release of ADH. These effects may be partly due to a reduction in renal blood flow, and urine output during thiopental anaesthesia is approximately 0.1 mL min^{-1} (about 10% of normal).

Distribution

High concentrations of thiopental are present in the brain and other well-perfused tissues within 1 minute of intravenous administration. The rapid emergence from sleep after a single dose is due to redistribution from the brain into less vascular regions, particularly skeletal muscle and skin. These tissues become saturated with thiopental within 15–30 minutes. Consequently, the plasma concentration rapidly falls, drug diffuses out of the brain and consciousness returns. In contrast, the fat depots, which have a poor blood supply, may require several hours to take up significant amounts and reach saturation. The concentration in blood, skeletal muscle and fat at various times after its administration is consistent with a classical physiological model with a central blood pool and six tissue compartments (Chapter 2).

Metabolism

Thiopental is extensively metabolized by the liver, and only trace amounts are eliminated in urine (normally <1% of the dose). Drug metabolism is relatively slow (10–15% of the amount remaining in the body is metabolized per hour) and is mainly due to ω-oxidation of thiopental to the inactive metabolite thiopental carboxylic acid (Table 7.2). Thiopental is also metabolized by (ω − 1) oxidation to hydroxythiopental, and by desulphuration to its oxybarbiturate analogue pentobarbital, which has a longer half-life than thiopental. When large doses of thiopental are used in cerebral resuscitation, metabolism becomes non-linear

Table 7.1 Pharmacological properties of induction agents.

	Onset of action	Recovery	Cardiovascular effects	Other effects
Thiopental	Rapid	Relatively rapid Complete recovery delayed	BP ↓ CO ↓	Extravascular complications Arterial thrombosis Laryngospasm and bronchospasm Enzyme induction ↑↓ICP
Propofol	Rapid	Rapid	BP ↓ CO ↓	Pain on injection Enzyme inhibition Delayed recovery after prolonged administration
Etomidate	Rapid	Moderately rapid	Minimal	Pain on injection Thrombophlebitis Excitatory effects Adrenocortical suppression
Ketamine	Slow	Slow	BP ↑ CO ↑ HR ↑	Analgesia ICP ↑ CBF ↑ Psychotomimetic effects

BP, blood pressure; CO, cardiac output; HR, heart rate; ICP, intracranial pressure; CBF, cerebral blood flow.

(zero-order) due to saturation of hepatic enzyme systems, leading to delayed recovery.

Pharmacokinetics

After intravenous administration, there is a triexponential decline in the plasma concentration of thiopental. The initial rapid disposition phase (half-life = 2–4 min) reflects the distribution of the drug to well-perfused organs such as the brain and liver and is followed by a slower disposition phase (half-life = 45–60 min) due to uptake by muscle and skin. Finally, the elimination of the drug from the body is reflected by the terminal decline in plasma concentration (half-life = 5–10 h). The volume of distribution of thiopental at steady state is slightly greater than total body water (1–4 L kg^{-1}), whilst its clearance is approximately 20% of liver blood flow (i.e. 1–5 mL min^{-1} kg^{-1}) (Table 7.2). Clearance is greater in infants and children than in adults, but is significantly decreased in obese patients and elderly subjects.

Table 7.2 Pharmacokinetic properties of intravenous anaesthetic agents.

	Terminal half-life (min)	Clearance (mL min^{-1} kg^{-1})	Apparent volume of distribution (L kg^{-1})	Metabolites
Thiopental	300–600	1.4–5.7	1.0–4.0	thiopental carboxylic acid hydroxy-thiopental pentobarbital
Propofol	300–700	21.4–28.6	3.3–5.7	2,6-diiso-propylphenol glucuronide 2,6-diiso-propylquinol glucuronide
Etomidate	60–90	10.0–24.3	2.2–4.3	1-(α-methyl-benzyl)- imidazole-5-carboxylic acid ethyl alcohol
Ketamine	150–200	17.1–20.0	2.9–3.1	norketamine hydroxy-norketamine hydroxy-ketamine glucuronide hydroxy-norketamine glucuronide

Unwanted effects

Thiopental is undoubtedly a safe and reliable induction agent as long as certain precautions are observed. Facilities for artificial ventilation and oxygenation must always be available. Deep levels of anaesthesia induced by thiopental can reduce smooth muscle tone in the gut and depress reflex laryngeal activity, and the risk of the aspiration of gastric contents must always be recognized. In particular, the usual recommended dose ($4–5$ mg kg^{-1}) may need to be considerably reduced in elderly, debilitated and hypovolaemic patients. The relatively slow elimination of thiopental (terminal half-life $= 5–10$ h) requires care and supervision during the prolonged recovery. Patients should be advised not to drive or operate machinery for at least 24 hours after anaesthesia, and to avoid alcohol and sedative drugs.

Extravascular administration

Although thiopental injection is usually painless, inadvertent extravascular administration can cause complications ranging from slight pain to extensive tissue necrosis. These effects are probably due to local tissue irritation produced by precipitation of insoluble thiopental at pH 7.4. Dispersal of thiopental by local injection of hyaluronidase and topically applied demulcents may be useful in the treatment of local complications.

Intra-arterial administration

Inadvertent intra-arterial injection of thiopental causes immediate and severe shooting pain usually followed by signs of arterial spasm, with blanching of the limb, increasing cyanosis and disappearance of the pulse, and the onset of unconsciousness may be delayed. These effects are due to the precipitation of thiopental crystals at pH 7.4, which are then transported in a progressively narrowing vascular bed and aggregate in small arterioles. Initial vascular spasm is followed by an intense chemical endarteritis, which rapidly involves the endothelial tissues. In addition, blood vessels may be occluded by crystals of thiopental and by erythrocyte and platelet aggregation, resulting in arterial thrombosis and gangrene. After intra-arterial injection of thiopental, immediate treatment is essential. If the needle is still in situ in the artery, injection of a vasodilator (either papaverine or procaine, $80–120$ mg) is required. Temporary sympathetic blockade by continuous axillary block or repeated stellate ganglion block will open up the collateral circulation, and heparin is often useful.

Porphyria

In subjects with acute intermittent porphyria and porphyria variegata, thiopental and other barbiturates induce hepatic synthesis of cytochrome P450, and thus increase porphyrin synthesis by the liver (Chapter 6). Although barbiturates do not always precipitate acute porphyria in susceptible patients, an acute attack may be fatal, and all barbiturates must be avoided in all forms of porphyria.

Anaphylactoid and anaphylactic reactions

Thiopental may induce transient urticarial or erythematous rashes, which are usually due to histamine release from mast cells and may be related to the dose and rate of injection. True hypersensitivity or anaphylactic responses are extremely rare, with a prevalence between 1 in 14,000 and 1 in 20,000. They usually present as bronchospasm, hypotension, generalized oedema or peripheral vascular collapse, and may be fatal.

Clinical use

Thiopental is still widely used as an induction agent and for the maintenance of anaesthesia (either by intermittent administration or by infusion). In addition, thiopental may be the drug of choice for the treatment of status epilepticus that does not respond to conventional anticonvulsant therapy, particularly when controlled ventilation is practicable. It has a more rapid onset of action than diazepam, which may be a considerable advantage.

Thiopental and other barbiturates have also been used to protect the brain from the effects of hypoxia after stroke and head injury. Although the haemodynamic effects of thiopental tend to reduce cerebral blood flow, the depression of cerebral metabolism reduces brain oedema and intracranial pressure, so that cerebral perfusion actually improves. Meticulous care of the airway and the monitoring of cardiovascular parameters and intracranial pressure are mandatory. In the UK, the use of barbiturates for cerebral resuscitation is controversial.

Propofol

Chemistry

Propofol (2,6-di-isopropyl phenol) is a chemically inert phenolic derivative with anaesthetic properties. Although propofol is almost insoluble in water at pH 7.0, forming a colourless or pale straw-coloured liquid, it is highly lipid soluble. The original preparation contained the solubilizing agent Cremophor EL (polyethoxylated castor oil), but was discarded due to the anaphylactoid potential of this agent. Since 1985, propofol has been normally administered as a 1% ($10\,\mathrm{mg\,mL^{-1}}$) isotonic emulsion, which contains 10% soya oil (as long chain triglycerides), sodium hydroxide, purified egg phosphatide and water. A 2% preparation of propofol, which is primarily used in continuous infusion techniques, is also available. Both preparations support bacterial growth, and outbreaks of postoperative infection have been related to the use of propofol in unsterile conditions and to the repeated use of single dose ampoules. Syringes containing propofol should be used immediately after their preparation, and any unused drug should be discarded. In addition, previously opened ampoules of the drug should not be allowed to stand at ambient temperatures. Attempts have been made to supplement formulations with EDTA (ethylene diamine tetraacetic acid) or sodium metabisulphite, although the latter may affect the stability of the emulsion. Prolonged infusion of the bisulphite preparation has been associated with a single fatal case of cardiovascular collapse.

In some patients, conventional preparations of propofol may increase plasma triglyceride concentrations. A formulation with long and medium chain triglycerides is now available in the UK (Propofol-Lipuro), and may modify the rise in plasma triglycerides as well as decreasing the prevalence of pain on injection. Preparations containing 5% soya oil have also been used in an attempt to modify the rise in lipid concentration.

Propofol is chemically unique when compared with other induction agents, since it is an achiral compound.

Mode of action

Propofol produces general anaesthesia by selective modulation of the activity of the $GABA_A$ receptor (Fig. 7.2). It mainly affects amino acid residues in the β_2- or β_3-subunits of the receptor adjacent to the chloride channel. Its site of action appears to be relatively insensitive to GABA itself and is quite distinct from the modulatory site for barbiturates and benzodiazepines. None of the effects of propofol are modified by the benzodiazepine antagonist flumazenil. In addition, propofol may affect two other receptor types in the CNS:

- Glycine receptors
- Nicotinic acetylcholine receptors

There is some evidence that propofol enhances the activity of strychnine-sensitive glycine receptors in the CNS. In addition, it may inhibit the activity of excitatory nicotinic acetylcholine receptors, although its effects may be limited to receptors that contain β-subunits. Effects at both these sites require higher concentrations than those required to produce anaesthesia. There is no evidence that propofol affects other ligand-gated ion channels, or voltage-gated channels.

Effects on the central nervous system

The normal induction dose of propofol ($1.5\text{–}2.5\,\mathrm{mg\,kg^{-1}}$) produces rapid loss of consciousness due to the immediate uptake of the lipid-soluble drug by the CNS. In general, closure of the eyes is slower than with thiopental, and the loss of verbal contact may be a more precise endpoint for loss of consciousness. Induction of anaesthesia produces an initial reduction in EEG frequency with an increase in amplitude. As the level of anaesthesia deepens, β- and δ-waves predominate. Spontaneous movements that may occur during induction appear to be associated with the δ-waves. Propofol also causes a reduction in cerebral blood flow and a decrease in cerebral oxygen consumption. Although there is a significant increase in cerebrovascular resistance, there is an overall reduction in intracranial pressure and cerebral perfusion pressure. After intravenous administration, the plasma concentration of propofol rapidly decreases due to the distribution of the drug throughout the body and its uptake by peripheral tissues. As the plasma concentration falls, propofol diffuses from the CNS to the systemic circulation. When bolus doses of the drug are used to induce anaesthesia there is a rapid recovery of full consciousness and awareness due to the rapid redistribution of the drug.

Effects on respiration

Propofol induces dose-related respiratory depression, with a decrease in both tidal and minute respiratory volumes, and apnoea may be observed. Although this is usually transient, it may be prolonged when doses at the higher end of the recommended range are used, or when other respiratory depressants are used concomitantly.

Nausea and vomiting

Postoperative nausea and vomiting appear to be extremely uncommon, particularly when propofol is used as the sole anaesthetic agent. The replacement of a standard inhalational anaesthetic by propofol reduces postoperative nausea and vomiting by approximately the same extent as a single dose of an antiemetic. These advantageous properties have undoubtedly contributed to its current popularity as an induction agent for short procedures and day-case surgery.

Effects on the cardiovascular system

Propofol frequently causes a significant reduction in systemic blood pressure, particularly in hypovolaemic patients, which may fall to 70–80% of the preoperative level. Hypotension is related to the dose and rate of injection and is usually maximal within 5–10 minutes. The fall in blood pressure is principally due to a decrease in systemic vascular resistance and is not usually accompanied by reflex tachycardia (Table 7.1). It has been suggested that propofol causes resetting of the baroreceptors in the aortic arch and carotid body, so that slower heart rates are associated with a given reduction in blood pressure. Alternatively, propofol may act as a calcium channel-blocking agent, or promote the release of nitric oxide from the endothelium. Cardiac output also falls and recent studies indicate that propofol may depress cardiac output in a similar manner to thiopental.

Distribution

After intravenous administration, propofol is rapidly and widely distributed in the body due to its high lipid solubility, and its volume 06 of distribution is 20–80 times greater than total body water (Chapter 2). As the plasma concentration falls due to extensive tissue uptake and rapid hepatic metabolism, propofol is progressively removed from the brain and dose-dependent recovery usually occurs within 10–20 minutes. Propofol is highly (96–97%) bound to albumin, so that its total plasma concentration may be significantly greater than the level of the unbound drug.

Metabolism

Propofol is rapidly eliminated by the liver mainly as a glucuronide conjugate, which is subsequently eliminated in urine. The remainder is metabolized by cytochrome P450 isoforms, particularly CYP 2B6 and CYP 2C9, to 2,6-diisopropylquinol and subsequently eliminated in urine as glucuronide and sulphate conjugates (Table 7.2). The presence of quinolic metabolites is responsible for the green-coloured urine that is occasionally seen after prolonged infusions. Additional trace metabolites can also be detected in urine and less than 1% of the drug is excreted unchanged.

The elimination of propofol is sensitive to changes in liver blood flow, but is unaffected by alterations in protein binding or enzyme activity. The clearance of propofol is greater than liver blood flow, and there is some evidence that extrahepatic metabolism of the drug occurs. Propofol hydroxylation can occur in the lungs, and glucuronide conjugation may take place in the enteric circulation. Furthermore, significant amounts of propofol glucuronide have been recovered from urine during the anhepatic phase of liver transplantation.

Propofol also inhibits drug metabolism by various isoforms of cytochrome P450, particularly CYP 1A1, CYP 2A1 and CYP 2B1. It decreases the clearance and may prolong the duration of action of fentanyl, alfentanil and propranolol, possibly due to inhibition of drug metabolism.

Propofol does not induce enzymes involved in porphyrin synthesis and its use is not contraindicated in this disease. However, experimental studies suggest that, in common with many inhalation anaesthetic agents, it can depress the chemotactic activity of leukocytes.

Pharmacokinetics

After an intravenous bolus dose ($1–4 \text{ mg kg}^{-1}$) the decline in the plasma concentration of propofol is usually consistent with a triexponential decline. The plasma concentration rapidly decreases during the first 10 minutes (half-life = 1–3 min) and is followed by a slower decline for 3–4 hours (half-life = 20–30 min). Both these phases reflect the almost immediate distribution of propofol from plasma and its uptake by tissues. They are followed by a slower decline in plasma concentration due to hepatic metabolism, which is constrained by the slow return of the drug from the periphery. In pharmacokinetic models, the decline in the plasma concentration of propofol is usually interpreted by an open three-compartment model (Chapter 2).

Estimated values for the derived pharmacokinetic constants are extremely variable. Some initial studies suggested that the terminal half-life of propofol was 1–5 hours, and that its total apparent volume of distribution was approximately 10 times greater than total body water. More recent studies suggest that the terminal half-life may be extremely long (40–50 h), and that the drug can be detected in plasma for up to 3 days after its administration. The clearance of propofol is about 20% greater than liver blood flow, probably due to significant extrahepatic metabolism.

Unwanted effects

Unwanted effects of propofol include
- Pain on injection
- Excitatory effects
- Bradycardia and hypotension
- Allergic reactions

Pain on injection

Pain on injection commonly occurs when propofol is injected into small veins on the dorsum of the hand or wrist. Pain may present at more proximal sites (upper arm and shoulder) during injection. The pain is transitory and thrombophlebitic sequelae are extremely rare. The incidence of pain is lessened if large veins in the antecubital fossa are used for administration, or if a small dose of lignocaine (10–20 mg) is given immediately before or added to propofol. Other drugs have also been used to alleviate or modify the pain on injection, including fentanyl, alfentanil and tramadol. Preparations of propofol containing long- and medium-chain triglycerides (e.g. Propofol-Lipuro) or the addition of long-chain triglycerides to generic propofol may reduce the prevalence of pain on injection, presumably due to a reduction in the concentration of the drug in the aqueous phase.

Excitatory effects

Excitatory side effects, including myoclonus, opisthotonos and convulsions, are sometimes associated with the administration of propofol and may occur during the recovery period. There is a risk of convulsions occurring if propofol is used in epileptic patients, and their onset is sometimes delayed.

Bradycardia and hypotension

Profound bradycardia occasionally occurs after administration of propofol and may require treatment with an antimuscarinic agent (e.g. atropine). Unexpected deaths have occurred in children during long-term sedation with propofol in an intensive care unit. The presenting clinical features were increasing metabolic acidosis, bradycardia and progressive myocardial failure. Although the cause is obscure, both the drug and the lipid content of the solvent have been implicated.

Allergic reactions

The initial use of propofol with Cremophor EL resulted in a number of hypersensitivity responses, which were attributed to the solubilizing agent. The present formulation in soya oil has been associated with more than 30 cases involving allergic or anaphylactoid phenomena. However, there has not been any direct immunological evidence to incriminate propofol per se, and the concomitant use of other drugs, particularly neuromuscular blocking agents, has been implicated in some of these reactions.

The safety margin of propofol is generally considered to be lower than that of etomidate but greater than thiopental, both in relation to undesirable side effects and to hypersensitivity responses.

Clinical use

Propofol is widely used to induce and maintain anaesthesia, to supplement anaesthetic techniques during diagnostic procedures and to provide prolonged sedation in adults during intensive care. It is also used in adults to maintain anaesthesia by means of target-controlled computer systems. Induction of anaesthesia usually requires doses of 1.5–2.5 mg kg^{-1}, administered at a rate of 20–40 mg every 10 seconds. The dose should be reduced in patients aged 55 or over. In intensive care situations, doses of 0.5–1 mg kg^{-1} are initially used to induce sedation, followed by an infusion of 0.5–4 mg kg^{-1} h^{-1}, although larger doses may be needed in agitated patients. Propofol should not be used to produce sedation in patients under the age of 17 years. The use of propofol is usually precluded in obstetric anaesthesia, due to its high placental transfer and the associated neonatal depression, although views on its use in this context are changing.

The main advantage of propofol in clinical practice is that rapid recovery of consciousness and full awareness occurs when bolus doses are used to induce anaesthesia, and that significant cumulation does not occur after repeated administration or infusion of the drug. Consequently, propofol is widely used in day-case anaesthesia. Respiratory side effects (e.g. cough, laryngospasm) are rarely encountered during induction and propofol is usually the agent of choice for the insertion of the laryngeal mask airway (LMA). Nevertheless, a number of studies suggest that the drug has a relatively long half-life, and prolonged infusions and multiple doses should be used with caution, particularly in younger patients.

Propofol should be used with caution in patients with disorders of lipid metabolism, since prolonged infusions may cause increases in plasma lipid concentrations.

Target-controlled infusion systems

Computer-controlled programmed infusion devices have been widely used in the UK to produce constant, reproducible plasma concentrations of propofol, and to maintain them within the therapeutic range (usually 2–4 $\mu g\ mL^{-1}$). The procedure is based on the use of the bolus, elimination and transfer method and an appropriate compartmental pharmacokinetic model (Chapter 2). A bolus of drug sufficient to fill the central compartment to the required concentration is administered, followed by a continuous infusion at an exponentially declining rate to compensate for the disappearance of the drug from the central compartment and its transfer to one or more peripheral compartments. The parameters of a three-compartment model are normally used as the input for a pharmacokinetic simulation program that controls a conventional intravenous infusion system, and a variety of different algorithms are now available to regulate the infusion rate. These systems rapidly achieve and maintain steady-state plasma concentrations, which can then be modified in a controlled manner according to the individual pharmacodynamic response. In more recent developments, the effect-site concentration can be predicted or targeted, and used to determine the onset of anaesthesia.

Pharmacokinetic data obtained during paediatric anaesthesia has also been used to derive a different model for the target-controlled infusion of propofol in children, with a larger central compartmental volume. A closed loop system, using a derivative of the EEG to assess hypnotic activity and provide feedback control of the infusion rate, has been used to maintain a constant level of sedation and anaesthesia.

Etomidate

maintain them within the therapeutic range (usually 2–4

tant effects, but can produce adverse effects if its elimination is impaired, and may interact with some other drugs (e.g. disulfiram, metronidazole). Etomidate has recently been prepared as an emulsion with medium- and long-chain triglycerides ('Etomidate-Lipuro'), thus reducing the prevalence of some of the adverse effects of the drug (Table 7.1).

Etomidate has a chiral centre in its methylbenzyl side chain. Unlike other induction agents, it is prepared and used as a single R(+)-isomer, which is about 10 times more potent than its S-enantiomer.

Mode of action
Recent evidence suggests that etomidate produces anaesthesia by direct and relatively specific effects on the $GABA_A$ receptor. Etomidate modifies the activity of a small number of amino acids in the β-subunits of the receptor, probably by regulating an allosteric site within the chloride channel (Fig. 7.2). Similar selective effects can be demonstrated for the structurally related compound lorecrezole, which opposes the proconvulsant effects of picrotoxin.

Effects on the central nervous system
Normal induction doses of etomidate (0.3 mg kg^{-1}) produce immediate loss of consciousness. The duration of action is dose-dependent and the drug shows little or no tendency to cumulate even with repeated dosage. Changes in the EEG pattern during the onset of anaesthesia mimic those of the intravenous barbiturates and involuntary muscle movement is not associated with abnormal EEG activity. The most significant advantage of etomidate is its relatively high safety margin. There is a 30-fold difference between the anaesthetic dose and the lethal dose, which compares favourably with the 4- to 5-fold difference for thiopental and propofol.

Effects on the cardiovascular system
Etomidate has little effect on the cardiovascular system (Table 7.1). It usually causes a slight fall in peripheral resistance and blood pressure. In most organs, blood flow is unchanged or slightly increased and myocardial contractility, oxygen consumption and coronary blood flow are usually unaffected. Etomidate reduces cerebral blood flow and intracranial pressure, and hypnotic doses cause respiratory depression, as assessed by the changes in ventilation produced by alterations in inspired $PaCO_2$.

Chemistry
Etomidate (R-(+)-1-(α-methylbenzyl)-imidazole-5-ethyl-carboxylate sulphate) is an ethylcarboxylate ester with an imidazole nucleus. The drug is usually prepared and used as a 0.2% solution (2 mg mL^{-1}). Although etomidate is highly water-soluble, forming a slightly alkaline solution, the commonest proprietary preparation contains propylene glycol (35% v/v). This alcoholic excipient improves the stability of the solution and reduces its local irri-

Metabolism

Etomidate is almost entirely eliminated from the body by metabolism, and only trace amounts of the unchanged drug (about 1–2% of the dose) are detected in urine and bile. It is primarily hydrolysed by non-specific hepatic esterases to a carboxylic acid metabolite (1-(α-methylbenzyl)-imidazole-5-carboxylic acid) and ethyl alcohol (Table 7.2). Etomidate may also be metabolized by cholinesterases and can inhibit plasma cholinesterase by competing with other substrates (e.g. suxamethonium, mivacurium) for the enzyme.

Pharmacokinetics

After intravenous injection of a bolus dose, there is usually a biexponential decline in the plasma concentration of etomidate. The initial fall in plasma concentration (half-life = 2–5 min) reflects the distribution of the drug to well-perfused tissues, and the subsequent slower decline is due to the elimination of the drug from the body (terminal half-life = 68–75 min). The apparent volume of distribution is slightly greater than total body water, and its clearance is about 50–80% of hepatic blood flow (Table 7.2). The relatively high extraction ratio is consistent with flow-limited hepatic clearance. Etomidate is bound to plasma albumin to a significant extent (70–80%), and the effects of the drug may be enhanced in the elderly and in low albumin states.

Unwanted effects

In spite of its advantages, the use of etomidate as an induction agent is restricted by several undesirable effects:

- Pain on injection
- Thrombophlebitis
- Involuntary muscle movements
- Postoperative nausea and vomiting
- Suppression of adrenocortical function

Pain on injection

Pain on injection occurs in 30–60% of patients. Although its precise cause is obscure, it is probably related to the use of propylene glycol as a solvent, since it is less common when etomidate is given with other solvents (triglycerides or cyclodextrins). It is often relieved by the concurrent use of opioid analgesics or lidocaine.

Thrombophlebitis

Thrombophlebitis occurs in up to 30% of patients within 2–3 days, particularly if etomidate is injected into small veins on the back of the hand. Some haemolysis may also occur, although this is often clinically insignificant. Both these effects are believed to be related to the solvent propylene glycol, since they are less common when etomidate is injected as a triglyceride emulsion.

Involuntary muscle movements

Etomidate commonly causes excitatory side effects, such as restlessness, spontaneous involuntary movements, hypertonicity of voluntary muscle and cough or hiccups. These phenomena can be modified by premedication with short-acting benzodiazepines or by opioid analgesics. The occurrence of convulsions has been occasionally reported in unpremedicated patients.

Postoperative nausea and vomiting

Postoperative nausea and vomiting occur in 25–30% of patients and is more commonly associated with etomidate than with other induction agents.

Suppression of adrenocortical function

Prolonged administration of etomidate by intravenous infusion may suppress adrenocortical function. Etomidate, like most other imidazole drugs, inhibits ferric haem enzymes and thus impairs the activity of mitochondrial cytochrome P450 isoforms in the adrenal cortex (particularly 11β-hydroxylase and 17α-hydroxylase), which are involved in the formation of corticosteroids. Consequently, the synthesis of both hydrocortisone (cortisol) and aldosterone may be suppressed. Etomidate may also inhibit cytochrome P450 isoforms in the liver, and thus affect the metabolism of other drugs. Consequently, the drug should not be given by continuous infusion, or used for the maintenance of anaesthesia.

Porphyria

In experimental conditions, continuous infusion of etomidate increases the activity of δ-amino-laevulinic acid synthetase, which is involved in porphyrin synthesis. It has also been implicated in attacks of acute intermittent porphyria, and its use is therefore contraindicated in all patients with porphyria.

Anaphylactic and anaphylactoid reactions

Both anaphylactic and anaphylactoid reactions are uncommon. Occasionally, histamine release from mast cells causes skin rashes during the induction of anaesthesia. Although severe reactions such as generalized erythema, hypotension and bronchospasm have occurred when etomidate was used with suxamethonium and alcuronium, the muscle relaxants were usually implicated as the causal factor. Indeed, some authorities consider that etomidate is the safest induction agent in susceptible patients and may be the drug of choice when a hypersensitivity response is anticipated.

Clinical use

Etomidate is usually prepared and used as a 0.2% solution (2 mg mL^{-1}), either as a solution in propylene glycol (35%) or as a medium-chain/long-chain triglyceride emulsion. The usual dose is 0.3 mg kg^{-1}, which should be reduced in elderly subjects. In spite of its disadvantages, the drug is sometimes used to induce anaesthesia in patients with cardiovascular impairment or hypovolaemia, since it has no adverse effects on the systemic or cerebral circulation. It may still be the drug of choice in atopic patients with a history of drug hypersensitivity, and its margin of safety is probably greater than any other drug in current use. It should not be used by continuous infusion or prolonged administration due to the danger of adrenal suppression. Similarly, its use should be avoided in patients with adrenal insufficiency.

Ketamine

Chemistry

Ketamine ((2-chlorophenyl)2-(methylamino)-cyclohexanone hydrochloride) is chemically related to cyclohexamine and phencyclidine. The hydrochloride salt is freely soluble in water, forming an acidic solution (pH 3.5–5.5). Ketamine is a chiral drug and contains a single asymmetric carbon atom in its chemical structure. In the UK, it is currently used clinically as a racemic mixture.

Mode of action

Ketamine and other phencyclidine analogues are antagonists of the excitatory neurotransmitter glutamate at N-methyl-D-aspartate (NMDA) receptor sites in the CNS. Antagonism of NMDA receptors by ketamine is non-competitive, and its effects are probably due to ion channel blockade (Fig. 7.4). The inhibitory effects of ketamine on NMDA receptors probably accounts for 'dissociative anaesthesia' and the analgesic effects of the drug. There is some evidence that both nitrous oxide and xenon have similar effects on NMDA receptors.

Onset and duration of action

Ketamine has a relatively slow onset of action when compared with other induction agents, and its maximal effect does not occur within one arm–brain circulation time. There is commonly a latent period of 2 minutes or more after injection before any CNS effect is observed. This delay can be as much as 8 minutes after intramuscular administration. It can be difficult to determine the precise time of the onset of action, and patients may gaze into the distance for several minutes without closing their eyes.

The duration of action of ketamine is dependent on the dose of the drug. Normal intravenous doses (2–3 mg kg^{-1}) act for 10–20 minutes, although this may be difficult to determine accurately.

Effects on the central nervous system

Ketamine differs from other intravenous induction agents in several important respects. It is almost devoid of hypnotic properties, but produces a state of 'dissociative anaesthesia' characterized by sedation, immobility, anterograde amnesia, profound analgesia and dissociation from the environment. Ketamine also causes an increase in cerebral blood flow, oxygen consumption and intracranial pressure.

The effects on the CNS are associated with characteristic changes in the EEG, and the α rhythm is usually depressed and replaced by θ and δ wave activity. These changes may persist for the duration of analgesia.

Effects on the cardiovascular system

In contrast to most other anaesthetic agents, ketamine invariably produces tachycardia, increases cardiac output and raises plasma noradrenaline concentrations. Both systolic and diastolic pressures as well as pulmonary vascular resistance are usually increased by 20–40% (Table 7.1). These changes often occur within 5 minutes and last for 10–20 minutes and may be partly due to a direct action on neuronal pathways in the CNS. However, experimental evidence suggests that the positive inotropic effects of ketamine are mediated by activation of cardiac

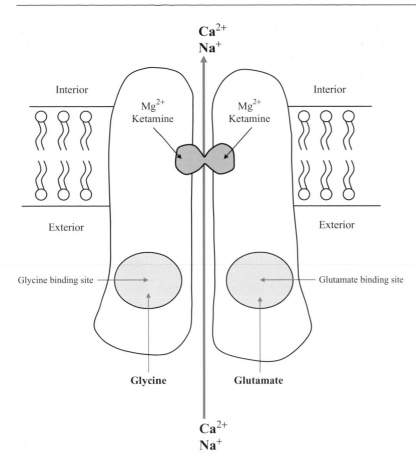

Fig. 7.4 The site of action of ketamine. NMDA receptors contain an intrinsic ion channel that is permeable to Na^+ and Ca^{2+}. Receptor activation depends on two agonists (glutamate and glycine), which are bound by different receptor subunits. The intrinsic ion channel is blocked by Mg^{2+}, ketamine and other phencyclidines, resulting in non-competitive blockade of the NMDA receptor.

β-adrenoceptors and that ketamine appears to have a depressant effect on denervated cardiac muscle.

Effects on the respiratory system
Respiratory activity is little affected, although the respiratory rate may slightly increase, and there is a normal response to alterations in $PaCO_2$. Coughing and laryngospasm are extremely rare, and experimental studies suggest that ketamine antagonizes the effects of histamine, acetylcholine and 5-HT on bronchial smooth muscle. The drug can be used safely in asthmatic patients. Although most reflex responses are not affected by ketamine, some depression of laryngeal reflexes may occur, which precludes its use for operations on the upper airway.

Effects on voluntary muscle
Hypertonus and spontaneous involuntary muscle movements, including tonic–clonic activity of the limbs, may occur during induction. Muscular relaxation is often poor, and the tone of the jaw muscles may be increased, causing obstruction of the airway.

Metabolism
Ketamine is primarily metabolized by cytochrome P450 (mainly by CYP 3A4) in the hepatic smooth endoplasmic reticulum. Its main demethylated metabolite (norketamine) has some hypnotic activity but is about 30% less potent than ketamine. Both ketamine and norketamine may be further metabolized to hydroxylated derivatives (hydroxyketamine and hydroxynorketamine), which are subsequently conjugated and eliminated in urine as glucuronides (Table 7.2). Only 2–3% of the drug is eliminated unchanged.

Pharmacokinetics
Ketamine is approximately 45% non-ionized at pH 7.4. After intravenous administration, the drug is rapidly

distributed in tissues and readily crosses the blood–brain barrier and the placenta. Plasma concentrations usually decrease in a biexponential manner, and the initial rapid fall in plasma concentration (half-life = 10–20 min) is followed by a slower decline (half-life = 150–200 min), which is due to the elimination of ketamine by hepatic metabolism. The apparent volume of distribution is 2–3 times greater than body water, and the clearance is approximately equal to liver blood flow. The relatively high extraction ratio is consistent with flow-limited hepatic clearance, and drugs that reduce liver blood flow can decrease the clearance of ketamine and prolong its terminal half-life. After intramuscular administration, ketamine is rapidly absorbed and maximum plasma concentrations are invariably present within 30 minutes.

Unwanted effects

Emergence phenomena

During recovery from ketamine anaesthesia there is a significant possibility of emergence phenomena, ranging from vivid dreams and visual images to hallucinations and delirium, which occur in about 30% of patients and may continue for 24 hours after administration. These psychotomimetic sequelae may be extremely unpleasant, and it has been suggested that they are related to the misperception or misinterpretation of sensory information, particularly visual or auditory stimuli. Emergence phenomena may be considerably modified by the use of appropriate premedication with opiates or benzodiazepines. Such problems tend to be commoner in women but are believed to be rare in children, particularly when their postoperative recovery is undisturbed. Nausea and vomiting are not infrequent during the postoperative period.

Cardiovascular effects

Ketamine increases heart rate, cardiac output, systolic and diastolic blood pressure, as well as intracranial pressure, cerebral blood flow and intraocular pressure (Table 7.1). Consequently, it is contraindicated in patients with raised intracranial and intraocular pressure. It should also be avoided in patients with tachycardia, hypertension or ischaemic heart disease.

Enantiomers of ketamine

Ketamine is a chiral drug, containing a single asymmetric carbon atom in its cyclohexanone ring. In the UK, ketamine is currently used as a racemic mixture of the S(+) and R(−) enantiomers, although in most European countries the drug is used as a single isomer preparation (S(+)-ketamine). There are important pharmacological differences between the two enantiomers, and the S(+) isomer has stereoselective effects on NMDA receptors *in vitro*. In clinical use, the S(+) enantiomer is approximately three times as potent as its R(−) antipode and is associated with significantly less psychotic emergence phenomena, agitated behaviour and postoperative pain, and superior intraoperative amnesia. The S(+) isomer has a larger volume of distribution and clearance, and a greater rate and extent of biotransformation than its enantiomer. In addition, the metabolism of S(+)-ketamine is inhibited by the R(−) isomer. These differences between the enantiomers probably reflect their different affinities for chiral receptors and enzymes, which are composed of L-amino acids with specific stereochemical requirements, so that one isomer has a better fit than the other. It is now generally accepted that ketamine has significant advantages when it is used as an S(+) isomer rather than as a racemic mixture.

Clinical use

In the UK, three different concentrations of ketamine hydrochloride (10, 50 and 100 mg mL^{-1}) are available for intravenous injection (1–4.5 mg kg^{-1}) or intramuscular administration (6.5–13 mg kg^{-1}). Ketamine has only a limited place in current anaesthetic practice due to its undesirable effects on the CNS and the cardiovascular system. It is usually avoided for patients with cardiac impairment, trauma or a history of psychotic illness. Nevertheless, the drug has a definite role in certain situations.

Paediatric practice

Ketamine is predominantly used in paediatric practice, when venepuncture is difficult or poorly tolerated, or when repeated anaesthesia is necessary. Its oral and rectal administration for sedation and premedication in small children has also been described. In these situations, ketamine appears to have a low bioavailability and to undergo significant first-pass metabolism.

Other indications

In adults, the indications for its use are more controversial and less well defined. It has been used to provide anaesthesia for cardiac catheterization, repeated burns dressings and other minor procedures (e.g. radiotherapy, bone marrow biopsy), and in the poor risk elderly patient. It is also useful in certain emergency situations when venous or airway access is impossible, particularly following road traffic or underground accidents. Ketamine has also been administered by intrathecal and extradural routes in the treatment of postoperative or neuropathic pain.

Adverse reactions to intravenous anaesthetic agents

Historical background

Since the first conclusive case of an adverse reaction associated with the use of thiopental was reported in 1952, there has been a progressive increase in the apparent prevalence of hypersensitivity reactions to intravenous anaesthetic agents. This coincided with the introduction and use of a number of non-barbiturate induction agents, and two of these agents (propanidid and althesin) have now been withdrawn because of their association with such adverse effects. Both these drugs contained the solubilizing agent Cremophor EL (polyethoxylated castor oil), which is a mixture of fatty acids with a molecular weight of approximately 3200, and was also present in some vitamin preparations and antifungal drugs. Although early studies suggested that Cremophor EL had no immunogenic or anaphylactoid potential, subsequent evidence indicated that it played an important role in the occurrence of adverse reactions to intravenous anaesthetic agents. Alternatively, its surfactant properties may have enhanced the immunogenic potential of propanidid and alphaxolone (the active steroid in althesin).

Prevalence

The current prevalence of anaphylactoid and hypersensitivity responses to anaesthetic agents has been estimated as 1 in 6000, and neuromuscular blocking agents appear to have been involved in at least 80% of the cases. The reported prevalence of responses associated with individual induction agents ranges from 1 in 14,000 to 1 in 450,000 (Table 7.3). The severity of hypersensitivity responses is difficult to assess and, although adverse reactions to thiopental appear to be relatively uncommon, approximately 10 deaths have been recorded. On the other hand, it is probable that many incidents are not reported, particularly those in which serious sequelae do not occur. The prevalence of reactions to propofol when used as an emulsion in soya bean oil and egg phosphatide is between 1 in 80,000 and 1 in 100,000, and many of them appear to be related to histamine release. In contrast, reactions to etomidate are extremely rare, and reactions to ketamine are almost unknown (Table 7.3).

Table 7.3 Prevalence of hypersensitivity responses associated with current induction agents.

Induction agent	Prevalence of reactions
Thiopental	1 in 14,000–1 in 20,000
Propofol	1 in 80,000–1 in 100,000
Etomidate	1 in 50,000–1 in 450,000
Ketamine	Extremely rare (2 cases)

In a number of instances, some undesirable effects (e.g. hypotension) may be due to the direct actions of the anaesthetic agent on the myocardium or on vascular smooth muscle, or an enhanced vasovagal response to venepuncture. In addition, mechanical problems with the airway, related to misplaced endotracheal tubes, may present as apparent bronchospasm. Anaesthetic techniques invariably involve some polypharmacy and the role of other drugs (e.g. muscle relaxants, colloid infusions) may be difficult to determine. Furthermore, the outcome of a hypersensitivity response can obviously depend on the early recognition of the problem and the ability to institute immediate therapeutic measures.

Clinical features

The clinical features of anaphylactoid and hypersensitivity reactions to induction agents may include bronchospasm, hypotension, peripheral vascular collapse, erythema, urticaria, oedema and abdominal pain. The clinical course of the reaction is variable, and in extreme cases bronchospasm occurs within seconds of injection, rapidly followed by cyanosis. The pulse may be impalpable and the blood pressure unrecordable, although the ECG may show an increase in heart rate. Localized or generalized oedema may subsequently develop. Occasionally, reactions to intravenous anaesthetics have a slower onset (over 10–90 min), their clinical features are often relatively benign and their cause may not be recognized.

Many of the presenting symptoms resemble the pharmacological effects of histamine in humans, or may be produced by other mediators, including bradykinin, 5-hydroxytryptamine, leukotrienes, prostaglandins and heparin.

Mechanism of adverse reactions

The mechanisms involved may be of several types (Chapter 6):

(1) Type I immediate hypersensitivity reactions, which depend upon previous exposure and sensitization to the drug, and the formation of IgE antibodies.

(2) Type II (cytotoxic) hypersensitivity responses have also been reported. In this mechanism, IgG or IgM antibodies bind to an antigen on the cell surface and activate the classical complement pathway.

(3) An anaphylactoid response due to the direct action of the drug on circulating basophils and mast cells, resulting in histamine release which appears to be related to the dose and speed of injection. Occasionally, it may involve the alternate complement pathway. Previous exposure to the drug is not a feature and systemic manifestations are usually mild.

Treatment

The diagnosis should be firmly established and airway obstruction must be excluded. Bronchospasm is usually the most life-threatening of the symptoms and treatment must primarily be aimed at preventing severe hypoxia. Endotracheal intubation and positive-pressure ventilation with 100% oxygen are often required. Intravenous adrenaline (1 in 10,000, i.e. 100 μg mL^{-1}) is the first-line drug of choice. In addition to its bronchodilator effect, adrenaline may prevent further release of histamine and improve peripheral vascular tone. In the most severe clinical circumstances, and with full cardiovascular monitoring facilities available, adrenaline may be administered by slow intravenous injection in aliquots of 3–5 mL (300–500 μg) and repeated at 5 minutes intervals until a satisfactory therapeutic response is achieved. If bronchospasm is less profound, smaller doses of adrenaline (i.e. 50–100 μg) may be effective. The development of glottic or subglottic oedema due to extravasation of fluid into the pharyngeal and laryngeal tissues may further compromise the airway. An H$_1$-receptor antagonist should be administered for the prophylaxis and treatment of this complication, and to inhibit the development of urticaria. Chlorphenamine (10 mg intravenously) is the drug of choice in this context.

Hydrocortisone hemisuccinate (up to 200 mg intravenously) should also be given. However, the maximum response may not occur for 1–6 hours and bronchospasm and hypotension may persist. The use of intravenous aminophylline or nebulized salbutamol may also be considered in cases of refractory bronchospasm. Crystalloid or colloid infusions should be used as plasma expanders, since 1–2 L of the circulating volume may have extravasated into the tissues.

Prevention of reactions

(1) The rate of injection and the dose of the induction agent should be carefully considered. The severity of many reactions is reduced by the slow administration of moderate doses of intravenous agents.

(2) Patients with a history of allergy or atopy (asthma, hay fever, eczema) may be especially sensitive to Type 1 hypersensitivity responses, particularly when there is evidence of increased IgE concentrations. The repeated exposure of these patients to induction agents known to produce such reactions is particularly hazardous. Alternative drugs or techniques involving local or regional anaesthesia should be considered.

(3) When general anaesthesia is required in such patients, premedication with an H$_1$ antagonist (e.g. chlorphenamine), an H$_2$ antagonist (e.g. ranitidine) and a corticosteroid is indicated. H$_1$ and H$_2$ antagonists may have complementary beneficial effects on the cardiovascular actions of histamine.

(4) It can be extremely important, for both therapeutic and medicolegal purposes, to distinguish between true hypersensitivity reactions and similar clinical manifestations. The latter may be associated with the enhanced pharmacological effects of the drugs involved, pharmacodynamic interactions or mechanical problems involving the airway. Plasma histamine levels can be measured by radioimmunoassay on blood samples taken after the event. Plasma levels of tryptase, a neutral proteolytic enzyme released from mast cell granules following activation and degranulation, may be elevated for approximately 6 hours after a hypersensitivity response (Chapter 6). Enhanced levels of the main metabolite of histamine, *N*-methylhistamine, may be detected in urinary samples and also aid in diagnosis. More specific investigations at a later stage may be useful to identify the responsible drug, including intradermal skin testing, estimations of IgE antibodies and possibly radioallergosorbent tests (RAST) for specific antibodies.

Total intravenous anaesthesia

Total intravenous anaesthesia (TIVA) is usually applied to techniques in which all anaesthetic agents are given intravenously during major surgical procedures. Thus, anaesthetics are used to induce hypnosis, opioids are given to prevent intraoperative pain and neuromuscular blockade is induced during controlled ventilation with oxygen-enriched air. In recent years, there has been considerable interest in TIVA due to environmental considerations and the introduction of drugs with suitable pharmacokinetic properties (e.g. propofol, alfentanil, atracurium). The use of continuous infusion techniques has considerable practical advantages, including minimal cardiovascular depression, rapid recovery and the avoidance of hazards of exposure to inhalational agents. Unfortunately, they are relatively expensive, since they usually depend on the accurate and controlled infusion of drugs with a short duration of action and a rapid recovery. In addition, they usually require precise pharmacokinetic data that have been previously collated from a defined patient population, as well as the determination and assessment of the various factors that are liable to influence the behaviour of drugs in the body. Thus, the concurrent administration of other drugs, as well as cardiovascular, renal and hepatic impairment, may affect the disposition and the activity of many intravenous agents. Present evidence suggests that there is considerable interindividual variability in the metabolism and elimination of anaesthetic drugs, at least some of which may be determined by genetic factors. Awareness and intraoperative dreaming are also problems of concern with TIVA. In spite of the obvious ecological advantages of this technique, a greater knowledge of potential drug interactions and more accurate methods of assessment of cerebral function are required before TIVA becomes a generally accepted practice. Recent studies on computer-controlled infusions of propofol has resulted in the development of target-controlled infusion systems, that can maintain appropriate plasma concentrations of propofol during surgery, and vary dose requirements to the required depth of anaesthesia. This technique has also been applied to other anaesthetic agents (e.g. remifentanil).

Suggested reading

Briggs, L.P., Clarke, R.S.J., Dundee, J.W., *et al.* (1981) Use of di-isopropylphenol as main agent for short procedures. *British Journal of Anaesthesia* **53**, 1197–1202.

Doenicke, A. (1974) Etomidate: a new intravenous hypnotic. *Acta Anaesthesiologica Belgica* **25**, 307–315.

Doenicke, A.W., Roizen, M.F., Hoernecke, R., *et al.* (1999) Solvent for etomidate may cause pain and adverse effects. *British Journal of Anaesthesia* **83**, 464–466.

Domino, E.F., Chodoff, P. & Corssen, G. (1965) Pharmacologic effects of CI 581, a new dissociative anesthetic in man. *Clinical Pharmacology and Therapeutics* **6**, 279–290.

Dundee, J.W. & Wyant, G.M. (1988) *Intravenous Anaesthesia.* Edinburgh: Churchill Livingstone.

Firestone, L.L., Quinlan, J.J. & Homanics, G.E. (1995) The role of gamma-amino butyric acid Type-A receptor subtypes in the pharmacology of general anaesthesia. *Current Opinion in Anesthesiology* **8**, 311–314.

Fryer, J.M. (2001) Intravenous induction agents. *Anaesthesia and Intensive Care Medicine* **2**, 277–281.

Hocking, G. & Cousins, M.J. (2003) Ketamine in chronic pain management: an evidence-based review. *Anesthesia and Analgesia* **97**, 1730–1739.

Laroche, D., Vergnaud, M.C., Sillard, B., *et al.* (1991) Biochemical markers of anaphylactoid reactions to drugs: comparison of plasma histamine and tryptase. *Anesthesiology* **75**, 945–949.

Liljeroth, E. & Akeson, J. (2005) Less local pain on intravenous infusion of a new propofol emulsion. *Acta Anaesthesiologica Scandinavica* **49**, 248–251.

Lingren, L. (1994) Anaesthetic activity and side effects of propofol. *Current Opinion in Anesthesiology* **7**, 321–325.

Lundy, J.S. (1935) Intravenous anesthesia: preliminary report of the use of two new thiobarbiturates. *Proceedings of Staff Meetings of the Mayo Clinic* **10**, 534–543.

Mirakhur, R.K. & Morgan, M. (1998) Intravenous anaesthesia: a step forward. *Anaesthesia* **53**(Suppl 1), 1–3.

Nau, C. & Strichartz, G.R. (2002) Drug chirality in anaesthesia. *Anesthesiology* **97**, 497–502.

Parke, T.J., Stevens, J.E., Rice, A.S.C., *et al.* (1992) Metabolic acidosis and fatal myocardial failure after propofol infusion in children: five case reports. *British Medical Journal* **305**, 613–615.

Sneyd, J.R. (2004) Recent advances in intravenous anaesthesia. *British Journal of Anaesthesia* **93**, 725–736.

Tanelian, D.L., Kosek, P., Mody, I. & MacIver, M.B. (1993) The role of GABA$_A$ receptor/chloride channel complex in anaesthesia. *Anesthesiology* **78**, 757–776.

Theilen, H.J., Adam, S., Albrecht, M.D. & Ragaller, M. (2002) Propofol in a medium and long-chain triglyceride emulsion: pharmacological characteristics and potential beneficial effects. *Anesthesia and Analgesia* **95**, 923–929.

Tomlin, S.L., Jenkins, A., Lieb, W.R., *et al.* (1998) Stereoselective effects of etomidate optical isomers on gamma-aminobutyric acid Type A receptors and animals. *Anesthesiology* **88**, 708–717.

Trotter, C. & Serpell, M.G. (1992) Neurological sequelae in children after prolonged propofol infusion. *Anaesthesia* **47**, 340–342.

Veroli, P., O'Reilly, B., Bertrand, F., *et al.* (1992) Extrahepatic metabolism of propofol in man during the anhepatic phase of orthoptic liver transplantation. *British Journal of Anaesthesia* **68**, 183–186.

Vuyk, J., Schnider, T.P. & Engbers, F. (2000) Population pharmacokinetics of propofol for target-controlled infusion (TCI) in the elderly. *Anesthesiology* **93**, 1557–1558.

White, P.F., Ham, J., Way, W.L. & Trevor, A.J. (1980) Pharmacology of ketamine isomers in surgical patients. *Anesthesiology* **52**, 231–239.

Yamakura, T., Bertaccini, E., Trudell, J.R. & Harris, R.A. (2001) Anesthetics and ion channels: molecular models and sites of action. *Annual Review of Pharmacology and Toxicology* **41**, 23–51.

8 Inhalational Anaesthetic Agents

History

Although the introduction of inhalational anaesthetics revolutionized operative surgery, their general acceptance by the medical profession was relatively slow. The effects of nitrous oxide on sensation and voluntary power were described by Joseph Priestley as early as 1772. Although the gas was first used clinically by Horace Wells in 1844, its value was only slowly acknowledged, and it was not generally used as an analgesic or an inhalational anaesthetic until the 1870s. Diethyl ether and chloroform were also introduced in the 1840s, but were more rapidly accepted. There were few further significant advances until 1934, when trichlorethylene and cyclopropane were introduced. Both these drugs possessed significant disadvantages and are now only of historical interest (Table 8.1). Some 20 years later, halothane was synthesized by Charles Suckling and studied by James Raventós and Michael Johnstone. Its introduction was a notable advance in inhalational anaesthesia, and for many years (1958–1985) it was the standard inhalational anaesthetic of choice. Its clinical use in the UK has markedly declined during the past two decades, mainly due to the extremely rare complication of 'halothane hepatitis'.

The introduction of halothane was followed by the introduction and clinical use of other fluorinated agents. Methoxyflurane was introduced by Artusio in 1959, but had significant disadvantages, such as a slow induction and recovery and its extensive metabolism and related nephrotoxicity. Enflurane was synthesized by R.C. Terrill in 1963, and was widely used for several decades, but has recently been superseded by other fluorinated agents. The only inhalational agents that are used in current practice are
- Nitrous oxide
- Halothane
- Isoflurane
- Sevoflurane
- Desflurane

The latter three drugs are all fluorinated ethers and were developed after halothane (a fluorinated hydrocarbon) was introduced into anaesthetic practice. Although halothane is still considered as the classical standard with which all other fluorinated agents are compared, it is now seldom used in the UK.

Mode of action

All inhalational anaesthetics have a relatively rapid onset of action, and their effects are readily reversible. It therefore seems improbable that their action depends on the formation of stable, covalent chemical bonds in the CNS. Inhalational anaesthesia is more likely to be related to the physical properties of individual agents, or to the formation of rapidly reversible, low energy, intermolecular forces, including Van der Waals forces, dipole–dipole interactions and ionic and hydrogen bonds.

Physicochemical properties

Most inhalational anaesthetics have certain physicochemical and biological properties in common. They are either gases or simple aliphatic hydrocarbons or ethers with 1–4 carbon atoms and have boiling points less than 90°C. They have varying anaesthetic potencies, which are closely related to their lipid solubility in organic solvents (Fig. 8.1). In addition, their anaesthetic potencies are additive, and their effects are usually modified or reversed by the application of pressure. Many simple and relatively inert chemical agents can behave as inhalational anaesthetics in appropriate circumstances, including some gases, hydrocarbons, ethers and organic solvents. Most of these agents cannot be used clinically due to their side effects or toxicity. Some compounds only produce anaesthetic effects at high partial pressures, as demonstrated by nitrogen, which requires a pressure of approximately 30 atmospheres. Consequently, the anaesthetic effects of nitrogen gas are only evident during scuba diving or similar activities.

Table 8.1 Inhalational anaesthetic agents of historical interest.

Agent	Introduction	Advantages	Disadvantages
Nitrous oxide	Horace Wells (1844)	Rapid induction and recovery No effect on cardiovascular system Not metabolized	Low potency Inactivation of vitamin B_{12} Neutropenia
Diethyl ether	William Morton (1846)	Cardiovascular stability Increased sympathetic tone Relaxation of voluntary muscle	Slow induction and recovery Irritant vapour ($\uparrow$ respiratory secretions) Postoperative nausea and vomiting Inflammable and explosive
Chloroform	James Young Simpson (1847)	High potency Non-irritant vapour Non-inflammable and non-explosive	Cardiac arrhythmias (ventricular extrasystoles and cardiac arrest during induction) Delayed hepatic necrosis (24–48 h after administration)
Trichlorethylene	Jackson (1933) Langton Hewer (1941)	Cardiovascular stability Non-irritant vapour Non-inflammable and non-explosive Potent analgesic	Slow induction and recovery Cardiac arrhythmias during induction Extensively metabolized Unstable in light and air $\rightarrow$ carbon monoxide and phosgene Reacts with soda lime $\rightarrow$ dichloracetylene
Cyclopropane	Waters and Schmidt (1934)	Rapid induction and recovery Non-irritant vapour Increased sympathetic tone	Cardiac arrhythmias (ventricular extrasystoles and ventricular tachycardia during induction) Inflammable and explosive
Halothane	Johnstone (1958)	Rapid induction and recovery Potent anaesthetic Non-inflammable and non-explosive	Halothane hepatitis (Type II hypersensitivity reaction) Cardiac arrhythmias Poor analgesic
Methoxyflurane	Artusio (1959)	Cardiovascular stability Non-irritant vapour Potent analgesic Non-inflammable and non-explosive	Slow induction and recovery Extensively metabolized (65%) Nephrotoxicity (metabolism to inorganic fluoride)
Enflurane	Terrill (1963)	Rapid induction and recovery Potent anaesthetic Non-inflammable and non-explosive	EEG effects Nephrotoxicity

Effects on synaptic transmission

Although their precise site or sites of action is uncertain, it has been recognized for many years that inhalational anaesthetics primarily affect synaptic transmission in the brain and the spinal cord. They have little or no effect on neuronal threshold potentials or axonal propagation, and many are believed to act by enhancing inhibitory postsynaptic transmission. At most synaptic junctions in the CNS, postsynaptic cell membranes are approximately 10 nm in diameter and consist of a bimolecular layer of phospholipid with intercalated molecules of protein (Fig. 1.1). Some protein molecules are receptors or ion channels that traverse the membrane, and their opening results in ionic changes that affect neuronal activity. The phospholipids immediately surrounding the ion channels (boundary lipids) are believed to modify their activity and may influence the transference of ions across the membrane.

Consequently, if inhalational agents produce anaesthesia by acting on postsynaptic membranes, they may affect either the phospholipid or the protein component of the membrane. Until 1980, it was widely believed that inhalational anaesthesia was due to biophysical changes in membrane phospholipids, although it is now considered that it is produced by effects on various protein targets in the CNS.

Phospholipid theories of anaesthesia

In 1899–1901, Meyer and Overton independently showed that the potency of many anaesthetics and hypnotics was closely related to their solubility in olive oil, relative to their aqueous solubility. Since this time, many hypotheses have been based on the correlation between anaesthetic potency and lipid-solubility, as assessed by the oil–gas partition coefficient at 37°C (Fig. 8.1). Most early theories of anaesthesia suggested that inhalational agents mainly produced their effects by acting on phospholipids in neuronal membranes. Inhalational anaesthetics were believed to initially dissolve in membrane phospholipids and change

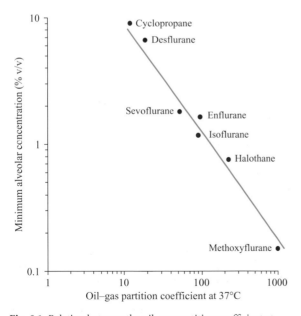

Fig. 8.1 Relation between the oil–gas partition coefficient at 37°C and the minimum alveolar concentration (% v/v) of different anaesthetic agents.

their physical properties, such as fluidity, volume, surface tension or lateral surface pressure, and thus modify the degree of order or disorder within the membrane. Alterations in the physical properties of boundary lipids were considered to have secondary effects on membrane proteins, resulting in conformational changes, which modified their activity. These changes reduced or prevented the release of neurotransmitters, or increased the volume and width of neuronal membranes, so that ion channels did not function effectively. According to these concepts, phospholipids were considered to be the primary targets of anaesthetic action, and modification of their physical properties then produced secondary effects on enzymes, receptors and ion channels. Nevertheless, it was difficult to understand how alterations in the physical properties of membrane phospholipids were primarily responsible for anaesthesia, since clinically relevant concentrations had little or no effect on pure lipid bilayers. Significant effects on lipid membranes are only produced by much higher concentrations of inhalational agents.

Pressure reversal of anaesthesia

A related hypothesis suggested that inhalational anaesthetics affected phospholipids in an inert manner, and physically modified the relationship between pressure and volume in the neuronal membrane. This theory was based on the 'pressure reversal' of anaesthesia, since numerous studies with luminous bacteria, tadpoles and mice showed that anaesthesia was reversed when external environmental pressures are increased. The pressure reversal of anaesthesia was explained by the 'critical volume hypothesis', which proposed that anaesthetics and pressure act at the same site, and by means of a common mechanism. It was considered that anaesthesia occurred when the volume of non-polar constituents expanded beyond a certain critical amount, and that when this volume was restored by changes in temperature or pressure, anaesthesia is reversed. Subsequent modifications of this hypothesis were proposed, e.g. the 'mean excess volume hypothesis' and the 'multi-site expansion hypothesis', which suggested that anaesthesia (and the pressure reversal of anaesthesia) were produced by actions at more than one type of molecular site and varied with different agents. Consequently, each anaesthetic agent produces its own pattern of CNS depression and activation.

These hypotheses are not now generally accepted. Recent experimental evidence suggests that pressure reversal is highly specific and selective, and may be due to effects on pressure-sensitive glycine channels, which play an important role in mediating inhibitory tone in the CNS. It therefore seems unlikely that anaesthesia and pressure act by means of a common mechanism. The pressure reversal of anaesthesia may be related to the high pressure neurological syndrome, which is characterized by tremor, convulsions and periods of microsleep. This condition occurs in many animals and humans at pressures above 30 atmospheres.

Protein theories of anaesthesia

Until 1980, membrane proteins were not considered to be a primary target of inhalational agents, since their well-constrained structure seemed unlikely to be modified in an identical manner by different anaesthetic molecules. Nevertheless, recent evidence suggests that inhalational agents may primarily interact with receptor proteins, producing conformational changes in their molecular structure, which affect the function of ion channels or enzymes.

In recent years, preparations of purified and soluble proteins have been used to study the effects of inhalational anaesthetics on receptors and enzymes in a lipid-free environment. Many soluble proteins and enzyme systems, including glycolytic enzymes and most voltage-gated ion channels, are unresponsive or resistant to clinical concentrations of inhalational anaesthetics. The phosphatidyl-inositol system, cyclic nucleotides and regulatory G proteins are also relatively resistant to inhalational agents. Some proteins such as haemoglobin and albumin bind to inhalational agents, and appear to undergo reversible conformational changes without any alteration in their physiological roles.

In contrast, the functional properties of other proteins, including GABA$_A$, glycine, glutamate and nicotinic receptors can be selectively modified by clinical concentrations of inhalational agents. Recent evidence suggests that fluorinated ethers and anaesthetic gases affect different receptors in the CNS. Consequently, these two groups of drugs may not produce anaesthesia in an identical manner.

Fluorinated anaesthetics

Fluorinated anaesthetics are believed to produce their effects by enhancing inhibitory transmission at postsynaptic GABA$_A$ and glycine receptors. It has been suggested that the drugs are bound by a specific binding pocket with a fixed molecular volume within these inhibitory receptor proteins. The anaesthetic binding site is formed within the second and third transmembrane domains (TM2 and TM3) of GABA$_A$ and glycine receptor subunits, approx-

imately 3 nm from the extracellular space, i.e. one third of the distance across the membrane. Two amino acids that are in adjacent positions in TM2 and TM3 (serine 19′ and alanine 40′) are believed to be specifically involved in the binding pocket, and studies with mutant receptors are consistent with their role in mediating the effects of inhalational anaesthetics.

Fluorinated agents also produce neuronal hyperpolarization in the CNS by activation of a specific background K$^+$ channel in the axonal membrane, thus affecting the resting membrane potential. There is an approximate correlation between neuronal hyperpolarization and anaesthetic potency, and although the net effect of fluorinated agents is small, it is sufficient to impair the initiation of postsynaptic action potentials in many neurons. For instance, isoflurane produces activation of K$^+$ channels in thalamocortical projection neurons, causing hyperpolarization and inhibition of tonic action potentials.

Thus, at present the balance of evidence suggests that fluorinated anaesthetics primarily affect inhibitory GABA$_A$ and glycine receptors, as well as a subgroup of potassium channels, resulting in the postsynaptic inhibition of neuronal activity and thus inducing anaesthesia.

Anaesthetic gases

The anaesthetic gases have little or no direct effect on GABA$_A$ or glycine receptors, and thus may produce anaesthesia in a fundamentally different manner. Most of the evidence suggests that they act by antagonism of glutamate at NMDA receptors (Fig. 7.4), but have little or no effect on kainate or AMPA[1] receptors, or on metabotropic glutamate receptors.

Consequently, anaesthetic gases, unlike fluorinated agents, appear to interfere with the excitatory postsynaptic neuronal currents that are normally mediated by glutamate at NMDA receptors.

Analgesia induced by nitrous oxide may increase inhibition by descending pathways from the periaqueductal gray matter to adrenergic α_2- and GABA$_A$-dependent interneurons in the spinal cord, thus inhibiting the primary nociceptive pathway.

Clinical studies

Clinical studies have also attempted to define the possible role of receptor or ion channel proteins in the pro-

---

[1] AMPA = α-amino-3-hydroxy-5-methyl-4-isoxazole proprionic acid.

Table 8.2 Some factors that affect the minimum alveolar concentration (MAC) of inhalational anaesthetics.

	Effect on MAC
Physiological and metabolic factors	
Age	
Infancy and childhood	↑
Maturity and old age	↓
Hyperthermia (>40°C)	↑
Hyperthyroidism	↑
Hypothermia (<30°C)	↓↓
Hypotension	↓
Hypothyroidism	↓
Pregnancy	↓
Postpartum period	↓
Epinephrine and norepinephrine	
Increased	↑
Decreased	↓
Pharmacological factors	
Opioid analgesics	
Acute dosage	↓
Chronic dosage	↑
α_2-Adrenoceptor agonists	↓
Sedatives and tranquillisers	↓↓
Ethyl alcohol	
Acute dosage	↓
Chronic dosage	↑
Lithium	↓
Amphetamines	
Acute dosage	↑↑↑
Chronic dosage	↓

↑ or ↓, 0–30% change; ↑↑ or ↓↓, 30–60% change; ↑↑↑, >60% change.

duction of inhalational anaesthesia. In these studies, the effects of receptor agonists or antagonists on anaesthetic potency have been assessed, as measured by changes in the minimum alveolar concentration (MAC) values of individual anaesthetics. Alterations in the MAC values of inhalational agents suggest (but do not prove) that the receptor or ion channel protein may play a part in the production of anaesthesia. For example, α_2-adrenoceptor agonists such as clonidine, azepexole and dexmedetomidine reduce the MAC values of most inhalational agents (Table 8.2) and can be used to partially replace them. These effects can be reversed or prevented by α_2-adrenoceptor antagonists (e.g. tolazoline, yohimbine), suggesting that these receptors may play an important role in the induction of anaesthesia.

Limitations of protein theories of anaesthesia

Although it is now widely accepted that inhalational anaesthetics produce their effects by interacting with protein targets in the CNS, the limitations of this approach should be recognized. It is not entirely clear how these theories account for the relationship between anaesthetic potency and lipid solubility, or the additive effects of inhalational anaesthetics that appear to have different mechanisms of action. Most drugs that act on enzymes or receptors are relatively potent, specific and stereoselective, and can be competitively or non-competitively inhibited by other drugs. Inhalational agents have none of these properties. Although there are differences in the experimental and clinical potencies of the enantiomers of isoflurane, these are much less than those usually observed with other stereoselective drugs that act on enzymes or receptor systems. In addition, it is very difficult to understand how inert or relatively inert gases such as nitrous oxide and xenon produce anaesthesia by interacting with proteins or receptors.

Site of action

Analysis of evoked cortical responses during anaesthesia shows that inhalational agents affect neuronal excitability and the conduction of impulses at many sites between the peripheral nervous system and the cerebral cortex. Although high anaesthetic concentrations can produce reversible electrical silence in the CNS, specific neuronal circuits show marked variability in their sensitivity. Excitability and synaptic transmission in the primary afferent pathway is modified, but there are also variable effects on the reticular activating system, the thalamus and basal ganglia, the hippocampus, the cerebellum, medullary centres and motor pathways in the spinal cord. Consequently, the neurological manifestations of anaesthesia appear to be due to multiple actions at different synaptic sites in the CNS.

It is generally accepted that analgesia and inhibition of responses to noxious stimuli is mainly due to selective depression of the primary afferent pathway at a spinal level, and fluorinated anaesthetics are known to directly inhibit the excitability of spinal motor neurons. In contrast, amnesia may be due to the effects of anaesthetics on the hippocampus and the limbic system, while unconsciousness may reflect effects on the thalamus and its efferent pathways, since many halogenated agents are known to depress the excitability of thalamocortical neurons.

Potency

MAC values

Inhalational anaesthetics vary greatly in potency, i.e. the alveolar concentration that is required to produce a given anaesthetic effect. Nitrous oxide is a relatively non-potent anaesthetic, and even concentrations of 80% in oxygen are usually insufficient to maintain anaesthesia. By contrast, concentrations of 15% cyclopropane, 5–10% diethyl ether or desflurane, or 1–4% of halothane, isoflurane or sevoflurane will produce general anaesthesia. These differences between inhalational anaesthetics are primarily related to their lipid-solubility. The potency of inhalational anaesthetics is traditionally expressed in terms of their MAC, i.e. the minimum steady-state concentration in oxygen that produces no reaction to a standard surgical stimulus (skin incision) in 50% of subjects at atmospheric pressure.

MAC values and lipid solubility

When the MAC (% v/v) of different inhalational agents is plotted against their lipid solubility (as expressed by their oil–gas partition coefficients at 37°C), a linear relationship is obtained (Fig. 8.1). Although this relationship was first established with olive oil, it is now known that the solubility of inhalational anaesthetics in purified solvents of rather greater polarity such as octanol or lecithin provides a better correlation with their potency, as expressed by their MAC values, and may be more representative of the presumptive site of action of inhalational anaesthetics. The Meyer–Overton correlation (page 131) suggests that ideal anaesthetic agents are amphipathic, and have both hydrophobic (non-polar) and hydrophilic (polar) properties.

Additive MAC values

When two different inhalational anaesthetics are administered simultaneously, their activities expressed as MAC values are additive (Fig. 8.2). Thus, 0.5 MAC of nitrous oxide (52%, v/v) and 0.5 MAC of halothane (0.37%, v/v) have an equal effect to 1.0 MAC of either, or of any other inhalational agent. The additive potencies of combinations of inhalational agents have been used to determine the MAC of nitrous oxide (104% v/v) and suggest that all anaesthetics may act in a similar manner (although this is clearly inconsistent with other evidence). In practice, there may be slight deviations from exact additivity, as with combinations of nitrous oxide and isoflurane. These

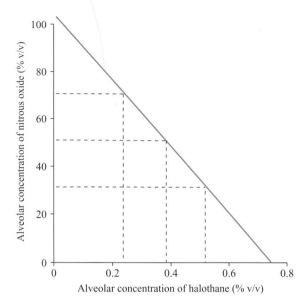

Fig. 8.2 A graph (or isobole) showing equi-effective concentrations of halothane and nitrous oxide. Each axis on the graph corresponds to the alveolar concentration of halothane or nitrous oxide. The MAC values of each agent are plotted on the coordinates of the graph and are joined by a straight line between the axes. Equi-effective combinations of the two agents (with an effect of 1 MAC) correspond to points on this line. Consequently, the potency of individual inhalational agents is additive (when expressed as MAC values).

deviations are generally considered to reflect patient variability.

The concept of MAC values has been recently extended to cover other responses to various clinical and anaesthetic endpoints. The MAC$_{awake}$ is the MAC of the anaesthetic at which response to verbal commands is lost in 50% of patients and appears to correspond to the anaesthetic concentration that produces amnesia and loss of awareness. It is invariably less than the MAC required to prevent movement in response to skin incision. In contrast, the MAC$_{intubation}$ is the MAC required to inhibit any response to tracheal intubation in 50% of patients and is invariably greater than the MAC$_{skin incision}$. The MAC$_{BAR}$ is the MAC that prevents the autonomic response to skin incision.

The MAC$_{skin incision}$ of inhalational anaesthetic agents is affected by many physiological and pharmacological factors (Table 8.2). MAC values are highest during childhood (less than 3 years of age) and progressively decline with increasing age, at the rate of approximately 0.5% per year (Fig. 8.3). They are increased in hyperthermia and hyperthyroidism, but are decreased in hypothermia by 50%

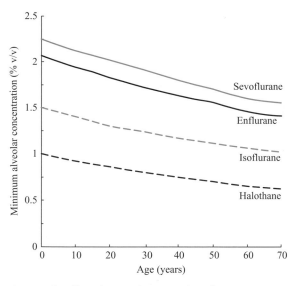

Fig. 8.3 The effect of age on the MAC value of some inhalational anaesthetics. In all instances, there is a progressive decline in MAC values with advancing age.

or more, due to the increasing solubility of inhalational anaesthetics at reduced temperatures. They are also decreased in hypotension, hypothyroidism, pregnancy and for several weeks after childbirth. Many drugs decrease the MAC values of inhalational anaesthetics, including opioid analgesics, α_2-adrenergic agonists, sedatives and tranquillisers, ethyl alcohol and lithium (Table 8.2).

Onset of action

General anaesthesia occurs when the concentration of the inhalational agent in the brain, which is reflected by its partial pressure or tension, is sufficiently great to induce loss of consciousness. The uptake and elimination of volatile anaesthetics can be considered as a series of exponential processes. During the induction of anaesthesia by the inhalation of a constant concentration of an anaesthetic agent, a series of diffusion gradients are established. These diffusion gradients occur
- between the concentration of inspired gas or vapour and its tension in pulmonary alveoli
- between the alveolar tension and the pulmonary capillary blood tension
- between the pulmonary capillary blood tension and the cerebral blood tension

- between the cerebral blood tension and the tension of the anaesthetic in the brain.

In practice, the main factor that determines the rapidity of action is the rate at which the alveolar tension (F_A) increases and approaches the inspired gas or vapour tension (F_I) (Fig. 8.4). A rapid increase in F_A produces a large diffusion gradient between the alveoli and the pulmonary capillary blood, so that its tension also rises rapidly and drives the other diffusion gradients. When equilibrium is achieved, the partial pressure of the anaesthetic in the alveoli is approximately equal to its tension in the brain.

These changes are reversed during recovery from inhalational anaesthesia. The inspired gas tension falls to zero and a series of diffusion gradients are established between the partial pressure of anaesthetic in the CNS and the exhaled vapour. The speed of recovery is mainly dependent on the rapidity with which the alveolar tension decreases, and thus produces a large diffusion gradient between pulmonary capillary blood and the alveoli. Consequently, factors that affect the onset of action of inhalational agents also affect recovery to an equal and opposite extent.

The main factors that determine the rate at which alveolar tension (F_A) increases and approaches the inspired gas or vapour tension (F_I) are
- Blood–gas partition coefficient

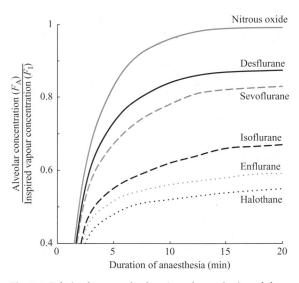

Fig. 8.4 Relation between the duration of anaesthesia and the rate of approach of alveolar concentration (F_A) to the inspired gas or vapour concentration (F_I). Inhalation anaesthetics that are less soluble in blood show a rapid rise in alveolar concentration, so that the ration F_A/F_I approaches unity.

- Pulmonary ventilation
- Inspired anaesthetic concentration
- Miscellaneous factors.

Blood–gas partition coefficient

The potency of inhalational anaesthetic agents, when expressed as their MACs, is closely related to their lipid solubility, as reflected by their oil–gas partition coefficients (Fig. 8.1). In contrast, the rate of onset of action is mainly determined by a different physical property, i.e. their solubility in blood. This is expressed numerically as the blood–gas partition coefficient at 37°C, and defined as the ratio of the amount of anaesthetic in blood and gas when the two phases are of equal volume and in equilibrium (i.e. at equal partial pressures). The blood–gas partition coefficient ranges from 0.20 (xenon) to 12.0 (diethyl ether and methoxyflurane), and is numerically equal to the Ostwald solubility coefficient (λ) in blood at 37°C.

Inhalational anaesthetics with a low blood–gas partition coefficient are poorly soluble in blood and have a rapid onset of action. During the induction of anaesthesia their alveolar concentration rapidly increases and approaches the inspired gas or vapour concentration (Fig. 8.4), and diffusion into pulmonary capillaries causes a rapid rise in their partial pressure in blood. Consequently, diffusion into the CNS occurs quickly and the onset of anaesthesia is rapid. In contrast, agents with a high blood–gas partition coefficient are more soluble in blood and have a slower onset of action. Although they are extensively removed from the alveoli due to solution in pulmonary capillary blood, their partial pressure in the alveoli and the vascular system remains relatively low. The onset of anaesthesia is therefore slower, since the diffusion gradient between cerebral blood and the CNS is relatively small. Changes in albumin and haemoglobin levels may also affect the blood–gas partition coefficient. All inhalational anaesthetics in current use in the UK have a low blood–gas partition coefficient, are poorly soluble in blood and have a rapid onset of action.

Pulmonary ventilation

In non-rebreathing systems, hyperventilation increases the rate of rise in alveolar tension of inhalational anaesthetics, resulting in the more rapid onset of anaesthesia by enhancing the diffusion gradient between cerebral blood and the CNS. Conversely, any reduction in pulmonary ventilation decreases the rate of rise in alveolar tension during inhalation of the anaesthetic. The effects of changes in ventilation are most obvious when anaesthesia is induced with a soluble agent, i.e. an agent with a high blood–gas partition coefficient, and all the anaesthetic that enters the lung is taken up by pulmonary capillary blood. In these conditions, doubling alveolar ventilation doubles anaesthetic uptake.

The functional residual capacity (FRC) of the lung also affects the alveolar tension of inhalational anaesthetics, since it acts as a buffer between the inspired concentration of a gas or vapour and its alveolar concentration. A reduction in the FRC enhances the rate at which the alveolar concentration rises, while an increase in FRC significantly slows the rate of rise in alveolar tension. Abnormal ventilation–perfusion ratios may also alter alveolar partial pressure and anaesthetic uptake, either by increasing end-tidal anaesthetic concentrations (dead-space effect), or by reducing arterial transfer (shunting effect).

Inspired anaesthetic concentration

Any increase in the inspired gas or vapour tension raises alveolar partial pressures and produces more rapid onset of anaesthesia. During induction, higher initial concentrations and higher gas flow rates than those required for the maintenance of anaesthesia are commonly used to accelerate its onset ('overpressurization'), and patients can be rapidly anaesthetized by any of the modern inhalational agents by means of this technique. It should be recognized that overpressurization in patients with a low cardiac output may result in extremely high alveolar concentrations of anaesthetic agents, which may have consequential side effects.

Miscellaneous factors

Other factors also affect the speed of induction of isoflurane and desflurane anaesthesia. For example, both drugs have a pungent, ethereal smell and may cause irritation of the upper airway, which can delay the onset of anaesthesia.

Concentration effect

The concentration effect is only observed with nitrous oxide, since this is the only agent in current use that is administered in sufficiently high volumes. When high concentrations of nitrous oxide are inhaled, the rate of rise of its arterial tension is more rapid than with lower concentrations. In an adult subject breathing an inspired concentration of 60% nitrous oxide, the uptake in the first few minutes is usually more than 1 L min^{-1}. The cause of this phenomenon is obscure.

Second gas effect

When two inhalational anaesthetics are given simultaneously, the uptake of large volumes of one agent may increase the alveolar tension of the other, thus accelerating the induction of anaesthesia. During the onset of anaesthesia, nitrous oxide is absorbed from the alveoli more rapidly than nitrogen diffuses from blood, and this phenomenon may increase the alveolar partial pressure of other anaesthetic agents. For example, when a constant concentration of halothane is inspired, the rise in its alveolar concentration is accelerated by the concurrent administration and uptake of nitrous oxide. The second gas effect lasts for approximately 10 minutes and terminates when the body is saturated with nitrous oxide.

Both the concentration effect and the second gas effect may have minor effects in accelerating the onset of anaesthesia during the first few minutes of inhalation.

Cardiac output

Changes in cardiac output may affect pulmonary capillary transit time during the induction of anaesthesia. Although a low cardiac output reduces anaesthetic uptake, it accelerates the rise in alveolar tension and the onset of anaesthesia.

These effects are only important when anaesthetic agents with a high blood–gas partition coefficient are used. When complete equilibration occurs, i.e. when the tension in the alveoli and pulmonary capillary blood are equal, diffusion ceases and no anaesthetic uptake occurs. In practice, complete equilibration is unlikely to occur since most anaesthetics are partly removed from the body by metabolism and excretion. Consequently, inhalational anaesthesia can be regarded as a state of partial equilibrium.

Anaesthetic circuit

The inspired gas or vapour tension, and the alveolar partial pressure, may be altered by the absorption of inhalational agents by various components of the anaesthetic circuit. All halogenated anaesthetics are partly soluble in rubber, and some may react with soda lime. Consequently, the concentration leaving the vaporizer and the inspired concentration may be different. In the past, the release of inhalational agents from rubber has influenced the course of subsequent anaesthesia. Since the introduction of single-use plastic breathing tubes, this problem no longer arises.

In circle breathing systems, some halogenated anaesthetics may also be taken up or react with soda lime or baralyme, especially when the absorbent is dry and warm.

In these conditions, the use of halogenated anaesthetics containing the difluoromethyl ($-CHF_2$) group (e.g. isoflurane, desflurane) may result in the formation of carbon monoxide, and the conversion of haemoglobin to carboxyhaemoglobin. This reaction does not occur in the presence of moisture, or if the soda lime (or baralyme) is normally (6–19%) hydrated.

The effect of ventilation on the uptake of inhalational agents is also influenced by anaesthetic systems. In non-rebreathing systems, anaesthetic uptake is primarily dependent upon ventilation, since the inspired concentration is set by the vaporizer. By contrast, in a circle system the inspired concentration depends upon the expired concentration, as well as the anaesthetic in the fresh gas supply. When anaesthetic uptake is low due to hypoventilation, higher concentrations are expired. Nevertheless, more anaesthetic is still added to the system, thus increasing the inspiratory concentration, the alveolar–arterial gradient and anaesthetic uptake. This will tend to compensate for any reduction in alveolar ventilation. In contrast, the effect of changes in cardiac output on alveolar concentration is greater in circle systems, since the uptake of anaesthetics by the blood has a greater effect on the residual concentration in the circuit.

Effects of chronic exposure to inhalational anaesthetics

In recent decades, there has been considerable interest in the effects of chronic occupational exposure to small concentrations of inhalational anaesthetics. Hospital staff working in operating theatres may be continually exposed to trace amounts of inhalational anaesthetics, and small concentrations of volatile agents or their metabolites can be detected in plasma, urine and exhaled air for several days after exposure. The hazards of chronic occupational exposure are poorly defined, although a number of epidemiological studies have attempted to assess the possible risks in female anaesthetists. It was concluded that there is no significant evidence that exposure to or administration of inhalational anaesthetics during pregnancy increases the risk of miscarriages or fetal malformations.

In other studies, abnormal liver function tests have been observed in anaesthetists chronically exposed to low concentrations of halogenated anaesthetics. In some instances, this was associated with hepatitis which resolved when exposure to inhalational agents ceased. The subacute and chronic effects of nitrous oxide have also been of particular concern (pages 142–143).

Although the hazards of trace concentrations of inhalational anaesthetics appear to be extremely small, large numbers of hospital staff may be chronically exposed to these agents. Consequently, efficient monitoring and scavenging systems are now widely used in operating theatres in most developed countries. Despite their high cost, these systems minimize the hazards of exposure to inhalational anaesthetics in the operating theatre. Similarly, the use of low-flow anaesthesia tends to reduce occupational exposure to inhalational agents.

In the UK, a series of Occupational Exposure Standards were adopted in 1996. During an 8-hour reference period the maximum average exposure to anaesthetic agents should be: nitrous oxide, 100 ppm; isoflurane, 50 ppm; halothane 10 ppm. These concentrations are about 20% of the levels known to have no effects in experimental animals.

Metabolism of inhalational anaesthetics

Since the 1960s, it has been generally recognized that most inhalational anaesthetics are metabolized to a variable extent. Metabolism mainly occurs in the liver and is dependent on the chemical structure of the individual agents. All of the halogenated anaesthetics in current use contain more than one carbon–halogen bond (C–F, C–Cl, or C–Br), which differ in their susceptibility to drug metabolism. In general, C–F bonds are highly stable, so the trifluoromethyl group (CF_3) in halothane, isoflurane, desflurane and sevoflurane is not significantly metabolized. In contrast, the C–Cl and C–Br bonds in halothane are less stable, and are extensively metabolized.

Because of these considerations, the metabolism of individual fluorinated agents declines in the order halothane (20%) > sevoflurane (3%) > isoflurane (0.2%) > desflurane (0.02%). The carbon–halogen bonds are broken down by oxidative enzymes, resulting in the release of reactive metabolites and halogen ions (F^-, Br^- or Cl^-).

Inhalational anaesthetics are mainly metabolized by the cytochrome P450 enzyme system in the liver. One of the isoforms of this enzyme system (CYP 2E1) is responsible for the defluorination of most common inhalational anaesthetics. Enzyme induction with ethanol or isoniazid (but not barbiturates or phenytoin) increases the rate of defluorination, and CYP 2E1 may also be induced by fasting, obesity and diabetic ketosis. Halothane is metabolized by this enzyme system, although it is not significantly defluorinated, except in hypoxic conditions.

In general, the toxicity of inhalational anaesthetics appears to be related to their metabolism. Anaesthetic agents that are significantly metabolized by hepatic enzyme systems are particularly associated with renal and hepatic toxicity. This factor has played a major role in the replacement of these drugs by more modern fluorinated agents, which are only metabolized to a limited extent, and are not significantly affected by most enzyme inducing agents. All current fluorinated agents are relatively potent and have low blood and tissue solubilities, which will tend to limit their accumulation in the body. Consequently, the toxic hazards associated with the metabolism of inhalational anaesthetics have progressively declined since the introduction of newer inhalational anaesthetics into clinical practice.

Metabolism of halothane
The metabolism of halothane may be oxidative or reductive, depending on the prevalent oxygen tension in the hepatocyte.

Oxidative metabolism
In oxidative conditions, approximately 20–25% of halothane is metabolized by CYP 2E1 to trifluoroacetic acid, chloride and bromide ions, which are slowly excreted in urine. There is little or no defluorination of halothane, and fluoride ions are not formed. Bromide ions may be detected in the body for several weeks after prolonged anaesthesia, and their concentration may be high enough to cause significant postoperative sedation.

Reductive metabolism
During hypoxia, halothane is partly reduced, resulting in the formation of fluoride and other reduced metabolites (chlorotrifluoroethane and chlorodifluoroethylene), which are excreted in a conjugated form in urine. The reductive metabolism of halothane is believed to be responsible for the mild and transient liver damage that occurs in approximately 25% of patients within 3 days of administration, and is associated with increases in aminotransferases but few abnormal clinical signs or abnormalities. This relatively common type of hepatic dysfunction appears to be related to slight hypoxia, particularly in the centrilobular region of hepatic lobules, and is normally associated with the reductive metabolism of halothane.

Hepatotoxicity (halothane hepatitis)
Postoperative jaundice and death after exposure to halothane were first reported soon after its introduction

in 1958. Halothane anaesthesia occasionally causes fulminant hepatic necrosis with a high mortality rate (typically, 50–80%). The condition usually occurs within 5 days of exposure to the drug and is accompanied by a large increase in aminotransferase levels. The duration of exposure is not usually critical, and many cases occurred after relatively short procedures. The overall incidence of hepatic necrosis is approximately 1 in 10,000 (range: 1 in 7000 to 1 in 35,000). It is commoner, and has a higher mortality, after repeated anaesthesia with halothane, with a maximum susceptibility interval of 28 days between successive exposures. It is generally considered to be impossible to entirely eliminate the risk of halothane hepatitis, except by avoiding the use of the drug.

In recent years, the immunological basis of halothane hepatitis has been clarified, and the condition is now considered to be a Type II hypersensitivity reaction. One of the oxidative metabolites of halothane, trifluoroacetyl chloride, is covalently bound to lysine residues on hepatic proteins (including isoforms of cytochrome P450). In susceptible individuals, the trifluoroacetylated proteins initiate an immune response, inducing the formation of antibodies that react with liver cells. Serum antibodies to trifluoroacetyl–lysine residues can be detected in about 70% of patients with halothane hepatitis, and antibody titres usually persist for 1–5 years. For unknown reasons, only a small percentage of individuals are sensitive to the antigen.

Halothane is normally metabolized to trifluoroacetic acid by the enzyme isoform CYP 2E1, which is inhibited by disulfiram. It has been suggested that this drug may decrease the formation of trifluoroacetyl chloride, and may thus prevent the occurrence of halothane hepatitis. Other fluorinated agents are converted to trifluoroacetate but do not appear to produce hepatitis, presumably due to their less extensive hepatic metabolism.

Properties of individual anaesthetic agents

The biological and physical properties of individual anaesthetic agents are summarized in Tables 8.3 and 8.4.

Nitrous oxide

In 1772, Joseph Priestley prepared nitrous oxide and described its subjective and objective effects on sensation and voluntary power. Approximately 20 years later Humphrey Davy suggested that its analgesic properties might be useful in the management of pain during operative surgery. Nevertheless, its potential advantages as an analgesic and inhalational anaesthetic were ignored for many years, and its acceptance by the medical profession was extremely slow. In 1844, Horace Wells, an American dentist, first used nitrous oxide to facilitate dental extraction, but his clinical demonstration of its effects was unsuccessful and disastrous, and its use fell into disrepute for about 20–30 years.

In the 1870s, it was recognized that nitrous oxide was a useful analgesic but had a relatively low anaesthetic potency, and that adequate oxygenation was required during anaesthesia. Since then, the gas has been frequently used as an adjuvant and as a vehicle for the administration of more potent agents during inhalational anaesthesia. It is also used to provide analgesia (particularly in obstetric practice) as an equal mixture of nitrous oxide and oxygen (50%:50%, v/v; Entonox).

General properties

At ambient temperatures and pressures, nitrous oxide is a colourless and odourless gas that boils at $-88°C$ and is heavier than air (specific gravity = 1.54). Although it is non-flammable, it strongly supports combustion. It is usually prepared by heating ammonium nitrate at 240°C, and if the reaction temperature is not precisely controlled, higher oxides of nitrogen are formed. Nitrous oxide normally contains small concentrations of nitric oxide (approximately 5 parts per billion), which can improve oxygenation, but its contamination by higher oxides of nitrogen (e.g. nitrogen dioxide) can have fatal effects in anaesthetized patients. After preparation, compressed nitrous oxide is cooled to $-40°C$, cleaned and then stored as a liquid under pressure in tanks or steel cylinders.

Nitrous oxide is a relatively insoluble agent with a low blood–gas partition coefficient (0.46). It has a lower lipid solubility than other anaesthetics, and its oil–gas solubility coefficient is only 1.4.

Induction and recovery

Both induction and recovery from anaesthesia are extremely rapid, and its alveolar concentration rapidly approaches the inspired gas concentration (Fig. 8.4).

Table 8.3 Biological properties of inhalational anaesthetics in current use in the UK.

Properties	Nitrous oxide	Halothane	Isoflurane	Sevoflurane	Desflurane
Onset/offset of action	Extremely rapid	Less rapid	Rapid	Extremely rapid	Extremely rapid
Analgesic properties	Marked	Poor	Moderate	Moderate	Moderate
Effect on respiration	Non-irritant Respiratory rate ↑ Tidal volume ↓ Pa_{CO_2} normal (enters air spaces)	Non-irritant Respiratory rate ↑ Tidal volume ↓↓ Pa_{CO_2} ↑	Slightly irritant Respiratory rate ↑ Tidal volume ↓↓ Pa_{CO_2} ↑	Non-irritant Respiratory rate ↑ Tidal volume ↓↓ Pa_{CO_2} ↑	Pungent and irritant Respiratory rate ↑ Tidal volume ↓↓ Pa_{CO_2} ↑
Effect on cardiovascular system	Little or no effect Cardiac sensitivity to catecholamines ↑ / ↓	Heart rate ↓↓ BP ↓↓ Cardiac output ↓↓ Peripheral resistance → Cardiac sensitivity to catecholamines ↑↑↑	Heart rate ↑↑ BP ↓↓ Cardiac output ↓ Peripheral resistance ↓↓ Cardiac sensitivity to catecholamines ↑ Coronary steal ?	Heart rate ↑ / ↓ BP ↓↓ Cardiac output ↓ (slight) Peripheral resistance ↓ Cardiac sensitivity to catecholamines ↑ Coronary steal ?	Heart rate ↑ BP ↓↓ Cardiac output ↓ Peripheral resistance ↓↓ Cardiac sensitivity to catecholamines ↑ Coronary steal ?
Effects on electroencephalogram	None	Decreased voltage Burst suppression	Decreased voltage Burst suppression	Decreased voltage Burst suppression	Decreased voltage Burst suppression
Cerebral blood flow	↑	↑↑↑	↑	↑	↑
Potentiation of non-depolarizing blockade	None	Moderate	Marked	Marked	Marked
Effect on uterus	None	Slight relaxation	Slight relaxation	Slight relaxation	Slight relaxation
Metabolism (%)	Minimal	15–25	0.2	3	0.02
Fluoride production	None	Minimal	Minimal	Significant	Minimal
Toxicity and hypersensitivity reactions	Inactivation of vitamin B_{12} Neutropenia	Hepatic damage (rare)	None	Renal toxicity?	None

↑ or ↓, minimal change; ↑↑ or ↓↓, moderate change; ↑↑↑, marked change; ↑ / ↓, no change.

Table 8.4 Physical properties of inhalational anaesthetics that are currently available in the UK.

	Boiling point at atmospheric pressure (°C)	Vapour pressure at 20°C (kPa)	MAC in O$_2$ (% v/v)	MAC in 70% N$_2$O (v/v)	Oil–gas partition coefficient	Blood–gas partition coefficient
Nitrous oxide	−88	5200	104		1.4	0.46
Halothane	50.2	32.4	0.75	0.26	224	2.3
Isoflurane	48.5	31.9	1.17	0.41	98	1.4
Sevoflurane	58.5	21.3	1.8	0.62	53	0.65
Desflurane	23.5	88.3	6.6	2.3	19	0.42

During induction, nitrous oxide may cause exhilaration and euphoria. In the nineteenth century, it became generally known as 'laughing gas', as subjects who inhaled it became jovial and boisterous. Unpremedicated patients solely anaesthetized with nitrous oxide and oxygen may also experience bizarre dreams during surgery.

Although nitrous oxide has a low blood solubility, it diffuses across membranes some 15 times more rapidly than oxygen, and 25 times more rapidly than nitrogen. Consequently, nitrous oxide diffuses across the alveolar epithelium into pulmonary capillaries more rapidly than oxygen, and the alveolar oxygen tension may therefore temporarily increase during induction (page 137). Reverse changes may occur during recovery from anaesthesia, due to the rapid diffusion of nitrous oxide from pulmonary capillary blood into the alveoli and its less rapid replacement by atmospheric nitrogen, and may cause temporary hypoxia ('diffusion hypoxia'). Nitrous oxide diffuses through tissues more readily than other anaesthetics, and in the average adult, the percutaneous diffusion rate is about 10 mL min^{-1}.

Since nitrous oxide is more diffusible than oxygen or nitrogen, it rapidly enters enclosed air-containing spaces more rapidly than oxygen or nitrogen can leave. These spaces include the cuff of an endotracheal tube, the bowel, pneumothoraces and air emboli, and nitrous oxide will increase their volume by an amount that is related to its alveolar concentration. During prolonged intra-abdominal procedures, distension of the gut may adversely affect operating conditions and make wound closure more difficult. Similarly, administration of 75% nitrous oxide doubles the size of a pneumothorax in 10 minutes, and triples it in 30–45 minutes. Nitrous oxide may also cause pressure changes in some non-compliant spaces, such as the middle ear, nasal sinuses and the eye.

Potency

Nitrous oxide is not a potent anaesthetic, due to its low lipid solubility, and its MAC is 104% v/v at atmospheric pressure.[2] The low potency of nitrous oxide restricts its use as an inhalational anaesthetic, and when the inspired concentration of nitrous oxide is more than 70%, arterial and tissue hypoxia may occur. A mixture of nitrous oxide and oxygen (usually 65% : 5%) is widely used as a carrier gas for more potent inhalational agents, or is administered with other drugs.

Analgesia

Nitrous oxide is a powerful analgesic, and inhalation of 20–50% mixtures in oxygen may have similar effects to standard doses of morphine or pethidine. A mixture of nitrous oxide and oxygen containing equal volumes of both gases (Entonox) is widely used in obstetric practice to relieve pain during childbirth and in minor surgical procedures. The explanation for the analgesic effects of nitrous oxide is uncertain. Recent evidence suggests that nitrous oxide produces analgesia by acting on central opioid receptors in the periaqueductal grey matter in the brain stem. This pathway projects to the dorsal horn of the spinal cord, where it acts via α$_2$-adrenergic receptors to inhibit pain. Analgesia induced by nitrous oxide is partially reversed by opioid antagonists e.g. naloxone. In addition, nitrous oxide can antagonize glutamate at NMDA receptors, and interferes with the excitatory postsynaptic neuronal currents that are normally mediated by this neurotransmitter.

---

[2] The MAC of nitrous oxide can be determined by hyperbaric techniques, or by the additive potencies, when expressed as MAC values, of individual inhalational agents; thus, 0.5 MAC halothane + 0.5 MAC nitrous oxide is equivalent to 1.0 MAC of either agent.

Respiratory effects

In anaesthetic concentrations, nitrous oxide tends to increase the respiratory rate, and thus compensates for any decrease in tidal volume, so that alveolar ventilation and Pa_{CO_2} are maintained at normal levels. However, nitrous oxide depresses the ventilatory response to increased Pa_{CO_2} or hypoxaemia, in a similar manner to other anaesthetic agents. Nitrous oxide anaesthesia is associated with a reduction in FRC, an increased incidence of atelectasis and a reduced Pa_{O_2} during the postoperative period. It also depresses mucociliary function and has a depressant effect on neutrophil motility.

Cardiovascular effects

Although nitrous oxide slightly reduces myocardial contractility, it increases sympathetic activity by its central effects. In most patients, the increase in sympathetic activity counteracts the direct myocardial depressant effects, and may also reduce the depressant effects of other inhalational agents. Consequently, administration of 70% nitrous oxide usually has no significant effect on haemodynamic performance, even in patients undergoing coronary artery surgery. Heart rate is generally unaffected by nitrous oxide, but systemic vascular resistance may increase slightly due to sympathetic stimulation. Extrasystoles or ectopic rhythms are only rarely induced and there is no evidence that sensitivity to endogenous or exogenous catecholamines is modified. Thus, nitrous oxide is not contraindicated in patients with serious cardiac disease.

Nitrous oxide increases cerebral blood flow and may also potentiate similar responses to halogenated inhalational agents. Consequently, it is sometimes avoided in subjects with serious intracranial pathology. In other patients, these effects are relatively minor and of little practical importance.

Metabolism

There is no evidence that significant amounts of nitrous oxide are metabolized in man. In this respect, the anaesthetic may differ from some other inhalational agents. Extremely small amounts may be converted to nitrogen during the oxidation of vitamin B_{12}, and some may also be reduced to nitrogen by intestinal bacteria.

Methionine synthase inhibition and DNA synthesis

The prolonged administration of nitrous oxide inhibits methionine synthase and thus interferes with the formation of methionine, with subsequent effects on deoxythymidine and DNA synthesis (Fig. 8.5). Nitrous

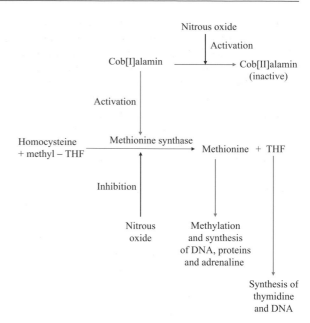

Fig. 8.5 Metabolic pathways that are affected by nitrous oxide. The active form of Vitamin B_{12} (cob[I]alamin) is the cofactor of methionine synthase and activates the enzyme. Nitrous oxide oxidizes the cobalt ion in vitamin B_{12} from this active monovalent form (cob[I]alamin) to an inactive divalent form (cob[II]alamin), thus reducing the activity of methionine synthase. Nitrous oxide also directly inactivates the enzyme, possibly due to the production of free radicals. The resultant inhibition of methionine synthase impairs the synthesis of methionine and tetrahydrofolate (THF) and has subsequent effects on DNA and protein synthesis.

oxide oxidizes the cobalt ion in vitamin B_{12} from the monovalent form [Cob(I)alamin] to the divalent form [Cob(II)alamin], which is relatively inactive. Since monovalent vitamin B_{12} is the cofactor of methionine synthase, the oxidation of vitamin B_{12} impairs the activity of this enzyme system. Nitrous oxide also directly inactivates methionine synthase, possibly due to the production of free radicals.

Clinical effects of methionine synthase inhibition

The clinical effects of impaired vitamin B_{12} metabolism and methionine synthesis are relatively rapid, and exposure to nitrous oxide for 2–24 hours may have effects on DNA synthesis and cause megaloblastic changes in bone marrow. More prolonged exposure to nitrous oxide (4–6 days) results in agranulocytosis, although some patients are relatively resistant. These effects are accompanied by a decrease in serum methionine. After exposure to nitrous oxide has ceased, the marrow gradually returns to normal within approximately 1 week. Recovery can be accelerated by folinic acid, which acts as an alternative source of tetrahydrofolate and restores normal thymidine synthesis within several hours. Administration of methionine, even in large dosages, is less effective. Although vitamin B_{12} may assist recovery, the time required for the formation of new methionine synthase (2–3 days) appears to be the main rate-limiting factor. Intermittent or repeated exposure to nitrous oxide within a short period may not allow sufficient time for enzyme activity to recover.

Nitrous oxide has little or no effect on vitamin B_{12} or methionine synthase at inhaled concentrations of 450 ppm or less, regardless of the duration of exposure. Concentrations in a scavenged operating theatre are approximately 50 ppm and the possible hazards of occupational exposure to nitrous oxide are relatively slight. Hospital staff working in unscavenged operating theatres are exposed to concentrations between 200 and 400 ppm, but have normal serum methionine levels. In contrast, prolonged exposure to nitrous oxide in heavily contaminated and unscavenged environments (e.g. dental surgeries) can produce neurological syndromes resembling subacute combined degeneration of the spinal cord, and their occurrence presumably reflects the chronic deficiency in vitamin B_{12} induced by nitrous oxide.

Teratogenic effects

In experimental animals, nitrous oxide is a mild teratogen when administered in concentrations of 50% or more for several days. These effects can be prevented by pretreatment with folinic acid, suggesting their relationship to impaired DNA synthesis. There is very little convincing evidence that exposure to nitrous oxide in early pregnancy (either as a patient or as a hospital employee) results in any adverse effects, in spite of the very large numbers of women that have been exposed over many years. Nevertheless, it may be considered prudent to avoid exposure to nitrous oxide during the first 6 weeks of pregnancy or to cover the anaesthetic with folinic acid.

Isoflurane

Chiral centre

Isoflurane (1-chloro-2,2,2-trifluoroethyl difluoromethyl ether) was synthesized by R.C. Terrell during the 1960s, and is now widely used as an inhalational agent in the UK and most developed countries. Isoflurane is a chiral drug, which is administered clinically as a racemic mixture of R(−) and S(+) isoflurane. In some *in vitro* and *in vivo* studies, the S(+) enantiomer is 40–100% more active than the R(−) enantiomer.

General properties

Isoflurane is a volatile colourless liquid that boils at 48.5°C and is not flammable at normal anaesthetic concentrations. It is extremely stable at ambient temperatures and does not decompose in the presence of light or react with hydrated soda lime. Its oil–gas partition coefficient at 37°C is 98, and its MAC value at 40 years of age is 1.17% v/v in oxygen (Fig. 8.3).

Isoflurane is relatively insoluble and has a low blood–gas partition coefficient (1.4). Consequently, the induction of anaesthesia is usually rapid and the level of anaesthesia is easily controlled. Unfortunately, isoflurane may cause problems (e.g. breath-holding) during the induction of anaesthesia. Inhaled concentrations of 2–4% are required for induction, and 1–2% for the maintenance of anaesthesia. Isoflurane has analgesic properties when administered in subanaesthetic concentrations (0.5%) and has been used to provide analgesia for burns dressings.

Respiratory effects

During spontaneous ventilation, isoflurane causes respiratory depression, which is usually reversed by surgical stimulation. The respiratory rate rises, tidal volume decreases and the minute volume is reduced. In spontaneously breathing subjects, Pa_{CO_2} increases and the ventilatory response to carbon dioxide is diminished. Respiratory responses to hypoxia and hypoxic pulmonary vasoconstriction are also depressed.

Isoflurane has a slightly pungent and ethereal odour; it irritates the upper airway, but does not cause bronchoconstriction in normal subjects. Isoflurane has mild bronchodilator effects and causes a reversible depression in mucus production.

Cardiovascular effects

Heart

Isoflurane has little or no direct effect on the heart, and anaesthetic concentrations (1–1.5 MAC) only cause a slight fall in myocardial contractility and stroke volume. Isoflurane causes peripheral vasodilatation and lowers blood pressure, but has only slight depressant effects on baroreceptor function. Consequently, reflex sympathetic activity is increased, and there is a variable rise in pulse rate, which usually maintains cardiac output above preoperative levels. In younger subjects, there may be considerable tachycardia. In the elderly, baroreceptor reflexes are often depressed and little or no change in pulse rate may occur. In these conditions, cardiac output may fall.

In general, isoflurane does not affect AV conduction or cardiac rhythm, although it may prolong the increased conduction time produced by β-adrenergic blockade or calcium channel blockers. In addition, isoflurane does not significantly sensitize the heart to adrenaline or other catecholamines.

Peripheral blood vessels

Isoflurane decreases peripheral resistance and is a potent vasodilator (particularly at higher concentrations). In many vascular beds, it maintains or increases blood flow and therefore allows better tissue oxygenation. In the cerebral circulation, low concentrations of isoflurane (<1 MAC) do not increase cerebral blood flow or intracranial pressure, although significant vasodilatation may occur with higher concentrations. There is little or no impairment of cerebral autoregulation or CO_2 responsiveness, and isoflurane is commonly used as an inhalational agent in neurosurgery.

Coronary blood vessels

The use of isoflurane in patients with coronary artery disease is controversial. Isoflurane is a potent coronary vasodilator, and it has been suggested that the drug may cause redistribution of blood in the coronary circulation ('coronary steal'), and thus induce myocardial ischaemia. In this phenomenon, blood is diverted from a myocardial area with inadequate perfusion to an area with relatively normal perfusion by dilatation of the coronary vasculature. Studies in experimental animals with stenosed coronary vessels suggest that isoflurane reduces blood flow through the stenosed segment, but increases perfusion in normal vasculature. Nevertheless, isoflurane appears to have little or no effect on the overall incidence of ischaemic episodes or mortality associated with bypass surgery.

Other factors modify myocardial blood flow and thus affect the incidence of intraoperative ischaemia. Hypotension and tachycardia may induce myocardial ischaemia, particularly if the ratio of mean blood pressure to heart rate falls to less than 1. These effects are not uncommon during isoflurane anaesthesia due to peripheral vasodilatation and the reflex increase in heart rate. Consequently, isoflurane is sometimes avoided in patients with severe coronary artery disease, particularly when associated with left ventricular failure. In susceptible patients, it is clearly important that the blood pressure is maintained, and that tachycardia is avoided.

Other effects

Isoflurane causes relaxation of voluntary muscle and enhances the effects of non-depolarizing muscle relaxants. The phenomenon is due to central effects, as well as its peripheral actions on voluntary muscle. Potentiation rapidly disappears when the anaesthetic is discontinued.

Isoflurane depresses cortical EEG activity and does not induce abnormal electrical activity or convulsions. It also causes relaxation of uterine smooth muscle, but can be used in low concentrations (0.5–0.75%) to prevent awareness during Caesarean section.

Metabolism and toxicity

Isoflurane is mainly eliminated unchanged and only 0.2% of the dose is metabolized by hepatic enzyme systems (mainly CYP 2E1). The main metabolites are trifluoroacetic acid, fluoride ions and small amounts of other fluorinated compounds. Peak inorganic fluoride levels are approximately $5 \, \mu\text{mol L}^{-1}$. Even when hepatic enzyme-inducing agents are also given, they are never high enough to cause renal damage.

Sevoflurane

$$F - \overset{\overset{\displaystyle H}{|}}{\underset{\underset{\displaystyle H}{|}}{C}} - O - \overset{\overset{\displaystyle CF_3}{|}}{\underset{\underset{\displaystyle H}{|}}{C}} - CF_3$$

Sevoflurane (1-trifluoromethyl-2,2,2-trifluoroethyl monofluoromethyl ether) was synthesized in the 1970s, but its introduction into clinical practice was delayed, due to the occurrence of toxicity in experimental animals. It was originally used as an inhalational agent in Japan and is now widely used in the UK, particularly in paediatric practice.

General properties

Sevoflurane is a volatile colourless liquid that boils at 58.5°C, and its vapour pressure at 20°C is 160 mm Hg (21.3 kPa). It is non-flammable in air and relatively stable at ambient temperatures.

Sevoflurane is relatively insoluble in blood and has a low blood–gas partition coefficient (0.65); it is slightly more soluble than nitrous oxide and desflurane. Since its tissue–blood partition coefficients are also low, induction and recovery from anaesthesia are extremely rapid, and the level of anaesthesia is easily controlled. Sevoflurane is less soluble than isoflurane in the plastic and rubber components of anaesthetic circuitry, which is an advantage in low flow systems.

Sevoflurane has an oil–gas partition coefficient at 37°C of 53, and its MAC value at age 40 is 1.80% v/v in oxygen (Fig. 8.3). Consequently, it is less lipid-soluble and less potent than isoflurane. Inhaled concentrations of 5–7% are required for induction, and 1–3% for the maintenance of anaesthesia. When administered in subanaesthetic concentrations, sevoflurane has analgesic properties.

Unlike other fluorinated agents, sevoflurane is partially hydrolysed on prolonged contact with water, or on exposure to strong bases. The degradation of sevoflurane by soda lime and baralyme is temperature dependent, and results in the formation of five breakdown products (compounds A, B, C, D and E). Only compounds A and B are produced in conditions encountered in clinical practice. Compound A (pentafluoroisopropenyl fluoromethylether, PIFE) may cause renal tubular necrosis when administered to rats in concentrations of 50 ppm for 3 hours, or 200 ppm for 1 hour. These concentrations are approximately 2–8 times greater than the equivalent levels produced in anaesthetic circuits during anaesthesia. Increased amounts of compound A are produced by high temperatures, raised concentrations of sevoflurane and low-flow anaesthesia. They are also higher with baralyme than with soda lime due to the higher temperatures that are present. Compound A is conjugated with cysteine and subsequently broken down in the kidney by β-lyase, resulting in the formation of a toxic metabolite. During clinical anaesthesia, compound B (pentafluoromethoxyisopropyl fluoromethylether, PMFE) is also produced by soda lime or baralyme. In closed circuit anaesthesia, compound B can be detected in 70% of patients, although only trace amounts are present (less than 1.5 ppm).

Sevoflurane is a chemical analogue of isoflurane and contains 7 fluorine atoms per molecule. Unlike most other fluorinated agents, it is an achiral compound and has no optical activity.

Respiratory effects

Sevoflurane is a respiratory depressant and has similar effects to other inhalational anaesthetics. It produces a rise in the respiratory rate, with a decrease in the tidal volume and minute volume. In spontaneously breathing subjects $PaCO_2$ increases, and the ventilatory response to increases in CO_2 is depressed. Respiratory depression is usually reduced or diminished by surgical stimulation. Sevoflurane has a pleasant smell and does not irritate the airway.

Cardiovascular effects

Heart

Sevoflurane has little or no direct effect on the heart. Although cardiac contractility is occasionally depressed, cardiac output is usually maintained at preoperative levels. Heart rate is normally stable and tachycardia is uncommon. Cardiac rhythm and AV conduction are usually unaffected and arrhythmias are extremely rare. Nevertheless, sevoflurane may prolong the increased conduction time produced by β-adrenergic blockade or calcium channel blockers. Like other fluorinated ethers, it does not significantly sensitize the heart to adrenaline or other catecholamines.

Peripheral blood vessels

Sevoflurane reduces systemic vascular resistance and lowers blood pressure. Blood flow is maintained or increased in the splanchnic and renal circulation. Cerebral vascular resistance is also decreased, and cerebral blood flow may increase slightly. Sevoflurane also increases coronary blood flow although it does not appear to cause coronary steal.

Other effects

Sevoflurane causes relaxation of voluntary muscle and enhances the effects of non-depolarizing muscle relaxants. The effects on the neuromuscular junction are similar to equipotent concentrations of isoflurane. This phenomenon is due to both central and peripheral effects, and potentiation rapidly disappears when the anaesthetic is discontinued. Sevoflurane, like other inhalational anaesthetics, may be a triggering agent for malignant hyperpyrexia in susceptible individuals. Sevoflurane also causes relaxation of uterine muscle, although small concentrations are used during elective Caesarean section.

Sevoflurane suppresses EEG activity and does not cause epileptiform activity during normocapnia or hypocapnia. Higher concentrations (>2 MAC) may increase intracranial pressure and decrease the cerebral metabolic rate by approximately 50%. In children, restlessness, agitation and increased coughing may occur.

Metabolism and toxicity

Sevoflurane is more extensively metabolized than other fluorinated ethers, and approximately 3–5% of the inhaled anaesthetic is converted to carbon dioxide, inorganic fluoride and hexafluoroisopropanol by the liver. The metabolism is dependent on CYP 2E1, which can be induced by ethyl alcohol or isoniazid, and possibly phenobarbitone. Enzyme induction increases the formation of the metabolites of sevoflurane.

Significant plasma fluoride concentrations (approximately 20–50 μmol L^{-1}) may occur during anaesthesia or the early postoperative period. Levels are usually maximal at 1–2 hours and return to normal within 24–48 hours. The main organic fluoride metabolite is hexafluoroisopropanol, which is rapidly converted to a glucuronide conjugate with a relatively long half-life (about 55 h). Fluoride production can be decreased by disulfiram (a selective inhibitor of CYP 2E1).

Desflurane

$$H-\overset{\displaystyle F}{\underset{\displaystyle F}{C}}-O-\overset{\displaystyle H}{\underset{\displaystyle F}{C}}-\overset{\displaystyle F}{\underset{\displaystyle F}{C}}-F$$

Chiral centre

Desflurane (1-fluoro-2,2,2-trifluoroethyl difluoromethyl ether) was synthesized in the 1960s, although clinical studies of its suitability as an inhalational anaesthetic only began in 1987. It is closely related chemically to isoflurane. Desflurane is also a chiral compound and is administered clinically as an equal mixture of two stereoisomers.

General properties

Desflurane is an extremely volatile and colourless liquid that boils at 23.5°C, and its vapour pressure at 20°C is 669 mm Hg (88.3 kPa). Consequently, it cannot be given by conventional means, and a heated and pressurized vaporizer is required for its administration. It is non-flammable and extremely stable at ambient temperatures and does not decompose in the presence of light or react with hydrated soda lime or baralyme. Desflurane is relatively insoluble in blood and has a lower blood–gas partition coefficient than

any other inhalational anaesthetic (0.42). Thus, induction and recovery from anaesthesia should be more rapid than with other inhalational agents, and the level of anaesthesia should be easier to control. Unfortunately, its clinical use is associated with several disadvantages.

The oil–gas partition coefficient of desflurane at 37°C is 19, and its MAC value in oxygen is 6.6% v/v, so it is less potent than other fluorinated agents. Inhaled concentrations of 6–9% are required for induction, and 4–6% for the maintenance of anaesthesia. When administered in subanaesthetic concentrations, desflurane has analgesic properties.

Respiratory effects

Desflurane is a respiratory depressant, and has similar effects on respiration as other inhalational anaesthetics, although it is less potent than isoflurane. There is a rise in respiratory rate and a decrease in tidal volume and minute volume. In spontaneously breathing subjects Pa_{CO_2} increases, and the ventilatory response to CO_2 is depressed. Respiratory depression is usually reduced or diminished by surgical stimulation.

Desflurane has a pungent, ethereal odour, to a greater extent than isoflurane or other inhalational agents, and often causes irritation of the airway that limits the rate of induction of inhalational anaesthesia. Consequently, desflurane frequently causes increased salivation, breathholding, coughing or laryngospasm, and may increase the incidence of hypoxaemia during induction. For these reasons, desflurane is rarely used to induce inhalational anaesthesia in children.

Cardiovascular effects

Heart

The effects of desflurane on the heart and the circulation are similar to isoflurane. There is often a rise in heart rate, which maintains cardiac output at preanaesthetic levels, and may be associated with the increased secretion of catecholamines. Occasionally, cardiac contractility is depressed during anaesthesia and may produce cardiovascular collapse. Desflurane does not usually affect AV conduction or cardiac rhythm, or sensitize the heart to adrenaline or other catecholamines.

Peripheral blood vessels

Desflurane causes peripheral vasodilatation and lowers blood pressure by decreasing systemic vascular resistance. Consequently, blood flow is maintained or increased in the splanchnic and renal circulation. Cerebral vascular resistance is also reduced, and cerebral blood flow may increase (depending on the concurrent effects on systemic blood pressure). Desflurane also increases coronary blood flow.

Other effects

Desflurane causes relaxation of voluntary muscle and enhances the effects of non-depolarizing muscle relaxants. It is approximately equi-potent with other fluorinated ethers. The relaxation of voluntary muscle is due to both central and peripheral effects, and potentiation rapidly disappears when the anaesthetic is discontinued. Desflurane also causes relaxation of uterine smooth muscle and has approximately the same potency as isoflurane.

Metabolism and toxicity

Desflurane contains six relatively stable C–F bonds, and only minute amounts (approximately 0.02%) are metabolized in man. After inhalation, there is a small increase in serum and urine trifluoroacetate concentrations (although the levels are only 10–20% of those observed after isoflurane). There are also slight but insignificant increases in inorganic and organic fluorides. The limited metabolism is entirely mediated by CYP 2E1, and enzyme induction with ethanol or isoniazid increases the formation of fluoride.

Since desflurane is almost entirely eliminated unchanged, its ability to produce hepatic or renal toxicity is extremely limited, and there is no evidence that it is associated with any cellular or organ toxicity. In experimental animals treated with enzyme inducing agents, repeated and prolonged desflurane anaesthesia does not produce any significant histological or histochemical changes.

Xenon

Xe

Xenon (atomic number = 54; atomic weight = 131.3 Da) is an inert gas, which is a mixture of nine naturally occurring isotopes, and has been used as an inhalational anaesthetic in both experimental animals and man. Xenon appears to produce anaesthesia by antagonism of glutamate at NMDA receptors (Fig. 7.4), but has little or no effect on kainate or AMPA receptors, or on metabotropic glutamate receptors. It may therefore interfere with the excitatory postsynaptic currents that are mediated by glutamate at NMDA receptors.

Xenon has similar effects to nitrous oxide, but is more potent (MAC in oxygen = 65–70% v/v), and mixtures of the inert gas with oxygen can produce anaesthesia without the risk of hypoxia. It has an extremely rapid onset and offset of action (blood–gas solubility coefficient = 0.2) and is also a potent analgesic. Like nitrous oxide, it may accumulate in air-filled spaces. In addition, it is odourless, non-irritant, non-inflammable, non-explosive and is not metabolized.

Although Xenon has considerable advantages over nitrous oxide as an analgesic and inhalational anaesthetic, it is not available for routine clinical use due to its cost. Nevertheless, it may well have a role as an inhalational agent in the future.

Suggested reading

Antognini, J.F. & Carstens, E. (2002) *In vivo* characterisation of clinical anaesthesia and its components. *British Journal of Anaesthesia* **89**, 156–166.

Belelli, D., Pistis, M., Peters, J.A. & Lambert, J.J. (1999) General anaesthetic action at transmitter-gated inhibitory amino acid receptors. *Trends in Pharmacological Sciences* **20**, 496–502.

Daniels, S. & Smith, E.B. (1993) Effects of general anaesthetics on ligand-gated ion channels. *British Journal of Anaesthesia* **71**, 59–64.

Eger, E.I., II (ed.) (1974) *Anesthetic Uptake and Action*. Baltimore: Williams and Wilkins.

Eger, E.I., II. (1994) New inhaled anesthetics. *Anesthesiology* **80**, 906–922.

Eger, E.I., II, Saidman, L.J. & Bandstater, B. (1965) Minimum alveolar concentration: a standard of anesthetic potency. *Anesthesiology* **26**, 756–763.

Franks, N.P. & Lieb, W.R. (1994) Molecular and cellular mechanisms of general anaesthesia. *Nature* **367**, 607–614.

Harper, N. (2001) Inhalational anaesthetics. *Anaesthesia and Intensive Care Medicine* **2**, 241–245.

Hatch, D.J. (1999) New inhalation agents in paediatric anaesthesia. *British Journal of Anaesthesia* **83**, 42–49.

Hess, W., Kannmacher, J. & Kruse, J. (2004) Contamination of anaesthetic gases with nitric oxide and its influence on oxygenation: study in patients undergoing open heart surgery. *British Journal of Anaesthesia* **93**, 629–633.

Jones, R.M., Cashman, J.N., Eger, E.I., II, Damask, M.C. & Johnson, B.H. (1990) Kinetics and potency of desflurane (I-653) in volunteers. *Anesthesia and Analgesia* **70**, 3–7.

Kharasch, E.D., Hankins, D., Mautz, D. & Thummel, K.E. (1996) Identification of the enzyme responsible for oxidative halothane metabolism: implications for prevention of halothane hepatitis. *Lancet* **347**, 1367–1371.

Mapleson, W.W. (1996) Effect of age on MAC in humans: a meta-analysis. *British Journal of Anaesthesia* **76**, 179–185.

Murat, I., Dubois, M.C. & Piat, V. (1995) Sevoflurane. *Annales Francaises d'Anesthesie et de Reanimation* **14**, 489–501.

Nunn, J.F. (1987) Clinical aspects of the interaction between nitrous oxide and vitamin B_{12}. *British Journal of Anaesthesia* **59**, 3–13.

Nunn, J.F., Chanarin, I., Tanner, A.G. & Owen, E.R.T.C. (1986) Megaloblastic bone marrow changes after repeated nitrous oxide anaesthesia. *British Journal of Anaesthesia* **58**, 1469-1470.Priebe, H.J. (1989) Isoflurane and coronary hemodynamics. *Anesthesiology* **71**, 960–976.

Smith, I., Nathanson, M. & White, P.F. (1996) Sevoflurane – a long-awaited volatile anaesthetic. *British Journal of Anaesthesia* **76**, 435–445.

Stoetling, R.K. & Eger, E.I., II. (1969) An additional explanation for the second gas effect: a concentrating effect. *Anesthesiology* **30**, 273–277.

Terrell, R.C. (1984) Physical and chemical properties of anaesthetic agents. *British Journal of Anaesthesia* **56**, 3S–7S.

Urban, B.W. (2002) Current assessment of targets and theories of anaesthesia. *British Journal of Anaesthesia* **89**, 167–183.

9 Local Anaesthetics

Local anaesthetic agents can be defined as drugs that are used clinically to produce reversible inhibition of excitation and conduction in peripheral nerve fibres and nerve endings, and thus produce the loss of sensation in a circumscribed area of the body. Many agents with different chemical structures, including chlorpromazine, propranolol and pethidine, that are primarily used for other purposes, have local anaesthetic properties. Only a small number of tertiary amines (esters or amides) are commonly used to induce local anaesthesia. Some of these may also be used as antiarrhythmic agents and have occasionally been used as anticonvulsants.

History of local anaesthetics

It has been recognized for many years that some naturally occurring substances can produce local or generalized changes in sensory appreciation and motor power. During his voyages of discovery in the eighteenth century, Captain James Cook tasted 'puffer fish' in the South Seas and graphically described its subjective effects on the nervous system. It is now recognized that these phenomena were due to tetrodotoxin poisoning. This substance is present in octopi, salamanders, newts and amphibia, as well as the Japanese puffer fish (*Spheroides spengleri*), and is probably produced by microbial biosynthesis. An unrelated series of biotoxins (the saxitoxins) are produced by the dinoflagellates (flagellated unicellular organisms which contaminate shellfish). Although both tetrodotoxin and saxitoxin are extremely potent substances, they are relatively polar compounds that do not readily penetrate cell membranes. Consequently, they are not used as local anaesthetics and are of no clinical importance.

The naturally occurring alkaloid cocaine was the first local anaesthetic used in clinical practice. It is derived from a shrub (*Erythroxylon coca*) that grows in the foothills of the Andes, and for many centuries its leaves were chewed by Peruvian Indians for its mood elevating and stimulant properties. Pure cocaine was first isolated by Niemann in

1860, who confirmed its effects on sensation, and its pharmacological actions were studied by Von Anrep between 1870 and 1880. The drug was introduced into clinical practice by Freud and Köller in 1884. Sigmund Freud used cocaine in an attempt to treat a morphine-dependent colleague, but converted him into a cocaine addict. He also took cocaine himself for a period of 10 years (while he was writing 'The Interpretation of Dreams'). Karl Köller[1] initially used cocaine to produce corneal anaesthesia in experimental animals and rapidly appreciated its potential advantages. He introduced it into ophthalmological practice as a surface anaesthetic, and its use for infiltration, conduction and spinal anaesthesia soon followed.

Unfortunately, its potential for producing drug dependence was not initially appreciated. Nevertheless, by 1890, its dangers were well recognized, and a search began for newer and safer drugs. Procaine, the first synthetic local anaesthetic, was introduced by Einhorn in 1905. Many other synthetic local anaesthetic esters were subsequently investigated. Most of these have now been discarded and are solely of historical interest. However, the local anaesthetic ester tetracaine is still widely used to produce topical anaesthesia.

An important milestone occurred in 1943 when lidocaine was synthesized by Lofgren and subsequently introduced into anaesthetic practice. This aminoacylamide was the prototype of a new group of local anaesthetic drugs. Since the advent of lidocaine, other amides have been introduced, some of which have been developed as single stereoisomers with significant clinical advantages.

Local anaesthetic agents that are currently used in the UK are

Esters:
Cocaine
Procaine

---

[1] An apocryphal story suggests that the enthusiasm of Karl Köller for cocaine anaesthesia led to the use of the soubriquet 'Coca Köller' by his friends and acquaintances, which was subsequently transliterated and employed in a rather different context.

Tetracaine
Amides:
Articaine
Lidocaine
Mepivacaine
Prilocaine
Bupivacaine
Ropivacaine
Levobupivacaine

Articaine and mepivacaine are only used in dental practice and are not considered in detail in this chapter. Etidocaine is an extremely potent amide anaesthetic, which has been used clinically in many countries (but not the UK). Some local anaesthetics (lidocaine and bupivacaine) have also been used experimentally as liposomal preparations[2] in order to prolong the duration of local anaesthesia and reduce systemic toxicity.

Structure and function of nerve fibres

Structure

Peripheral nerves consist of the dendrites and axons of sensory and/or motor nerves, which are bound together and surrounded by connective tissue. Layers of longitudinally arranged collagen surround individual nerve fibres (the endoneurium) or groups of nerve fibres (the perineurium). An outer connective tissue sheath (the epineurium) surrounds the nerve trunk and carries its blood vessels and lymphatics. Each nerve fibre is connected with a central cell body from which it receives its metabolic and nutritional requirements and is surrounded by a sheath of Schwann cell cytoplasm.

Unmyelinated fibres are usually enclosed in groups by the sheath of a single Schwann cell (which may be up to 0.5 mm long), which is in contact with the cytoplasm of adjacent Schwann cells. In contrast, each myelinated fibre is enclosed by the cytoplasm of a single Schwann cell, with its phospholipid cell membrane wound spirally around the fibre to form the myelin sheath (Fig. 9.1). Between individual Schwann cells the myelin sheath is absent, and the resultant junctions between adjacent cells are known as the nodes of Ranvier. The internodal distance is related to the size of the Schwann cells and the diameter of the nerve fibres. In large myelinated nerves, the internodal distance may be 1–2 mm.

---

[2] Liposomes are vesicles with a diameter of 50 nm–10 μm; they consist of an aqueous phase surrounded by a phospholipid bilayer. Drugs can be incorporated in either the lipid or the aqueous phase.

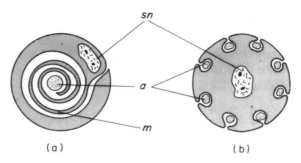

Fig. 9.1 Diagram showing transverse section of (a) myelinated nerve fibres and (b) unmyelinated nerve fibres. a, axon or dendrite; m, myelin sheath; sn, nucleus of Schwann cell.

Individual nerve fibres consist of a central core (the neuroplasm), which is enclosed by a limiting cell membrane (the neurilemma). The neuroplasm contains mitochondria, microtubules and neurofilaments, which are required for normal nutrition and metabolism. In contrast, the neurilemma is a characteristic phospholipid membrane and contains integral proteins (Fig. 1.1). Some of these proteins contain pores or ion channels, which play an important role in neuronal function.

Physiology

In the inactive state, there is a difference in potential of 60–90 mV across the neurilemma, i.e. the inside is electronegative relative to the outside. This potential difference (the resting potential) mainly reflects the selective permeability of the neurilemma to K^+. In resting conditions, the membrane is impermeable to Na^+, but K^+ can slowly diffuse from the neuroplasm. This process is opposed by the negative charge on intracellular proteins, which tends to prevent K^+ diffusion. The balance between these two forces represents the resting membrane potential, an electrochemical gradient which is closely related to the ratio K_i^+/K_o^+ (Fig. 9.2).

During activity, characteristic changes occur in the membrane potential. Initially, there is a slow phase of depolarization as the cell becomes progressively less negative. When the threshold potential (about -50 mV) is reached, there is a rapid and transient depolarization to approximately $+25$ mV, followed by a return to the resting value (repolarization). These changes are referred to as the action potential and occur within 1–2 milliseconds (Fig. 9.3).

The ability to generate an action potential depends on the presence of voltage-sensitive Na^+ channels in the

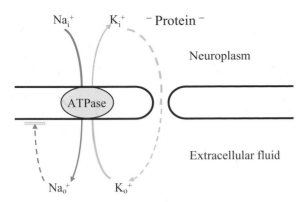

Fig. 9.2 The origin of the resting membrane potential. The enzyme Na^+/K^+ ATPase maintains a high internal K^+ concentration (K_i^+) and a high external Na^+ concentration (Na_o^+). In the resting state, the membrane is effectively impermeable to Na^+ (···▶), although K^+ can passively diffuse from the neuroplasm to extracellular fluid (···▶). The tendency for K^+ to leave the fibre is opposed by the ionic charges on intracellular proteins ($^-$protein$^-$), giving rise to the resting membrane potential.

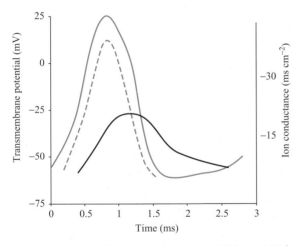

Fig. 9.3 Changes in the transmembrane potential (——), Na^+ conductance (– – –) and K^+ conductance (——) during a nerve action potential.

membrane. During excitation, Na^+ channels open and Na^+ rapidly diffuse across the neurilemma, causing the transient reversal in the membrane potential. After 1–2 milliseconds, K^+ slowly diffuses across the neurilemma, resulting in repolarization. During the refractory period, these ionic changes are reversed by the enzyme Na^+/K^+ ATPase in the membrane, which extrudes 3 Na^+ in exchange for the entry of 2 K^+.

Calcium ions are also present in the neuronal membrane and can affect the function of voltage-sensitive Na^+ channels. In experimental conditions, the threshold potential required for Na^+ channel opening is reduced (i.e. becomes more negative) when the local concentration of Ca^{2+} decreases, although the resting membrane potential is unaltered.

In unmyelinated fibres, activation and depolarization produces a local flow of current in the neurilemma, which decreases the membrane potential of the adjacent nerve. Voltage-sensitive Na^+ channels are activated and impulses are propagated along the nerve fibre. Retrograde conduction cannot occur due to the rapid inactivation of Na^+ channels in the wake of the impulse.

In contrast, in myelinated fibres current flows from one node of Ranvier to the immediate precedent and adjacent node. Since the internodal distance may be 1–2 mm, saltatory[3] conduction in myelinated fibres is much more rapid (up to approximately 120 m s^{-1}).

Molecular structure of sodium and potassium channels

In recent years, the detailed structure of Na^+ and K^+ channels in neuronal membranes has been clarified by biochemical, biophysical and molecular biological techniques.

Sodium channels

Voltage sensitive Na^+ channels are integral proteins that cross neuronal membranes and surround an aqueous pore (Fig. 1.1). Most Na^+ channels consist of three subunits (α, β_1 and β_2). The largest subunit (the α unit) has a molecular weight of 260 kDa and consists of a single long peptide chain (1950 amino acids) containing four hydrophobic regions (domains I–IV), which cross the membrane and symmetrically surround the pore (Fig. 9.4). The four domains are connected to each other by intracellular bridges.

Each domain consists of six membrane-spanning segments (S1–S6). The S4 segment is a voltage sensor, and the short loop between S5 and S6 forms part of the lining of the outer pore of the channel. The intracellular bridge between two of the regions (III and IV) is the fast inactivation gate. This gate is responsible for the rapid inactivation of Na^+ channels.

---

[3] Saltare: to leap, jump or skip.

(a)

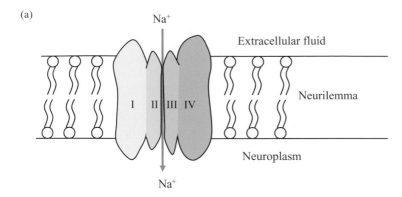

(b)

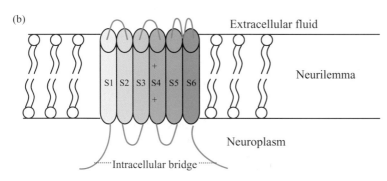

Fig. 9.4 (a) Structure of the α-subunit of voltage-sensitive Na^+ channels in the neurilemma. The α-subunit consists of a single long peptide chain containing four hydrophobic regions (I–IV), which cross the neuronal membrane. The four hydrophobic regions symmetrically surround the aqueous pore of the Na^+ channel; (b) The detailed structure of one of the hydrophobic regions. Each region consists of six transmembrane segments (S1–S6), and S4 is a voltage sensor (+). The short loops between S5 and S6 form part of the lining of the Na^+ channel, and intracellular bridges connect S1 and S6 to adjacent regions. Local anaesthetics are believed to block the channel near tyrosine and phenylalanine residues in the S6 segment of region IV.

Potassium channels

Potassium channels are a large and heterogeneous group of membrane proteins. Many different types of K^+ channel have been recognized and serve a variety of physiological functions. Some K^+ channels are voltage-sensitive, while others respond to neurotransmitters, intracellular Ca^{2+} or ATP. They may or may not inactivate after membrane depolarization. Since the equilibrium potential for K^+ is -100 mV, all open K^+ channels tend to cause neuronal repolarization and reduce membrane excitability.

In many respects, K^+ channels have structural similarities with Na^+ channels. Most voltage-sensitive K^+ channels consist of four distinct subunits, each of which is equivalent to a single domain of the Na^+ channel. Voltage-sensitive K^+ channels also contain a sensor in the S4 segment, and some of them slowly inactivate due to occlusion by the terminal region of each subunit.

Mode of action

Physicochemical factors

Most local anaesthetic agents are tertiary amine bases (B), which are administered as water-soluble hydrochlorides

(B.HCl). In this form, they readily dissolve to form acidic solutions:

$$B.HCl \rightleftarrows BH^+ + Cl^-$$

After injection into tissues, a proportion of the ionized basic form (BH^+) is converted to the non-ionized basic form (B) at the pH of extracellular fluid:

$$BH^+ + HCO_3^- \rightleftarrows B + H_2O + CO_2$$

Consequently, local anaesthetics are present in tissues in both an ionized form (BH^+) and a non-ionized form (B). The relative proportions of the two forms depend on the difference between their dissociation constants (pK_a value)[4] and extracellular pH. Only the non-ionized form

---

[4] The dissociation constant or pK_a value of a local anaesthetic is defined by a modification of the Henderson–Hasselbalch equation:

$$pK_a = pH + log_{10} \frac{[BH^+]}{[B]}$$

and is equal to the pH at which the concentration of the ionized base (BH^+) and the non-ionized base (B) are equal. It can be used to calculate the proportion of the two forms that are present in solution at different pH values (Table 9.1).

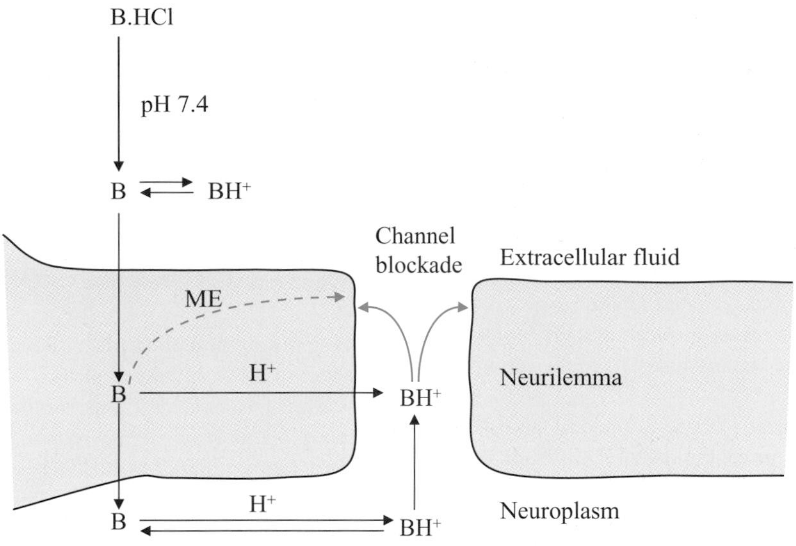

Fig. 9.5 Mode and site of action of local anaesthetics in Na^+ channels. Local anaesthetics are administered as hydrochloride salts (B.HCl) which release the unionized base (B) in extracellular fluid. Only the unionized form B diffuses across the neurilemmal membrane, attracts H^+ in the neuroplasm, and then gains access to its site of action in the open Na^+ channel, causing its blockade. The unionized form B can also directly diffuse to the Na^+ channel through the neurilemma, and attract H^+ in the Na^+ channel. It may also cause channel blockade by 'membrane expansion' (ME), i.e. by causing swelling of the lipoprotein membrane. Tetrodotoxin and saxitoxin directly block the Na^+ channel from the exterior of the membrane, close to the external pore.

(B) is lipid-soluble and can diffuse through the nerve sheath, perineuronal tissues, and the neurilemma to reach the neuroplasm, where it attracts H^+ and reverts to the cationic form (BH^+).

Effects on sodium channels

In the ionized form BH^+, local anaesthetics in the neuroplasm enter the Na^+ channel from its inner aspect, and physically occlude the Na^+ channel from the inside. They are believed to interact with phenylalanine (1764) and tyrosine (1771) residues in the S6 segment of domain IV, which are approximately one third of the distance along the channel (Fig. 9.4). Local anaesthetics presumably block the Na^+ channel in a non-specific manner, since all tertiary bases with pK_a values between 7.5 and 9 appear to have some local anaesthetic activity. Since the diffusion of local anaesthetics (as BH^+) through the inner pores of Na^+ channels is essential for them to reach their site of action, nerve blockade is often dependent on the frequency of stimulation ('use-dependent blockade' or 'phasic blockade').

Convincing evidence to support this rather complex mechanism of action (Fig. 9.5) was provided by exper-

iments in which lidocaine and its *N*-ethylated quaternary derivative were applied to different sides of the neurilemma. Lidocaine produces local anaesthesia when applied to the inside or the outside of the neurilemma. In contrast, its quaternary derivative is only effective when applied to the inner aspect of the membrane.

Membrane expansion

Certain local anaesthetics (e.g. benzocaine) are only present in the body as uncharged tertiary bases and must therefore act in a rather different way. They are believed to cause conduction blockade by 'membrane expansion' (i.e. by causing swelling of the lipoprotein matrix of the Na^+ channel). To some extent, other local anaesthetics which are partly present in the neurilemma as the uncharged base (Fig. 9.5) may act in this manner.

Local anaesthesia is influenced by the availability of the free base (B), since this is the form that readily diffuses through connective tissue and crosses the neurilemma. Local anaesthetics are relatively inactive when injected into tissues with an acid pH (e.g. pyogenic abcesses). This is presumably due to the reduced availability of the free base for diffusion, and to the more rapid removal of local anaesthetic due to the increase in tissue vascularity.

Carbonated solutions

Factors that increase the conversion of the free local anaesthetic base (B) to the active form (BH$^+$) in the neuroplasm increase the diffusion gradient and the concentration of BH$^+$ in the Na$^+$ channel. In these conditions, the speed of onset and the depth of local anaesthesia may be enhanced. In isolated preparations, CO_2 rapidly diffuses across the neurilemma and decreases intracellular pH, enhancing the conversion of the tertiary base (B) to the active form (BH$^+$).

Although carbonated solutions of local anaesthetics have been used to improve the speed of onset and quality of blockade, it is doubtful whether they have any advantages in clinical practice. When carbon dioxide diffuses across the neurilemma, it is rapidly buffered by intracellular proteins, so that changes in pH are minimal. In addition, carbonated solutions are unstable, the local anaesthetic may be precipitated and any added vasoconstrictor is more easily hydrolysed. Consequently, carbonated solutions of local anaesthetics are not widely used in current practice. Other agents (e.g. sodium bicarbonate, various dextrans) have also been added to local anaesthetic solutions, in order to modify the proportion of the free base that is present in solution and increase the intensity and duration of action.

Antiarrhythmic effects

Local anaesthetics produce their effects by blockade of Na$^+$ channels, and thus retard or prevent depolarization. Similar effects may be produced in other excitable tissues, particularly in the heart. In atrial and ventricular muscle, the depolarization of myocardial cells from -80 mV to approximately $+30$ mV during phase 0 of the cardiac action potential is mainly due to the rapid influx of Na$^+$. Local anaesthetics reduce Na$^+$ entry and the rate of depolarization of ventricular muscle, and some of them (e.g. lidocaine) have a recognized role as antiarrhythmic drugs (Chapter 15).

Effects on other ion channels

Local anaesthetics can also affect other ion channels (particularly K$^+$ and Ca^{2+} channels), although they have a reduced affinity at these sites. They do not usually modify the neuronal resting potential, except in extremely high concentrations. Similarly, they do not alter the threshold potential required for impulse propagation, although the rates of depolarization and repolarization are decreased, and conduction velocity is diminished. Nevertheless, it is usually considered that the toxic effects of bupivacaine on the heart are partially related to its effects on K$^+$ and Ca^{2+} channels.

Effect on different sensory modalities

During conduction blockade, different modalities may be affected to an unequal extent by local anaesthetics. The sensation of pain usually disappears before touch and pressure, while motor fibres may remain functional although sensory pathways are blocked. These differences may be partly related to the diameter of nerve fibres that mediate different sensations.

Small diameter unmyelinated C fibres are usually most susceptible to local anaesthetics, since they have a relatively large surface area, due to the absence of a myelin sheath. In contrast, myelinated fibres have a relatively small surface area, are only susceptible to blockade at the nodes of Ranvier, and sequential blockade of 2–3 nodes may be required to interrupt impulse conduction. Since the internodal distance is usually related to nerve fibre diameter, smaller Aβ and Aγ myelinated fibres are usually more susceptible than the larger (Aα) fibres. Consequently, pain (which is partly mediated by unmyelinated C fibres) is commonly blocked before touch and pressure (mediated by Aβ and Aγ fibres), which in turn are blocked before proprioception and motor function (which are dependent on Aα fibres).

Nevertheless, these considerations do not adequately explain several clinical observations. For instance, myelinated fibres of the Aδ group, which conduct the sensation of fast or first pain, may be blocked before some nonmyelinated C fibres. This phenomenon may reflect the anatomical distribution of nerve fibres and their accessibility to drugs.

Physicochemical factors may also account for the differential effects of local anaesthetics on sensory and motor function. For instance, low concentrations of bupivacaine and ropivacaine may readily affect unmyelinated C fibres due to their high lipid-solubility. In contrast, they may not readily diffuse across myelinated Aα fibres and cause motor blockade (due to their relatively high pK$_a$ value). Consequently, these drugs may possess the optimal physicochemical characteristics required for differential sensory and motor blockade.

Local anaesthetic preparations

Most local anaesthetics are bases that are almost insoluble in water. Consequently, their hydrochloride salts, which are extremely water-soluble, are usually dissolved in saline to form acidic solutions (pH 4.0–6.5). Preparations with added adrenaline often contain a reducing agent (e.g. sodium metabisulphite), in order to prevent the oxidation and enhance the stability of the vasoconstrictor. Some local anaesthetic preparations (particularly multidose vials) also incorporate a preservative/fungicide (e.g. methyl *p*-hydroxybenzoate). Most local anaesthetic solutions are extremely stable and usually have an effective shelf-life of more than 2 years.

Vasoconstrictors

Many local anaesthetics have vasodilator effects and are rapidly absorbed after local injection. Consequently, they are often used with added vasoconstrictors, which enhance their potency and prolong their duration of action. Vasoconstrictors also decrease the systemic toxicity and increase the safety margin of local anaesthetics by reducing their rate of absorption, which is mainly dependent on local blood flow. Nevertheless, the effectiveness of added vasoconstrictors is extremely variable. In most infiltration procedures and in conduction blockade, vasoconstrictors usually prolong and enhance local anaesthesia. In contrast, they may have little effect on the duration of extradural blockade.

Adrenaline is the most commonly used vasoconstrictor and is added to local anaesthetic solutions in concentrations ranging from 1 in 500,000 (2 µg mL^{-1}) to 1 in 200,000 (5 µg mL^{-1}). Higher concentrations may have toxic effects on the cardiovascular system, peripheral nerves and the spinal cord. In addition, vasoconstrictors must not be used with local anaesthetic solutions that are injected into digits or appendages, as they may induce ischaemic necrosis. Although other sympathomimetic drugs have been used as vasoconstrictors, adrenaline is more effective than phenylephrine or noradrenaline in decreasing the rate of absorption of most local anaesthetics.

Vasoconstrictors in dentistry

Local anaesthetic preparations containing higher concentrations of adrenaline (e.g. 1 in 80,000; 12.5 µg/mL) are commonly used in dental practice. Preparations containing noradrenaline have been used in the past, but are now avoided due to their pressor effects. Some solutions of prilocaine (3%) that are licensed for dental use contain the vasoconstrictor felypressin (0.03 i.u./mL). Felypressin is a noncatecholamine vasoconstrictor that is chemically related to vasopressin, the posterior pituitary hormone. It is a synthetic octapeptide that only affects peripheral blood vessels and has no action on the heart. Although it produces less marked vasoconstriction than adrenaline, it may be useful for patients with ischaemic heart disease when the use of catecholamines is undesirable.

Chemical structure and physicochemical properties

All local anaesthetics have certain chemical features in common. They are almost all weak bases that are partially ionized at physiological pH values, and consist of an aromatic lipophilic group, an intermediate ester (–CO.O–) or amide (–NH.CO–) chain, and a hydrophilic secondary or tertiary amine group. The intermediate chain is the basis of the usual classification of local anaesthetics into esters or amides.

There are important practical differences between these two groups of local anaesthetics. Esters are relatively unstable in solution and are rapidly hydrolysed in the body by butyrylcholinesterase (BChE) as well as some other esterases. Para-aminobenzoic acid (PABA) is usually one of the hydrolytic products and is sometimes associated with allergic reactions. By contrast, amides are relatively stable in solution and are slowly broken down by amidases in the liver. In addition, hypersensitivity reactions to amide local anaesthetics are almost unknown. In the UK, tetracaine is the only ester currently used to produce local anaesthesia.

Physicochemical properties

The chemical structure and physicochemical characteristics of local anaesthetics affect their clinical properties. In particular, these are modified by
- Lipid solubility
- Protein binding
- Dissociation constant (pK$_a$ value)

Lipid solubility

There is a close correlation between their lipid-solubility and anaesthetic potency (particularly in *in vitro* conditions). The lipid solubility of different anaesthetics governs their ability to penetrate perineuronal tissues and the neuronal membrane, and reaches their site of action in the neuroplasm. For instance, in many clinical situations bupivacaine, levobupivacaine and ropivacaine are approximately 3–4 times as potent as lidocaine or prilocaine, due to differences in their lipid-solubility (Table 9.1).

Protein binding

Tissue protein binding primarily affects the duration of action of local anaesthetics. For example, procaine is not extensively bound to tissue proteins and normally has a short duration of action. In contrast, bupivacaine, levobupivacaine and ropivacaine are extensively bound to plasma and tissue proteins and have prolonged effects. Lidocaine and prilocaine are moderately bound to tissue proteins and have an intermediate duration of action (Table 9.1).

Dissociation constant (pK$_a$ value)

The dissociation constant of local anaesthetics is the most important factor affecting the rapidity of their onset of action. The pK$_a$ value governs the proportion of the local anaesthetic that is present in a non-ionized form at physiological pH values and is therefore available to diffuse across tissue barriers to its site of action (pages 152–153). Low pK$_a$ values are associated with a rapid onset of blockade, since more of the drug is present as the unionized base at pH 7.4. In contrast, higher values are associated with a slower onset, since less of the drug is present as the non-ionized base at pH 7.4.

For example, both lidocaine and prilocaine have a pK$_a$ value of approximately 7.7. At pH 7.4, about one third (33%) of these drugs is present in solution as the non-ionized base B and is available to diffuse across the nerve sheath. In contrast, bupivacaine and ropivacaine have a pK$_a$ value of 8.1, and at pH 7.4 only 17% is present in solution as a non-ionized, diffusible base. These differences are responsible for the more rapid onset of action of lidocaine and prilocaine, and the slower onset of action of ropivacaine and bupivacaine (Table 9.1).

Despite these considerations, the rapidity of onset and latency of action of local anaesthetics can also be modified by unrelated factors, such as the dose and the resultant concentration of the drug in tissues.

Chirality

Most ester local anaesthetics are achiral compounds. In contrast, most of the amides, with the exception of lidocaine, are chiral drugs (Chapter 3, Appendix II). Some chiral local anaesthetics are administered clinically as racemic mixtures, while others have been developed and used as single enantiomers. Although individual enantiomers have approximately equal local anaesthetic activity, the (S)-enantiomers have important advantages in other respects. For example, they may produce vasoconstriction and thus prolong local anaesthetic activity. They may also reduce the intensity and duration of motor blockade and are associated with a reduced risk of cardiotoxicity. In addition, there are also significant differences in their metabolism and pharmacokinetics.

Tachyphylaxis to local anaesthetics

When lidocaine is given by extradural administration, tachyphylaxis, i.e. the development of rapid drug tolerance, may occur. Repeated, identical doses tend to produce progressively decreasing effects, so that increasing doses are required to maintain the same degree of blockade. Tachyphylaxis is uncommon with other local anaesthetics that have a longer duration of action. It is been suggested that tachyphylaxis is related to the local changes in pH produced by the introduction of relatively acidic solutions of lidocaine (pH 4–5) into the extradural space. Since the volume and buffering capacity of extradural tissues is limited, local anaesthetic solutions may decrease its effective pH and thus reduce the relative concentration of free base that is available for diffusion into the intradural spinal nerve roots. In these conditions, there may be a progressive decrease in the extent and duration of sensory blockade and analgesia.

Alternatively, it has been proposed that tachyphylaxis is related to the increased sensitization of the spinal cord to chronic painful stimuli and may be due to the modification of central synaptic pathways. In experimental conditions, the recurrence of pain appears to have an important role in the development of tachyphylaxis, and its development can be prevented by NMDA antagonists or by inhibitors of nitric oxide synthase.

Systemic absorption

Significant absorption of local anaesthetics occurs from their site of injection. The amount of local anaesthetic absorbed and the peak plasma concentration will be dependent on the dose, and may also be modified by the presence or the absence of a vasoconstrictor, particularly during infiltration or conduction anaesthesia. The site of

Table 9.1 Physicochemical properties and pharmacological effects of some local anaesthetic agents.

	pK$_a$ value	Relative lipid solubility	Relative potency	Protein binding (%)	Onset of action	Duration of action	Clinical use	Properties
Procaine	8.9	1	1	6	Slow	Short	Limited Vascular spasm Diagnostic procedures	Vasodilatation Allergenic
Tetracaine	8.5	200	8	75	Slow	Long	Topical anaesthesia	Systemic toxicity
Lidocaine	7.7	150	2	65	Fast	Moderate	Infiltration anaesthesia Peripheral nerve block Extradural anaesthesia IVRA	Versatile Moderate vasodilatation
Prilocaine	7.7	50	2	55	Fast	Moderate	Infiltration anaesthesia Peripheral nerve block IVRA	Methaemoglobinaemia Low systemic toxicity
Bupivacaine	8.1	1000	8	95	Moderate	Long	Infiltration anaesthesia Peripheral nerve block Extradural anaesthesia Spinal anaesthesia	Separation of sensory and motor blockade Cardiotoxicity
Levo-bupivacaine	8.1	1000	8	95	Moderate	Long	Infiltration anaesthesia Peripheral nerve block Extradural anaesthesia Spinal anaesthesia	Separation of sensory and motor blockade Reduced cardiotoxicity
Ropivacaine	8.1	400	6	94	Moderate	Long	Infiltration anaesthesia Peripheral nerve block Extradural anaesthesia	Separation of sensory and motor blockade Reduced motor block

injection is also important, and higher blood levels may be attained after intercostal and caudal blockade than with lumbar epidural or brachial plexus blockade. Thus, for every 100 mg lidocaine injected in an adult, the peak venous plasma concentration ranges from 1.5 μg mL^{-1} (intercostal blockade), 1.2 μg mL^{-1} (caudal and paracervical blockade), 1.0 μg mL^{-1} (epidural blockade), 0.6 μg mL^{-1} (brachial plexus blockade) to 0.4 μg mL^{-1} (intrathecal blockade). This range of concentrations is mainly due to differences in vascularity, although other factors (e.g. uptake by tissue lipids) may also be involved. In these conditions, adherence to dose limits for local anaesthetics may obscure potential differences in systemic toxicity, depending on the site of injection. Clearly, identical doses of local anaesthetics may be more toxic in certain injection sites than in others.

Many local anaesthetics are also well absorbed from mucous membranes. The rate of uptake is closely related to the surface area available for absorption. Thus, it is extremely rapid when local anaesthetic sprays are applied to the tracheobronchial tract. In addition, the inherent effects of drugs on vascular smooth muscle tone may affect their rate of absorption. Cocaine prevents the neuronal uptake of catecholamines (Uptake$_1$) and inhibits the enzyme monoamine oxidase, thus producing vasoconstriction and delaying drug absorption. Most other local anaesthetics have a biphasic action on vascular smooth muscle, and in concentrations that are used clinically tend to produce some degree of vasodilatation (usually in the order procaine > prilocaine > lidocaine > mepivacaine > bupivacaine). Both levobupivacaine and ropivacaine have a lesser effect and may even produce some vasoconstriction. These differences may affect the rate of absorption of individual drugs. Procaine, chloroprocaine and related esters are potent vasodilators, are readily absorbed, and are rapidly broken down in tissues and plasma by esterase enzymes. The inactivation of procaine by enzymes in mucous membranes accounts for its relative lack of surface anaesthetic activity.

The (S)-isomers of prilocaine, mepivacaine and bupivacaine produce less vasodilatation than the R-enantiomers, and the (S)-forms of chiral local anaesthetics often have a longer duration of action than their antipodes.

Plasma protein binding and placental transfer

The reversible binding of local anaesthetics by plasma proteins may affect their pharmacokinetic behaviour and pharmacodynamic effects. In general, esters are not significantly bound by plasma proteins (i.e. 5–10% or less). In contrast, amides are mainly bound by α_1-acid glycoprotein, in the order prilocaine < lidocaine < ropivacaine < bupivacaine = levobupivacaine (Table 9.1). The extent ranges from 55 to 95%, and does not appear to restrict the uptake of local anaesthetics by most tissues and organs. Protein binding is influenced by changes in the concentration of α_1-acid glycoprotein, which may occur in infancy, pregnancy, old age, myocardial infarction, renal failure, malignant disease and after operative surgery. In these conditions, binding is increased and the free (unbound) concentration of drugs is reduced.

The binding of local anaesthetics may also affect their placental transfer. In general, highly protein-bound drugs have a low umbilical vein–maternal blood (UV:M) concentration ratio, while less protein-bound drugs have a higher UV:M ratio. Thus, for bupivacaine and ropivacaine the UV:M ratio is approximately 0.2, and for lidocaine and prilocaine, the UV:M ratio is 0.5. These values do not necessarily reflect the relative safety of the local anaesthetics in pregnancy and labour, since they do not take account of differential α_1-acid glycoprotein binding in maternal and foetal blood. Nevertheless, it is generally accepted that the placental transfer of bupivacaine and ropivacaine is less than lidocaine and prilocaine, and this has obvious advantages in pregnancy and labour.

Pharmacokinetics

After absorption from the site of injection, the plasma concentration of local anaesthetics depends on their rate of distribution in tissues and their elimination from the body. The prolonged absorption of local anaesthetics may preclude or obscure the investigation of their pharmacokinetics.

After intravenous administration, the plasma concentration of all local anaesthetics usually declines in a biexponential manner. There is an initial rapid distribution phase (half-life = 1–3 min), associated with their rapid uptake by highly perfused organs (e.g. lung, liver, kidney, skeletal muscle). Subsequently, there is a slower decline in plasma concentration, which represents the removal of the local anaesthetic by metabolism and excretion.

The terminal half-life of most ester anaesthetics is relatively short (approximately 10 min) due to their rapid hydrolysis by plasma cholinesterase. In contrast, the terminal half-life of the amides ranges from 100 minutes (lidocaine) to 200 minutes (bupivacaine). Their volume

Table 9.2 Pharmacokinetics and metabolism of local anaesthetics.

	Terminal half-life (min)	Clearance (mL min^{-1} kg^{-1})	Apparent volume of distribution (L kg^{-1})	Metabolites
Cocaine	48	31	2.0	Norcocaine Ecgonine Benzoylated derivatives
Procaine	8	60	0.7	Diethylaminoethanol p-aminobenzoate
Tetracaine	15	47	1.0	Butyl-aminobenzoate Dimethyl-aminoethanol
Lidocaine	100	15	1.3	Monoethylglycine-xylidide Ethylglycine 2,6-xylidine 4-hydroxy-2,6-xylidine
Prilocaine	100	34	2.7	N-propylamine o-toluidine
Bupivacaine	200	9	1.1	Pipecolic acid Pipecolyl-xylidide
Levobupivacaine	200	9	1.1	Pipecolic acid Pipecolyl-xylidide
Ropivacaine	110	7	0.7	3-Hydroxy-ropivacaine 3-Hydroxy-ropivacaine glucuronide 4-Hydroxy-ropivacaine

of distribution is rather greater than total body water, while their plasma clearance is usually less than liver blood flow (Table 9.2). Pathological conditions may alter the pharmacokinetics of local anaesthetics. In particular, cardiovascular disease and hepatic cirrhosis may decrease the clearance and volume of distribution of local anaesthetics, with variable effects on the terminal half-life. In neonatal life, the clearance of local anaesthetics is decreased and their half-life is prolonged.

Metabolism and elimination

The metabolism of local anaesthetics depends on their chemical structure, and esters and amides are usually metabolized in different ways.

Esters

Most ester local anaesthetics are rapidly broken down by plasma cholinesterase, and only small amounts of the unchanged drugs are eliminated in urine. In certain tissues, they are also broken down by other esterases.

Cocaine

Cocaine is extensively metabolized in the liver, and only trace amounts (approximately 1% of the dose) are excreted unchanged in urine. Studies using radiolabelled cocaine suggest that the drug is converted to several metabolites, i.e. norcocaine, ecgonine and their benzoylated analogues, and that some of them may be responsible for the stimulant effects of cocaine on the CNS. Cocaine is relatively resistant to hydrolysis by plasma cholinesterase.

Procaine

Procaine is extensively hydrolysed by plasma cholinesterase to para-aminobenzoic acid and diethylaminoethanol, which itself is further metabolized by alcohol dehydrogenase to diethylglycine. Little or none of the drug is excreted unchanged in urine.

Tetracaine

Tetracaine is also hydrolysed by plasma cholinesterase to butyl-p-aminobenzoic acid and dimethylaminoethanol, which is also converted to glycine.

Amides

In contrast to most ester anaesthetics, the amides are extensively metabolized by hepatic enzymes, particularly by amidases that are associated with the cytoplasm and the smooth endoplasmic reticulum.

Lidocaine

Lidocaine is extensively metabolized by the liver, and after oral administration only trace amounts gain access to the systemic circulation, i.e. it has an extremely high first-pass effect. Less than 10% of the dose is excreted unchanged in urine. The drug is initially de-alkylated to acetaldehyde and monoethylglycine-xylidide, which is then hydrolysed to N-ethylglycine and 2,6-xylidine. This compound is subsequently converted to 4-hydroxy-2,6-xylidine, which is the main metabolite eliminated in urine (Table 9.2).

Some of the metabolites of lidocaine have local anaesthetic activity, while others appear to have convulsive properties (e.g. monoethylglycine-xylidide). Glycine-xylidide (a minor metabolite of lidocaine) is a CNS depressant, has a relatively long half-life, and may take several days to be eliminated from the body.

Prilocaine

Prilocaine is more rapidly metabolized than other amide anaesthetics. Although it is mainly metabolized by the liver, it may also be broken down by the kidney and the lung. Its principal metabolites are N-propylamine and o-toluidine (Table 9.2), and the latter is probably responsible for the methaemoglobinaemia and cyanosis, which can occur 5–6 hours after large doses of prilocaine. Although this usually resolves spontaneously, it may be treated with reducing agents (ascorbic acid or methylene blue). Prilocaine is administered clinically as a chiral mixture, and R-prilocaine is more rapidly metabolized than S-prilocaine, and may produce higher plasma concentrations of o-toluidine.

Bupivacaine

Bupivacaine is slowly metabolized by the liver, and only 6% of the dose is eliminated unchanged in urine. Bupivacaine is mainly hydrolysed to pipecolic acid, although about 5% of the dose is converted to a dealkylated metabolite (pipecolylxylidide). Both these metabolites are eliminated in urine (Table 9.2).

Levobupivacaine is metabolized and eliminated in a similar manner.

Ropivacaine

Ropivacaine is predominantly metabolized by the liver to 3-hydroxy-ropivacaine, which is then conjugated and eliminated in urine. Minor amounts of 4-hydroxy-ropivacaine and other metabolites are also formed, and subsequently excreted in urine. Only 1–2% of the drug is eliminated unchanged.

Unwanted effects of local anaesthetics

Unwanted effects of local anaesthetics may be
• Caused by overdosage
• Occur as part of the therapeutic procedure
• Due to the vasoconstrictor
• Specific effects

Effects caused by overdosage

Local anaesthetics and their metabolites are weak bases, and cross the blood–brain barrier relatively easily. Severe and occasionally fatal CNS toxicity may occur with gross overdosage, and cardiovascular toxicity occurs when large doses inadvertently reach the heart and circulation.

Central nervous system

As long as the injection is not too rapid, early signs of CNS toxicity are often recognized before more serious effects occur. Local anaesthetics characteristically produce biphasic effects on the CNS. Signs of central excitation usually follow the absorption of significant amounts of local anaesthetics, although small doses of lidocaine have anticonvulsant effects, and have been used in the treatment of status epilepticus. Increasing plasma concentrations of local anaesthetics are usually associated with numbness of the tongue and mouth, lightheadedness, visual disturbances, slurring of speech, muscular twitching and tremors, restlessness and irrational conversation. Grand mal convulsions may occur at plasma concentrations of 9 μg mL^{-1} (lidocaine) or 2 μg mL^{-1} (bupivacaine). The threshold for convulsions is influenced by the presence of other drugs that affect the CNS, and by acidosis and hypoxia. Some local anaesthetics (e.g. procaine) are relatively free from convulsant activity. The excitatory effects of local anaesthetics are probably due to the selective depression of inhibitory cortical pathways, and may be followed by signs of cortical and medullary depression (coma, apnoea).

Convulsions should be treated by maintaining adequate ventilation and oxygenation, and controlled by anticonvulsant drugs. Diazepam (10–20 mg intravenously, repeated if necessary) is unlikely to potentiate the phase of CNS depression. Alternatively, thiopental (150–250 mg intravenously) may be used.

Accidental injection of large volumes of local anaesthetics into the CSF during epidural or paravertebral block can produce 'total spinal' anaesthesia. Total spinal anaesthesia usually presents as complete respiratory paralysis, due to motor and medullary involvement and hypotension, due to autonomic blockade. Treatment includes mechanical ventilation and circulatory support, and the use of a vasopressor may be indicated.

Cardiovascular system

Overdosage with local anaesthetics may cause profound hypotension, bradycardia, bradyarrhythmias and even cardiac arrest, and usually follows signs of CNS toxicity. High systemic concentrations of bupivacaine are particularly associated with significant cardiotoxicity. In addition to producing prolonged blockade of Na^+ channels, bupivacaine affects myocardial Ca^{2+} and K^+ channels, and is preferentially bound by cardiac muscle. Myocardial contractility and conduction in junctional tissues is depressed, with widening of the QRS complex and distortion of the ST segment. High concentrations of bupivacaine predispose to the development of re-entrant phenomena and ventricular arrhythmias, which are potentiated by hypoxia, acidosis and hyperkalaemia. Arrhythmias and bradycardia may respond to intravenous atropine (1.2–1.8 mg), and colloid or crystalloid infusions may be required to expand plasma volume.

In the UK, the use of racemic bupivacaine during IVRA (Bier's block) has been associated with significant cardiotoxicity, including at least five deaths. Current evidence suggests that the use of local anaesthetic enantiomers with the (S)-configuration reduce the risks of cardiac depression and cardiotoxicity, and ropivacaine (an S-isomer) and levobupivacaine (S-bupivacaine) may have significant advantages compared to racemic bupivacaine.

When local anaesthetics are used to produce analgesia in labour, foetal bradycardia and other signs of foetal distress may occur after paracervical blockade, due to the rapid drug absorption from this site.

As part of the therapeutic procedure

When multiple intercostal blocks are performed, respiratory insufficiency may occur due to the unavoidable paralysis of some motor fibres. During spinal anaesthesia, a variable degree of hypotension due to autonomic blockade is not uncommon, and extradural analgesia during labour may potentiate the effects of hypotension related to inferior vena caval compression. Preloading with crystalloids or colloids usually minimizes these complications, although symptomatic treatment with ephedrine or phenylephrine may be required.

Due to the added vasoconstrictor

The unwanted effects of added vasoconstrictors are usually due to their accidental intravascular injection. When sympathomimetic amines are used, cardiac arrhythmias and hypertensive responses are predictable side effects, although the local anaesthetic itself may have some protective effect on the heart.

Vasoconstrictor agents must not be added when local anaesthetics are used for the blockade of digital nerves or other extremities, as the intense ischaemia produced may lead to gangrene. Similarly, these solutions must never be given by intravenous administration.

Specific effects

Allergic responses to most currently used local anaesthetics are extremely rare. Skin reactions following repeated handling of esters have been most frequently reported, although anaphylactic responses occasionally occur. The metabolite *para*-aminobenzoic acid (PABA) probably acts as a hapten and induces an immunological response. Allergic reactions associated with the amide group are much less common, and cross-sensitization between amide and ester local anaesthetics is almost unknown. Some reactions may occur when multidose ampoules are used (possibly due to the added preservative).

Procaine and related esters are hydrolysed to PABA, and thus may antagonize the effects of sulphonamides, and the concurrent use of esters and preparations containing sulphonamides (e.g. co-trimoxazole) is undesirable.

Methaemoglobinaemia formation may occur when high doses of prilocaine are given (e.g. more than 600 mg), probably due to the accumulation of its main metabolite (*o*-toluidine). The foetus is at special risk, since its erythrocytes are deficient in methaemoglobin reductase (the enzyme that reduces methaemoglobin to haemoglobin).

When necessary, methylene blue (5 mg kg^{-1}) is an immediate and effective antidote in the mother and the child.

Clinical use of local anaesthetics

Esters
Cocaine

Cocaine is a powerful vasoconstrictor and inhibits both monoamine oxidase and the uptake of catecholamines by sympathetic nerves. Consequently, it is a useful agent when both the reduction of bleeding and local anaesthesia are required. Its main indication in current practice is to provide surface anaesthesia for intranasal procedures. Aqueous solutions and pastes containing 4–10% cocaine are commonly used for this purpose, and adrenaline (1 in 1000) has sometimes been added. In the past, cocaine has been used to produce corneal anaesthesia, although its desiccating effect is a marked disadvantage and may led to corneal ulceration.

Cocaine inhibits the uptake of adrenaline and noradrenaline by central and peripheral sympathetic nerve endings (Uptake$_1$), and thus enhances the effects of sympathetic nerve stimulation. In the CNS, it increases neuronal activity in sympathetic pathways in the hypothalamus and the medulla. Consequently, it may produce mental stimulation, euphoria, hallucinations, vasoconstriction, pupillary dilatation and hypertension, as well as tachycardia and cardiac arrhythmias. It is a Class A controlled drug, due to its propensity to produce dependence and addiction.

Procaine

In current practice, procaine is rarely used as a local anaesthetic. Nevertheless, it is an extremely effective and short-acting vasodilator, and is sometimes used in the management of vascular spasm associated with inadvertent intra-arterial injections, trauma and surgery.

Procaine is also an ideal diagnostic agent, due to its relatively short duration of action (15–45 min) and its localized effects (which are due to its poor diffusion properties). In the treatment of chronic pain it has been used to block somatic or autonomic fibres, so that the efficiency

of permanent neurolytic blockade can be more easily assessed.

At one time, intravenous procaine (1% in saline) was used as a supplement to general anaesthesia, to produce analgesia for burns dressings and to relieve postoperative pain. Its action was rather unpredictable and side effects were not uncommon. It is rarely if ever used for this purpose in current anaesthetic practice.

Procaine decreases the excitability of atrial and ventricular muscle, and at one time was used as an antiarrhythmic agent. Its short duration of action led to the development of its close analogue procainamide, which is not broken down by cholinesterase and was widely used in the management of ventricular and supraventricular arrhythmias (Chapter 15). Procaine has also been used as a component of cardioplegic solutions during cardiopulmonary bypass.

Procaine forms less soluble conjugates with some other drugs (e.g. penicillin), producing slow-release preparations. It can also be added to other drugs to reduce the pain of intramuscular injections.

Tetracaine

In recent years, tetracaine gel (4%) has been widely used to produce surface anaesthesia prior to venepuncture or venous cannulation. When applied to the skin under an occlusive dressing, it has a moderate onset (30–45 min) and a long duration of action (4–6 h), and produces some vasodilatation. It is an excellent topical anaesthetic and is also used in ophthalmological practice to produce corneal anaesthesia before minor surgical procedures.

Tetracaine is an effective, potent, but extremely toxic local anaesthetic, which is rapidly absorbed from most mucous membranes. It should never ever be used to provide topical anaesthesia for tracheal intubation, bronchoscopy or cystoscopy, since significant absorption occurs from vascular areas, and fatalities have followed the application of extremely small doses to mucosal surfaces.

In the past, tetracaine was widely used to produce spinal anaesthesia, since it has a rapid onset and a relatively prolonged duration of action.

Benzocaine

$$NH_2 \longrightarrow \bigcirc \longrightarrow CO \cdot O \cdot C_2H_5$$

Benzocaine is the ethyl ester of aminobenzoic acid and is a non-ionized local anaesthetic with low potency (and toxicity). It is incorporated into various ointments, creams, gels and sprays that are used for the symptomatic relief of muscle strains, pruritis and painful fissures. It is also an ingredient of various lozenges and sprays that are used in the local treatment of oral ulceration.

Amides
Lidocaine

$$\bigcirc \begin{array}{c} CH_3 \\ \\ CH_3 \end{array} NH \cdot CO \cdot CH_2 \longrightarrow N \begin{array}{c} C_2H_5 \\ \\ C_2H_5 \end{array}$$

Lidocaine is an extremely versatile local anaesthetic and was the first aminoacyl amide to be introduced into clinical practice (in 1948). It remains a popular and widely used agent due to its potency, rapid onset and intermediate duration of action. The maximum safe dose is generally considered to be 200 mg in plain solutions, and 500 mg in solutions containing adrenaline, although these dose limits are sometimes modified depending on the site of administration.

Topical anaesthesia
Lidocaine is a widely used topical agent, and numerous preparations are available as aqueous solutions (2–4%) or in water-miscible bases as gels, ointments, creams and sprays (2–10%). Preparations may be applied to the skin, the eye, the ear, the nose and the mouth, as well as other mucous membranes. Lidocaine spray (4%) is frequently used to produce anaesthesia of the tracheobronchial tract prior to endotracheal intubation or bronchoscopic examination, and a lidocaine/chlorhexidine gel is sometimes used to produce anaesthesia of the urethra during diagnostic urological procedures. Sprays containing lidocaine may be applied to mucosal surfaces to provide anaesthesia for suturing of episiotomy wounds, minor lacerations or dental injections. In these conditions, lidocaine has a rapid onset of action (3–5 min) and a moderate duration of action (30–60 min).

The absorption of lidocaine through intact skin is slow and unreliable, and high concentrations (e.g. 30–40%) may be required to produce any significant anaesthesia. Nevertheless, the crystalline tertiary bases of lidocaine and prilocaine can be combined to form a eutectic mixture, which is widely used to produce cutaneous anaesthesia in the form of EMLA cream (page 164).

Infiltration anaesthesia
Infiltration techniques are frequently employed in dentistry and to provide anaesthesia for minor surgical procedures. Solutions of lidocaine (1%) are commonly used for this purpose. Its site of action is at the unmyelinated nerve endings, and provides satisfactory operating conditions in over 90% of cases. The onset of action is almost immediate after submucosal or subcutaneous injection, and in these situations lidocaine usually has a moderate duration of action (70–140 min). Residual anaesthesia persists rather longer after intradermal injection (4–7 h) than after submucosal injection (1–3 h), presumably due to differences in vascularity and absorption. The addition of adrenaline (1 in 200,000, 5 μg mL^{-1}) may increase the quality and prolong the duration of anaesthesia.

Conduction anaesthesia
Lidocaine is commonly used to produce conduction anaesthesia of both moderately accessible minor nerve trunks (e.g. ulnar, radial, intercostal nerves), as well as major nerve trunks with a wide dermatomal distribution (e.g. sciatic nerve, brachial plexus). Solutions containing vasoconstrictors are commonly administered in these techniques.

When used to produce blockade of minor nerve trunks, lidocaine has a relatively rapid onset of action (3–6 min) and a moderate duration of action (1–2 h), which can be increased to 4–5 hours by the addition of adrenaline (1 in 200,000, 5 μg mL^{-1}). Lidocaine is sometimes mixed with other drugs (e.g. bupivacaine), in order to combine a rapid onset with a prolonged duration of action.

In major nerve blockade, the onset of action of lidocaine is more variable, mainly due to anatomical factors, which can restrict the access of the local anaesthetic to its site of action. In this situation, the use of a nerve stimulator can be of value in the accurate localization of the injection site. During brachial plexus or sciatic nerve blockade, lidocaine and other local anaesthetics may be placed outside the fascial planes or connective tissues that surround nerve trunks. In this situation, lidocaine must diffuse across extensive connective tissue barriers as well as the myelin sheaths of nerve trunks, and may be also taken up by the surrounding adipose tissue and by muscle. Consequently, the onset and duration of action of lidocaine is rather variable, although it usually acts within 15 minutes, and analgesia persists for 3–4 hours. Persistent paraesthesia after nerve blockade is probably due to mechanical trauma, rather than to any pharmacological effects.

Spinal and extradural anaesthesia

In the UK, lidocaine is not commonly used alone to produce spinal or extradural anaesthesia. Although it produces rapid and dense sensory anaesthesia and complete motor blockade, the localization and duration of action of single doses is often unsuitable, and tachyphylaxis may occur (page 156).

Other indications

Lidocaine produces blockade of Na^+ channels in myocardial and junctional tissues, in a similar manner to its effects on peripheral nerves. Blockade of Na^+ channels in cardiac muscle decreases the rise time of phase 0 of the cardiac action potential (V_{max}) in a dose-dependent manner. It is commonly used in the treatment of ventricular arrhythmias, which occur after myocardial infarction or during anaesthesia (Chapter 15).

Intravenous lidocaine has also been used to produce systemic analgesia in both acute postoperative and chronic neuropathic pain, although its mode of action is uncertain. In current practice, it is rarely if ever used for this purpose.

Prilocaine

Prilocaine is a local anaesthetic similar to lidocaine, although it produces less vasodilatation, and in most situations it can be used without an added vasoconstrictor. The maximum recommended dose is 400 mg. Large doses of prilocaine may produce methaemoglobinaemia and cyanosis, due to its metabolite o-toluidine, which can oxidize haemoglobin (Fe^{2+}) to methaemoglobin (Fe^{3+}).

Infiltration anaesthesia

Prilocaine (1%, 10 mg mL^{-1}) is often used to produce infiltration and conduction anaesthesia. In this situation, it has a similar onset and duration of action to lidocaine (page 163).

In addition, prilocaine is a constituent of EMLA cream and is frequently used as a dental anaesthesic. It is also the standard drug used to produce intravenous regional analgesia (IVRA).

EMLA cream

The absorption of lidocaine and prilocaine through intact skin is usually slow and unreliable, and high concentrations (e.g. 40%) are required. In recent years, a eutectic mixture of local anaesthetics (EMLA) has been widely used to produce surface anaesthesia prior to venepuncture, particularly in paediatric practice. The crystalline tertiary bases of lidocaine and prilocaine melt to form an oil at temperatures greater than 16°C (a eutectic mixture). In these conditions, the droplet concentration of the local anaesthetics in an oil-in-water emulsion is high enough (approximately 80%) to produce effective surface anaesthesia. The eutectic mixture contains equal proportions (25 mg mL^{-1}) of the tertiary bases of lidocaine and prilocaine, and is used as an emulsion, which can be applied as a cream to the skin. The preparation may cause transient skin blanching and erythema. An occlusive dressing is often necessary to ensure cutaneous contact, and at least 60 minutes is usually required to demonstrate significant surface analgesia.

Dental anaesthesia

Prilocaine (4%) is sometimes used to provide local anaesthesia prior to dental surgery. In infiltration anaesthesia, its site of action is at the unmyelinated nerve endings, and usually provides satisfactory operating conditions. It usually has a rapid onset and a similar duration of action to lidocaine (70–140 min).

Some preparations of prilocaine (3%) that are intended for dental use contain the vasoconstrictor felypressin (0.03 i.u./mL). Felypressin (octapressin) is a non-catecholamine vasoconstrictor that is chemically related to vasopressin, a posterior pituitary hormone. It is a synthetic octapeptide that only affects peripheral blood vessels and has no action on the heart. Although it produces less marked vasoconstriction than adrenaline, it may be useful for patients with ischaemic heart disease when the use of catecholamines is undesirable.

Intravenous regional analgesia

Prilocaine (or lignocaine) is commonly used to produce IVRA and can provide analgesia for minor surgical procedures. This procedure was first described by August Bier in 1908, but only became widely used about 35 years ago. In this technique, prilocaine or lignocaine is slowly injected over 2–3 minutes into the vein of a limb that has been previously exsanguinated by an Esmarch bandage and occluded by an orthopaedic tourniquet inflated to 100 mm Hg above systolic blood pressure. Application of the tourniquet may produce some discomfort or pain after 20–30 minutes. This may be avoided by the use of a double tourniquet.

After injection of the local anaesthetic, paraesthesia and the onset of analgesia are almost immediate, and complete sensory blockade usually develops within 10 minutes. The quality and duration of analgesia are dependent on the dose of local anaesthetic administered, the efficiency of exsanguination, the period of ischaemia prior to injection and the site of injection. It may also be influenced by the effects of local acidosis and vasodilatation due to CO_2 accumulation. The site of action is probably the unmyelinated nerve terminals, which prilocaine or lidocaine reach by retrograde spread in the vascular bed. Nerve conduction is not usually affected, although motor paralysis and muscle relaxation usually occur within 15–20 minutes, due to the presynaptic and postsynaptic effects of the local anaesthetics at the neuromuscular junction.

Prilocaine or lidocaine (200 mg, or 40 mL of a 0.5% solution) is commonly used to produce regional anaesthesia in the arm. Larger doses are required for the lower limb and the results are less satisfactory. If the tourniquet is not released until 15–20 minutes after injection, plasma concentrations of lidocaine or prilocaine are unlikely to be significant, although minor symptoms of local anaesthetic toxicity (e.g. paraesthesia, tinnitus) are not uncommon. Systemic toxicity is usually associated with the accidental or inadvertent deflation of the tourniquet.

Both prilocaine and lignocaine produce effective local anaesthesia, and the period of residual analgesia usually ranges from 30 to 120 minutes. Nevertheless, IVRA is not normally used for procedures that last longer than an hour. Although nerve damage is extremely rare, it is associated with prolonged tourniquet times.

Bupivacaine, levobupivacaine and ropivacaine must not be used to produce IVRA.

Bupivacaine

Bupivacaine has a relatively slow onset of action (approximately 30 min) but a prolonged duration of action. These features are related to its physicochemical characteristics (particularly its pK_a value and extensive protein binding, page 156). Its main advantage compared to lidocaine and prilocaine is its prolonged duration of action, and it is commonly used to produce infiltration and conduction anaesthesia. In addition, it is the standard drug that is used to produce extradural lumbar and thoracic blockade and to produce spinal subarachnoid anaesthesia.

The main disadvantage of bupivacaine is its ability to cause significant cardiotoxicity, and high doses of the drug may cause ventricular arrhythmias and cardiac arrest. Although bupivacaine has similar effects to lidocaine on Na^+ channels in the heart, it is bound by them with far greater avidity. It is also bound by Ca^{2+} and K^+ channels, and consequently affects the myocardium to a far greater extent than other local anaesthetics. High doses and concentrations are associated with significant cardiotoxicity and can result in sudden death.

Infiltration anaesthesia

Bupivacaine (0.25%) can be used to provide anaesthesia for minor surgical procedures. In this situation, it has a relatively rapid onset and a long duration of action (approximately 200 min), which can be further prolonged by the addition of adrenaline (1 in 200,000, 5 $\mu g\ mL^{-1}$). Residual anaesthesia persists longer after intradermal injection (4–7 h) than after submucosal injection, presumably due to differences in vascular absorption.

Conduction anaesthesia

Bupivacaine is commonly used to produce blockade of both minor and major nerve trunks. When bupivacaine (0.25%) is used to produce minor nerve blockade, it has a relatively rapid onset of action (3–6 min), and a long duration of action (2–6 h). Its action can be further prolonged by increasing the dose of the local anaesthetic, or by the addition of a vasoconstrictor (e.g. adrenaline 1 in 200,000, i.e. 5 $\mu g\ mL^{-1}$). Mixtures of bupivacaine with other local anaesthetics (lidocaine, prilocaine) are commonly used to combine a rapid onset with a prolonged duration of action.

Bupivacaine is also frequently used to produce brachial plexus or sciatic nerve blockade. In these conditions, its onset of action is more variable, mainly due to the presence of connective tissue barriers, which restrict access to its site of action. The use of a nerve stimulator may assist the accurate localization of the site of injection. When bupivacaine is used to produce major nerve blockade, it has a relatively slow onset of action (20–25 min), but sensory anaesthesia usually persists for 4–10 hours, and occasionally lasts for 24 hours. Persistent paraesthesia after nerve blockade is probably due to mechanical trauma, rather than to other factors.

Extradural anaesthesia

The administration of local anaesthetics in the extradural space between the dura mater and the periosteum lining of the vertebral canal is widely used to provide analgesia in labour and the postoperative period, and is usually given in the thoracolumbar region of the spinal cord. After injection, local anaesthetic solutions spread widely in all directions, and produce conduction blockade of the intradural spinal nerve roots. The spread of local anaesthetic solutions is more extensive in parturient women, since the peridural venous plexus is distended due to compression of the inferior vena cava, and the volume of the potential space is reduced. Consequently, the dose of local anaesthetic required to produce extradural blockade in pregnancy is usually reduced. Similar considerations apply to arteriosclerotic patients and the elderly due to the impairment of vascular absorption from the extradural space.

In the UK, bupivacaine (0.25–0.5%, 12–20 mL) is the standard drug used to produce extradural anaesthesia. Its administration is normally preceded by a test dose of local anaesthetic to exclude intravascular placement or subarachnoid administration. Although bupivacaine has a relatively slow onset of action (10–20 min), it usually provides analgesia for several hours, and its high lipid-solubility and protein binding usually delay absorption into the systemic circulation. For similar reasons, only small amounts of the drug cross the placenta and reach the foetal circulation. Lower concentrations (0.1%) provide sensory analgesia with minimal motor blockade, allowing patients to be ambulatory (with assistance). Higher concentrations (i.e. 0.25% and above) have a longer duration of action with a moderate degree of motor blockade. Adrenaline (1 in 200,000–1 in 300,000; 3.3–5 μg mL^{-1}) is sometimes added to solutions of bupivacaine. Although the duration of blockade is unaffected, peak plasma concentrations of bupivacaine are reduced and its presence may give an early indication of inadvertent intravascular uptake. Anaesthesia can be prolonged by repeated dosage through an extradural catheter using patient controlled devices or continuous infusion techniques.

The quality and extent of extradural blockade is determined by the volume and concentration, as well as the total dose of the local anaesthetic. Raised volumes increase the spread of the solution in the extradural space and the extent of blockade, while higher concentrations reduce the onset time and increase the intensity of anaesthesia (and motor blockade). Higher total doses increase the duration of blockade. Other important factors are the site of injection, the speed of administration and the position of the patient. A lateral posture encourages the development of sensory and motor blockade on the dependent side.

Extradural blockade above the lower thoracic region (T10) may be associated with significant hypotension, i.e. a reduction in systolic blood pressure >30 mm Hg, due to the blockade of sympathetic vasoconstrictor pathways in the spinal cord and autonomic ganglia. Vascular dilatation in splanchnic blood vessels results in the pooling of blood in capacitance vessels and a substantial reduction in venous return. Hypotension can be prevented or minimized by preloading with crystalloid or colloid solutions, or treated with ephedrine (10–15 mg).

Other drugs are sometimes given by extradural administration. For instance, opioids (e.g. fentanyl, diamorphine), α_2-receptor agonists (e.g. clonidine, dexmedetomidine) or benzodiazepines (midazolam) are sometimes used extradurally for the relief of acute or chronic pain, either alone or with local anaesthetics.

Caudal anaesthesia

Caudal blockade is a form of extradural anaesthesia and is commonly used to produce blockade of the lower lumbar and sacral nerve roots. The nerves of the cauda equina descending in the sacral canal are blocked by local anaesthetics inserted via a needle in the sacral hiatus, producing sacral or perineal anaesthesia. Local anaesthetic agents do not need to traverse a dural sleeve or the dura (which ends at the lower border of S2).

Bupivacaine (0.5%, 20–30 mL) is usually used to produce caudal blockade, in particular to provide supplementary analgesia after haemorrhoidectomy and perineal surgery in adults. The slow onset of blockade and the significant failure rate are probably due to considerable vascular absorption into the sacral and vertebral venous plexuses, and the wide distribution of the drug through the various sacral foramina. The extent of blockade may be affected by the position of the patient and the dose and speed of injection.

Spinal anaesthesia

Introduction of bupivacaine into the subarachnoid space and the CSF produces spinal (subarachnoid) anaesthesia. The central attachments of ventral and dorsal nerve roots are unmyelinated, and local anaesthetics are rapidly taken up by the nerve roots, dorsal root ganglia and the spinal cord. Consequently, the potency of bupivacaine after subarachnoid injection is 10–15 times greater than after extradural administration, and motor blockade is more pronounced. In addition, the onset of anaesthesia is more rapid, since bupivacaine does not need to penetrate extensive tissue or diffusion barriers in order to reach its site of action. Because of the smaller dose of bupivacaine that is used, the duration of subarachnoid anaesthesia is usually shorter than extradural anaesthesia. The quality and extent of blockade is related to the dose of bupivacaine administered, the speed of injection, the position of the patient and the specific gravity of the solution injected (when compared with the specific gravity of CSF, i.e. 1.003–1.006). An increase in the dose of bupivacaine improves the quality and intensity of anaesthesia, prolongs its duration, and may increase the spread of the local anaesthetic. The effect of the position of the patient depends on the specific gravity of the solution injected.

In the UK, 'heavy' bupivacaine (0.5% in 8% dextrose; specific gravity = 1.026) is most commonly used to produce spinal subarachnoid blockade. Moderate doses (10–20 mg, i.e. 2–4 mL) have an onset within 5–15 minutes and a duration of action of approximately 2–3 hours. Bupivacaine and dextrose are not metabolized in the CSF, but are taken up by the spinal cord or absorbed by branches of the spinal arteries, which form a vascular network in the pia mater.

The spread of hyperbaric 'heavy' bupivacaine (0.5% in 8% dextrose) in the CSF is affected by gravity and by posture. When hyperbaric bupivacaine is injected in the mid-lumbar region (L2–L3 or L3–L4) and the patient is placed supine, blockade usually spreads to the mid-thoracic level (T4–T7). When the patient remains in the sitting position after injection, blockade only extends to T7–T10. When injected at L4–L5 and the patient remains sitting, a 'saddle' blockade is produced, which can be used for perineal surgery. The spread of hyperbaric bupivacaine in the CSF is also affected by age, height, spinal curvature and the volume and capacity of the subarachnoid space. Thus, compression of the inferior vena cava in pregnancy or by intra-abdominal tumours distends the vertebral venous plexus and decreases the volume of the subarachnoid space. In these conditions, the spread of the local anaesthetic and the degree of analgesia are increased.

Hypobaric solutions of bupivacaine (0.25% or 0.5% bupivacaine in water, specific gravity = 1.003–1.006) tend to rise in the CSF. Their spread does not depend on the position of the patient, and their effects tend to be unpredictable. Although their duration of action is usually longer than hyperbaric bupivacaine, the blockade is frequently of variable quality. Isobaric solutions of bupivacaine are more physiological, and their spread in the CSF does not depend on posture. Unfortunately, their effects are also less predictable.

Spinal subarachnoid anaesthesia above the lower thoracic region (T10) may cause significant hypotension due to the blockade of sympathetic vasoconstrictor pathways in the spinal cord and autonomic ganglia. Vascular dilatation in splanchnic blood vessels results in the pooling of blood in capacitance vessels and a substantial reduction in venous return. Hypotension can be prevented or minimized by preloading with crystalloid or colloid solutions, or treated with ephedrine (10–15 mg).

Different sensory modalities do not have the same sensitivity to subarachnoid blockade, and the area of analgesia is usually greater than the area of anaesthesia. Similarly, the level of motor blockade is approximately two dermatomes lower than the level of sensory blockade.

Neurological complications of spinal anaesthesia are relatively uncommon and are usually related to CSF leakage, mechanical trauma and the introduction of infection or pre-existing pathology. However, the incidence of arachnoiditis and cauda equina syndromes is probably commoner when higher concentrations of bupivacaine are used.

Levobupivacaine

Chiral centre (S-configuration)

Levobupivacaine is the S(−)-isomer of bupivacaine. In experimental and human volunteer studies, it is approximately 30% toxic than racemic bupivacaine or R(+)-bupivacaine, probably due to its reduced affinity for the CNS and myocardial tissue. Consequently, its most important advantage is the reduction in the risk of cardiotoxicity when compared with the parent drug. Levobupivacaine also causes less negative inotropism and prolongation of the QT interval than racemic bupivacaine or R(+)-bupivacaine. In addition, it may cause enhanced vasoconstriction with a prolonged duration of action, and a reduction in the intensity and duration of motor blockade.

In accordance with a European Union directive, levobupivacaine is standardized in terms of the concentration of the active local anaesthetic base S(−)-bupivacaine per mL. In contrast, racemic bupivacaine is standardized in terms of the concentration of the local anaesthetic salt (bupivacaine hydrochloride) per mL. Consequently, solutions of levobupivacaine with the same nominal local anaesthetic concentrations as bupivacaine (2.5 mg mL^{-1} or 5 mg mL^{-1}) contain 11% more molecules of local anaesthetic. This is an important consideration when making comparisons between the two drugs.

In general, the clinical indications, uses and effects of levobupivacaine in infiltration anaesthesia, conduction anaesthesia, extradural anaesthesia and spinal anaesthesia are similar to racemic bupivacaine. Its use is contraindicated in intravenous regional anaesthesia (Bier's block) and paracervical obstetric blockade.

Infiltration anaesthesia

Levobupivacaine (0.25%, 2.5 mg mL^{-1}) has been used to produce infiltration anaesthesia (maximum dose = 60 mL, i.e. 150 mg). It has similar analgesic effects, and a comparable duration of action to racemic bupivacaine.

Conduction anaesthesia

Levobupivacaine can also be used to produce both minor and major nerve blockade (0.25% or 0.5%, maximum dose = 150 mg). The onset of action and characteristics of nerve blockade are similar to racemic bupivacaine, although the duration of sensory anaesthesia is slightly longer.

Spinal anaesthesia

Subarachnoid blockade has been produced by levobupivacaine (0.5%) prior to surgery of the lower limb. The usually recommended dose is 15 mg (3 mL), and the solutions in common use (0.5%) are slightly hypobaric. Although these solutions (like those of hypobaric bupivacaine) are more physiological, their spread in the CSF is less predictable. Consequently, their clinical effects are generally less satisfactory than after hyperbaric bupivacaine.

Extradural anaesthesia

Levobupivacaine has also been used to produce epidural anaesthesia prior to surgical anaesthesia (0.5–0.75%, 50–150 mg) and Caesarean section (0.5%, 75–150 mg). In general, the onset of action and the duration of sensory and motor blockade are similar to racemic bupivacaine. Lower concentrations (0.125–0.25%) of levobupivacaine can be used to produce analgesia during labour.

Ropivacaine

Chiral centre

Ropivacaine is the S(−)-propyl analogue of bupivacaine and is only prepared and used as a single enantiomer. It has several distinct advantages when compared with racemic bupivacaine. Ropivacaine is associated with a reduced risk of negative inotropism and cardiotoxicity due to its decreased affinity for cardiac Na$^+$ channels. In experimental studies, its toxicity is approximately 20–30% less than racemic bupivacaine or R-bupivacaine, due to its reduced affinity for myocardial tissue. When compared to bupivacaine, it decreases the intensity and duration of motor blockade, and produces better separation of motor and sensory blockade. In addition, ropivacaine has a shorter half-life than bupivacaine (Table 9.2).

Ropivacaine has a similar pK$_a$ value and rate of onset to bupivacaine, although its lipid solubility and protein binding are marginally lower (Table 9.1). Consequently, its potency and duration of action are usually slightly less than bupivacaine, although it may produce some local vasoconstriction which prolongs its duration of action.

Infiltration anaesthesia

Ropivacaine (0.2%, 2 mg mL^{-1}) has been used to produce infiltration anaesthesia and has similar analgesic effects and a prolonged duration of action (200 min or more) when compared to racemic bupivacaine. Some studies have suggested that the duration of cutaneous anaesthesia may be 2–3 times longer than racemic bupivacaine, and ropivacaine should probably not be used for infiltration in tissues without a collateral blood supply. Residual anaesthesia usually persists longer after intradermal injection than after submucosal injection, possibly due to differences in vascular absorption.

Conduction anaesthesia

Ropivacaine has been used to produce minor blockade of the ulnar, radial and intercostal nerves, as well as major blockade of the sciatic nerve or brachial plexus. In general, the duration of local anaesthesia is similar to bupivacaine, and minor nerve blockade usually occurs within 10–15 minutes and lasts for 2–6 hours. Major nerve blockade is less predictable, since ropivacaine must diffuse across extensive connective tissue barriers as well as the myelin sheaths of nerve trunks. Local anaesthesia usually occurs within 15–25 minutes and may last for up to 10 hours. In most studies, ropivacaine has a slightly more rapid onset of action than bupivacaine, but a very similar duration of action. Moderately concentrated solutions of ropivacaine (i.e. 5 mg mL^{-1} or 7.5 mg mL^{-1}) are usually required to produce effective and long-lasting local anaesthesia.

Spinal anaesthesia

In studies in which ropivacaine has been compared with racemic bupivacaine, it appears to produce similar sensory blockade, but a lesser degree of motor blockade. Nevertheless, it usually has a shorter duration of action and is less potent than bupivacaine, and the drug is not currently licensed to produce subarachnoid anaesthesia in the UK.

Extradural anaesthesia

Ropivacaine (0.75–1.0%, 7.5–10 mg mL^{-1}) is commonly used to produce extradural anaesthesia prior to general surgical procedures (although only concentrations of 7.5 mg mL^{-1} are currently licensed for use in obstetric anaesthesia). Its clinical use is normally preceded by a test dose of local anaesthetic to exclude intravascular placement or inadvertent subarachnoid administration. After extradural administration, the sensory blockade produced by equivalent doses of ropivacaine and bupivacaine has a similar onset and duration, although motor blockade is slower in onset, of shorter duration, and is less intense. Consequently, ropivacaine provides better separation of sensory and motor blockade than bupivacaine.

Ropivacaine is also widely used as a continuous epidural infusion to provide analgesia after surgical operations and during labour. Solutions of ropivacaine (0.2%, 2 mg mL^{-1}) are usually infused at the rate of 6–12 mL h^{-1}, and provide effective and long lasting analgesia without motor blockade.

Suggested reading

Bardsley, H., Gristwood, R., Baker, H., Watson, N. & Nimmo, W. (1998) A comparison of the cardiovascular effects of levobupivacaine and rac-bupivacaine following intravenous administration to healthy volunteers. *British Journal of Clinical Pharmacology* **46**, 245–249.

Bay-Nielsen, M., Klarskov, B., Bech, K., Andersen, J. & Kehlet, H. (1999) Levobupivacaine vs bupivacaine as infiltration anaesthesia in inguinal herniorrhaphy. *British Journal of Anaesthesia* **82**, 280–282.

Benhamou, D., Hamza, J., Eledjam, J.J., *et al.* (1997) Continual extradural infusion of ropivacaine 2 mg mL^{-1} for pain relief during labour. *British Journal of Anaesthesia* **78**, 748–750.

Brockway, M.S., Bannister, J., McClure, J.H., McKeown, D. & Wildsmith, J.A.W. (1991) Comparison of extradural ropivacaine and bupivacaine. *British Journal of Anaesthesia* **66**, 31–37.

Catterall, W.A. (1993) Structure and function of voltage-gated ion channels. *Trends in Neurosciences* **16**, 500–506.

Covino, B.G. (1986) Pharmacology of local anaesthetic agents. *British Journal of Anaesthesia* **58**, 701–716.

Cox, C.R., Faccenda, K.A., Gilhooly, C., Bannister, J., Scott, N.B. & Morrison, L.M.M. (1998) Extradural S(−) bupivacaine: comparison with racemic RS-bupivacaine. *British Journal of Anaesthesia* **80**, 289–293.

Denny, N.M. & Selander, D.E. (1998) Continuous spinal anaesthesia. *British Journal of Anaesthesia* **81**, 590–597.

Duncan, L. & Wildsmith, J.A.W. (1995) Liposomal local anaesthetics. *British Journal of Anaesthesia* **75**, 260–261.

Foster, R.H. & Markham, A. (2000) Levobupivacaine: a review of its pharmacology and use as a local anaesthetic. *Drugs* **59**, 551–579.

Kopacz, D.J., Allen, H.W. & Thompson, G.E. (2000) A comparison of epidural levobupivacaine 0.75% with racemic bupivacaine for lower abdominal surgery. *Anesthesia and Analgesia* **90**, 642–648.

Lyons, G., Columb, M., Wilson, R.C. & Johnson, R.V. (1995) Epidural pain relief in labour: potencies of levobupivacaine and racemic bupivacaine. *British Journal of Anaesthesia* **81**, 899–901.

McClure, J.H. (1996) Ropivacaine. *British Journal of Anaesthesia* **76**, 300–307.

McCrae, A.F., Jozwiak, H. & McClure, J.H. (1995) Comparison of ropivacaine and bupivacaine in extradural analgesia for the relief of pain in labour. *British Journal of Anaesthesia* **74**, 261–265.

Morrison, L.M.M., Emanuelsson, B.M., McClure, J.H., *et al.* (1994) Efficacy and kinetics of extradural ropivacaine: comparison with bupivacaine. *British Journal of Anaesthesia* **72**, 164–169.

Narahashi, T., Yamada, M. & Frazier, D.T. (1969) Cationic forms of local anesthetics block action potentials from inside the nerve membrane. *Nature* **223**, 748–749.

Reynolds, F. (1987) Adverse effects of local anaesthetics. *British Journal of Anaesthesia* **59**, 78–95.

Santos, A.C., Karpel, B. & Noble, G. (1990) The placental transfer and fetal effects of levobupivacaine, racemic bupivacaine and ropivacaine. *Anesthesiology* **90**, 1698–1703.

Scott, D.B. (1986) Toxic effects of local anaesthetic agents on the central nervous system. *British Journal of Anaesthesia* **58**, 732–735.

Tucker, G.T. (1986) Pharmacokinetics of local anaesthetics. *British Journal of Anaesthesia* **58**, 717–731.

Wahedi, W., Nolte, H. & Kline, P. (1996) Ropivacaine in spinal anaesthesia. *Anaesthetist* **45**, 737–744.

Wann, K.T. (1993) Neuronal sodium and potassium channels: structure and function. *British Journal of Anaesthesia* **71**, 2–14.

Whiteside, J.B., Burke, D. & Wildsmith, J.A.W. (2001) Spinal anaesthesia with ropivacaine 5 mg mL^{-1} in glucose 10 mg mL^{-1} or 50 mg mL^{-1}. *British Journal of Anaesthesia* **86**, 241–244.

Whiteside, J.B. & Wildsmith, J.A.W. (2001) Developments in local anaesthetic drugs. *British Journal of Anaesthesia* **87**, 27–35.

10 Drugs that Act on the Neuromuscular Junction

Structure of the neuromuscular junction

Motor nerve fibres are the axons of nerve cells that originate in the anterior horn of the brain stem and the spinal cord. The axon terminals branch extensively, and each anterior horn cell normally innervates 10–150 muscle fibres (the motor unit). As each terminal branch approaches skeletal muscle it loses its myelin sheath, and the neuromuscular junction (the 'final common pathway' of Charles Sherrington) commences at the non-myelinated nerve ending that is distal to the last node of Ranvier.

Focal innervation

Most axon terminals are situated in a junctional fold on the surface of the muscle fibre (the motor endplate). In most mammalian muscles, each muscle fibre has a single motor endplate near its midpoint (focal innervation). This usually forms an elevation on the surface of the fibre, which is called an *en plaque* neuromuscular junction. These fibres are supplied by fast conducting Aα axons, and have rapid rates of contraction and relaxation.

Multiple innervation

A minority of muscle fibres are densely innervated at numerous sites by slower conducting Aγ axons. Multiple innervation occurs in extraocular, intrinsic laryngeal and some facial muscles where the termination of motor nerves resembles a bunch of grapes, and is called an *en grappe* neuromuscular junction. These fibres are unable to propagate action potentials and require a series of impulses to produce a muscle response. The resultant contraction and subsequent relaxation is thus slower than in focally innervated fibres, and is sometimes described as a contracture.

The motor endplate

The essential features of focally innervated motor endplates can be revealed by electron microscopy (Fig. 10.1). The axon terminal, which is enveloped by processes of Schwann cell cytoplasm, lies in a cleft in the sarcolemmal membrane and contains numerous mitochondria and synaptic vesicles. Many of these vesicles are associated with specialized zones in the axon membrane that correspond to sites of neurotransmitter release. The synaptic vesicles are synthesized in anterior horn cells of the spinal cord and are transported to the motor nerve terminal by the microtubular system. The terminal axolemmal membrane is separated from the postsynaptic membrane by the synaptic gap, which is approximately 50 nm wide. The synaptic gap includes a basement lamina approximately 20 nm wide, which mainly consists of mucopolysaccharides.

Acetylcholine receptors are primarily present in discrete groups on the shoulders of the junctional folds. Their maximum density at these sites is approximately 10,000 per square micrometre (μm^2). The distal valleys contain acetylcholinesterase (AChE), which has a globular structure and is predominantly present in the synaptic gap. The enzyme is firmly attached to the basement membrane by collagen fibres. Both acetylcholine receptors and AChE are also present at presynaptic sites on the motor nerve terminal.

Physiology of neuromuscular transmission

The synthesis, storage and release of acetylcholine

Neuromuscular transmission depends on the synthesis, storage and release of acetylcholine by the motor nerve terminal. At the motor endplate, choline is partly derived from plasma and partly produced by the hydrolysis

171

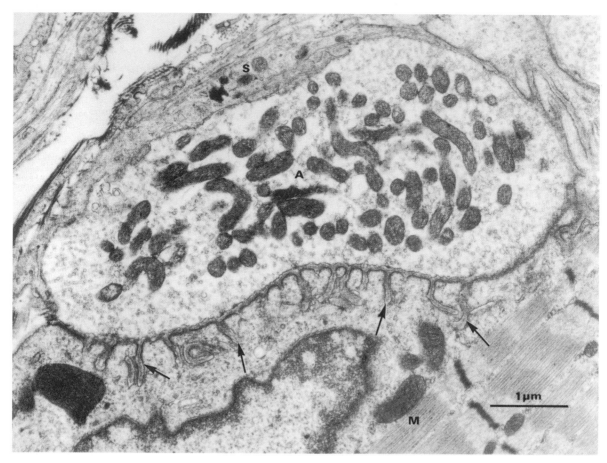

Fig. 10.1 Electron micrograph of part of a normal neuromuscular junction. The axonal terminal (A) lies in a deep indentation of the sarcolemmal membrane and contains abundant mitochondria and synaptic vesicles. The external surface of the axon is covered by processes of Schwann cell cytoplasm (S). There are numerous infoldings (arrowed) of the sarcolemma beneath the axon, and basal lamina material lies between nerve and muscle (M) and fills these subneural folds (×30,000). (Courtesy of Professor L.W. Duchen)

of acetylcholine. Choline is transported from extracellular fluid into the axoplasm by a high affinity carrier system that is present in all cholinergic nerves (Fig. 10.2). The active transport of choline across the neurolemma is usually the rate-limiting step in the synthesis of acetylcholine by choline acetyltransferase, according to the reaction:

choline + acetyl-coenzyme A → acetylcholine

+ coenzyme A

The synthesis of the neurotransmitter in the axoplasm is increased by its release, and it is not usually possible to cause depletion of acetylcholine by rapid rates of nerve stimulation or by choline deficiency.

Approximately 50% of acetylcholine synthesized in the axoplasm is transferred to small synaptic vesicles about 50 nm in diameter and stored as molecular packages or quanta. Each synaptic vesicle contains 10,000–12,000 molecules of acetylcholine, as well as Ca^{2+}, ATP and various protoglycans. Some of the remaining acetylcholine leaks across the axonal membrane and may be present in significant amounts in Schwann cells and in the sarcoplasm of muscle fibres, although its function at these sites is unknown. A few large dense-core vesicles can also be detected at motor nerve endings, and contain calcitonin gene-related peptide (CGRP), which is released into the synaptic gap following high frequency stimulation.

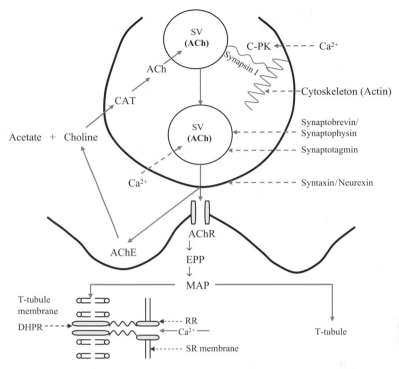

Fig. 10.2 Diagrammatic representation of neuromuscular transmission. Acetylcholine (ACh) is synthesized in the axoplasm by choline acetylase (CAT) and is then stored in the synaptic vesicles (SV), which are anchored to cytoskeletal elements by Synapsin I. After depolarization Ca^2 enters the axoplasm (via P/Q channels) and activates a Ca^{2+}/calmodulin-dependent protein kinase (C-PK), causing the phosphorylation of Synapsin I and the release of SVs from the cytoskeleton. SVs migrate to the axonal membrane, and vesicular proteins (synaptotagmin, synaptobrevin and synaptophysin) are bound by docking sites in the membrane (syntaxin and neurexin). Synaptotagmin is activated by Ca^{2+} entry, resulting in the release of ACh into the synaptic gap. ACh is rapidly hydrolysed by acetylcholinesterase (AChE) and the choline formed is recycled by active transport. Released ACh combines with binding sites on the α-subunits of the acetylcholine receptor (AChR), opening the ion channel. Na^+ entry results in an endplate potential (EPP), and a muscle action potential (MAP) is propagated along the muscle fibre. At the end of the sarcomere, the MAP depolarizes the T-tubule membrane and activates a dihydropyridine receptor (DHPR) in the membrane. This in turn activates the ryanodine receptor (RR), the Ca^{2+} release channel of the sarcoplasmic reticulum (SR). The released Ca^{2+} is rapidly bound by Troponin-C, resulting in myosin–actin interaction and muscle contraction.

About 1% of the acetylcholine vesicles are located at release sites on the axolemma of the motor nerve terminal, and constitute the 'easily available' store of the neurotransmitter (Fig. 10.1). The remaining vesicles are distributed throughout the axoplasm, where they are bound to microtubules, actin filaments and other cytoskeletal elements, forming a large reserve store. They can be rapidly mobilized and can readily migrate to docking sites on the terminal axolemmal membrane during repetitive nerve activity. After the release of the neurotransmitter, synaptic vesicles are retrieved and recycled by endocytosis.

Integral proteins contained in the nerve terminal appear to play an important role in the docking of vesicles at the release site, and in the formation of an extrusion pore, which allows the escape of acetylcholine into the synaptic gap. Several integral proteins are involved in this process:

• Synapsin I is a phosphoprotein which encircles synaptic vesicles in the axoplasm and anchors them to cytoskeletal elements. After depolarization of the terminal plasma membrane, calcium P/Q channels open, allowing Ca^{2+} to enter the axoplasm and combine with calmodulin. This results in the activation of a Ca^{2+}/calmodulin-dependent protein kinase that phosphorylates serine residues in the tail of synapsin I, resulting in the release of the vesicles (Fig. 10.2).

• Synaptobrevin, synaptotagmin and synaptophysin are vesicular membrane proteins that are bound by specific receptor docking sites (e.g. syntaxin, neurexin) in the presynaptic membrane. Synaptotagmin appears to be activated by Ca^{2+} entry, allowing it (and the synaptic vesicles) to combine with the presynaptic docking proteins, and to release quanta of acetylcholine into the junctional gap.

Acetylcholine receptors

During the past 40 years, there has been considerable progress in the isolation and purification of acetylcholine receptors, and their precise structure has been determined by molecular biological techniques. Similar receptors are present in abundance in the electroplaque organs of certain fishes, such as the South American freshwater eel and the giant electric ray. These receptors are irreversibly bound by the toxins of certain snakes, such as α-bungarotoxin derived from the Taiwan banded krait and α-cobra toxin. Consequently, they can be isolated and purified by affinity chromatography. In addition, receptors have been sequenced and inserted into artificial and amphibian oocyte membranes by molecular biological techniques.

Postsynaptic receptors

The acetylcholine receptor on the postsynaptic membrane of the neuromuscular junction is an integral membrane protein with a molecular weight of approximately 250 kDa. It is the classical example of a receptor that contains an intrinsic ion channel. In adults, it consists of five glycoprotein subunits (α_1, α_1, β, ε, δ), which cross the postsynaptic membrane and surround a central cation channel (Fig. 10.3).[1] The α-subunits have a molecular weight of approximately 40 kDa, and each contains an acetylcholine-binding site at the interface with a different subunit (ε or δ). Each acetylcholine-binding site is adjacent to specific amino acid residues (cysteines 192 and 193, tyrosines 93 and 190 and tryptamine 149), and the phospholipid composition of the surrounding membrane may influence combination of the α-subunits with acetylcholine and subsequent receptor activation.

---

[1] In the fetus, denervated muscle, and many other species the ε-subunit is replaced by the γ-subunit, which has a lower ionic conductance but a longer channel opening time.

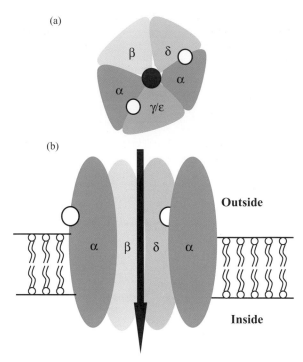

Fig. 10.3 Diagrammatic representation of the nicotinic receptor at the neuromuscular junction. The receptor consists of five subunits (α_1, α_1, β, γ or ε, and δ) surrounding the central transmembrane ion channel. It has two binding sites for acetylcholine (at the α–γ/ε and α–δ interfaces). (a) View of the receptor from above; (b) vertical cross-section of the receptor in the muscle cell membrane. Acetylcholine-binding sites (○); ion channel (●, ↓).

Presynaptic receptors

Acetylcholine receptors at the neuromuscular junction are also present on the presynaptic motor nerve terminal and the most distal node of Ranvier, although their molecular structure is slightly different, consisting of α_3-, α_3-, β-, ε- and δ-subunits. Presynaptic receptors on the motor nerve terminal play an important part in maintaining transmitter output at high rates of nerve stimulation ('positive feedback'), and their blockade by non-depolarizing agents is responsible for the phenomenon of decrement or fade (page 183). In contrast, acetylcholine receptors on the most distal node of Ranvier can induce retrograde (antidromic) firing of the motor nerve. The injection of acetylcholine into the popliteal artery of experimental animals not only produces activity of the appropriate muscle groups, but also gives rise to antidromic nerve action potentials that are conducted in a retrograde direction, and can be recorded from ventral nerve roots by appropriate electrophysiological methods. Similar effects are produced by anticholinesterase drugs and suxamethonium, indicating that drugs acting at the neuromuscular junction may also affect the motor nerve terminal.

Neuromuscular transmission
Miniature endplate potentials
In the absence of nerve impulses, postsynaptic receptors display spontaneous electrical activity. This occurs as discrete, randomly distributed miniature endplate potentials (MEPPs), which have an amplitude of 0.5–1.5 mV. Each MEPP is considered to arise from the release of a single molecular packet or quantum of acetylcholine, and reflects the random spontaneous activity of isolated vesicles that have collided or lined up with extrusion sites on the membrane.

Acetylcholine release
When a nerve action potential reaches the axon terminal, the contents of 200–300 synaptic vesicles, each containing 10,000–12,000 molecules of acetylcholine, are released from the terminal into the synaptic gap. The released acetylcholine diffuses across the synaptic cleft and combines with the α-subunits close to their α/δ and α/ε interfaces, resulting in conformational changes that open the ion channel. The probability of this occurring is considerably increased when both sites are occupied by acetylcholine ('positive cooperativity').

Ion channel opening
Ion channel opening is an extremely rapid 'all or none' phenomenon that results in the entry of 10,000–20,000 cations (mainly Na^+, but also K^+ or Ca^{2+}) during the 1–2 milliseconds that each channel is open.[2] These ionic changes result in multiple single channel currents, each of which has an amplitude of approximately 4 pA (4×10^{-12} A), which summate to produce an endplate current. If the small and localized endplate potential reaches a critical amplitude (a depolarization of $\approx$10–15 mV), voltage-sensitive Na^+ channels open, and a muscle action potential (MAP) is propagated along the muscle fibre. The amount of acetylcholine released is normally greater than that required to produce minimal endplate depolarization, i.e. there is a considerable safety margin in neuromuscular transmission.

[2] In practice, the ion channel opens for about 0.4 milliseconds, and then briefly closes 4–5 times during this 1–2 millisecond interval.

MAPs and excitation–contraction coupling
The MAP is conducted as a wave of depolarization along the sarcolemma, and enters the transverse or T-tubular system at the end of the sarcomere. Depolarization of the T-tubular system, which is perpendicular to the sarcolemma, results in conformational changes in the dihydropyridine receptor in the T-tubular membrane. These allosteric changes activate the Ca^{2+} release channel in the adjacent sarcoplasmic reticulum (the ryanodine receptor), and the subsequent release of Ca^{2+} from the sarcoplasmic reticulum initiates contraction of the muscle fibre (Fig. 10.2). The released Ca^{2+} are bound by troponin C, resulting in conformational changes in troponin I, troponin T and tropomyosin. Cross-bridges are then formed between myosin and actin, resulting in the phenomenon of muscle contraction. The sequence of physiological and biochemical changes between depolarization of the T-tubular system and muscle contraction are known as excitation–contraction coupling.

Acetylcholinesterase
The action of acetylcholine at the motor endplate is rapidly terminated by the hydrolytic enzyme AChE. The enzyme is predominantly associated with the basement membrane in the distal valleys of the synaptic space, where it is anchored by connective tissue fibres (collagen Q). AChE combines with acetylcholine at two sites approximately 0.5 nm apart, called the anionic and the esteratic site (Fig. 10.4). The anionic site mainly consists of a negatively charged glutamate group, which forms a reversible ionic bond with the positively charged quaternary nitrogen in acetylcholine. The esteratic site consists of the amino acids serine and histidine. The terminal hydroxyl group in serine attacks and splits acetylcholine at its ester link, resulting in the release of choline and the transient acetylation of the serine residue in AChE (Fig. 10.4). The acetylated enzyme reacts with water extremely rapidly (half-life of hydrolysis = 40 μs) resulting in the regeneration of AChE and the release of the acetate group (as acetic acid).

AChE is present at all cholinergic junctions and is probably synthesized at these sites. It is also found in red blood cells and in many regions of the CNS. Erythrocyte AChE may play an important part in the hydrolysis of certain drugs (e.g. diamorphine, esmolol).

Butyrylcholinesterase
In contrast, butyrylcholinesterase (BChE), also known as plasma cholinesterase or pseudocholinesterase, is synthesized in the liver, and is also present in many other tissues.

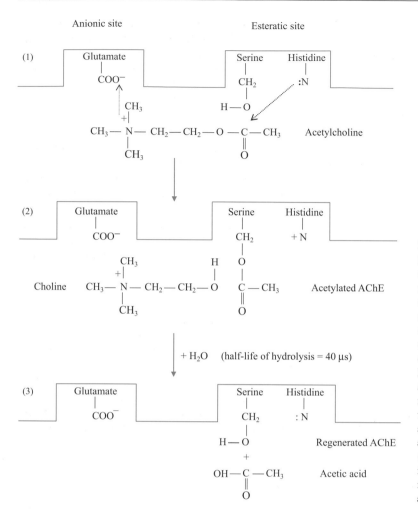

Fig. 10.4 The hydrolysis of acetylcholine by AChE. (1) The quaternary nitrogen atom in acetylcholine (N^+) forms a reversible ionic bond with the negatively charged glutamate group (COO^-) at the anionic site, and electron donation occurs from histidine to the carbonyl carbon atom in acetylcholine at the esteratic site ($\swarrow$); (2) The terminal hydroxyl group in serine attacks and splits acetylcholine at its ester link, resulting in the formation of choline and the transient acetylation of the esteratic site; (3) Choline is released, and the acetylated enzyme is rapidly hydrolysed (half-life of hydrolysis = 40 μs) resulting in the regeneration of AChE and the release of the acetate group (as acetic acid).

Although BChE can slowly metabolize acetylcholine, it may have a more important function in the regulation and hydrolysis of other choline esters that are present in the gut wall (e.g. propionylcholine, butyrylcholine). In anaesthetic practice BChE has an essential role in the hydrolysis of certain muscle relaxants (e.g. suxamethonium, mivacurium) which are unaffected by AChE. Genetic variants of BChE can prolong the action of suxamethonium and mivacurium (Chapter 6). BChE also contains two binding sites, and the serine group at the esteratic site combines with choline esters in a similar manner to AChE (Fig. 10.4). However, at the anionic site, BChE forms a dipolar bond rather than an ionic bond with many substrates.

Drugs that inhibit the synthesis of acetylcholine

The synthesis of acetylcholine is dependent on the active transport of choline from the extracellular fluid to the axoplasm. Several drugs, including hemicholinium and triethylcholine, inhibit this process and impair the synthesis of acetylcholine. In addition to its effects on choline transport, triethylcholine is also converted by choline acetyltransferase to a 'false transmitter' (acetyltriethylcholine), which is stored in synaptic vesicles and released by nerve stimulation, but does not produce depolarization of the motor endplate. The experimental drug vesamicol also impairs neuromuscular transmission by preventing the uptake of acetylcholine by synaptic vesicles.

Although all of these drugs have been extensively investigated, none of them have any clinical applications.

Drugs that modify the release of acetylcholine

Several drugs can modify the release of acetylcholine from the motor nerve terminal, including:
- Drugs that affect calcium entry
- Local anaesthetics
- General anaesthetics
- Neurotoxins
- Guanidine and aminopyridine
- Miscellaneous drugs

Drugs that modify calcium entry

The release of acetylcholine from the motor nerve terminal is dependent upon the passive entry of Ca^{2+} through P/Q Ca^{2+} channels, which is induced by depolarization of the neuronal membrane (Fig. 10.2). Consequently, alterations in extracellular Ca^{2+} might be expected to affect neurotransmitter release. In practice, although hypocalcaemia and hypercalcaemia have important effects on the excitability of tissues and cardiac contraction, they do not usually modify acetylcholine release, except in experimental conditions.

Nevertheless, drugs that prevent Ca^{2+} entry into the motor nerve terminal can impair neuromuscular transmission and prolong non-depolarizing neuromuscular blockade. This phenomenon has been mainly reported with the aminoglycosides and polymyxins, but may also occur with various other antibiotics (e.g. colistin, tetracyclines, lincomycin). In the past, neuromuscular function was occasionally impaired in patients on long-term streptomycin therapy for tuberculosis, and neostigmine-resistant curarization sometimes occurred after abdominal surgery when large doses of aminoglycosides were insufflated to the peritoneal cavity. Similar problems have been observed when antibiotics are given to patients with myasthenia gravis.

Although this problem is rarely encountered in current anaesthetic practice, calcium salts (e.g. calcium gluconate) can reverse antibiotic-induced neuromuscular blockade. Less commonly, anticholinesterase drugs are useful.

Magnesium salts can also prolong non-depolarizing blockade, since Mg^{2+} compete with Ca^{2+} for transport into the motor nerve terminal, and thus decrease the release of acetylcholine. Parenteral magnesium sulphate or magnesium-containing antacids may reduce neurotransmitter release and prolong the action of muscle relaxants, particularly in patients with renal failure.

Local anaesthetics

Local anaesthetics decrease Na^+ entry into motor nerve fibres and prevent conduction of the nervous impulse (Chapter 9). Consequently, they decrease Ca^{2+} entry into the motor nerve terminal and prevent the release of acetylcholine. After systemic administration or absorption, they affect conduction in unmyelinated nerve endings, and conduction blockade of major or minor nerve trunks may prevent transmission of nerve impulses from anterior horn cells.

Inhalational anaesthetics

Inhalational anaesthetic agents may also decrease the release of acetylcholine and can profoundly affect the degree of neuromuscular blockade. They induce depression of the CNS, decrease the generation of nerve impulses and have direct effects on the muscle cell membrane. The cardiovascular effects of inhalational anaesthetics may also modify the pharmacokinetic behaviour of muscle relaxants.

Neurotoxins

Certain neurotoxins can prevent the release of acetylcholine, for example:
- α-Latrotoxin
- Botulinus toxin
- β-Bungarotoxin

α-Latrotoxin

Latrotoxin is a constituent of black widow spider venom and affects the release of acetylcholine from all cholinergic nerves. At the neuromuscular junction, α-latrotoxin initially produces the irreversible fusion of synaptic vesicles with the terminal axonal membrane. Subsequently, the vesicles become disorganized and lose their ability to concentrate newly synthesized acetylcholine, partly due to disruption of the vesicular membrane protein synaptotagmin, which fuses synaptic vesicles to the docking proteins in the nerve terminal.

Botulinus toxin

Botulinus toxin, which also affects all cholinergic nerves, is a zinc endopeptidase. The toxin consists of a number of distinct enzymes that break down synaptobrevin and synaptotagmin and thus prevent the release of acetylcholine from synaptic vesicles (although the neurotransmitter content of the motor nerve terminal is unaffected). Botulinus toxin typically causes progressive parasympathetic and motor paralysis (botulism), resulting in a high mortality due to respiratory failure. Although botulinus antitoxin may be lifesaving, it must be administered before the appearance of any clinical signs of botulism in order to be of therapeutic value. β-Bungarotoxin has a similar action to botulinus toxin.

Guanidine and aminopyridine

Both guanidine and aminopyridine prolong the duration of the neuronal action potential and increase the calcium channel opening time. Consequently, they increase Ca^{2+} entry into the motor nerve terminal and thus facilitate the release of acetylcholine. Their mode of action is slightly different, since guanidine delays the inactivation of Na^+ channels, while aminopyridine tends to inactivate K^+ channels and thus prevent repolarization. Both drugs have been used to increase the release of acetylcholine from the motor nerve terminal in botulism and the Eaton–Lambert syndrome, a rare disorder of neuromuscular transmission usually associated with a small cell carcinoma of the bronchus. Unfortunately, both guanidine and aminopyridine readily cross the blood–brain barrier and can cause convulsions, and this has severely restricted their clinical use.

Other drugs

Theophylline and other xanthine derivatives can enhance the release of acetylcholine, either by adenosine receptor blockade or by phosphodiesterase inhibition and accumulation of cAMP. This phenomenon may also explain the improvement that occurs in myasthenia gravis when sympathomimetic drugs (e.g. ephedrine) are administered.

Drugs that modify the action of acetylcholine

Drugs that modify the action of acetylcholine by combining with postsynaptic cholinergic receptors are traditionally referred to as neuromuscular blocking agents or muscle relaxants. They are commonly divided into two groups:
- Depolarizing agents
- Non-depolarizing agents

Depolarizing agents

Suxamethonium chloride is the only depolarizing agent that is in current clinical use. In the past, decamethonium was used but is now only of historical interest. As their name implies, these drugs produce depolarization of the motor endplate immediately before the onset of neuromuscular blockade.

Suxamethonium

$$CH_3-\overset{\overset{\displaystyle CH_3}{|+}}{\underset{\underset{\displaystyle CH_3}{|}}{N}}-CH_2-CH_2-O-\overset{\overset{\displaystyle}{}}{\underset{\underset{\displaystyle O}{\parallel}}{C}}-CH_2-CH_2-\overset{\overset{\displaystyle}{}}{\underset{\underset{\displaystyle O}{\parallel}}{C}}-O-CH_2-CH_2-\overset{\overset{\displaystyle CH_3}{|+}}{\underset{\underset{\displaystyle CH_3}{|}}{N}}-CH_3$$

Suxamethonium is a quaternary amine ester consisting of two molecules of acetylcholine linked by their acetyl groups at their non-quaternary ends. It is a slender, elongated and flexible molecule (a leptocurare) with three methyl groups attached to each quaternary head, which are separated by a distance of approximately 1.2 nm.

The ability of suxamethonium to produce depolarization blockade in humans was first recognized in 1949–1951, although its pharmacological properties were initially investigated in curarized animals in 1906. After the intravenous injection of suxamethonium, profound muscle relaxation preceded by observable muscle fasciculations normally occurs within 1 minute. The duration of neuromuscular blockade after normal doses (1.0–1.5 mg kg^{-1}) is usually 4–6 minutes.

It is usually the agent of choice for rapid sequence induction and this remains the main indication for its clinical use.

Mode of action

Since suxamethonium is not hydrolysed by AChE, it can produce prolonged and repetitive depolarization of the motor endplate. Depolarization activates voltage-sensitive Na^+ channels in the adjacent muscle fibre, resulting in the generation and propagation of MAPs and producing muscle fasciculations. However, the persistent depolarization produced by suxamethonium is rapidly followed by the generation of local current circuits in the adjacent muscle fibre, which cause conformational changes in voltage-sensitive Na^+ channels, resulting in their inactivation.

These changes occur within several milliseconds, and produce a zone of electrical inexcitability that surrounds the motor endplate and extends for 1–2 mm along the muscle fibre membrane. This zone will not transmit or propagate impulses, although the remainder of the muscle fibre is normally excitable by direct stimulation.

Anticholinesterase drugs may increase the depth and duration of suxamethonium blockade, since the drug is normally metabolized by BChE (plasma cholinesterase). In addition, inhibition of AChE results in the accumulation of acetylcholine in the synaptic cleft, and thus augments depolarization blockade.

Effects of indirect stimulation

Suxamethonium causes a progressive decrease in the electromyographic or mechanical response of muscle at slow rates of nerve stimulation (e.g. 0.1 Hz), reflecting the balance of activity in muscle fibres that are unaffected by neuromuscular blockade and those that are refractory. At more rapid rates of intermittent stimulation (e.g. a 'train of four', 2 Hz for 2 s), there is no evidence of decrement or fade, since acetylcholine output is maintained. The absence of decrement or fade probably reflects the positive effects of suxamethonium and released acetylcholine on presynaptic receptors that normally preserve transmitter output at high rates of impulse conduction ('positive feedback').

Effects of tetanic stimulation

During suxamethonium blockade, tetanic stimulation does not affect the amplitude of the response or result in post-tetanic potentiation. Tetanic stimulation of motor nerves normally results in a progressive decrease in acetylcholine release per stimulus, which is rapidly followed by enhanced synthesis and transmitter mobilization. Consequently, when the tetanus ends, acetylcholine output per stimulus is increased. In the presence of suxamethonium, this has little or no effect on neuromuscular function, and post-tetanic changes are not observed on the electromyogram or mechanomyogram.

Unwanted effects

The clinical use of suxamethonium may be associated with a number of adverse effects, including:

• Muscle fasciculations
• Postoperative myalgia
• Hyperkalaemia
• Tachyphylaxis and dual blockade
• Increased introcular pressure
• Parasympathomimetic effects
• Malignant hyperpyrexia

Muscle fasciculations

Neuromuscular blockade is preceded by muscle fasciculations, which may be slight (usually involving the small muscles of the hand and the facial muscles), moderate (affecting larger muscle groups in the limbs) or severe and generalized. Moderate and severe fasciculations can facilitate venous return and cause an increase in cardiac output, a rise in blood pressure and increased intracranial tension. Fasciculations that involve the abdominal muscles may cause an increase in intragastric pressure.

Muscle fasciculations are incoordinated contractions due to the repetitive firing of muscle fibres and are associated with increased electromyographic activity. It is generally considered that fasciculations are due to the effects of suxamethonium on presynaptic cholinergic receptors, resulting in the firing of antidromic impulses from the axon or motor unit. Reflex effects that are mediated by cholinergic receptors in muscle spindles may play a secondary role.

Postoperative myalgia

Postoperative muscle pain is a frequent complication of suxamethonium, and occurs chiefly in the subcostal region, the trunk and the shoulder girdle. Women are more susceptible than men, and symptoms are more frequent in patients who are mobilized soon after surgery and in those unaccustomed to muscular exercise. The prevalence of postoperative myalgia varies between 6 and 60%. The concentration of creatine phosphokinase is significantly raised and myoglobinuria occasionally occurs, suggesting that suxamethonium myalgia may be related to muscle damage caused by drug-induced fasciculations. Nevertheless, in many studies the incidence of muscle fasciculations is not directly related to the occurrence of postoperative pain.

Hyperkalaemia

Suxamethonium results in depolarization of the motor endplate and the adjacent sarcolemma, and repolarization causes the efflux of K^+ into extracellular fluid. In normal conditions, plasma K^+ levels are elevated by ≈ 0.5 mmol L^{-1}, an increase which is rarely of clinical significance.

In contrast, in patients with severe burns or certain neurological disorders, much greater rises in serum K^+ concentrations (e.g. 4–9 mmol L^{-1}) have been reported. In neurological conditions, the major hyperkalaemic response occurs in venous blood draining paralysed or injured limbs. A latent period (usually 1–2 weeks) may occur between the time of injury and significant hyper-kalaemia.

It is usually considered that abnormal hyperkalaemic responses are due to 'denervation supersensitivity'. In den-ervated or severely damaged muscle (and during fetal life), acetylcholine receptors on the postsynaptic membrane are not just localized to the motor endplate, but extend along the entire surface of the muscle fibre. These acetylcholine receptors (with α-, α-, β-, γ- and δ-subunits) have a rapid turnover time (24–48 h) and a prolonged opening time, a smaller channel conductance and are depolarized more readily. In these conditions, the increased loss of K^+ from muscle is related to the extensive area of the muscle mem-brane containing these receptors that is depolarized by suxamethonium.

Cardiac arrest has been reported following the use of suxamethonium in patients with severe burns and neuro-logical conditions, usually between 20 and 60 days after the initial injury. Although clear evidence of muscle dam-age or denervation may not be present, hyperkalaemia is probably the main causal factor. Hypovolaemia, acidosis and autonomic imbalance may also be involved. The use of suxamethonium in patients with pre-existing hyper-kalaemia, as in renal failure or severe acidosis, may result in cardiac arrhythmias.

Tachyphylaxis and dual blockade
Suxamethonium (particularly in excessive doses) may be associated with the development of tachyphylaxis and dual neuromuscular blockade. Tachyphylaxis is usually recog-nized by a progressively decreased response to successive doses of the drug, and often precedes the gradual devel-opment of non-depolarizing blockade (dual or phase II block). In humans, this is most commonly seen when large doses or prolonged infusions of suxamethonium are used, or when drug elimination is compromised by genetic ab-normalities in BChE or by anticholinesterase drugs.

The precise explanation for the development of tachy-phylaxis and dual block is unclear. It may reflect the con-tinual presence of suxamethonium at the motor endplate, resulting in a prolonged channel opening time, which al-lows the drug to enter the ion channel and produce non-competitive blockade. Alternatively, it may be related to receptor desensitization (Chapter 3).

Increased intraocular pressure
Suxamethonium causes a rise in intraocular tension, which may last for several minutes. Consequently, the drug should be used with caution in patients with penetrating eye injuries, and during open ocular surgery.

In humans the extrinsic muscles of the eye are multiply innervated by slowly conducting Aγ axons. In this respect, the innervation of extraocular muscles is similar to avian muscles, in which suxamethonium characteristically pro-duces a slow and sustained contraction (contracture) of voluntary muscle. Similar effects are probably produced in human extraocular muscles.

Parasympathomimetic effects
Suxamethonium is a close chemical analogue of acetyl-choline and has cholinergic effects at muscarinic recep-tors. Bradycardia or AV nodal rhythms may occur after a large single dose, or with repeated administration (es-pecially in children). These effects may be enhanced by digoxin or by other drugs that alter autonomic balance in favour of parasympathetic activity (e.g. β-adrenoceptor antagonists).

Other muscarinic effects are not uncommon. Increased production of bronchial and salivary secretions is fre-quently observed, especially with repeated dosage. Gastric tone is also increased, and a rise of intragastric pressure occurs (although this is partly related to fasciculations involving the abdominal muscles). Repeated doses of sux-amethonium may cause a marked increase in uterine tone during Cesarean section. All these parasympathetic effects can be prevented or attenuated by premedication with atropine or other antimuscarinic drugs.

Malignant hyperpyrexia
Malignant hyperpyrexia is a genetic disorder that affects sarcoplasmic Ca^{2+} regulation and can be triggered by sux-amethonium in susceptible individuals (Chapter 6). The initial dose may fail to produce muscle relaxation, and cause generalized muscle rigidity and a rapidly rising tem-perature within several minutes. Suxamethonium proba-bly precipitates the release of Ca^{2+} from the calcium re-lease channel in the sarcoplasmic reticulum of susceptible individuals (the ryanidine receptor), leading to sustained contraction and subsequent muscle damage.

Metabolism of suxamethonium
Suxamethonium is rapidly hydrolysed in plasma by BChE, and a single dose of suxamethonium usually has a short duration of action (4–6 min). The breakdown of the drug occurs in two stages. Suxamethonium is initially converted to succinylmonocholine, which has weak neu-romuscular blocking activity ($\approx$10% of the potency of suxamethonium). Succinylmonocholine is subsequently broken down to succinic acid and choline. Delayed or prolonged metabolism of suxamethonium may cause pro-longed paralysis and apnoea, as well as tachyphylaxis and

Table 10.1 Drugs that inhibit BChE and that may prolong the action of suxamethonium.

Edrophonium
Neostigmine
Pyridostigmine
Pancuronium
Trimetaphan
Local anaesthetic esters
Aprotinin
Bambuterol
Cimetidine
Cyclophosphamide
Metoclopramide
Tetrahydroaminacrine
Organophosphorus compounds

the increased likelihood of phase II block, and is usually due to

• genetic polymorphism of BChE (Chapter 6)
• severe hepatic dysfunction, causing abnormally low BChE concentrations
• renal failure and renal dialysis
• interactions with other drugs that inhibit BChE

In the past, some inhibitors of BChE (tetrahydroaminacrine and hexafluorenium) have been intentionally used to prolong neuromuscular blockade, although their action is unpredictable. In addition, many other drugs inhibit BChE and can prolong the action of suxamethonium (Table 10.1).

Non-depolarizing agents

All non-depolarizing or competitive agents contain one or more quaternary amine groups and have a bulky molecular structure ('pachycurares'). Non-depolarizing muscle relaxants primarily produce neuromuscular blockade by competition with acetylcholine for receptor sites on the postsynaptic membrane, and they all produce similar effects at the neuromuscular junction.

History
Curare

Curare is a generic term for various South American arrow poisons and is correctly used to describe the crude extracts obtained from certain species of the plants *Chondrodendron* and *Strychnos*. Impure extracts of these plants contain several different alkaloids and were used for many centuries by South American Indians as an arrow or blowdart poison in order to paralyse and kill their prey. The preparation of curare was shrouded in mystery and ritual, and the samples of the drug which first reached civilization were classified by the containers in which they had been transported. Tube curare was preserved in bamboo tubes, pot curare was carried in earthenware jars and calabash curare was kept in gourds. Scientific interest in curare dates from the classical observations of Claude Bernard in 1856, when he correctly localized the paralytic effects of curare to the neuromuscular junction, since the drug did not affect nerve conduction or the response of voluntary muscle to direct stimulation.

The clinical use of curare dates from 1932, when purified fractions were first used in the treatment of tetanus and spastic disorders. The drug was later used to control pentylenetetrazole-induced convulsions during the treatment of psychiatric disorders. The purified alkaloid d-tubocurarine was first used as a muscle relaxant during anaesthesia by Griffith and Johnson in Canada in 1942, and by Gray and Halton in Liverpool in 1945.

Tubocurarine

The introduction of tubocurarine revolutionized the practice of anaesthesia and for many years the drug was the main non-depolarizing relaxant in clinical use. Its semisynthetic derivative dimethyltubocurarine was also widely used in the USA. Unfortunately, tubocurarine had a relatively long and somewhat unpredictable duration of action, and significant histamine releasing properties that could contribute to hypotension and hypersensitivity responses. The introduction of safer relaxants (and the high cost of production) led to a decline in its use, and d-tubocurarine is no longer commercially available in the UK.

Gallamine

Gallamine triethiodide was the first synthetic non-depolarizing relaxant and was introduced by Bovet in 1947. It is a tris-quaternary amine, and for many years it was the only available alternative to tubocurarine. Although gallamine has a rapid onset and an intermediate duration of action, it commonly induces tachycardia and is almost entirely eliminated unchanged in urine. Consequently, in renal failure its clearance is greatly decreased and its terminal half-life is prolonged 10–20 times. Because of these disadvantages and its relative expense, gallamine is rarely used in current practice.

Alcuronium

Alcuronium is a semisynthetic derivative of the curare alkaloid toxiferine and was first used in the UK in 1962. It had a relatively long duration of action, it was commonly implicated in atopic and hypersensitivity responses and its elimination was dependent on renal function. These factors (as well as problems in its manufacture) have led to the withdrawal of the drug.

The muscle relaxants in common use can be divided into two groups:
• Aminosteroids (pancuronium, vecuronium and rocuronium)
• Benzylisoquinolinium derivatives (mivacurium, atracurium and cisatracurium)

Mode of action

All non-depolarizing agents produce neuromuscular blockade by competition with acetylcholine for its binding sites on the α_1-subunits of the postsynaptic cholinergic receptor. Most muscle relaxants have different affinities for the two α_1-binding sites on each cholinergic receptor. The acetylcholine binding site on the α/ϵ-subunit interface has a 5- to 10-fold greater affinity for non-depolarizing agents than the comparable site on the α/δ-subunit. Nevertheless, blockade of only one of these binding sites is required in order to produce neuromuscular blockade. Non-depolarizing agents are often referred to as 'competitive' neuromuscular blocking drugs, although not all their effects are due to competitive antagonism at postsynaptic sites. For example, most of these drugs can produce ion channel blockade, but this is of little pharmacological importance due to the restricted channel opening time (1–2 ms).

The combination of non-depolarizing agents with postsynaptic receptors decreases the number of sites that are available for binding by acetylcholine, but does not change membrane conductance or ionic permeability. Consequently, depolarization by acetylcholine is progressively diminished, due to a reduction in the number of available receptors. The amplitude of the endplate potential gradually decreases and eventually fails to generate a propagated MAP, resulting in neuromuscular blockade (Fig. 10.5). Normal neuromuscular function is restored when adequate redistribution and/or elimination of the muscle relaxant occurs, or when acetylcholine accumulates at unblocked postsynaptic receptors.

In normal conditions, the amount of acetylcholine released by nerve stimulation exceeds that required to produce an endplate potential and the subsequent MAP. Consequently, there must be considerable receptor occupation by non-depolarizing agents before there is evidence of any neuromuscular blockade. Experimental evidence suggests that at least 80% of postsynaptic receptors must be occupied before there is any effect on neuromuscular trans-

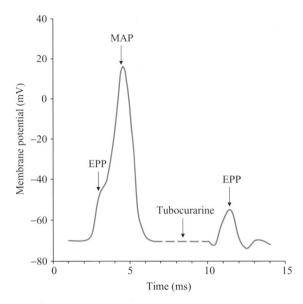

Fig. 10.5 The effect of non-depolarizing relaxants on the endplate potential (EPP) and the muscle action potential. Microelectrode recordings were made at the mammalian motor endplate. In normal conditions, the EPP generates (and is subsequently eclipsed by) the MAP. After tubocurarine and other muscle relaxants, the EPP progressively declines until it fails to generate the MAP.

mission, and that 90–95% receptor occupation may be required for complete blockade.

In addition to their postsynaptic effects, non-depolarizing agents combine with presynaptic receptors on the motor nerve terminal. These receptors are normally responsible for the maintenance of transmitter output at high rates of nerve stimulation and are normally activated by released acetylcholine. Consequently, when the motor nerve is stimulated during partial neuromuscular blockade, the amount of acetylcholine released from the axon terminal is progressively diminished by the presynaptic effects of muscle relaxants, resulting in decrement or fade. Non-depolarizing relaxants may also physically occlude ion channels at presynaptic sites.

These presynaptic actions may account for the effectiveness of 'precurarization' i.e. the ability of small doses of non-depolarizing agents to prevent or ameliorate the fasciculations and muscle pain induced by suxamethonium. Prejunctional depolarization and local axon reflexes are prevented or attenuated by the non-depolarizing agent, and the rate of firing of motor units is reduced. These effects are also responsible for the phenomenon of decrement or fade.

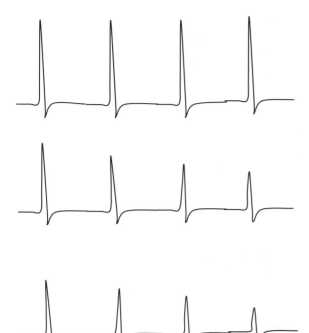

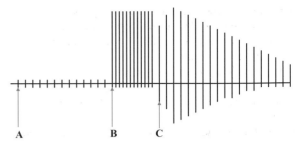

Fig. 10.7 Post-tetanic potentiation during partial recovery from non-depolarizing blockade. (A) Compound muscle action potentials evoked by repetitive indirect stimulation; (B) Conditioning tetanus (the amplitude is due to the presence of a stimulus artefact); (C) Post-tetanic potentiation after reversion to the original rate of indirect stimulation.

Effect of tetanic stimulation

Tetanic stimulation of motor nerves results in a progressive decrease in the release of acetylcholine per stimulus, which is rapidly followed by its enhanced synthesis and mobilization. Consequently, when the tetanus ends, acetylcholine output per impulse is increased at less rapid rates of stimulation for 10–15 seconds. During non-depolarizing blockade, the increase in acetylcholine output per stimulus allows the neurotransmitter to temporarily displace non-depolarizing relaxants from postsynaptic and presynaptic sites, resulting in post-tetanic potentiation (Fig. 10.7). During profound neuromuscular blockade, the 'post-tetanic count' can be used to monitor the effects of muscle relaxants on the motor endplate.

Distribution

Since all non-depolarizing relaxants are quaternary amines, they are not absorbed from the gut. After intravenous administration, they are mainly distributed in extracellular fluid and may be partly bound to plasma proteins. Many *in vitro* techniques, including plasmapheresis, equilibrium dialysis and ultrafiltration, have been extensively used to assess the protein binding of individual muscle relaxants. Although there are many inconsistencies, most of the results suggest that 20–60% of pancuronium are bound by IgG and by albumin, but only minor amounts of other relaxants are significantly bound by plasma proteins. Changes in the binding of muscle relaxants to plasma proteins in pathological conditions are probably of little practical significance. Subjects with raised IgG concentrations, as in severe burns and liver disease, are occasionally resistant to pancuronium, although it is unclear whether this phenomenon is related to altered plasma protein binding or other factors.

Fig. 10.6 Muscle action potentials evoked by indirect nerve stimulation during the induction of non-depolarizing neuromuscular blockade. A train-of-four supramaximal impulses was used to stimulate the ulnar nerve, and electromyographic recordings were made from the motor point of adductor pollicis with surface electrodes. The figure shows the gradual decline in the amplitude of the first response in each train, and the presence of decrement or fade during the induction of non-depolarizing blockade.

Effect of indirect stimulation

Non-depolarizing relaxants progressively decrease the electromyographic or mechanical response at slow rates of nerve stimulation (e.g. 0.1 Hz). At more rapid rates of nerve stimulation (e.g. a 'train of four' stimulus of 2 Hz for 2 s) they cause the characteristic phenomenon of decrement or fade (Fig. 10.6). During non-depolarizing blockade there is a progressive decrease in the quantal release of acetylcholine during 'train-of-four' stimulation, which is probably related to blockade of presynaptic receptors on the nerve terminal. Since postsynaptic receptors are also partially blocked, the 'safety factor' of neuromuscular transmission is compromised, resulting in decrement or fade. The progressive decline in the electrical or mechanical response to indirect stimulation reflects the decreased output of acetylcholine from the motor nerve terminal.

Because of their chemical structure, non-depolarizing relaxants do not cross the blood–brain barrier or the placental barrier in appreciable amounts. Nevertheless, small concentrations of most muscle relaxants (usually less than 1% of the maternal level) can be detected in the fetal circulation or cord blood after administration to the mother. Foetal apnoea is only rarely associated with the use of these drugs during anaesthesia for Cesarean section, although paralysis has occurred following repeated dosage during long-term ventilation in pregnancy. Gallamine is more liable to cross the placenta than other muscle relaxants.

Pharmacokinetics

After administration of a non-depolarizing agent, there is a rapid fall in plasma concentration during the first 2–10 minutes, mainly due to its rapid distribution in extracellular fluid, as well as its uptake by renal and hepatic cells. Only small concentrations are localized at the motor endplate, or are non-specifically bound at anionic sites in the junctional cleft and the basement membrane of muscle fibres. After 10–15 minutes, there is a further slower phase of exponential decline, which reflects the removal of muscle relaxants by renal or biliary excretion, or by metabolism. This terminal decline is more rapid with the benzylisoquinolinium derivatives than with the aminosteroids.

Consequently, the disposition of most muscle relaxants has usually been represented in terms of two or three compartment models. Constants derived from these models can be used to calculate pharmacokinetic parameters, or they may be derived by model-independent methods (Chapter 2). The total apparent volume of distribution of most muscle relaxants is similar to extracellular fluid volume and usually ranges from 150 to 350 mL kg^{-1}. Their clearance is more variable, ranging from 1.2 to 5.5 mL min^{-1} kg^{-1}, with the notable exception of mivacurium. Differences in the terminal half-lives of muscle relaxants usually reflect this range of clearance values and correspond to their relative duration of action (Table 10.2). In most instances there is a close relationship between their steady-state plasma concentration and the degree of neuromuscular blockade.

The pharmacokinetics of muscle relaxants may be modified by renal and hepatic disease. In renal failure, the terminal half-lives of pancuronium and gallamine are prolonged due to a reduction in their clearance. The half-lives and clearance of vecuronium and rocuronium are affected to a lesser extent, while the clearance of benzylisoquinolinium derivatives is usually unaffected. In hepatic disease, the pharmacokinetics of muscle relaxants that are mainly eliminated by the liver (e.g. vecuronium, rocuronium) may be modified.

Aminosteroid muscle relaxants

Pancuronium

Pancuronium is a bisquaternary aminosteroid that was introduced in 1967 and is a chemical derivative of malouétine (a plant alkaloid from the periwinkle family with neuromuscular blocking activity). After conventional doses (50–100 μg kg^{-1}) the drug has a slow onset (3–4 min) and a long duration of action (60–90 min), which may be further prolonged in elderly patients. Pancuronium often produces tachycardia and may increase blood pressure and cardiac output, due to its antimuscarinic effects and the potentiation of noradrenaline release and inhibition of catecholamine reuptake (Uptake$_1$). For similar reasons, it may cause tachyarrhythmias in patients on tricyclic antidepressant drugs. Pancuronium may also inhibit BChE. In recent years, the clinical use of pancuronium has significantly declined.

Elimination

Pancuronium is mainly eliminated unchanged in urine (and can cumulate in renal failure), although 15–40% may be metabolized by the liver to three deacetylated compounds (3-hydroxypancuronium, 17-hydroxypancuronium and 3,17-dihydroxypancuronium). At least one of these metabolites (3-hydroxypancuronium) has some neuromuscular blocking activity and has been used as a muscle relaxant (dacuronium). Only trace amounts of pancuronium are eliminated in bile.

Vecuronium

Table 10.2 Pharmacological differences between non-depolarizing relaxants.

	Onset of action	Histamine release	Cardiovascular effects	Duration of action	Plasma protein binding (%)	Volume of distribution (mL kg^{-1})	Clearance (mL min^{-1} kg^{-1})	Terminal half-life (min)	Elimination
Aminosteroids									
Pancuronium	Moderate	Rare	Tachycardia	Long	20–60	190	1.5	130	Metabolized to three deacetylated metabolites (30%) Eliminated in urine (70%)
Vecuronium	Moderate	Rare	None	Short	<20	240	5.2	70	Metabolized to three deacetylated metabolites (20%) Eliminated in bile and urine (80%)
Rocuronium	Rapid	Rare	None	Medium	<20	180	2.9	85	Metabolized to deacetylated metabolites (10%) Eliminated in bile (55%) and urine (35%)
Benzylisoquinolinium agents									
Atracurium	Moderate	Moderate	None	Short	<20	120	5.5	20	Metabolized to laudanosine, a quaternary acrylate, acid and alcohol (95%) Eliminated unchanged (5%)
Mivacurium	Moderate	Moderate	None	Short	<20				Metabolized by plasma BChE to quaternary alcohol and quaternary acid (95%) Eliminated unchanged (5%)
cis-cis						320	5.5	55	
cis-trans						210	90	2	
trans-trans						210	90	2	
Cisatracurium	Moderate	Rare	None	Short	<20	140	5.2	22	Metabolized to laudanosine, a quaternary acrylate, acid and alcohol (95%) Eliminated unchanged (5%)
Other agents									
Gallamine	Rapid	Rare	Tachycardia	Medium	<20	230	1.2	150	Eliminated unchanged in urine (100%)

Values for the volume of distribution, clearance and terminal half-lives are median values obtained from patients with normal hepatic and renal function.

Vecuronium is the monoquaternary analogue of pancuronium and was introduced in 1980. The drug is relatively unstable in aqueous solution and is presented as a lyophilized powder, which is dissolved immediately before injection. After conventional doses ($50-100\ \mu g\ kg^{-1}$) the drug has a slow onset (3–4 min) and an intermediate duration of action (20–30 min), which is not usually prolonged in renal or hepatic disease. Because of its monoquaternary structure, the drug does not affect the cardiovascular system and histamine release is extremely rare. Vecuronium is often considered as the relaxant of choice for patients with a history of atopy or previous hypersensitivity responses.

Elimination

Vecuronium is partly eliminated unchanged in bile (30–40%), and the remainder is converted to three deacetylated metabolites, which are eliminated in bile and in urine. At least one of these metabolites (3-hydroxyvecuronium) has some neuromuscular blocking activity and is approximately 50–60% as potent as the parent compound.

Rocuronium

Rocuronium is an aminosteroid that was introduced into clinical practice in 1995. It is structurally related to vecuronium, but is only 10–15% as potent as the parent drug. After conventional doses ($0.6\ mg\ kg^{-1}$) it has a rapid onset (60–90 s) but an intermediate duration of action. The rapid onset of action is its main clinical advantage, and is usually considered to be due to its low potency, since the higher doses required for neuromuscular blockade will enhance the diffusion gradient between plasma and the neuromuscular junction. Although rocuronium has little effect on the cardiovascular system, it may have mild vagolytic effects but does not cause histamine release.

Elimination

Rocuronium is mainly eliminated unchanged in bile (55%) and urine (35%), although some deacetylated metabolites may be produced. Its effects and duration of action may be slightly prolonged in renal failure and hepatic cirrhosis.

Benzylisoquinolinium muscle relaxants

Atracurium

Atracurium is a *bis*-benzylisoquinolinium ester with four asymmetric centres (resulting in 16 potential stereoisomers), which was introduced in 1982. Because of the internal symmetry of the atracurium molecule, six of the isomers are not unique (i.e. they are identical to other configurations), so that the drug used clinically is a mixture of the 10 different stereoisomers.

Atracurium is usually stored at pH 3.5 and 4°C, since it is unstable at physiological pH values. Conventional doses ($0.3-0.6\ mg\ kg^{-1}$) have an onset within 3–4 minutes and a duration of action of 25–40 minutes, which is not modified by renal or hepatic disease. Higher doses may cause significant histamine release from mast cells. Although atracurium occasionally causes bradycardia, other cardiovascular side effects are rare.

Elimination

Atracurium has a chemical structure that was designed to cause its spontaneous degradation *in vivo* (Hofmann elimination). Although the drug is stable in acid conditions (pH 3) at 4°C, it is rapidly broken down in the body to the tertiary base laudanosine and a quaternary acrylate. Since atracurium is a bisquaternary ester, it is also metabolized by lung and plasma esterases to a monoquaternary alcohol and a monoquaternary acid. Although laudanosine has effects of its own and is a glycine antagonist, its accumulation in renal or hepatic disease is unlikely. The spontaneous recovery from the effects of atracurium is a marked advantage, and the drug is often the relaxant of choice for patients with renal or liver disease.

Mivacurium

Mivacurium was introduced in 1993 and rapidly achieved a role in day-case surgery and for other short elective procedures requiring endotracheal intubation. Mivacurium is a *bis*-benzylisoquinolinium ester that consists of a mixture of three stereospecific geometric isomers, all with the R–R configuration (*cis–cis* mivacurium 6%, *cis–trans* mivacurium 36%, and *trans–trans* mivacurium 58%). The *cis–cis* stereoisomer is only 10% as potent as the other isomers, but is not subject to enzymatic hydrolysis, as shown by the pharmacokinetic data (Table 10.2). In conventional doses ($70–250\ \mu g\ kg^{-1}$) mivacurium has a relatively slow onset (3–5 min) and a short duration of action (15–20 min), which is not usually extended by increasing the dose or by renal failure. Mivacurium does not significantly affect the cardiovascular system, although it sometimes causes histamine release.

Elimination

The two principal stereoisomers in mivacurium (*cis–trans* and *trans–trans*) are rapidly hydrolysed by BChE, as reflected by their high clearance rates ($90\ mL\ min^{-1}\ kg^{-1}$). Consequently, genetic variants (Chapter 6), particularly in the atypical enzyme, may prolong their duration of action. Similar effects are produced by liver disease due to reduced enzyme synthesis, and by drugs that inhibit BChE (Table 10.1). The clearance of *cis–cis* mivacurium, which is not metabolized by BChE, appears to be reduced in renal failure but this is of little clinical significance.

Cisatracurium

Cisatracurium (R-*cis*, R-*cis* atracurium) was introduced in the UK in 1997. It is usually stored at pH 3–4 and 4°C. It is the principal and most active stereoisomer in atracurium and is 3–5 times more potent than the parent drug. Conventional doses ($150\ \mu g\ kg^{-1}$) have a predictably slower onset of action than atracurium, and a slightly longer duration of action (35–45 min). There is no evidence of accumulation after repeated dosage. Because of the lower doses that are used, cisatracurium is less likely to cause histamine release or haemodynamic instability than atracurium.

Elimination

The pharmacokinetic profile of cisatracurium is similar to that of atracurium, and the drug is eliminated by both Hofmann elimination (to laudanosine and an acrylate) and by ester hydrolysis (to a quaternary acid and a quaternary alcohol). Because of the lower doses that are used, the amount of metabolites that are formed is about 75% less than with atracurium.

Newer drugs

It is generally accepted that the ideal muscle relaxant would be a non-depolarizing agent, which would allow optimal conditions for intubation within 1 minute. Total paralysis should last 5–10 minutes and complete spontaneous recovery (to 95% of initial twitch height and a train-of-four value >0.9) should occur within 15–20 minutes of drug administration. Neuromuscular blockade should be rapidly antagonized, when necessary, by anticholinesterase drugs. The ideal agent would not cause histamine release and would be devoid of significant haemodynamic effects. Interactions with other drugs would not occur, and the pharmacological effects of the muscle relaxant would not be influenced by metabolic dysfunction or pH disturbances.

Many studies have suggested that the rapid onset of non-depolarizing blockade can only be achieved by using large doses of muscle relaxants. If relatively potent drugs are used, this advantage can only be gained at the expense of a prolonged duration of blockade, while with less potent drugs, commercial factors and the propensity to produce side effects may be of more importance.

These points have been recently illustrated by studies with the muscle relaxant rapacuronium (Org 9847). Although this novel drug has a rapid onset of action (60–90 s) and a short duration of action (15–20 min), its clinical use is associated with significant histamine release, bronchospasm and vagolytic effects. Although the drug was used for a short time in the USA, it has now been withdrawn.

Anaphylactoid reactions to neuromuscular blocking agents

Anaphylactoid reactions do not require previous exposure to drugs, and their clinical presentation is usually less severe than that of true anaphylactic responses. In common with many other basic drugs (e.g. opioid analgesics), some muscle relaxants can release histamine and other autacoids from mast cells, either by displacement or by exocytosis. Benzylisoquinolinium relaxants are particularly associated with histamine release from mast cells. Localized effects (a wheal and flare response, resulting in oedema, erythema and vasodilatation) are sometimes observed in the hand and arm after intravenous atracurium, and are usually considered to be due to high local drug concentrations, resulting in the displacement of histamine from basophils or endothelial mast cells in the adjacent vessel wall. These phenomena are rarely associated with any systemic manifestations. Although similar effects may be produced by mivacurium, they are unusual after cisatracurium, since this agent is 3–5 times more potent than atracurium. Consequently, it is less likely to be associated with histamine release or haemodynamic instability. Similarly, the aminosteroids do not usually cause histamine release or anaphylactoid reactions.

Anaphylactic reactions

Generalized hypersensitivity reactions, sometimes leading to life-threatening bronchospasm and hypotension, are occasionally associated with the use of muscle relaxants in anaesthetic practice. In most cases, these reactions are due to Type I hypersensitivity reactions, and a history of atopy, previous exposure to the drug and the subsequent detection of specific IgE antibodies with positive responses to intradermal testing are common features. Although these reactions are extremely rare, they may occur with any muscle relaxant (including suxamethonium, which is not infrequently incriminated).

In many cases, the polypharmacy inevitably associated with anaesthetic practice inhibits the identification of the responsible drug. The treatment of hypersensitivity responses occurring in anaesthetic practice is discussed in Chapter 6.

Anticholinesterase drugs

Anticholinesterase drugs combine with and inhibit the enzyme AChE, and thus prevent the rapid hydrolysis of released acetylcholine by AChE. Consequently, they cause the accumulation of acetylcholine at all cholinergic synapses where they gain access. All anticholinesterase drugs produce effects on neuromuscular transmission and the autonomic nervous system. In addition, physostigmine and most organophosphates cross the blood–brain barrier and produce central effects. Anticholinesterase drugs also inhibit BChE, and may prolong the effects of suxamethonium.

Anticholinesterase drugs are usually classified into three main groups:

- Edrophonium
- Carbamate esters
- Organophosphorus compounds

Edrophonium

Edrophonium is a phenolic quaternary amine with a simple chemical structure and is a reversible competitive inhibitor of AChE. The quaternary group is attracted to the anionic site on AChE and forms an ionic bond with the enzyme. Hydrogen bonding between the hydroxyl group and the esteratic site also occurs, producing a rapidly reversible complex (Fig. 10.8).

Following intravenous injection, edrophonium characteristically causes muscle fasciculations (due to inhibition of AChE at the motor endplate), which are frequently associated with muscarinic effects (e.g. bradycardia, increased secretions). Since edrophonium is a quaternary amine, it does not cross the blood–brain or placental barriers. After intravenous injection, the plasma concentration of edrophonium rapidly declines due to its distribution in extracellular fluid and its subsequent elimination by glucuronide conjugation and renal excretion (terminal half-life = 25–45 min). As the plasma concentration falls, AChE inhibition is rapidly reversed (Fig. 10.8), so that the effects of edrophonium are usually transient. Edrophonium (2–10 mg intravenously) has been widely used as a diagnostic test in suspected cases of myasthenia gravis, and to distinguish between myasthenic and cholinergic crises in the established disease. In anaesthetic practice, edrophonium has been used to reverse non-depolarizing blockade produced by atracurium and mivacurium. In these conditions, relatively large doses are required (0.5–1.0 mg kg^{-1}) to ensure that enzyme inhibition persists for long enough to prevent recurarization. Edrophonium has also been used to establish or exclude the development of dual blockade after the administration of suxamethonium.

Carbamate esters

Carbamate esters may be quaternary amines (neostigmine and pyridostigmine) or tertiary amines (physostigmine). All of them are ionized at physiological pH values and

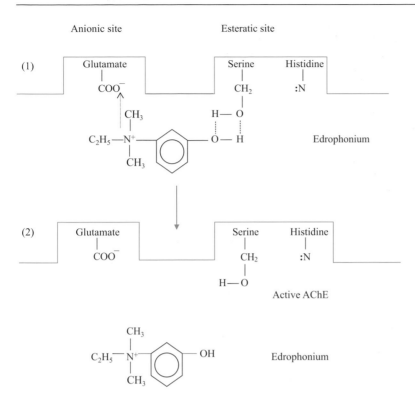

Fig. 10.8 The inhibition of AChE by edrophonium. (1) The quaternary nitrogen atom in edrophonium (N^+) forms a reversible ionic bond with the negatively charged glutamate group (COO^-) at the anionic site, and weak reversible ionic bonds are also formed at the esteratic site (O….H). Consequently, acetylcholine is not hydrolysed by AChE and accumulates at the motor endplate; (2) As the plasma concentration of edrophonium decreases, the quaternary amine rapidly diffuses away from the endplate and AChE immediately recovers from reversible enzyme inhibition.

inhibit AChE in a similar manner. Carbamates are sometimes referred to as oxydiaphoretic (acid-transferring) or time-dependent inhibitors of AChE.

Neostigmine

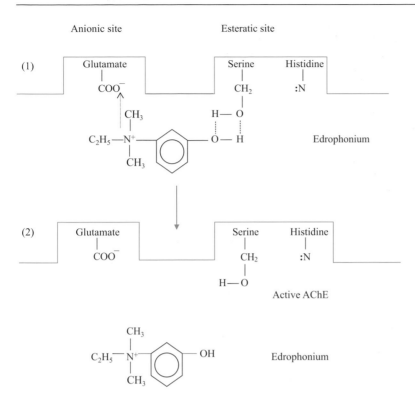

Neostigmine combines with AChE at both anionic and esteratic sites, which are approximately 0.5 nm apart (Figs. 10.3 and 10.9). The anionic site mainly consists of a negatively charged glutamate group, while the esteratic site consists of the amino acids serine and histidine. At the anionic site, the positively charged quaternary nitrogen in neostigmine is attracted by the glutamate group, forming a reversible ionic bond (in a similar manner to edrophonium). At the esteratic site, the hydroxyl group in serine combines with neostigmine at its ester linkage, resulting in the release of a quaternary phenol

(hydroxyphenyltrimethylammonium) and the formation of a dimethylcarbamyl enzyme (Fig. 10.9). Consequently, the combination of neostigmine with AChE is essentially similar to the reaction of acetylcholine with the enzyme. However, the hydrolysis of the dimethylcarbamyl enzyme by water (half-time of hydrolysis = 30–40 min) is about 50 million times slower than the parallel reaction with the acetylated enzyme (half-time of hydrolysis = 40 μs), so that enzyme inhibition by neostigmine persists until significant amounts of AChE are regenerated (and the drug is removed from the motor endplate). Its relatively long duration of action, which far exceeds its removal from plasma, probably reflects the slow hydrolysis of inhibited AChE in the synaptic gap. At least 80–90% inhibition of AChE is normally required to interfere with or prevent the hydrolysis of acetylcholine at the motor endplate.

In addition to its effects on AChE, neostigmine also inhibits plasma cholinesterase (BChE) and can prolong the effects of suxamethonium. Although it may also prolong the half-life of mivacurium, it will antagonize its effects on neuromuscular transmission. In certain conditions, it also has a direct effect on the motor endplate and on autonomic ganglia, due to its chemical similarity to acetylcholine.

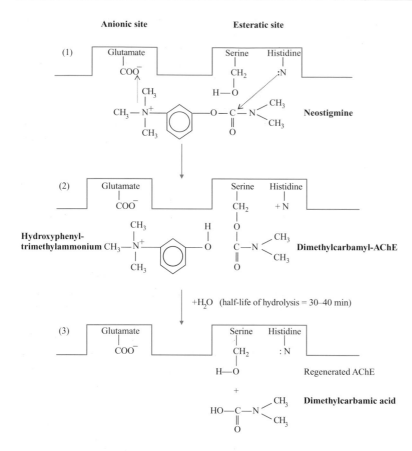

Fig. 10.9 The inhibition of AChE by neostigmine. (1) The quaternary nitrogen atom in neostigmine (N^+) forms a reversible ionic bond with the negatively charged glutamate group (COO^-) at the anionic site, and electron donation occurs from histidine to the carbonyl carbon atom in neostigmine at the esteratic site; (2) The terminal hydroxyl group in serine attacks and splits neostigmine at its ester link, resulting in the formation of a quaternary phenol (hydroxyphenyltrimethylammonium) and dimethylcarbamyl-AChE; (3) The quaternary phenol is released, and the dimethylcarbamyl-AChE is slowly hydrolysed (half-life of hydrolysis = 30–40 min) resulting in the slow regeneration of AChE and the formation of dimethylcarbamic acid. The slow hydrolysis accounts for the duration of action of neostigmine in man.

Since neostigmine is a quaternary amine, its absorption from the gut is relatively poor and its potency after oral administration is only 10–20% of its parenteral potency. After absorption, neostigmine is mainly distributed in extracellular fluid and does not cross the blood–brain or the placental barrier in significant amounts. It is partly metabolized by the liver to a phenolic glucuronide and is also eliminated unchanged in urine. After intravenous administration, it has an onset of action within 1–2 minutes, and a maximal effect at 5–7 minutes. It inhibits AChE and prevents acetylcholine hydrolysis for approximately 30 minutes.

In anaesthetic practice, neostigmine is the standard drug used to antagonize non-depolarizing neuromuscular blockade. Atropine or glycopyrronium is usually given before or with neostigmine, in order to prevent muscarinic side effects.

Neostigmine is also used, by oral administration, in the long-term management of myasthenia gravis. Because of its autonomic effects, it is often given with antimuscarinic drugs. In some patients tolerance to these effects may oc-

cur, and concurrent therapy with antimuscarinic drugs is not always necessary. Neostigmine has also been used in the management of supraventricular tachycardias, and to improve smooth muscle activity in the bladder and the bowel, particularly in the postoperative period.

Pyridostigmine

Pyridostigmine is a quaternary amine and a close chemical analogue of neostigmine. It inhibits AChE in an identical manner, but is 4–5 times less potent than neostigmine, since its quaternary nitrogen atom is enclosed in a pyridine (C_5H_5N) ring.

Pyridostigmine does not cross the blood–brain or the placental barrier, and has similar but less pronounced effects than neostigmine on AChE, neuromuscular transmission and the autonomic nervous system. It is more slowly absorbed than neostigmine, and has less first-pass metabolism, so that its oral bioavailability is rather greater (20–30%). Pyridostigmine is metabolized more slowly than neostigmine, so its duration of action is rather longer.

Pyridostigmine is often used in the long-term management of myasthenia gravis. It is often better tolerated than neostigmine, since its autonomic effects are less marked and its duration of action is rather longer. In some patients tolerance to its autonomic side effects occurs, and concurrent therapy with antimuscarinic drugs is not always necessary.

Distigmine is a combination of two molecules of pyridostigmine, linked by a methylene chain at their non-quaternary ends. Distigmine has a relatively long duration of action and is sometimes used in the management of postoperative paralytic ileus or urinary retention.

Physostigmine

Physostigmine (eserine) is a tertiary amine that is derived from the Calabar bean and was once used by native tribes in West Africa in 'trial by ordeal'. It is well absorbed from the gastrointestinal tract and penetrates most cellular membranes, and also crosses the placenta and the blood–brain barrier. It has been used in the treatment of poisoning with anticholinergic drugs (e.g. tricyclic antidepressants). In the past, physostigmine eye drops have been used to produce miosis in narrow angle glaucoma.

Organophosphorus compounds

Organophosphorus compounds inhibit AChE by phosphorylation of the esteratic site of the enzyme (Figs. 10.3 and 10.8), forming an extremely stable complex with serine that is resistant to hydrolysis or reactivation. In some instances, chemical changes take place after phosphorylation which prevent the reactivation of AChE (ageing). Consequently, recovery from the effects of inhibition is mainly dependent on the synthesis of new enzyme, and organophosphorus agents are considered to be irreversible

inhibitors of AChE. Most of these drugs are also potent inhibitors of BChE.

The classical organophosphorus compounds are diisopropyl-fluorophosphonate (DFP; dyflos) and tetraethylpyrophosphate (TEPP). Many of their analogues have been widely used as insecticides, and a number of volatile and lipid-soluble agents were synthesized during World War II as chemical warfare agents. These compounds are readily absorbed by the lungs and through the skin. Exposure leads to numerous toxic manifestations, including nicotinic effects (muscle weakness, paralysis and hypotension) and muscarinic effects (increased smooth muscle tone and secretomotor activity). In addition, excitation of the CNS occurs causing tremors and convulsions, and may be followed by CNS depression, with coma and respiratory paralysis.

Organophosphorus poisoning is treated with reactivators of AChE (e.g. pralidoxime, obidoxime), which promote the hydrolysis of the phosphorylated enzyme. Repeated administration of atropine (2–4 mg) and anticonvulsant drugs, and mechanical ventilation of the lungs may also be necessary. Pretreatment with carbamates has a protective effect against organophosphorus poisoning. Chronic exposure to organophosphorus agents may lead to the development of severe polyneuritis.

Drugs that interfere with excitation–contraction coupling

Normal voluntary muscle contraction depends on the release of Ca^{2+} from the sarcoplasmic reticulum by the ryanodine receptor, and its subsequent binding by Troponin C. The binding of Ca^{2+} causes conformational changes in the troponin–tropomyosin complex, resulting in the interaction of myosin and actin, and muscle contraction (page 175). In genetically susceptible patients, the administration of depolarizing muscle relaxants or halogenated anaesthetic agents may lead to the excessive release of Ca^{2+} from the sarcoplasmic reticulum, resulting in potentially fatal malignant hyperpyrexia (Chapter 6). Prominent signs and symptoms include a rapidly rising body temperature, muscular rigidity and contracture, tachycardia and both respiratory and metabolic acidosis.

In recent years, it has been possible to reverse many of these changes by the use of dantrolene sodium, which acts by inhibiting the release of Ca^{2+} from the sarcoplasmic reticulum and thus prevents excitation-contraction coupling and abnormal heat production. An intravenous preparation of the drug (sodium dantrolene with mannitol and sodium hydroxide) is available as a powder for reconstitution with water. The initial dose ($1\ mg\ kg^{-1}$) may be repeated at 5–10 minutes intervals to a maximum dose of $10\ mg\ kg^{-1}$.

Dantrolene sodium is also available as an oral preparation for the treatment of spasticity associated with chronic neurological disorders, including cerebrovascular accidents, multiple sclerosis, spinal cord injury and cerebral palsy. Central effects (e.g. dizziness, weakness) are not uncommon, and occasional hepatotoxicity may occur. The drug should be administered in gradually increasing doses until the optimum effect is attained.

Practical considerations

Choice of relaxant

Suxamethonium remains the drug of choice to provide optimal conditions for rapid endotracheal intubation and is also indicated for short procedures (e.g. electroconvulsive therapy). During longer procedures, suxamethonium has also been administered by intermittent or continuous infusion. This technique is now rarely used, since the development of phase II blockade may occur when the total dose used is more than $7–8\ mg\ kg^{-1}$ during nitrous oxide–opioid anaesthesia, and with considerably smaller doses in the presence of volatile anaesthetic agents.

An antimuscarinic drug may be given prior to suxamethonium at the discretion of the anaesthetist, but is usually precluded in obstetric anaesthesia. However, atropine should always be administered if repeated dosage is contemplated, or in the presence of significant β-adrenoceptor blockade. Small doses of a non-depolarizing relaxant (e.g. atracurium 5 mg, pancuronium 1 mg) are frequently given prior to suxamethonium in order to reduce the muscle fasciculations and subsequent muscle pains, or to modify the sustained activity in the extraocular muscles in cases of penetrating eye injury. In these circumstances, the dose of suxamethonium should be increased by 50%.

Contraindications to the use of suxamethonium include:

- Major burns and neurological injuries
- Hyperkalaemic states (e.g. renal failure)
- Myasthenic and myotonic diseases
- Major qualitative abnormalities of BChE
- A family history of susceptibility to malignant hyperpyrexia

In particular, careful consideration should be given to the use of suxamethonium in children. Reports from the USA and Germany indicate a significant incidence of masseteric muscle spasm, which is sometimes a prelude to malignant hyperthermia, associated with the administration of suxamethonium. Furthermore, there is a possibility of hyperkalaemic cardiac arrest in children with previously undiagnosed myopathies following depolarization blockade.

For a number of years, the choice of a non-depolarizing drug in anaesthetic practice was principally determined by the expected duration of the surgical procedure, with secondary considerations being given to the condition of the patient. However, there is little doubt that the safety factor of cisatracurium and atracurium, i.e. spontaneous degradation *in vivo* by Hofmann elimination, coupled with its relative lack of significant side effects (particularly with cisatracurium) has led to their widespread use in clinical practice at the present time. Cisatracurium is probably the drug of choice in renal disease, hepatic impairment and in frail and elderly subjects. Cisatracurium and vecuronium have a relatively short duration of action and may have advantages over atracurium if hypersensitivity responses to anaesthesia are predicted or when cardiovascular stability during anaesthesia is particularly important. Vecuronium is mainly eliminated in bile and does not cumulate in renal failure. Both drugs have been used to provide neuromuscular blockade for patients with myasthenia gravis undergoing surgical procedures, since other muscle relaxants may produce prolonged apnoea in this condition. They may be administered by single or repeated dosage or by continuous infusion techniques. In recent years, they have been widely used to assist long-term ventilatory control (e.g. in the management of tetanus or status epilepticus), since these drugs do not cumulate and offer the advantage of flexibility.

In the past, pancuronium has been a logical alternative, although some tachycardia may be expected, particularly in association with the use of inotropic drugs. Other advantages of individual drugs include the use of pancuronium in hypovolaemic patients, mivacurium in day case surgery and rocuronium when a rapid onset of activity is required.

Reversal of neuromuscular blockade

Neostigmine (usually $0.07\ mg\ kg^{-1}$, with a maximum dose of 5 mg) is the standard drug that is used to reverse nondepolarizing neuromuscular blockade. Atropine (0.02 mg

kg^{-1}, with a maximum dose of 1.2 mg) is normally administered simultaneously, in order to control the muscarinic effects of neostigmine. However, secretomotor activity appears to be more favourably modified if atropine is given 5 minutes previously. Full oxygenation and efficient pulmonary ventilation should be maintained during the administration of these drugs, as hypoxia and hypercarbia increase the risk of cardiac arrhythmias. To minimize the possibility of recurarization, neostigmine should not be administered less than 20–30 minutes after full doses of the non-depolarizing muscle relaxants, and preferably when there is some evidence of return of muscle tone.

In the past, clinical evaluation of ventilatory activity and muscle strength have been used to assess recovery from neuromuscular blockade. The classical clinical signs of adequate reversal include an efficient tidal volume, return of the cough reflex, the absence of a tracheal tug, the return of jaw tone, the ability to protrude the tongue and a head lift, which can be sustained for at least 5 seconds. These signs are often correlated with at least 75% recovery in the electrical or mechanical activity in voluntary muscles induced by indirect stimulation.

Nevertheless, it should be recognized that clinical signs of reversal are potentially unreliable and may be difficult to elicit in patients recovering from general anaesthesia without the risk of awareness. Undoubtedly, the use of a nerve stimulator is the method of choice in the assessment of any residual neuromuscular blockade. It is now generally recognized that recovery from neuromuscular blockade is only complete when the train-of-four ratio is 0.9 or above, i.e. when the amplitude of the final response to a train-of-four supramaximal stimuli is at least 90% of the amplitude of the first response.

The reversal of neuromuscular blockade is considerably influenced by the pharmacokinetic properties of the muscle relaxant that is used, the amount of drug that is given and the timing of its administration. The advent of newer agents with a short duration of action and novel routes of elimination (page 186) often allows a reduction in the standard dosage of neostigmine or even spontaneous recovery, and this may have considerable advantages. There is little doubt that the prolonged muscarinic effects of neostigmine on gastrointestinal smooth muscle contribute to postoperative pain and may increase the incidence of postoperative nausea and vomiting. In addition, the development of postoperative bradycardia may be partly or entirely due to the muscarinic effects of neostigmine. In these conditions, antimuscarinic drugs with a longer duration of action than atropine (e.g. glycopyrronium, 10–15 $\mu g\ kg^{-1}$) may be useful.

In recent years, sugammadex (a modified α-cyclodextrin) has been used to reverse rocuronium-induced neuromuscular blockade. Cyclodextrins are complex cyclic carbohydrates that can incorporate steroidal muscle relaxants within their molecular structure, and thus effectively remove them from the circulation. This novel approach to the reversal of neuromuscular blockade may reduce the use of anticholinesterase drugs (and the concurrent use of atropine or glycopyrronium).

Monitoring of neuromuscular blockade

Individual responses to muscle relaxants vary widely and may be modified by age, body temperature, plasma and extracellular pH, electrolyte changes, the presence of other drugs and pathological conditions. Consequently, in individual patients the response to muscle relaxants or their antagonists may be unpredictable, and the effects of some drugs may change rapidly during recovery from neuromuscular blockade. Methods of monitoring the effects of muscle relaxants are therefore desirable, and in certain circumstances may be essential. The most commonly used methods depend on indirect supramaximal stimulation of the ulnar nerve, and the recording of the MAP or the mechanical twitch response of the adductor pollicis. A square wave stimulus of short duration (0.1–0.2 ms) is frequently employed in order to prevent repetitive muscle firing. In anaesthetized patients, tetanic rates of stimulation (>50 Hz) may be used, although a train-of-four stimulus (2 Hz for 2 s) is more commonly employed. Neuromuscular blockade may be monitored by comparing the amplitude of the first response in the train (T1) with the control response before the administration of the relaxant (T0). This ratio (T1/T0) is probably the most accurate measurement of postsynaptic neuromuscular blockade. More commonly, transmission is monitored by observing the amplitude (or presence, absence or reappearance) of the fourth response (T4) compared to the first response (T1) within a train of four stimuli (i.e. the ratio T4:T1). This method avoids the necessity for a control response, although it may reflect the presynaptic effects of non-depolarizing muscle relaxants rather than their postsynaptic actions. In practice, the difference may be unimportant, since there is usually a close relation between the ratios T1:T0 and T4:T1.

Suggested reading

Berg, H., Roed, J. & Viby-Mogensen, J., *et al.* (1997) Residual neuromuscular block is a risk factor for postoperative pulmonary complications. A prospective, randomised, and blinded study of postoperative pulmonary complications after atracurium, vecuronium and pancuronium. *Acta Anaesthesiologica Scandinavica* **41**, 1095–1103.

Bevan, D.R. (1994) Succinylcholine. *Canadian Journal of Anaesthesia* **41**, 465–468.

Caldwell, J. (1995) New muscle relaxants. *Current Opinion in Anaesthesiology* **8**, 356–361.

Calvey, T.N. (1984) Assessment of neuromuscular blockade by electromyography: a review. *Journal of the Royal Society of Medicine* **77**, 56–59.

Changeux, J.-P., Giraudat, J. & Dennis, M. (1987) The nicotinic acetylcholine receptor: molecular architecture of a ligand-regulated ion channel. *Trends in Pharmacological Sciences* **8**, 459–465.

Fleming, N.W. & Lewis, B.K. (1994) Cholinesterase inhibitors do not prolong neuromuscular block produced by mivacurium. *British Journal of Anaesthesia* **73**, 241–243.

Kopman, A.F., Klewicka, M.M., Kopman, D.J. & Neuman, G.G. (1999) Molar potency is predictive of the speed of onset of neuromuscular block for agents of intermediate, short, and ultrashort duration. *Anesthesiology* **90**, 425–431.

Lee, C. (2001) Structure, conformation, and action of neuromuscular blocking drugs. *British Journal of Anaesthesia* **87**, 755–769.

Martyn, J.A. (1999) Succinylcholine hyperkalemia after burns. *Anesthesiology* **91**, 321–322.

O'Sullivan, E.P., Williams, N.E. & Calvey, T.N. (1988) Differential effects of neuromuscular blocking agents on suxamethonium-induced fasciculations and myalgia. *British Journal of Anaesthesia* **60**, 367–371.

Paton, W.D.M. & Waud, D.R. (1967) The margin of safety of neuromuscular transmission. *Journal of Physiology* **191**, 59–90.

Pollard, B.J. (2005) Neuromuscular blocking agents and reversal agents. *Anaesthesia and Intensive Care Medicine* **6**, 189–192.

Rosenberg, H. & Gronert, G.A. (1992) Intractable cardiac arrest in children given succinylcholine. *Anesthesiology* **77**, 1054.

Roy, J.J. & Varin, F. (2004) Physicochemical properties of neuromuscular blocking agents and their impact on the pharmacokinetic–pharmacodynamic relationship. *British Journal of Anaesthesia* **93**, 241–248.

Sardesai, A.M. & Griffiths, R. (2005) Monitoring techniques: neuromuscular blockade. *Anaesthesia and Intensive Care Medicine* **6**, 198–200.

Stenlake, J.B., Waigh, R.D., Urwin, J., Dewar, G.H. & Coker, G.G. (1983) Atracurium: conception and inception. *British Journal of Anaesthesia* **55**(Suppl I), S3–S10.

Sudhof, T.C. & Jahn, R. (1991) Proteins of synaptic vesicles involved in exocytosis and membrane recycling. *Neurone* **6**, 665–667.

Tolmie, J.D., Joyce, T.H. & Mitchell, G.D. (1967) Succinylcholine danger in the burned patient. *Anesthesiology* **28**, 467–470.

Ward, J.M. & Martyn, J.A. (1993) Burn injury-induced nicotinic acetylcholine receptor changes on muscle membrane. *Muscle Nerve* **16**, 348–354.

Wareham, A.C. (2005) Neuromuscular function and transmission. *Anaesthesia and Intensive Care Medicine* **6**, 203–205.

Wareham, A.C. (2005) Muscle. *Anaesthesia and Intensive Care Medicine* **6**, 209–212.

Whittaker, V.P. (1986) The storage and release of acetylcholine. *Trends in Pharmacological Sciences* **7**, 312–315.

Wong, S.F. & Chung, F. (2000) Succinylcholine associated postoperative myalgia. *Anaesthesia* **55**, 144–152.

Zhang, M.Q. (2003) Drug-specific cyclodextrins: the future of rapid neuromuscular reversal? *Drugs Future* **28**, 347–354.

11 Analgesic Drugs

Anatomy and physiology of pain transmission

Pain pathways

Peripheral nociceptive receptors do not have a distinct histological structure, but are interwoven plexiform arrangements of free nerve endings that are widely distributed in interstitial tissues and around blood vessels. They respond specifically to painful stimuli of chemical, mechanical or thermal origin.

Two types of pain have been described. Fast pain allows the injury to be identified in time and space, initiates the rapid reflex withdrawal from the painful stimulus, and is of short duration. Slow pain occurs after fast pain, is less localized and more persistent.

Afferent pain fibres can be divided into two groups:
• Small myelinated Aδ fibres are 2–5 μm in diameter and have a moderate conduction velocity (2.5–20 m s^{-1}). They conduct first or fast pain and enter the deeper part of the dorsal horn (Rexed laminae IV and V).
• Unmyelinated C fibres are less than 2 μm in diameter and have a higher threshold and lower conduction velocity (less than 2.5 m s^{-1}). They transmit second or slow pain and synapse in the superficial area of the dorsal horn (Rexed laminae I and II).

Primary nociceptive pathway

The transmission of impulses from these two types of fibres is modified by intraneuronal activity in the substantia gelatinosa, and this may influence the quality and intensity of pain that is experienced. The input of nociceptive impulses is also modulated by impulses from collateral branches from larger A fibres which ascend in the posterior columns. These conduct other sensory impulses and have a lower threshold of activity and a greater conduction velocity than Aδ or C fibres.

Second-order neurons from Aδ and C fibres originate in the dorsal horn, decussate in the spinal cord and ascend in the spinothalamic tract and more diffuse spinoreticular pathways. They eventually terminate in the ventral and medial nuclei of the thalamus and synapse with cells whose axons project to the somatosensory cortex. The medial thalamic nucleus responds to noxious peripheral stimuli and is probably the main region associated with the appreciation of pain. However, further projections to the postcentral gyri are undoubtedly associated with the localization of nociceptive impulses, while connections with the cingulate cortex, prefrontal and temporal lobes, and the limbic areas are related to the affective component and the memory of pain. Consequently, it is not surprising that pain has been described as an unpleasant emotional state rather than as a simple sensory modality.

Descending pathways

Descending pathways from central grey matter activate cells in the SG, which are mainly short inhibitory interneurons projecting to laminae I and V. Many of these pathways originate in the periaqueductal grey matter (PAG), which receives neuronal input from the cortex, thalamus and hypothalamus, and its fibres mainly project to the nucleus raphe magnus (NRM) in the medulla. The principal descending pathways from the NRM are the reticular formation and the reticulospinal tract, which synapse with and activate inhibitory cells in the SG (Fig. 11.1). The main neurotransmitter in this pathway is 5-HT, although the descending tracts also have abundant opioid receptors and are believed to be an important site of analgesic action. The NRM also receives neuronal input from the spinothalamic tract (via the paragigantocellular reticular nucleus). In addition, a noradrenergic pathway originates in the locus caeruleus (LC) in the floor of the fourth ventricle, and also activates synaptic transmission in the substantia gelatinosa, resulting in inhibition of the primary nociceptive pathway.

These neuronal pathways form a regulatory feedback circuit that modulates the activity of the SG, which forms a 'gate control' of nociceptive input. This may partially

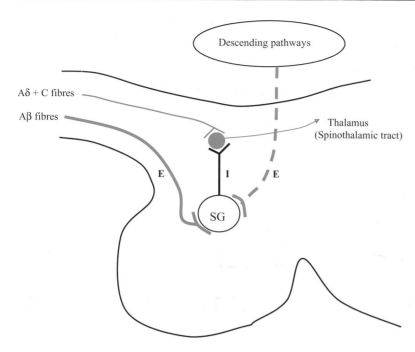

Fig. 11.1 The role of the substantia gelatinosa (SG) in modulation of the primary nociceptive pathway in the dorsal horn of the spinal cord. Excitatory pathways (——— **E**, — — **E**); inhibitory pathways (——— **I**). The primary nociceptive pathway carries pain impulses via Aδ and C fibres, synapses in the dorsal horn and carries pain impulses to the thalamus via the spinothalamic tract. Cells in the SG inhibit the activity of the primary pathway via short interneurons. Activity of SG cells is facilitated by impulses from large sensory Aβ fibres (———), and by descending pathways from the PAG and the LC (— —).

explain why counter-irritation by heat or touch, or distraction of the individual, can reduce the intensity of a painful stimulus.

Pain production

Pain can be produced by
• mechanical or thermal damage to superficial or deep tissues
• ischaemia of somatic or visceral structures
• spasm of smooth or striated muscle
• dilatation of extracranial or occipital blood vessels.
Some endogenous chemical agents excite peripheral nerve endings, including H^+, K^+, histamine, 5-HT and bradykinin. Phosphate ions have also been implicated in the production of bone pain in malignant disease. Other endogenous agents such as many prostaglandins do not produce pain directly, but sensitize afferent nerve endings to the effects of bradykinin or lower the threshold of nociceptors. Various vanilloids that are present in plants, such as capsaicin and resiniferatoxin, are direct agonists at the vanilloid receptor VR1, which is a ligand-gated ion channel present on most nociceptive nerve endings. Many endogenous agents may cause pain by indirectly affecting VR1 receptors.

Post-traumatic, inflammatory and neurogenic pain

A complex series of events is initiated during the development of pain associated with trauma, inflammation and peripheral nerve damage. Some of these changes in peripheral sensitization and central excitability, which are sometimes described as increased 'neuroplasticity', may be partly obtunded by the use of 'pre-emptive' analgesia prior to surgical procedures.

Sensory neuropeptides

Afferent nerves produce sensory neuropeptides such as substance P, neurokinin A (substance K) and calcitonin gene-related peptide (CGRP). These neuropeptides, which are present in 25–47% of primary afferent nerve fibres, can migrate both centrally and peripherally. Their peripheral migration increases the excitability of sensory fibres and adjacent postganglionic sympathetic fibres, while their central migration enhances nociceptive transmission in the SG, via neurokinin (NK_1 and NK_2) receptors. Nerve growth factor (NGF) is released by Schwann cells following peripheral damage and causes cellular changes that facilitate the neuroplasmic transport of substance P, neurokinin A and CGRP. In addition, after trauma or chronic inflammation the genes encoding sensory neuropeptides are induced within approximately 2 weeks. These changes enhance the hyperexcitability of sensory neurons, so that light touch or pressure may induce a painful sensation that is mediated by large A fibres (allodynia). In addition, the endogenous expression of dynorphins, enkephalins and prostaglandins is also increased, but with a rather different time course. Prostaglandin synthesis is increased within 24–48 hours, although increases in dynorphin synthesis do not occur until 2–5 days after injury or inflammation.

Glutamate

The central transmission of nociceptive impulses in chronic pain may also be enhanced by an increase in glutamate-mediated transmission in the dorsal horn. Glutamate is released from the central terminals of primary afferent fibres and excites fast synaptic responses that are mediated by both AMPA[1] and NMDA[2] receptors (which are also upregulated during chronic inflammation). These changes increase the production of nitric oxide, which may have a role in pain transmission.

Cholecystokinin (CCK) can also influence pain pathways, and its synthesis in the dorsal horn in neuropathic pain may antagonize morphine analgesia.

Gene expression

Increased nociceptive sensitization within the CNS and the associated behavioural hyperalgesia in animals may be linked to the enhanced expression of immediate early genes, such as *c-fos* and *c-jun*. The number of *fos*-like neurons can be identified by immunoreactive techniques and used as an index to quantify the antinociceptive activity of drugs. Experimental evidence suggests that the prior administration of opioid analgesics, NMDA antagonists and α_2-agonists can suppress *fos*-like reactivity.

Opioid receptors

After trauma, inflammation or tissue damage, opioid receptors are synthesized in the cell bodies of sensory neurons and are transported in both central and peripheral directions. Their central migration results in the presence of presynaptic opioid receptors on C-fibre terminals in the SG, while receptors that migrate to the periphery are only activated after local tissue damage. Immunocompetent cells, which possess opioid receptors and the ability

[1] AMPA, α-amino-3-hydroxy-5-methyl-4-isoxazole proprionic acid.
[2] NMDA, *N*-methyl-D-aspartate.

to synthesize opioid peptides, also migrate to the site of tissue trauma.

Classification of analgesic drugs

Analgesic drugs can be divided into three main groups:
- Opioid analgesics
- Simple analgesics
- Other agents

Opioid analgesics
History

Opium was first obtained by the Sumerians and predynastic Egyptians from the capsules of the unripe Oriental poppy *Papaver somniferum* in the fourth century BC. Early writings suggested that it was principally used for its antidiarrhoeal activity, but by the sixteenth century the analgesic, sedative and antitussive properties of opium were widely recognized throughout Europe. Opium smoking became popular in the Orient during the eighteenth century. Crude opium contains 9–17% of morphine, and the invention of the hypodermic syringe and needle in 1853 led to the increased usage of morphine and other opium alkaloids in the treatment of battle injuries. In addition, the migration of Chinese labourers during the late nineteenth century contributed to the development of compulsive drug usage and drug dependence in western civilization.

The semisynthetic opioid heroin (diamorphine or diacetylmorphine) was produced at St Mary's Hospital in 1874, with the aim of curing dependence on morphine. It was many years before it was appreciated that it provided a cure by replacing morphine with a more powerful drug of addiction. During the past century, the search for agents with the analgesic effects of morphine, but without its drawbacks of dependence and tolerance, has been only partly successful. Pethidine was originally developed as a spasmolytic agent in 1939, and was subsequently found to have analgesic activity.

In contrast, methadone is a phenylpropylamine derivative that was originally synthesized by German chemists in the 1940s, and was initially used as an alternative to morphine during World War II. During the past 50 years many other semisynthetic and synthetic opioids have been developed, but almost all effective agents inevitably possess the tendency to induce drug dependence. It seems probable that this disadvantage will apply to all opioids that are synthesized in the future.

The mode of action of opioid analgesics remained unclear for many years. It was evident that these agents could significantly modify the reactive components of pain, such as anxiety, fear and suffering, and the ability of patients to tolerate painful conditions. In some clinical studies the pain threshold, i.e. the intensity at which a stimulus is first appreciated as pain, was only minimally affected by opioid analgesics.

Physiological and pharmacological background

Approximately 50 years ago it was suggested that morphine and other opioids produced analgesia by their interaction with specific opioid receptors in the CNS. This proposal was based on three main observations:

• Most opioid analgesics show considerable stereospecificity, with stereospecific indices of 10–100. Almost invariably, analgesic activity is associated with the levorotatory isomer.

• The chemical synthesis of extremely potent opioid analgesics such as etorphine.

• The development of pure opioid antagonists, whose actions were consistent with the displacement of opioids from receptor sites.

Meanwhile, nalorphine (*N*-allyl-normorphine) had been shown to antagonize the analgesic and respiratory depressant effects of morphine and to cause withdrawal symptoms in morphine-dependent individuals. When given alone, it was an active analgesic but caused dysphoria and other psychotomimetic effects, rather than euphoria and sedation. Its actions were explained by the concept of 'receptor dualism', which postulated the existence of two distinct receptors, one for morphine and another for nalorphine.

It was subsequently shown that a series of opioids produced different profiles of activity in *in vivo* conditions. The various syndromes produced were interpreted in terms of the actions of these drugs at three different receptor sites:

• μ-Receptors, mediating euphoria, supraspinal analgesia and morphine-like physical dependence. Morphine was considered to be the prototypical agonist.

• κ-Receptors were associated with spinal analgesia, sedation and signs of nalorphine-like dependence. Ketocyclazocine was the prototypical agonist.

• σ-Receptors produced mydriasis, tachypnoea, tachycardia, delirium and mania. *N*-allyl-normetazocine was the prototypical agonist.

δ-Opioid receptors were subsequently identified in the gut and the CNS. They were shown to be implicated in spinal analgesia, but not in supraspinal mechanisms.

In recent years, a further 'orphan' opioid receptor (N/OFQ receptor) has been identified, which has a high degree of structural similarity with the classical opioid receptors, although it does not specifically bind endogenous peptides and opioid analgesics. Nevertheless, it is now accepted as a member of the family of opioid receptors.

σ-Receptors are no longer classified as opioid receptors, since they do not show the stereoselectivity or antagonism of the classical receptors. They have high affinity binding for phencyclidine and ketamine, and the term 'σ-receptor' is sometimes used to describe the binding site for these agents on the ionotropic glutamate-NMDA receptor complex.

Nomenclature of opioid receptors

Present views suggest that three major classes of opioid receptors are present in the CNS, i.e. μ, κ and δ. The 'orphan' receptor was designated as ORL_1, but was subsequently known as the N/OFQ, or nociceptin/orphanin FQ receptor. At least three other different systems of nomenclature have been used (Table 11.1). The original traditional nomenclature is still the most widely accepted, and is the one that is used in this book.

Opioid receptor subtypes

There is some evidence suggesting that subtypes of opioid receptors may be present in the CNS. Studies with highly selective opioid antagonists led to the proposal that μ-receptors may exist as two distinct subtypes, μ_1 and μ_2. It was suggested that supraspinal analgesia was mediated by μ_1-receptors, while spinal analgesia and respiratory depression were due to activation of μ_2-receptors. Similarly, κ-receptors have been divided into κ_1, κ_2 and κ_3, and it was proposed that the κ_3-subtype corresponds to the original

Table 11.1 The nomenclature of opioid receptors.

Classical names	Other names			
μ-Receptor		OP_3	MOR	MOP
κ-Receptor		OP_2	KOR	KOP
δ-Receptor		OP_1	DOR	DOP
N/OFQ receptor	ORL_1	OP_4	NOR	NOP

nalorphine receptor. δ-receptors have also been classified as δ_1- and δ_2-subtypes.

The identification of opioid receptor subtypes has been primarily based on binding studies with poorly selective radioactive ligands, and there is at present no molecular or genetic evidence for their existence. Experimental studies with μ-opioid receptor knockout mice, i.e. animals that are engineered without μ-receptors, are consistent with this interpretation. Although opioid receptors are only subject to minimal alternative splicing, they may undergo post-translational modification or dimerization (molecular combination with each other), which is believed to be a relatively common phenomenon. Consequently, the identification of opioid receptor subtypes may be due to heterodimerization of opioid receptors with each other, or even with other receptors.

Localization of opioid receptors

The regional localization of opioid receptors has been extensively studied by autoradiographic and binding techniques, and they are widely present in peripheral tissues, including many sensory nerves.

In the spinal cord, they are mainly localized to the SG in the dorsal horn, which contains mainly μ-receptors (although κ- and δ-receptors are also present). In the brainstem, high concentrations have been identified in the PAG, the NRM and the NTS (which receives afferent vagal fibres). They are also present in the area postrema, the limbic system, the amygdaloid nuclei, the thalamus and the cerebral cortex. In the central and peripheral nervous system, they are most frequently situated at presynaptic sites.

The presence of opioid receptors outside the CNS accounts for some of the other effects of analgesic drugs, such as constipation and an increase in biliary pressure. Many central and peripheral physiological functions may be dependent on complex interactions between different opioid receptors.

Receptor transduction and effector mechanisms

All four opioid receptors have been cloned and their amino acid sequences determined, and all rely on the same signal transduction and effector mechanism. Receptor activation results in binding of the inhibitory G-protein G_i, GTP/GDP exchange and inhibition of adenylate cyclase, thus decreasing the synthesis of cAMP (Fig. 11.2). The dissimilar effects of μ-, κ- and δ-agonists are due to differences in receptor distribution, rather than to the subcel-

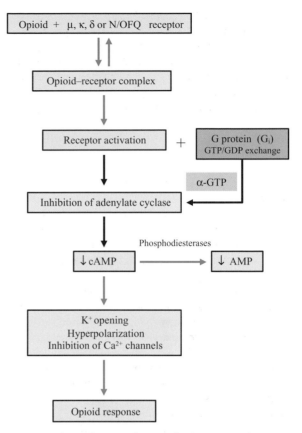

Fig. 11.2 The mechanism of action of endogenous and exogenous opioids at μ, κ, δ or N/OFQ receptors. Activation results in inhibition of adenylate cyclase, decreased synthesis of cAMP and an opioid response.

lular mechanisms involved in signal transduction. Opioid receptor activation and the resultant decreases in cAMP result in secondary changes, particularly in K^+ channel activation, hyperpolarization and the inhibition of voltage-sensitive Ca^{2+} channels. These ionic changes result in decreased central and peripheral neurotransmitter release.

Opioid receptors are subject to 'up-regulation' and 'down-regulation' by changes in agonist concentration, and receptor down-regulation may be an important cause of tolerance to opioids during chronic administration (Chapter 3).

In general, there is significant correlation between the analgesic potency of opioids and their affinity for μ-receptors, and experimental evidence suggests that significant analgesia may be produced by a limited degree of receptor occupation.

Table 11.2 Endogenous opioid peptides and their original gene products and precursor proteins.

Gene product	Precursor protein	Endogenous peptide
Prepro-opiomelanocortin (PPOMC)	Pro-opioimelanocortin (265) (POMC)	β-Endorphin (31) ACTH (39) → α-MSH (13)
Prepro-enkephalin	Pro-enkephalin (267)	[Met]-enkephalin (5) [Leu]-enkephalin (5)
Prepro-dynorphin	Pro-dynorphin (256)	Dynorphin A (17) Dynorphin A 1-8 (8) Dynorphin B (13) α-Neoendorphin (10) β-Neoendorphin (9)
Prepro-nociceptin/orphanin-FQ	Pronociceptin/orphanin-FQ	Nociceptin/orphanin-FQ (17)

The number of amino acid residues in each protein or peptide are shown in parentheses.

Endogenous opioid peptides

The identification and characterization of opioid receptors led to the discovery of their endogenous ligands, and three distinct families of opioid peptides (enkephalins, endorphins and dynorphins) were rapidly identified in various regions of the CNS, the gastrointestinal tract and at other peripheral sites.

The three classical families of opioid peptides are coded by three distinct genes, whose products are preproopiomelanocortin (PPOMC), preproenkephalin and preprodynorphin (Table 11.2). PPOMC is the precursor of β-endorphin (as well as ACTH and MSH), preproenkephalin gives rise to the enkephalins, while preprodynorphin is the precursor of dynorphin (and some endorphins). Nociceptin/orphanin FQ is derived from a fourth opioid precursor, prepronociceptin/orphanin FQ. Although these peptides and their derivatives are widely distributed in the CNS and are frequently found in the same region of the brain, they do not occur in the same groups of neurons.

Endogenous opioid peptides are currently classified as
- Enkephalins
- Endorphins
- Dynorphins
- Nociceptin/orphanin-FQ
- Endomorphins
- Other peptides

These endogenous peptides have different potencies and are preferentially but not exclusively bound by different opioid receptors. In general, enkephalins have the highest affinity for δ-receptors, endorphins mainly act at μ- and δ-receptors, while dynorphins have the highest affinity for κ-receptors. Nociceptin/orphanin-FQ has a high affinity for N/OFQ-receptors, but none for other receptors, while endomorphins have a high affinity and selectivity for μ-receptors.

Enkephalins

In 1972, two similar pentapeptides (methionine or met-enkephalin and leucine or leu-enkephalin) were isolated from brain extracts. They were shown to produce analgesia, and to compete with the opioid antagonist naloxone for some receptor sites in the brain. The initial pentapeptide sequence of many endogenous opioids contains the structure of met-enkephalin or leu-enkephalin (Table 11.3).

Subsequent studies showed that regional variations in enkephalin levels reflected the distribution of opioid receptors. Enkephalins are widely distributed throughout the CNS, particularly in the spinal cord, the hypothalamus, the posterior pituitary, the globus pallidus and the limbic system. They are also present in the gastrointestinal tract, sympathetic ganglia, the adrenal medulla and the skin. Enkephalins have a selective affinity for δ-receptors and are present in the CSF after some pain-relieving procedures including placebo analgesia, acupuncture and electrical stimulation of the PAG. Naloxone usually antagonizes the analgesia produced by these procedures.

All enkephalins are derived from the inactive precursor proenkephalin and fulfil the accepted criteria for a classical neurotransmitter. They are rapidly hydrolysed in the body, partly by specific peptidases such as the enzyme

Table 11.3 The amino acid sequences of some endogenous opioid peptides.

Opioid peptide	Amino acid sequence
[Met]-enkephalin	**Tyr-Gly-Gly-Phe-Met**
[Leu]-enkephalin	**Tyr-Gly-Gly-Phe-Leu**
β-Endorphin	**Tyr-Gly-Gly-Phe-Met**-Thr-Ser-Glu-Lys-Ser-Glu-Thr-Pro-Leu-Val-Thr-Leu-Phe-Lys-Asn-Ala-Ile-Ile-Lys-Asn-Ala-Tyr-Lys-Lys-Gly-Gln
Dynorphin A	**Tyr-Gly-Gly-Phe-Leu**-Arg-Arg-Iso-Arg-Pro-Lys-Leu-Lys-Trp-Asp-Asn-Glu
Dynorphin B	**Tyr-Gly-Gly-Phe-Leu**-Arg-Arg-Glu-Phe-Lys-Val-Val-Thr
α-Neoendorphin	**Tyr-Gly-Gly-Phe-Leu**-Arg-Lys-Tyr-Pro-Lys
β-Neoendorphin	**Tyr-Gly-Gly-Phe-Leu**-Arg-Lys-Tyr-Pro
Nociceptin/Orphanin-FQ	Phe-Gly-Gly-Phe-Thr-Gly-Ala-Arg-Lys-Ser-Ala-Arg-Lys-Leu-Ala-Asn-Glu
Endomorphin-1	Tyr-Pro-Trp-Phe–NH_2
Endomorphin-2	Tyr-Pro-Phe-Phe–NH_2

The pentapeptide sequence of [Met]-enkephalin and [Leu]-enkephalin that is present in other opioid peptides is indicated in bold type.

enkephalinase, and their action may be prolonged by some enzyme inhibitors (e.g. D-phenylalanine). A number of synthetic analogues with amino acid substitutions have been synthesized, although many of them, as well as the endogenous pentapeptides, may produce tolerance and dependence.

Endorphins

β-endorphin contains 31 amino acids and binds preferentially to μ- and δ-receptors. Its distribution in the CNS is more restricted than the enkephalins, and it is mainly limited to the hypothalamus, the pituitary gland and their connections. In general, the β-endorphins are far more potent and stable compounds than the enkephalins, and when injected into the CSF can produce profound and long-lasting analgesia. The endorphins appear to be independent of the enkephalins, since extirpation of the hypothalamo-pituitary axis in experimental animals does not lead to a decrease in enkephalin synthesis.

β-endorphins are derived from the inactive precursor pro-opiomelanocortin (POMC). In response to acute pain and stress, both ACTH and β-endorphin are secreted in increased concentrations. Although β-endorphin contains the same amino acid sequence as met-enkephalin, it does not act as its precursor.

Dynorphins

The dynorphins (and the neoendorphins) are derived from the inactive precursor prodynorphin, which is mainly present in the posterior pituitary and the hypothalamus. The dynorphins are a group of peptides containing 8–17 amino acids and are preferentially bound by κ-receptors. These peptides differ from other endogenous opioids, since they have no analgesic effects in the brain or the spinal cord. They appear to modulate the effects of other opioids such as analgesia, respiratory depression and cardiovascular depression. Some dynorphins may produce flaccid paralysis when injected intrathecally, and it is possible that they have a role in the pathophysiology of spinal cord injuries. Thus, experimental studies have shown that dynorphin levels in the CNS are increased after spinal trauma. Administration of dynorphins may prolong survival and improve neurological deficits after cerebrovascular accidents.

Nociceptin/orphanin FQ

The use of nucleic acid probes based on conventional opioid receptors identified a DNA sequence that encoded a previously unidentified receptor. Approximately 65% of its amino acid sequence is identical to the three classical receptors, although it does not specifically bind opioid analgesics and endogenous peptides. It was originally called the opioid-like orphan receptor (ORL_1), since it had no known endogenous peptide agonists. However, the specific ligand nociceptin/orphanin FQ was subsequently isolated, and its amino acid sequence was shown to be similar to the endogenous opioid peptides (Table 11.3). The substitution of phenylalanine for tyrosine at the N-terminus substantially affects its binding characteristics, and nociceptin/orphanin FQ has no significant affinity for μ-, δ- or κ-receptors. The N/OFQ receptor is present in many neuronal pathways, and a particularly dense concentration is present in superficial layers of the dorsal horn, sensory pathways of the trigeminal nerve and other areas associated with the perception of pain such as the PAG, dorsal raphe, hippocampus and amygdaloid nuclei. The functional significance of the N/OFQ receptor system is currently unclear, and various studies have indicated that it may involve analgesic, hyperalgesic and biphasic responses. In experimental conditions, locomotor impairment is observed when high doses of nociceptin/orphanin FQ are administered.

Endomorphins

During the past decade, two additional endogenous opioids have been isolated from the human brain. Both endomorphin-1 and endomorphin-2 are amidated tetrapeptides (Table 11.3) with a high affinity and selectivity for μ-receptors, and induce spinal and supraspinal analgesia in animals. It is not clear whether these are true endogenous peptides or are merely fragments of larger proteins produced during extraction.

Other peptides

Many other peptides are not derived from the four opioid precursor proteins but have some affinity and selectivity for opioid receptors. These atypical opioid peptides include the β-casomorphins, haemorphins, cytochrophins, dermophins and deltorphins. Some of these peptides have been identified in mammalian tissues, although their significance is unclear.

Endogenous morphine

Endogenous morphine has also been identified in mammalian tissues, although it is present in extremely low concentrations. In addition, SH-SY5Y human neuroblastoma cells can synthesize morphine *in vitro* by means of a process that is basically similar to its synthesis by *Papaver somniferum*.

Clinical significance of endogenous opioids

Current evidence suggests that endogenous opioids have important physiological roles in man, as well as their involvement in nociceptive pathways. These include:
- the regulation of body temperature
- immunity
- gastrointestinal motility
- renal and hepatic function
- behaviour patterns

- extrapyramidal activity
- cardiac and respiratory function
- stress responses
- appetite and thirst
- hypothalamic and pituitary function.

There are also high concentrations of μ- and κ-receptors in the vagal nuclei, and this may be related to the bradycardia frequently seen after the administration of opioids in anaesthetic practice.

Endogenous opioids have an important role in autonomic function, and there are similarities between the signs of opioid overdose and those of circulatory shock. Consequently, endogenous opioid peptides have been directly or indirectly linked to the manifestations of shock. Circulating levels of enkephalins and β-endorphin are elevated in experimental shock, and opioids inhibit the effects of catecholamines on myocardial contractility and heart rate. These effects may be related to interference with Ca^{2+} influx across myocardial cell membranes. Although the administration of large doses of opioid antagonists can elevate blood pressure in experimental animals and human volunteers, clinical experience in shocked patients is unimpressive, and there has been little or no change in survival rates in patients with circulatory shock who have received naloxone. Furthermore, there are many potential disadvantages, and complications of naloxone include grand mal seizure, pulmonary oedema and ventricular fibrillation, which may be related to activation of the sympathetic nervous system. At present, there is insufficient clinical evidence to support the routine use of naloxone for patients with shock.

Definitions

The term 'opioid' includes all naturally occurring or synthetic drugs which have stereospecific actions at opioid receptors, and whose effects can be antagonized by naloxone. In contrast, the term 'opiate' is less specific, but is not usually applied to endogenous peptides.

Opioid analgesics are considered in two groups:
- Pure agonists
- Agonist–antagonists

Pure agonists act predominantly at μ-receptors, but may also produce lesser effects on δ- and κ-receptors (Table 11.4). Many pure agonists have complex chemical structures, but a common structural feature of most drugs is the 'chair' or substituted piperidine ring, which is outlined in green in the formulae of individual drugs.

In contrast, agonist–antagonists have agonist or partial agonist effects on some opioid receptors, but antagonist effects on others.

Table 11.4 The principal sites of action of endogenous and exogenous opioids and their antagonists.

Receptor	Agonist	Partial agonist	Antagonist
Mu (μ)	β-Endorphin Endomorphins Morphine Pethidine Methadone Fentanyl	Buprenorphine	Naloxone Naltrexone Pentazocine Nalorphine
Kappa (κ)	Dynorphin Morphine† Pentazocine Nalorphine		Naloxone* Naltrexone
Delta (δ)	[Met]-enkephalin [Leu]-enkephalin Deltorphin II		Naloxone*

*Naloxone is a more effective antagonist at μ-receptors than at κ-receptors or δ-receptors.

†Morphine has a greater affinity for μ-receptors than for κ-receptors.

Table 11.5 The principal pharmacological effects of morphine.

Analgesia
Sedation
Relief of anxiety
Sedation
Euphoria/dysphoria
Respiratory depression
Depression of cough reflex
Nausea and vomiting
Smooth muscle spasm
Constipation
Histamine release
Pupillary constriction
Hormonal effects
Muscle rigidity (uncommon)
Tolerance
Dependence

Most of these effects are due to its agonist effects at μ-receptors. Some of them (e.g. respiratory depression) may be desirable or undesirable, depending on the circumstances in which the drug is used.

Pure opioid agonists

Morphine

Morphine is the principal active phenanthrene derivative in opium and is the standard analgesic agent with which all other opioids are compared. It was originally isolated by Sertürner in 1806, and was named after Morpheus, the Greek god of dreams. It was first produced by chemical synthesis in 1903. The main effects of morphine are almost entirely mediated by μ-receptors in the CNS (Table 11.5).

Analgesia. Although morphine relieves most forms of pain, it is most valuable for the treatment of continuous, dull, poorly localized pain arising from visceral and deeper structures, particularly when there are associated symptoms of fear and anxiety. Patients frequently report that the pain is still present, but that they feel more comfortable. Thus, morphine is most useful for the treatment of pain arising from acute abdominal catastrophes, postoperative pain, major trauma, myocardial infarction, and in the management of pain associated with malignant disease. It is less effective in experimentally induced pain, and in acute pain arising from superficial structures.

Sedation. Sedation and drowsiness usually occur after the administration of morphine. Sleep is less commonly induced, although there is a shift of the EEG towards increased voltage and lower frequencies (a δ rhythm), and REM sleep is suppressed. Some patients experience euphoria (an unrealistic sense of well-being), although dysphoria (an unpleasant sensation associated with mild anxiety or fear) may also occur, especially when morphine is administered in the absence of pain. In anaesthetic practice, this may be seen if the drug is administered a few minutes before the induction of anaesthesia.

Respiratory depression. Therapeutic doses of morphine will depress the rate and the depth of respiration by a direct effect on respiratory centres in the brainstem.

Maximal respiratory depression occurs within 7 minutes of intravenous administration, but up to 30 minutes after intramuscular injection, and may last for 4–5 hours. The responsiveness to CO_2 is decreased, as shown by a shift to the right and a flattening of the P_{CO_2}–ventilation curve. When hypoxia is the main stimulus to respiration, oxygen therapy may augment respiratory depression by suppressing reflex chemoreceptor activity. When other CNS depressants are used concurrently, marked bradypnoea and periodic breathing can occur. The foetal respiratory centre appears to be highly sensitive to morphine, and this precludes the use of the drug as an analgesic during labour.

Nausea and vomiting. These common and unpleasant side effects of morphine are primarily due to stimulation of dopamine and 5-HT$_3$ receptors associated with the CTZ in the area postrema of the medulla. The activity of the vomiting centre may actually be depressed, particularly after repeated doses of morphine. Effects on the vestibular apparatus and on the smooth muscle of the gut may also be involved.

Cardiovascular effects. After administration of morphine mild bradycardia often occurs, which may be due to the decreased sympathetic drive associated with sedation or a direct effect on the vagal nuclei. Hypotension may occur, but is not usually significant in normovolaemic supine patients. It is probably due to a reduction in sympathetic tone leading to peripheral vasodilatation, and to the release of histamine from mast cells. Morphine does not produce direct myocardial depression and doses up to 3 mg kg^{-1} are well tolerated during controlled ventilation for patients with aortic valve disease undergoing open heart surgery.

Morphine has a beneficial effect in paroxysmal nocturnal dyspnoea, since it produces sedation, reduces preload and depresses abnormal respiratory drive.

Histamine release. Morphine releases histamine from mast cells and may produce bronchospasm and hypotension in susceptible patients. Nasal itching (or even generalized pruritus) may occur and may be related to histamine release. Atropine may partially antagonize some of these effects.

Gastrointestinal effects. Morphine diminishes propulsive contractions and reduces secretory activity throughout the gut. However, the resting tone in smooth muscle is increased, particularly in most sphincters, and results in a prolonged gastric emptying time, delayed passage through the intestine and constipation. An important exception is

lower oesophageal sphincter tone, which is decreased by morphine in patients with pre-existing reflux.

Spasm of the smooth muscle of the biliary tract and the sphincter of Oddi can also occur. The resulting rise of intraluminal pressure may lead to the reflux of bile into the pancreatic duct, and elevated levels of serum amylase and lipase may occur after the administration of morphine. Therapeutic doses also increase the tone and amplitude of ureteric contractions.

Ocular effects. Miosis is due to stimulation of the Edinger–Westphal nucleus, depression of supranuclear pathways or effects on central sympathetic activity. Pinpoint pupils are characteristic features of morphine overdose.

Hormonal effects. The release of ACTH, prolactin and gonadotrophic hormones is inhibited by morphine, although ADH secretion is increased. These effects may be mediated via dopamine receptors in the hypothalamus.

Muscle rigidity. Morphine and other opioids occasionally produce rigidity of the thoracic wall, or even generalized muscle rigidity. These effects may be mediated via opioid receptors in the substantia nigra and corpus striatum interacting with dopaminergic and GABA pathways, and can resemble convulsions. However, true convulsions are uncommon and are usually associated with gross overdose of morphine.

Tolerance and dependence. Tolerance is characterized by decreased intensity and duration of the usual effects of morphine after repeated administration of the same dose. It may occur in subjects who have become socially habituated to the drug, or in patients who require continuous therapy for chronic pain. Although the pharmacokinetic parameters of morphine are not altered by its repeated use, a negative feedback system may result in decreased production of endogenous opioids, and there may also be down-regulation of opioid receptors. An increase in glutamate-mediated transmission via NMDA receptors is also considered to contribute to the development of tolerance.

The development of morphine dependence can be demonstrated when the drug is suddenly withdrawn after its repeated use. Various physical and psychological phenomena may develop, whose severity is related to the total amount administered. Symptoms and signs of withdrawal include restlessness and irritability, frequent yawning, excessive sweating, lacrimation and salivation, painful muscle cramps and intense and uncontrolled vomiting,

Table 11.6 Typical pharmacokinetic and physicochemical parameters of some opioid analgesics.

	Relative lipid solubility	Terminal half-life (h)	Clearance (mL min^{-1} kg^{-1})	Volume of distribution (L kg^{-1})	pK$_a$	% non-ionized (pH 7.4)
Morphine	1	3	15	3.5	7.9	24
Pethidine	28	4	12	4.0	8.7	5
Fentanyl	580	3.5	13	4.0	8.4	9
Alfentanil	90	1.6	6	0.8	6.5	89
Remifentanil	50	0.06	50	0.4	7.1	65
Tramadol	1	5.0	6	3.1	4.5	99

diarrhoea and urination. Mild symptoms have been reported after only 48 hours treatment.

Routes of administration. Morphine is usually administered by intramuscular injection, as a sulphate, tartrate or hydrochloride salt. It may also be given subcutaneously. Morphine is well absorbed from these sites, and produces blood levels which are almost as high as after intravenous administration. However, absorption may be prolonged if there is peripheral vasoconstriction associated with hypovolaemia, hypotension, hypothermia or severe pain. The normal adult dose is 10–15 mg, but this should be reduced in frail and elderly subjects, or in those with underlying respiratory disorders. After intramuscular administration, peak effects are achieved after 30–60 minutes, and its duration of action is approximately 3–4 hours. Its onset of action is only slightly more rapid following intravenous administration, as the main factor governing its latency is low lipid solubility and slow permeation of the blood–brain barrier. Morphine may also be administered orally. However, it undergoes extensive first-pass effects so that only 10–30% of an orally administered dose reaches the systemic circulation, and large doses have to be given to achieve adequate analgesia. Nevertheless, oral therapy with morphine solutions is commonly used in the long-term management of pain associated with malignancy. Slow release preparations and suppository forms of the drug are also available.

Pharmacokinetics. After administration of intravenous morphine, plasma concentrations decline in a triexponential manner. Distribution occurs rapidly at first, and then the plasma concentration declines more slowly. During this period, morphine enters the CNS gradually, due to its relatively low lipid solubility. These phases of drug distribution are followed by a slower phase of exponential

decline, which reflects the terminal half-life of approximately 3 hours (Table 11.6). Although the terminal half-life of morphine is shorter than pethidine or fentanyl, its duration of action is longer, because the decline in CNS concentration is slower, due to its lower lipid solubility. Its duration of action may also be related to the cumulation of active metabolites such as morphine 6-glucuronide in the CNS. There is no direct relationship between the plasma concentration of morphine and its clinical effects, such as respiratory depression.

Pharmacokinetic variability. Several factors may affect the pharmacokinetics of morphine. Neonates are more sensitive to its effects, as the conjugating capacity of the liver is not fully developed. In elderly patients, the volume of distribution is about half that of younger subjects, and plasma concentrations after a standard dose are considerably higher. In hepatic cirrhosis, morphine clearance may be unaltered, since glucuronidation in the endoplasmic reticulum is largely unaffected. Nevertheless, in severe liver disease morphine clearance is reduced by 50%, and its terminal half-life is doubled. In renal failure, sensitivity to morphine is increased, possibly due to the accumulation of morphine6-glucuronide.

Metabolism. Morphine is almost entirely metabolized by the gut wall and the liver to several active or inactive compounds, and more than 90% of the dose is excreted within 24 hours. The principal metabolite, accounting for 70% of the dose, is morphine-3-glucuronide. This metabolite is partly excreted in bile, but can be broken down by intestinal bacteria, so that morphine is released and reabsorbed by enterohepatic recirculation. Morphine is also metabolized to morphine-6-glucuronide, which appears to be similar to but more potent than the parent drug. When patients receive continuous oral morphine, high concentrations of morphine-6-glucuronide are present and may be principally responsible for the analgesic effects.

Papaveretum

Papaveretum was formerly known as Omnopon, and is a semisynthetic mixture of the hydrochlorides of three opium alkaloids (morphine, codeine and papaverine). Its morphine content is 65% of the prescribed or stated amount of papaveretum (usually 7.7–15.4 mg). Although papaveretum can be used for premedication or postoperative pain and may be given intravenously, intramuscularly or subcutaneously, errors in its administration are not uncommon and it is rarely used in current practice.

Diamorphine

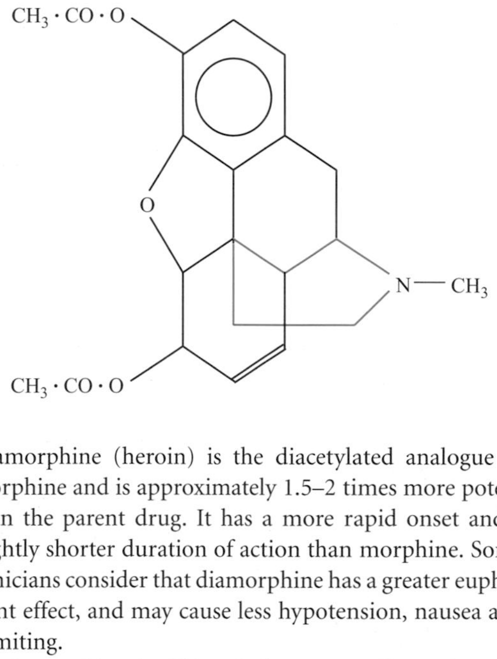

Diamorphine (heroin) is the diacetylated analogue of morphine and is approximately 1.5–2 times more potent than the parent drug. It has a more rapid onset and a slightly shorter duration of action than morphine. Some clinicians consider that diamorphine has a greater euphoriant effect, and may cause less hypotension, nausea and vomiting.

Diamorphine itself has little or no affinity for opioid receptors. It is rapidly and completely metabolized to monoacetylmorphine by red cell and tissue esterases, and its plasma half-life is extremely short (1–3 min). Both diamorphine and monoacetylmorphine are more lipid-soluble than morphine, penetrate the blood–brain barrier more easily, and are rapidly converted to morphine in the CNS. In many countries, the manufacture or importation of heroin, even for medical use, is illegal.

When patients with terminal malignant disease require large doses of morphine for pain relief, diamorphine can be administered in a smaller volume of solution than the equivalent dose of morphine. This is an important practical consideration for patients with malignant disease, muscle wasting and cachexia, and is the only significant advantage of diamorphine. In these conditions, the drug is given intramuscularly as the hydrochloride salt, or preferably by continuous subcutaneous infusion with a syringe driver.

Codeine

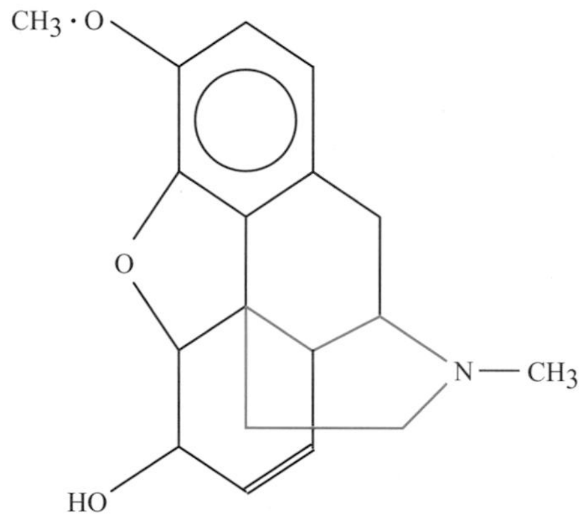

Codeine is the 3-methyl derivative of morphine. It has some analgesic and antitussive activity but a low abuse potential, and large doses tend to produce excitement rather than CNS depression. Its continual administration reduces intestinal activity, resulting in marked constipation. Codeine has a higher oral bioavailability than morphine due to the presence of the 3-methyl group, which protects the drug from the activity of conjugating enzymes. In most patients, approximately 10% is metabolized to the parent drug by O-demethylation, which depends upon the activity of the CYP 2D6 isoform (Chapter 1). This enzyme exhibits genetic polymorphism, and it has been suggested that poor metabolizers may experience little pain relief when codeine is used as an analgesic. It is currently considered that almost all the analgesic effects of codeine are due to its partial demethylation to morphine by CYP 2D6.

Varying doses of codeine (8–30 mg) are commonly incorporated with paracetamol, aspirin or NSAIDs in compound preparations that are used to treat pain of moderate intensity. It is also present in various antitussive and antidiarrhoeal preparations.

Dihydrocodeine, a related compound, is a valuable drug for the management of chronic pain. Oxycodone is even more effective, but has a higher abuse potential. The drug is available in suppository form for the management of pain in terminal care.

Pethidine

$$CO-O-CH_2-CH_3$$

$$N-CH_3$$

Pethidine was originally developed as an antimuscarinic agent, but was subsequently shown to have analgesic properties and was first used clinically in 1939. Despite its apparent chemical dissimilarity to morphine, it contains the characteristic piperidine ring (shown in green). The effects of equipotent doses of morphine and pethidine are generally similar with respect to analgesia, respiratory depression, nausea and vomiting, and tolerance and dependence. Nevertheless, there are certain differences between pethidine and morphine, and some of these may reflect its antimuscarinic effects. Sedation and miosis are less evident, and dry mouth and tachycardia sometimes occur. In addition, a significant fall in blood pressure may occur when pethidine is given to elderly patients.

Pethidine is more lipid-soluble than morphine, and penetrates the blood–brain barrier more readily. Consequently, it has a more rapid onset but shorter duration of action than morphine, although its terminal half-life is longer (Table 11.6). There is usually a clear relationship between the plasma concentration of pethidine and its analgesic effects.

Pethidine can produce serious adverse effects in patients receiving MAOIs, including coma, hypotension or hypertension, convulsions and hyperpyrexia. The mechanism of this interaction is uncertain, and may involve effects on the turnover of 5-HT in the CNS, although inhibition of pethidine metabolism by MAOIs has also been implicated. Consequently, the use of pethidine is absolutely contraindicated in patients receiving MAOIs.

Metabolism and pharmacokinetics. Pethidine has a greater oral bioavailability than morphine, and is extensively (70%) bound to plasma proteins, particularly α_1-acid glycoprotein. It is metabolized in the liver by demethylation to norpethidine, pethidinic acid and pethidine-*N*-oxide. A variable amount is also metabolized and cleared by the lungs. The clearance of pethidine is reduced in liver disease, in the elderly and during the perioperative period. Only 5–10% is excreted unchanged in urine in 24 hours, and this proportion is enhanced by urinary acidification, but reduced by alkalinization.

Norpethidine is a demethylated metabolite of pethidine which is normally eliminated unchanged in urine and has excitatory effects on the CNS. In patients with normal renal function, the terminal half-life of norpethidine is 14–21 hours. In renal failure, both pethidine and norpethidine accumulate, and this may be associated with certain neurological sequelae, including excitatory phenomena and grand mal seizures, particularly when the ratio of the metabolite to the parent compound is greater than one. The elimination of both pethidine and norpethidine is considerably prolonged in the neonate, and their terminal half-lives are about three times longer than in adults (mainly due to a reduction in their clearance).

Pethidine is still frequently used to provide analgesia during labour. However, it readily crosses the placenta, and significant amounts reach the foetus over a period of several hours. By contrast, little norpethidine or other metabolites of pethidine cross the placenta from the maternal circulation.

Fentanyl

$$CH_3 \cdot CH_2 \cdot CO-N$$

$$N-CH_2-CH_2$$

Fentanyl is approximately 100 times more potent than morphine and is widely used in anaesthetic practice. In small doses (1 $\mu g\ kg^{-1}$, intravenously) it has a rapid onset and a short duration of action (20–30 min), and produces mild sedation. By contrast, in high doses (50–150 $\mu g\ kg^{-1}$) profound sedation and unconsciousness occur, and fentanyl has been used as the sole anaesthetic agent, although awareness has been reported during surgery. When given in high doses muscular rigidity of the chest wall may occur.

Fentanyl, like other opioid analgesics, depresses respiration in a dose-dependent manner. Cardiovascular stability is present even when the drug is administered in high dosage, although bradycardia can occur and may require treatment with atropine. High dose fentanyl anaesthesia also reduces or eliminates the stress response to surgery.

Duration of action. Since fentanyl is highly lipid-soluble it rapidly crosses the blood–brain barrier, and concentrations in the CNS usually reflect those in plasma (with a time delay of ≈ 5 min). In small doses (1–2 $\mu g\ kg^{-1}$), its duration of action is short, since plasma and CNS concentrations fall below an effective level during the distribution phase. Consequently, there is rapid recovery from its effects. In contrast, after large or multiple doses of fentanyl, the distribution phase is completed while the plasma concentration of fentanyl is still higher than the minimum effective level. Recovery from the effects of the drug then depends on its relatively slow elimination from the body, and its duration of action is significantly prolonged. In these circumstances, profound respiratory depression may be present for several hours during the postoperative period.

Pharmacokinetics. There is considerable interindividual variation in the pharmacokinetics of fentanyl. After an intravenous bolus dose, plasma concentrations decline rapidly (distribution half-life $\approx$13 min). Its terminal half-life is 3–4 hours in normal subjects, but may be as long as 7–8 hours in some patients. The volume of distribution is relatively large ($\approx$4 L kg^{-1}) due to its high lipid solubility and extensive uptake by tissues, and clearance is slightly less than hepatic blood flow. Fentanyl is predominantly metabolized by N-dealkylation and hydroxylation in the liver, and metabolites can be detected in blood within 1–2 minutes. Approximately 70% of the drug is excreted in urine as inactive metabolites over several days.

Fentanyl is also available as lozenges or self-adhesive patches for palliative care. Lozenges contain 200 μg, and are used to control breakthrough pain in patients already receiving chronic opioid therapy. Fentanyl patches contain 25–100 μg, and may be applied for up to 72 hours in the management of intractable pain associated with malignant disease.

Alfentanil

Alfentanil is a synthetic opioid that is structurally related to fentanyl, but has approximately 10–20% of its potency, a more rapid onset and a shorter duration of action. It is a typical μ-agonist with similar effects on the respiratory and cardiovascular systems to fentanyl, and it is used in similar situations. However, small doses of the drug can cause apnoea in some patients. Although this is usually very brief it is unpredictable, and careful monitoring is essential, particularly in elderly patients who are more sensitive to respiratory depression.

Pharmacokinetics. There are important pharmacokinetic differences between alfentanil and fentanyl (Table 11.6). Although alfentanil has a much lower lipid solubility, its pK$_a$ value (6.5) is lower than fentanyl and 89% is present in plasma in a non-ionized form. It rapidly equilibrates with the CNS (half-time of equilibration = 0.9 min), so that its onset of action is extremely rapid. Its lower lipid solubility results in a smaller volume of distribution and its clearance is approximately half that of fentanyl. Consequently, alfentanil has a shorter distribution half-life (10–12 min) and a shorter terminal half-life (90–120 min). Its context-sensitive half-time (normally 36–60 min) may be significantly reduced by enzyme-inducing agents. Complete recovery from its effects is more rapid than with fentanyl, and alfentanil provides very little postoperative analgesia.

Alfentanil has a hepatic extraction ratio of 0.3–0.5 and is extensively metabolized in the liver by CYP 3A4. Less than 2% of the parent drug is excreted unchanged. Its clearance is unaffected by renal disease, but is prolonged in cirrhosis and in patients on inhibitors of CYT 3A4, such as cimetidine.

Administration. Alfentanil may be administered in either bolus doses or as a continuous infusion. Bolus doses (10 μg kg^{-1}) are used to attenuate the cardiovascular responses to intubation and stimulation during surgery. The pharmacokinetics of alfentanil is consistent with administration by continuous intravenous infusion, and it may be used as the sole anaesthetic agent, or for sedation in intensive care for patients on mechanical ventilation. Typically, a loading dose of 35–70 μg kg^{-1} is given, followed by an infusion of 0.2–2.0 μg kg^{-1} min^{-1}, according to the response.

Remifentanil

Ester link hydrolysed by red cell and tissue esterases

Metabolism and pharmacokinetics.. Remifentanil is a μ-agonist and a piperidine ester that is susceptible to rapid hydrolysis by red cell and tissue esterases at its ester bond. It is not metabolized by plasma cholinesterase, so that its action is unaffected by genetic abnormalities of BChE or the concomitant administration of anticholinesterase drugs. Remifentanil has a low volume of distribution

(400 mL kg^{-1}) but a large clearance (40–45 mL kg^{-1} min^{-1}), so that its elimination half-life is extremely short (8–10 min). Similarly, the offset of activity following continuous infusion of remifentanil is considerably more rapid than with fentanyl or alfentanil, and is not influenced by the duration of infusion (context-sensitive half time = 3–5 min). There is no evidence of delayed clearance or cumulation in renal or hepatic failure. Remifentanil rapidly equilibrates with the CNS (half-time = 1.3 min), so that its onset of action is also extremely rapid. The main metabolite of remifentanil is a carboxylic acid, which is also a μ-opioid agonist, but has only 0.02% of the activity of remifentanil. Although this metabolite accumulates in renal failure, this is of little or no clinical significance.

Administration. Since remifentanil has a rapid offset of action, it should always be given by continuous intravenous infusion. A loading dose of 50–100 μg over 10 minutes or as a bolus is commonly used to produce optimal effects during intubation, followed by an infusion of 0.5–1 μg kg^{-1} min^{-1}. A wider range of infusion rates (0.05–2 μg kg^{-1} min^{-1}) is used to provide analgesia and suppress respiratory activity during intensive care. Although apnoea may occur at higher dose levels or rapid rates of administration, there is little risk of residual respiratory depression. Severe muscle rigidity of the chest wall or the jaw may be induced by remifentanil as well as fentanyl and alfentanil, and may require treatment with muscle relaxants. During the past decade, remifentanil has achieved a definite role in anaesthetic practice and in intensive care. Because of its rapid offset of activity, alternative regimes must usually be established before the infusion is terminated, since there is little or no residual analgesia.

Other fentanyl derivatives
Although other fentanyl analogues have been investigated or used in other countries (carfentanil, lofentanil, mirfentanil, sufentanil and trefentanil), none of these drugs is currently available in the UK.

Methadone

Methadone is well absorbed after oral administration, and in contrast to many other opioids, has little or no first-pass effect. Consequently, it has a high oral bioavailability, and the oral and parenteral doses are usually similar (range = 5–15 mg). Methadone is highly bound to plasma proteins (90%), and has a slow onset but a long duration of action, with a terminal half-life of 15–20 hours. It produces typical opioid effects, and miosis and respiratory depression can usually be detected for more than 24 hours. The drug also binds avidly to tissue proteins, and cumulative effects may be observed with repeated dosage, especially in elderly patients who may experience marked sedation. Methadone is extensively metabolized in the liver by cytochrome P450 isoenzymes to N-demethylated and cyclic compounds. Enzyme inducing agents (e.g. rifampicin) can produce withdrawal symptoms in patients on chronic methadone treatment.

Tolerance develops more slowly to methadone than to morphine, and the drug is widely used as an adjunct in the treatment of morphine dependence. Thus, methadone may be substituted for morphine without precipitating an abstinence syndrome. However, the overall abuse potential of methadone is comparable to that of morphine, and this limits its use for this purpose.

Dipipanone

Dipipanone is a piperidine derivative that is chemically related to methadone. Both drugs have similar properties and potency, although the duration of action of dipipanone is shorter. It is well absorbed after oral administration with little or no first-pass effect, and is usually combined with the antiemetic drug cyclizine in an oral proprietary preparation (Diconal). In the past, dipipanone was widely used in the management of chronic pain associated with malignancy, but is not currently recommended for regular regimes of palliative care.

Dextropropoxyphene

Propoxyphene is a phenylpropylamine derivative that is synthesized as a racemic mixture, although only the d-isomer possesses analgesic activity and is about half as potent as oral codeine. It has been widely used in the UK as co-proxamol (Distalgesic), which contains paracetamol (325 mg) and dextropropoxyphene (32.5 mg). Co-proxamol has been prescribed for a wide variety of painful conditions. Unfortunately, dependence to dextropropoxyphene can occur, and overdosage or drug interaction with alcohol can cause profound respiratory depression and heart failure. Its use in current practice is actively discouraged, and it is likely to be withdrawn.

Tramadol

Mode of action. Tramadol is a derivative of cyclohexanol that is administered as a racemic mixture of two enantiomers (1R,2R and 1S,2S), which have different but complementary effects at opioid and non-opioid receptors. Tramadol is only slightly bound by κ- and δ-receptors, but has significantly higher affinity and agonist activity at μ-receptors. In addition, it inhibits the neuronal uptake of noradrenaline and 5-HT, and is believed to modulate pain by the indirect activation of central descending monoaminergic pathways which inhibit the transmission of nociceptive impulses to the brain. Consequently, analgesia is dependent on a mixture of opioid and monaminergic activity and is only partially antagonized by pure opioid antagonists.

Absorption and metabolism. Tramadol has a high oral bioavailability (70–80%) that can increase to 90–100% with repeated dosage. Thus, there is little difference between the dose requirements with oral or parenteral administration. Tramadol is only 20% bound to plasma proteins but has a high affinity for tissues, with a volume of distribution of 3.0–4.4 L kg^{-1} and a terminal half-life of 4–6 hours. It is predominantly converted by hepatic CYP 2D6 to N- and O-demethylated metabolites, and 1R,2R-(+)-O-desmethyltramadol is an agonist with a higher affinity for μ-receptors than the parent compound.

Both tramadol and its metabolites cumulate in chronic renal disease and hepatic failure, and dose requirements may be reduced by 50%. Conversely, the concurrent use of enzyme-inducing agents (e.g. carbamazepine) may considerably reduce its plasma concentration and analgesic efficacy.

Clinical use. Tramadol is sometimes used in the management of postoperative pain, and initial doses of 250 mg are given during the first hour, followed by 50–100 mg every 4–6 hours. It has a similar potency and efficacy to pethidine when both drugs are given intravenously using patient-controlled analgesia, but is less effective than other opioids in severe postoperative or neuropathic pain. Tramadol shares many of the common adverse effects of opioids such as nausea, vomiting, drowsiness and ambulatory dizziness, but is less liable to induce respiratory depression, constipation or dependence. Its use may be associated with increased operative recall. Tramadol should not be used for patients receiving MAOIs, and is contraindicated if there is a history of epilepsy. At the present time, it is not classified as a controlled drug.

Agonist–antagonists
Agonist–antagonist drugs can be defined as agents that do not produce full or complete agonism at all types of opioid receptor, and includes two distinct types of drugs:
• Drugs with a mixed agonist–antagonist profile produce analgesia by their agonist effects at κ-receptors, but are

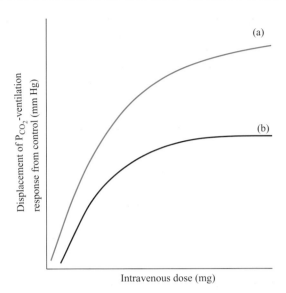

Fig. 11.3 The effect of (a) pure agonists and (b) partial agonists on the response of ventilation to changes in P_{CO_2}. The displacement of the curve from the control is an indication of respiratory depression. In the case of partial agonists, a plateau or ceiling effect occurs, so that further increases in dosage do not enhance respiratory depression.

antagonists at μ-receptors. Agents in this group can be classified as those in which κ-agonist or partial agonist activity predominates (e.g. pentazocine, meptazinol), and those in which μ-antagonist activity predominates (e.g. nalorphine).

• Drugs that are essentially partial agonists, but that may produce agonist or antagonist effects at μ-receptors in different clinical circumstances, due to their low intrinsic activity (e.g. buprenorphine).

The dose–response curve of true partial agonists generally shows a plateau or ceiling effect, with the top of the plateau representing the maximum possible effect (Fig. 11.3).

Pentazocine

Although pentazocine is usually classified as a benzomorphan, it is also a derivative of piperidine and has a mixed agonist–antagonist profile. It is a weak competitive antagonist at μ-receptors, but an agonist or partial agonist at κ- and δ-receptors. It has approximately 25% of the analgesic potency of morphine, but is not very effective in relieving severe pain, partly due to the absence of any euphoriant effects. Analgesia is mainly due to its agonist effects on κ-receptors, and sequential analgesia with pentazocine and pure opioid μ-agonists can produce unpredictable results.

Adverse effects. Intravenous administration invariably produces a rise in blood pressure and heart rate, and increases circulating catecholamine levels. A rise in pulmonary vascular resistance and mean pulmonary arterial pressure is not uncommon, and pentazocine should not be used after myocardial infarction, in pulmonary or systemic hypertension, or in patients with heart failure. Psychotomimetic sequelae including thought disturbances, hallucinations and bizarre dreams occur in about 6% of patients.

Drug dependence. Pentazocine has a much lower abuse potential than morphine, diamorphine or other piperidines. Because of its antagonist effects on μ-receptors, it may precipitate withdrawal syndromes in patients dependent on other opioids, and may also precipitate attacks of acute porphyria in susceptible patients. For these reasons and because of its adverse effects, it is only rarely used in current practice.

Meptazinol

Meptazinol is approximately 10% as potent as morphine and has a shorter duration of action (3–4 h). It has a high affinity for μ-receptors but is antagonized by naloxone, and can produce withdrawal symptoms in morphine dependent subjects. It is also bound with lower affinity by κ- and δ-receptors. Meptazinol facilitates central cholinergic transmission in the cerebellum, labyrinth and vestibular apparatus, which may contribute to its analgesic effects. For similar reasons, it is believed to produce less respiratory depression than other opioids. Although meptazinol rarely causes dysphoria, it often produces nausea and vomiting, which may be related to its cholinergic effects. The incidence of emetic complications can be reduced by antimuscarinic drugs, although the analgesic effects may also be diminished.

Buprenorphine

Buprenorphine is a partial agonist at μ-receptors and has lesser effects on κ- and δ-receptors. It is bound with high avidity by μ-receptors, but only slowly dissociates from them, so that its effects are long lasting and are not readily antagonized by naloxone. In addition, analgesia may also be partly related to its slight agonist activity at κ-receptors.

Metabolism and pharmacokinetics. Buprenorphine is an extremely lipid-soluble drug and is readily absorbed after sublingual administration. It has an extremely low oral bioavailability due to its high first-pass effect, and is extensively metabolized by the liver. Although its terminal half-life is similar to pethidine (3–4 h), it has a long duration of action due to its slow dissociation from the μ-receptor. The clearance of buprenorphine is not affected by renal failure.

Interactions with other opioids. When buprenorphine is given with morphine or other pure agonists, analgesia may be decreased to a ceiling level, but purely additive effects are more likely in the perioperative situation. Interactions with other opioids and their antagonists are highly dependent on the relative doses involved. A combination of buprenorphine and naloxone is currently used in the management of opioid dependence.

Administration. Buprenorphine is approximately 30 times more potent than morphine, so that 300 μg buprenorphine and 10 mg morphine produce the same degree of analgesia. It has a much longer duration of action than morphine and a single dose may produce effective analgesia for 6–8 hours. Buprenorphine is well absorbed sublingually, but can also be given by intramuscular and intravenous administration. It produces typical opioid adverse effects although dysphoria is uncommon, and unwanted haemodynamic effects mediated by CNS stimulation are rare.

Because of its high affinity for μ-receptors, the effects of buprenorphine are not completely reversed by naloxone or naltrexone. Although a plateau or ceiling effect has been described, respiratory depression can be clinically significant and should be managed with doxapram. Although it was initially believed to have a low abuse potential, dependence can occur and buprenorphine is classified as a controlled drug.

Spinal opioid analgesia

Opioid receptors in the dorsal horn of the spinal cord play an important part in modulating the appreciation of pain by the CNS. Spinal analgesia, produced by endogenous opioid peptides or analgesic drugs, is mediated via presynaptic and postsynaptic receptors, which are extensively present on interneurons and C-fibre terminals in lamina 1 and the SG. The discovery of opioid receptors in the spinal cord in the 1970s was soon followed by the use of analgesic drugs by intrathecal and extradural administration.

It was originally considered that the use of spinal opioids would have two main advantages over their systemic administration:
• Localized effects would be produced by relatively low doses, and these effects would be enhanced and prolonged by the absence of drug-metabolizing enzymes at these sites.
• Adverse effects would be minimal due to lack of any supraspinal activity.
Experimental studies using radiolabelled substrates showed that morphine was rapidly taken up by the laminae of the dorsal horn after intrathecal administration.

Subsequent clinical and experimental studies confirmed that a small dose produced prolonged and effective analgesia, and that equipotent doses of other opioids produced comparable effects. In general, the doses used were approximately 10% of the parenteral dose. However, supraspinal and systemic effects also occurred, which depended on the nature and properties of the individual agents, particularly their molecular size and lipid-solubility.

Intrathecal opioids
Although intrathecal opioids have not been widely used in the UK, small doses of fentanyl (5–25 μg), morphine (100–300 μg) or diamorphine (100–250 μg) are occasionally used with local anaesthetics to increase the intensity and duration of analgesia. Fentanyl has a short duration of action (1–6 h) and its effects resemble those seen after intravenous administration. Morphine and diamorphine have a longer duration of action (12–24 h), although their use may be limited by delayed onset respiratory depression, pruritis and urinary retention.

The administration of single doses of intrathecal opioids appears to provide little advantage over the use of more conventional routes, and continuous infusion techniques can present problems associated with spinal cord infection and catheter breakage. In addition, preservative-free preparations must always be used in order to avoid neurological sequelae.

Extradural opioids
The use of extradural opioids has become generally accepted. A significant increase in dosage is required when compared with intrathecal administration, and the availability of morphine, reflecting uptake from the extradural space to the CSF, has been reported as <5%. In many instances, opioids are used in combination with local anaesthetics, and their differential effects on the nociceptive pathway may produce additive effects. The reduced dose requirements of drugs in combination tend to diminish adverse effects, such as motor weakness and hypotension with local anaesthetic agents, and respiratory depression and vomiting induced by opioids.

The behaviour and effects of specific opioids in the extradural space are mainly related to their lipid-solubility, which influences the rate of uptake into peridural fat and adjacent veins, and diffusion into the subarachnoid space and CSF. Molecular size is a less important factor since the molecular weights of fentanyl (336 Da), morphine (285 Da) and diamorphine (369 Da) are similar. The influence of their relative lipophilicity can be illustrated by comparing the extradural administration of fentanyl and morphine.

Fentanyl
Fentanyl is extremely lipid-soluble (octanol–water partition coefficient = 810). Consequently, it crosses the dural membrane extremely rapidly and diffuses into the spinal cord within several minutes. At the same time vascular uptake via the peridural fat is relatively high, resulting in raised plasma levels and early peak concentrations. Thus, the effects of extradural fentanyl are similar to those seen after systemic administration, with any supraspinal effects such as respiratory depression, nausea and vomiting occurring at a relatively early stage.

Morphine
Morphine is relatively hydrophilic (octanol–water partition coefficient = 6), and has a delayed onset of action, due to its slower diffusion across the dura and uptake by the spinal cord. Consequently, there is less uptake into the systemic circulation, and peak CSF levels occur 1–2 hours after administration, with 50% still present after 12 hours. The prolonged presence of morphine in the CSF enhances rostral spread via convection, and results in the uptake of morphine at higher segmental levels. Thus analgesia occurs in higher dermatomes, and thoracic analgesia after lumbar extradural injection is more pronounced than after fentanyl. There is also an enhanced possibility of delayed supraspinal effects, and late-onset respiratory depression, pruritis and urinary retention may occur.

Diamorphine
Diamorphine is frequently administered by the extradural route. Although diamorphine has a slightly greater molecular weight than morphine, it is 50–100 times more lipid-soluble than morphine, and about one third as soluble as fentanyl. Thus, diamorphine may have immediate effects due to its rapid systemic and CNS uptake, but is rapidly hydrolysed to monoacetylmorphine and morphine, which are much less lipophilic, and only spread by convection in the CSF. Consequently, diamorphine usually has a rapid onset but a prolonged duration of action after extradural administration.

Adverse effects
Specific adverse effects are related to the administration of spinal opiates, particularly urinary retention and pruritus. Itching is not confined to the segmental area involved in analgesia, but also occurs in the head and neck. This

may be related to enhancement of C-fibre activity and activation of G_s proteins, although local release of histamine also occurs. The mechanisms that are involved in urinary retention are unclear, although its rapid onset in young men suggest there are spinal effects on the parasympathetic sacral outflow. Both pruritis and urinary retention are readily reversed by naloxone, although analgesia is similarly affected.

There is no conclusive evidence that extradural or intrathecal opioids provide analgesia that is qualitatively superior to that produced by more conventional routes of administration. An undisputed advantage is their ability to produce more prolonged analgesia, usually with lower doses of opioids. These techniques have been used with considerable success in the management of pain associated with surgery, myocardial infarction, chest injuries and in low dose combinations with local anaesthetics in the relief of pain during labour.

Opioid antagonists

Nalorphine

Nalorphine (*N*-allyl-normorphine) was the first opioid antagonist used in clinical practice. Although it is no longer available in the UK, it played an important part in the development of current concepts of opioid receptors. More than 60 years ago, nalorphine was shown to antagonize the analgesic and respiratory effects of morphine, and was used in the treatment of opioid overdosage. It was also shown to possess some analgesic activity when used alone, although its clinical use was associated with an unacceptable incidence of psychotomimetic side effects. It is now generally accepted that morphine antagonism is due to blockade of μ-receptors, while analgesia and dysphoria are due to its agonist effects on κ-receptors.

Naloxone

Naloxone (*N*-allyl-oxymorphone) is a pure opioid antagonist and has no agonist activity at receptor sites. It has a higher affinity for μ- than for κ- or δ-receptors, although it can displace most agonists from their binding sites. However, it may only partially reverse the effects of long-acting opioids, e.g. buprenorphine. Naloxone was originally considered to be devoid of any other inherent actions. However, it is now recognized that it may produce antanalgesic effects in opioid naive subjects, and hypotensive or hypertensive reactions, pulmonary oedema and ventricular arrhythmias can also occur. It is unclear whether these effects are related to antagonism of opioid receptors, or whether they reflect central excitation. Naloxone may produce beneficial effects in patients with thalamic pain, although its mechanism of action is obscure.

Metabolism and pharmacokinetics. Naloxone is readily absorbed from the small intestine, but is almost completely metabolized by glucuronide conjugation in the liver and predominantly excreted in bile. Consequently, only small amounts reach the CNS after oral administration, and the drug must be given parenterally. Because of its rapid metabolism, naloxone has a relatively short terminal half-life (0.5–2 h).

Clinical use. Naloxone is the current drug of choice for the treatment of opioid overdose. In mild or moderate cases, a single dose (100–400 μg) may be sufficient to antagonize the effects of opioid analgesics. However, the duration of effective antagonism may be limited to about 30–45 minutes, and since most μ-agonists outlast this effect further bolus doses or an infusion are required. Smaller doses (0.5–1.0 μg kg^{-1}) may be used to reverse respiratory depression without significantly affecting the level of analgesia. Nevertheless, large bolus doses (1–2 mg) may be required to antagonize severe opioid overdose. Naloxone has also been used in the treatment of septic shock.

Naltrexone

Naltrexone is also a pure opioid antagonist but produces mild pupillary changes. It can displace most agonists from their binding sites, but has a higher affinity for μ- than for κ- or δ-receptors.

Pharmacokinetics. Naltrexone has two important pharmacokinetic advantages compared to naloxone. It has a longer duration of action and is subject to less first-pass metabolism so that it is effective after oral administration. Naloxone has a terminal half-life of 7–9 hours, and is mainly metabolized to 6β-naltrexol, which has about 5% of its opioid antagonist activity. Both the unchanged drug and its metabolite are eliminated in urine as glucuronide conjugates. Consequently, a single oral dose of naltrexone (50 mg) remains active for at least 24 hours, and causes prolonged and severe withdrawal symptoms in opioid-dependent patients. It is used as maintenance therapy, usually three times weekly, for detoxified opioid-dependent subjects, and in relapsing cases it will block the euphoric effects of high doses of opioids.

Doxapram

Doxapram is not an opioid antagonist, but an analeptic that is sometimes used in the prevention or treatment of opioid-induced respiratory depression, particularly in the immediate postoperative period. It is also useful in respiratory depression caused by buprenorphine, whose effects are only partially antagonized by naloxone. Doxapram mainly acts by affecting reflex mechanisms mediated via chemoreceptors in the carotid body, but also directly stimulates the respiratory centre. Only very high doses produce cortical stimulation. It should be used cautiously for patients with hypertension, ischaemic heart disease, thyrotoxicosis and epilepsy.

Doxapram may antagonize opioid-induced respiratory depression without abolishing analgesia, and its use in combination with opioid analgesics reduces the incidence of postoperative chest complications. It has a short duration of action (5–12 min) and may need to be given by infusion. The usual intravenous dose ($1.0–1.5$ mg kg^{-1}) is administered over 30 seconds. It is also available as a ready-made solution (2 mg mL^{-1}) which should be infused at a rate of 2–3 mg min^{-1}. The drug may be of some value in the management of respiratory failure in chronic obstructive pulmonary disease.

Choice of analgesic

Acute pain

Acute pain states include abdominal catastrophes, major trauma, pain following myocardial infarction and pain associated with labour. In most cases, morphine is the drug of choice, although pethidine is preferred in obstetrics. Morphine should be administered by slow intravenous injection in the shocked patient to produce an optimal effect. For the undiagnosed acute abdomen, half the usual dose of morphine or pethidine is sometimes given, in order to produce some analgesia without masking vital signs.

Although diamorphine has been widely used to relieve the pain of myocardial infarction, its advantages are doubtful, although some clinicians consider that it produces more sedation and euphoria and less vomiting than other analgesics. Codeine and its derivatives are commonly used for the management of traumatic pain associated with head injury, since they are less likely to disturb levels of consciousness and have minimal effects on pupillary signs.

In general, agonist–antagonist drugs have significant disadvantages compared with pure agonists. The quality of analgesia is often inferior due to the ceiling effect, and dysphoria is more common. Furthermore, antagonist actions at the μ-receptor may complicate any subsequent change of therapy.

The perioperative period

When pain is present, morphine or pethidine is usually indicated for premedication. The value of pre-emptive analgesia on the course of postoperative pain suggests that the careful timing of opioid premedication, or the use of highly lipid-soluble analgesics at induction, may confer considerable advantages. Fentanyl, alfentanil and remifentanil are particularly useful during induction of anaesthesia, in order to suppress the cardiovascular responses to intubation.

Intravenous morphine is sometimes used to provide supplementary analgesia during surgery. Alternatively, fentanyl and alfentanil may be given intermittently or by continuous infusion in the intraoperative period, particularly in TIVA. The risks of delayed respiratory depression during recovery must be considered, and the rapid recovery from the effects of remifentanil may have considerable advantages.

Morphine and pethidine are still frequently used for the relief of postoperative pain. However, intramuscular injection is not the most effective way of ensuring good postoperative analgesia, and in recent years newer techniques have been developed in an attempt to provide more effective pain relief. Current methods now include spinally administered opioids, patient-controlled analgesia, computer-assisted infusions, and transdermal and transmucosal drug delivery by sublingual, buccal, gingival and nasal administration. The partial agonist buprenorphine has a longer duration of action than most other opioids, and may have possible advantages (as well as several disadvantages) as a postoperative analgesic.

Prolonged intermittent positive-pressure ventilation

During prolonged intermittent positive-pressure ventilation (IPPV), analgesics are often necessary, both to provide adequate pain relief and to facilitate compliance with mechanical ventilation. In recent years, alfentanil has been used for this purpose. When administered by infusion, it provides good analgesia and the rate of administration can be increased to cover periods of increased stimulation (e.g. physiotherapy). However, the effects of remifentanil decline more rapidly, particularly after prolonged infusions, and may have considerable advantages.

Chronic pain

Opioid analgesics are widely used for the management of intractable pain associated with malignant disease. In most situations, effective analgesia can be provided by oral or sublingual administration of drugs.

Morphine is the most useful opioid analgesic for the management of terminal pain. It may be given orally as an elixir (e.g. morphine hydrochloride in chloroform water, 4 hourly), or as slow-release tablets. The initial dose should be the minimum that is compatible with adequate pain relief, and frequent readjustment may be necessary. It is important to ensure that the drug is given at regular intervals and in sufficient dosage to prevent the return of severe pain. Respiratory depression is not usually a problem, although nausea and constipation may require concurrent treatment with other agents (e.g. phenothiazines, laxatives). The oral bioavailability of morphine is poor due to the large first-pass effect. Nevertheless, regular oral morphine may be remarkably effective in the management of terminal pain. It has been suggested that the first-pass effect of morphine gradually decreases with its chronic oral administration, or that accumulation of the active metabolite (morphine6-glucuronide) occurs. Although compound elixirs (e.g. cocaine and diamorphine elixir) have been widely used in the past, they have no significant advantages compared with oral morphine.

Other opioid analgesics are sometimes given by oral administration in terminal pain due to malignant disease. Tramadol can be used for moderate pain, or methadone may be useful since it has a relatively long half-life and a high oral bioavailability. Drugs that are effective by sublingual administration (e.g. buprenorphine) may be particularly useful due to their rapid onset of action.

In advanced malignant disease, problems with swallowing may occur. In these conditions, morphine suppositories can be used, or opioids can be given parenterally. Diamorphine, which is preferred to morphine because of its high aqueous solubility, can be given by continuous subcutaneous administration, using a battery-driven syringe driver. Fentanyl can also be administered as patches or lozenges, and may be useful in the control of breakthrough pain in malignant disease.

Simple analgesics

Simple analgesics, also known as antipyretic or non-opioid analgesics, are commonly used in the treatment of mild or moderate pain. Since most of them also possess some anti-inflammatory activity, they are frequently referred

Table 11.7 The analgesic, antipyretic and anti-inflammatory activity of some simple analgesic drugs.

Drug	Analgesic activity	Antipyretic activity	Anti-inflammatory activity
Aspirin (<3 g day^{-1})	2	2	0
Aspirin (>3 g day^{-1})	3	2	2
Paracetamol	2	2	0
Ibuprofen	1	1	1
Ketoprofen	1	1	2
Naproxen	1	1	2
Diclofenac	1	1	3
Ketorolac	3	1	1
Indometacin	1	1	3

0, absent; 1, slight; 2, moderate; 3, marked.

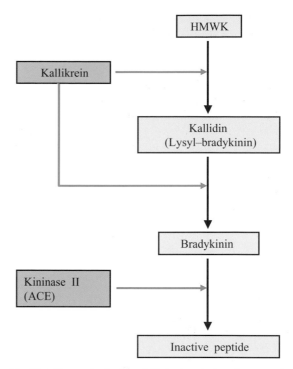

Fig. 11.4 The synthesis of bradykinin from its inactive precursor HMWK (high molecular weight kininogen). The active peptide bradykinin is rapidly degraded by kininase II (also known as angiotensin converting enzyme or ACE).

to as non-steroidal anti-inflammatory drugs (NSAIDs). However, paracetamol has little or no effect on inflammatory processes, and may not be as suitable when pain is associated with inflammation. Similarly, low doses of aspirin (<3g daily) will not produce anti-inflammatory effects (Table 11.7).

NSAIDs mainly act at peripheral sites and are usually administered orally. They are principally used in the treatment of mild or moderate pain associated with somatic structures and are of limited value in severe visceral pain. Nevertheless, some NSAIDs are used in renal colic and are increasingly employed in the control of postoperative pain. In minor surgery, they may eliminate the need for additional analgesia and significantly reduce opioid requirements after major procedures.

Mode of action

Most NSAIDs inhibit cyclooxygenase enzymes that mediate the conversion of arachidonic acid to cyclic endoperoxides, and thus prevent the synthesis of prostaglandins in many tissues. Although prostaglandins do not directly induce pain, they sensitize afferent C fibres to bradykinin, as well as histamine, 5-HT and other potent nociceptive peptides. Consequently, inhibition of prostaglandin synthesis usually produces analgesic effects.

Bradykinin

Bradykinin is rapidly synthesized during tissue injury from an α_2-globulin in plasma known as high molecular weight kininogen, which is then converted by the enzyme kallikrein to a decapeptide (kallidin or lysyl-bradykinin).

Subsequently, kallidin is converted to the active nonapeptide bradykinin (Fig. 11.4). Bradykinin has a half-life of about 10–20 seconds, and is rapidly broken down by angiotensin-converting enzyme (ACE), also known as kininase II. ACE inhibitors may significantly prolong the half-life of bradykinin.

The hyperaemia, pain and oedema of the inflammatory response are partly mediated by bradykinin and other polypeptides, such as substance P, neurokinin A and calcitonin gene-related peptide. High concentrations of bradykinin are present after tissue injury, as well as in inflammatory exudates and synovial fluid from osteoarthritic joints. Bradykinin stimulates most sensory nerve endings, and its subcutaneous administration in humans causes intense, evanescent pain, which is antagonized by aspirin. The analgesic effects of aspirin are due to inhibition of the synthesis of prostaglandins such as PGE$_2$, which sensitize nerve endings to the action of bradykinin.

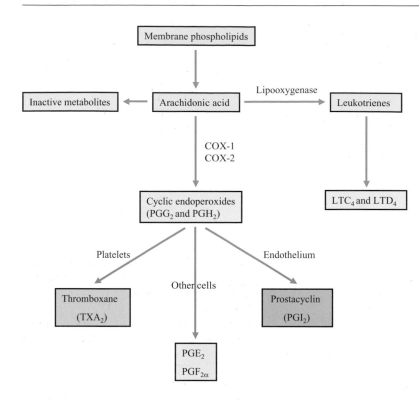

Fig. 11.5 The synthesis of prostaglandins, thromboxanes and leukotrienes. COX-1, cyclooxygenase-1; COX-2, cyclooxygenase-2. Phospholipids in cellular membranes are converted to arachidonic acid, which is subsequently metabolized to the cyclic endoperoxides (PGG$_2$ and PGH$_2$) and other prostaglandins.

Prostaglandin synthesis

In the 1930s, human seminal fluid was shown to cause contraction of isolated smooth muscle. Approximately 30 years later, prostaglandins were isolated from the prostate gland as a series of unsaturated fatty acid derivatives. They are also known as eicosanoids, since they are chemically related to the 20-carbon atom organic acid, eicosanoic acid. Prostaglandins have been isolated and identified in almost all tissues, and are synthesized after tissue injury or inflammation. Their inactive precursor arachidonic acid is present in the phospholipid membrane of most cells, and is released from phospholipids by the enzyme phospholipase A$_2$. It is subsequently converted by cyclooxygenase enzymes to the cyclic endoperoxides PGG$_2$ and PGH$_2$, which are the precursors of prostaglandins (Fig. 11.5).

Cyclooxygenase isoenzymes

Several cyclooxygenase isoenzymes have now been isolated and identified. Cyclooxygenase-1 (COX-1) is the constitutive physiological enzyme that is responsible for the production of prostaglandins that regulate rapid responses in platelets, vascular endothelium, the kidney and gas-

tric mucosa. Cyclooxygenase-2 (COX-2) is also present physiologically in some tissues, but is predominantly an inducible enzyme that is synthesized in response to tissue trauma and inflammation, via intermediates such as growth factors, cytokines and bacterial liposaccharides. In these conditions, COX-2 activity in monocytes and fibroblasts is significantly increased, and mediates the increased prostaglandin synthesis that occurs in inflammatory reactions. Cyclooxygenase-3 (COX-3) is present in the CNS, and is believed to be concerned with the modulation of central pathways, including inhibitory descending pathways that release 5-HT.

Effects of prostaglandins

In most tissues, the cyclic endoperoxides PGG$_2$ and PGH$_2$ are converted to prostaglandins of the D$_2$, E$_2$ and F$_{2\alpha}$ series, which have complex effects on inflammation, smooth muscle activity, glandular secretions, renal function, peripheral blood vessels and bone resorption.

In platelets, cyclic endoperoxides are converted by thromboxane synthetase to thromboxane A$_2$ (TXA$_2$), causing platelet adhesion and vasoconstriction. By contrast, in vascular endothelial cells, the endoperoxides

Table 11.8 Classification of non-steroidal anti-inflammatory drugs (NSAIDs).

Salicylates	Propionates	Acetates	Oxicams	Coxibs	Other agents
Aspirin	Fenbufen	Aceclofenac	Piroxicam	Lumaracoxib	Mefenamic acid
Diflunisal	Fenoprofen	Diclofenac	Tenoxicam	Celecoxib	Nabumetone
	Flurbiprofen	Etodolac	Meloxicam	Etoricoxib	
	Ibuprofen	Ketorolac		Parecoxib	
	Dexibuprofen	Sulindac			
	Ketoprofen	Indometacin			
	Dexketoprofen	Acemetacin			
	Naproxen				
	Tiaprofenic acid				

are converted by prostacyclin synthetase to prostacyclin (PGI_2), resulting in inhibition of platelet adhesion and vasodilatation. It is believed that the balance between the formation of thromboxanes (by the platelets) and PGI_2 (by the vascular endothelium) plays an important role in maintaining the integrity of platelets in circulating blood, and that when this balance is disturbed thrombosis may occur.

In gastric mucosal cells, PGI_2 and other prostaglandins are synthesized, and have a protective role in preventing mucosal damage. In leucocytes, various leukotrienes are directly synthesized from arachidonic acid by lipooxygenase (Fig. 11.5), and leukotrienes C_4 and D_4 play an important role in mediating bronchoconstriction in allergic and anaphylactic conditions.

Prostaglandin metabolism
Many prostaglandins are highly unstable, and have extremely short half-lives. Both TXA_2 and PGI_2 have half-lives of approximately 30 seconds, and PGE_2 and $F_{2\alpha}$ are almost entirely metabolized in a single passage through the pulmonary circulation.

Inhibition of prostaglandin synthesis
Most of the actions of NSAIDs can be explained by their inhibitory effects on prostaglandin synthesis. Their anti-inflammatory activity is mainly due to inhibition of COX-2 and decreased synthesis of PGE_2 and $PGF_{2\alpha}$. Effects on platelet adhesiveness are caused by inhibition of COX-1 and the resultant reduction in thromboxane synthesis, while adverse effects such as gastric irritation and ulceration may be related to decreased prostaglandin synthesis by gastric mucosal cells. Consequently, inhibition of COX-1 is mainly responsible for the gastric and haemor-

rhagic side effects of NSAIDs, whilst inhibition of COX-2 accounts for their anti-inflammatory properties. Individual NSAIDs have different effects on the two isoenzymes. Although naproxen and diclofenac affect both equally, indometacin and aspirin have a much greater effect on COX-1, which may account for their enhanced toxicity.

Selective COX-2 inhibitors
The development of selective inhibitors of COX-2 ('coxibs') appeared to offer significant therapeutic advantages, and a number of these drugs have been introduced and used for their anti-inflammatory effects (Table 11.8). Unfortunately, the clinical use of some of these agents has been associated with an increase in the incidence of cardiovascular and cerebrovascular adverse effects, and some selective COX-2 inhibitors have been withdrawn in the UK. In pathological conditions, the synthesis of endothelial PGI_2 may be critically dependent on COX-2 rather than COX-1, and its selective inhibition may increase the likelihood of myocardial infarction and strokes. In addition prostaglandins synthesized by COX-2 may play a crucial role in the maintenance of gastrointestinal mucosal integrity, particularly when the mucosa is damaged or inflamed.

Other effects of NSAIDs
The beneficial effects of NSAIDs in rheumatoid arthritis and related diseases may be due to direct inhibition of neutrophil activity and function. They may also have analgesic effects unrelated to cyclooxygenase inhibition, possibly involving an increase in plasma ß-endorphin and inhibition of phosphodiesterase. There is some experimental evidence suggesting that NSAIDs may also exert antinociceptive effects at thalamic levels.

Aspirin

$$COOH$$

$$-O-CO-CH_3$$

Aspirin is the acetylated derivative of salicylic acid, which is produced from the glycoside salicin obtained from willow bark. It was introduced into medicine in 1899, and is now one of the cheapest and most widely used drugs in the world. Most of its pharmacological actions are due to inhibition of cyclooxygenase isoenzymes.

Pharmacological effects

Aspirin is most commonly used for its analgesic, antipyretic and anti-inflammatory effects. It is most effective in low intensity somatic pain, rather than severe visceral pain. Aspirin also rapidly reduces body temperature in febrile patients. Bacterial pyrogens cause the release of the inflammatory cytokines IL-1 and TNF-α, increasing central PGE_2 production by COX-3. Aspirin inhibits COX-3 as well as COX-1 and COX-2, decreases prostaglandin synthesis in the hypothalamus, and thus reduces body temperature.

The anti-inflammatory effects of aspirin are due to the decreased synthesis of prostaglandins, particularly by COX-2, although relatively high doses are usually required. In general, dosage of 3–6 g day^{-1} usually decreases inflammatory responses, mainly due to its active salicylate metabolites, but may produce unacceptable gastrointestinal effects.

Aspirin irreversibly acetylates COX-1 in platelets, decreasing thromboxane synthesis and reducing their adhesiveness and aggregation, so that the bleeding time is prolonged. A new generation of platelets must be formed from megakaryocytes before normal thromboxane production is restored. Consequently, aspirin (75–325 mg daily) has an established role in the prophylaxis of thromboembolic disorders (Chapter 15). Doses of more than 3 g day^{-1} may result in inhibition of prothrombin synthesis, a marked decrease in plasma iron concentration and shortening of erythrocyte survival time. Aspirin also affects renal function, and even low doses may cause urate retention due to inhibition of tubular secretion. Higher doses inhibit the tubular reabsorption of urates.

Aspirin can also produce complex effects on carbohydrate metabolism. Therapeutic doses may lower blood glucose, due to an increase in tissue utilization, and can augment the effects of insulin or oral hypoglycaemic agents. Higher doses occasionally cause hyperglycaemia.

Toxic and hypersensitivity reactions

High doses of aspirin frequently cause salicylism, resulting in confusion, dizziness, tinnitus, deafness, sweating, tachycardia and hyperventilation. These effects are usually associated with doses of 5–6 g day^{-1} and plasma concentrations of 300 μg mL^{-1} or above. In particular, tinnitus is often associated with high therapeutic doses of aspirin.

Aspirin often produces gastric erosions and other gastrointestinal side effects, and may reactivate peptic ulceration. These effects may be related to the inhibition of COX-1 and PGI_2 production, or to the trapping of salicylate anions in the gastric mucosa (Chapter 1). In 70% of patients receiving aspirin, there is daily blood loss of 5–15 mL. Occasionally, aspirin causes severe gastrointestinal haemorrhage.

Hypersensitivity reactions to aspirin occasionally occur, most commonly in atopic individuals with a history of infantile eczema or asthma. These may present as bronchospasm, angio-oedema, skin rashes, or rhinitis, and occasionally blood dyscrasias and thrombocytopenia. Bronchospasm may be related to the facilitation of leukotriene synthesis.

The incidence of Reye's syndrome may be commoner in children with febrile illnesses who are given aspirin. Reye's syndrome is a rare condition that causes hepatic damage and encephalopathy, and has a high mortality rate. Consequently, aspirin should not normally be given to children under the age of 12 years.

Acute overdosage

In adults, acute overdosage with aspirin leads to an increase in metabolism and a rise in O_2 consumption and CO_2 production, due to abnormal cellular respiration. In addition, there are complex effects on acid–base balance. Toxic doses of aspirin produce a CSF acidosis, causing stimulation of the respiratory centre and increased ventilation, with a rise in pH and a fall in Pa_{CO_2}. Terminally, an acidotic state due to respiratory and metabolic changes may occur. This is a common presentation of severe aspirin overdosage.

In children, hyperventilation is rare, since the rise in plasma salicylate levels usually depresses the respiratory centre. In addition, metabolic changes occur, and overdosage usually presents as a combination of respiratory and metabolic acidosis.

Gastric lavage may be worthwhile for up to 12 hours after acute poisoning, and dilute sodium bicarbonate (1.26%, 150 mmol L^{-1}) is often infused to enhance the renal excretion of salicylate ions. Haemodialysis and charcoal haemoperfusion may also be used to increase the elimination of salicylates.

Absorption, distribution and elimination

Although aspirin is present in the stomach in a non-ionized form ($pK_a = 3.5$), absorption mainly occurs from the small intestine due to its larger surface area. It is then rapidly hydrolysed by esterase enzymes in the intestinal mucosa and the liver to salicylate, the form which is mainly present in the systemic circulation. Approximately 80–90% is bound to plasma albumin. Both aspirin and salicylates are rapidly distributed in tissues and readily cross most cellular barriers. They are metabolized in the liver to several glucuronide conjugates and salicyluric acid (a glycine conjugate). The conversion of salicylate to salicylurate is often saturated during acute overdosage.

Aspirin, salicylates and their metabolites are eliminated by the kidney, and their excretion is enhanced in alkaline urine. The terminal half-life of salicylate is approximately 4–12 hours, but increases in drug overdosage due to zero-order metabolism.

Clinical uses

Aspirin is often used to relieve pain of moderate intensity, and in the symptomatic management of painful conditions associated with inflammatory processes (e.g. rheumatic diseases, musculoskeletal disorders). Although its antipyretic effects provide some relief in febrile conditions, they are unlikely to alter the course of the underlying disease.

Aspirin is also widely and increasingly used for its antiplatelet effects in the secondary prevention of myocardial infarction and to prevent cerebrovascular strokes.

Aspirin and related drugs are sometimes used in the management of diarrhoea due to irradiation of pelvic tumours, or to bacterial toxins. In these conditions, there may be increased release of prostaglandins from the damaged gut wall. Similarly, certain malignant tumours may synthesize substantial amounts of prostaglandins and their derivatives. These compounds may influence the deposition of metastases in bone, with subsequent bone resorption and pain.

Administration

Whenever possible, aspirin should be used as dispersible tablets and dissolved in water before administration, preferably after meals. In these conditions, aspirin is readily dispersed in gastric secretions, rapidly passes into the small intestine, and is distributed over its large absorptive surface. Enteric-coated preparations that only dissolve in the higher pH of the small intestine are also available, although they have a slower onset of action. Compound tablets of aspirin with codeine, papaveretum, caffeine or other constituents are occasionally useful.

Drug interaction

Aspirin may interact with many other drugs that affect blood coagulation or haemostasis. Its interaction with warfarin is particularly important, and can lead to major haemorrhage (Chapter 4).

Other NSAIDs

Many other NSAIDs have been synthesized and used in the treatment of rheumatic conditions and other painful somatic disorders (Table 11.8). All of these drugs inhibit cyclooxygenases and have significant anti-inflammatory effects, but often have less analgesic and antipyretic activity than equivalent doses of aspirin. They were developed principally as alternatives to aspirin, but without its propensity to produce adverse effects, particularly those affecting the gastrointestinal tract. However, no drug in this group is completely harmless, and there is marked interindividual variability, both with regard to therapeutic responses and to the incidence of toxicity.

In general, NSAIDs should be avoided if possible in patients with a history of peptic ulceration, although many patients who develop ulcers when given NSAIDs have no previous history of dyspepsia. The incidence of gastrointestinal side effects may be reduced by the use of H_2 antagonists, and the prostaglandin analogue misoprostol may provide some measure of protection. NSAIDs should always be taken with food or milk. Gastrointestinal complications are much commoner in the over 60s, particularly in women.

Inhibition of prostaglandin synthesis by NSAIDs can reduce renal blood flow and glomerular filtration rate, and may cause hyperkalaemia and fluid retention, particularly in the elderly. Some individual NSAIDs are highly protein-bound and can enhance the action of anticoagulants, hydantoins, lithium and certain sulphonamides. In addition, various adverse effects such as blood dyscrasias and skin rashes may occur.

In the UK, approximately 20 of these drugs are currently available (Table 11.8). Ibuprofen, ketoprofen and naproxen are probably the most commonly used agents that are used to suppress pain and inflammation in osteoarthritis and other musculoskeletal disorders. Both ibuprofen and ketoprofen are normally administered as racemic mixtures of two enantiomers, but can also be administered as single active stereoisomers (dexibuprofen and dexketoprofen).

Ibuprofen is a relatively mild anti-inflammatory drug that produces fewer adverse effects than other NSAIDs. Although it is widely used as an analgesic in dental practice, it has a relatively low affinity for cyclooxygenase, and is not suitable for the management of conditions in which inflammation is a prominent feature (e.g. ankylosing spondylitis). Ketoprofen is a more effective but more toxic alternative.

Naproxen is also a more effective anti-inflammatory drug, and has a relatively low incidence of gastrointestinal side effects. Since it has a relatively long half-life, it can be given twice daily. It is commonly used in the treatment of acute gout.

Indometacin has marked anti-inflammatory effects, but frequently causes headaches and gastrointestinal side effects. It is sometimes used in the treatment of acute gout, and is also used in neonates to close a patent ductus arteriosus. It is occasionally used to inhibit labour in late pregnancy, although it may affect renal function in the foetus.

Selective inhibitors of COX-2 ('coxibs') are effective anti-inflammatory drugs, and are less likely to cause gastrointestinal side effects than non-selective agents. However, in some instances their clinical use has been associated with an increased incidence of cardiovascular and cerebrovascular complications, and some selective COX-2 inhibitors have been withdrawn. In general, they should not be used in patients with ischaemic heart disease or cerebrovascular disease.

NSAIDs in anaesthetic practice

In recent years, some NSAIDs have been widely used in anaesthetic practice, both as 'pre-emptive' analgesics before surgery and in the treatment of postoperative pain. They appear to be particularly useful in ENT, plastic and minor gynaecological surgery, in day-case surgery and in certain orthopaedic procedures, especially when supplementary local anaesthetic techniques are used. Diclofenac and ketorolac are commonly employed for this purpose, and can be given orally or parenterally. Both drugs have been incorporated as part of multi-modal analgesic regimes, and have been shown to be as effective as conventional doses of morphine or pethidine in mild or moderate postoperative pain. They should both be avoided in patients with acute porphyria.

Other NSAIDS may be equally effective, but are at present only available as oral preparations (Table 11.8).

Diclofenac

Diclofenac is a potent inhibitor of the cyclooxygenase pathway, but also decreases the production of leukotrienes, suggesting that it may reduce the availability of arachidonic acid or exhibit an inhibitory effect on the lipooxygenase pathway. It can be given orally, as an intramuscular or intravenous injection, or as a suppository. Parenteral diclofenac may be extremely painful and should always be given at deep intramuscular sites in the gluteal region.

Diclofenac is also commonly employed to provide analgesia in renal colic.

Although diclofenac is well absorbed after oral administration, it has a significant first-pass effect, but reaches peak concentrations within 1–2 hours. It has a short terminal half-life (1.5–2 h) and a relatively rapid clearance (3–5 mL kg^{-1} min^{-1}). Most of the drug is eliminated in urine within 12–24 hours, mainly as glucuronide and sulphate conjugates, and less than 1% is excreted unchanged.

Ketorolac

Ketorolac is a moderately potent analgesic, but has relatively little anti-inflammatory effect in the doses commonly used to relieve postoperative pain. In these conditions, it usually produces excellent analgesia, and has a longer duration of action than morphine or pethidine.

Ketorolac can be used as an oral preparation, or given by intramuscular or intravenous administration (usually 10–30 mg 4–6 hourly).

Ketorolac is rapidly and well absorbed after oral administration, producing peak plasma levels within 30–60 minutes. It has a relatively long terminal half-life (4–6 h) but a low clearance ($0.1–0.2$ mL kg^{-1} min^{-1}). Ketorolac is mainly metabolized by *para*-hydroxylation or glucuronide conjugation, and over 90% is eliminated in urine within 36–48 hours.

Advantages and disadvantages

NSAIDs have obvious advantages as analgesic drugs, in particular their lack of respiratory depression and the low incidence of nausea and vomiting when compared with conventional opioids. Although they are significantly bound to plasma proteins (95–99%), there appear to be no significant drug interactions with opioids that are used concurrently.

Nevertheless, the perioperative use of NSAIDs must be viewed with caution. Problems may be encountered when these drugs are given to patients with atopic tendencies or a history of asthma. NSAIDs must be used sparingly, if at all, when there is impairment of renal function, and the incidence of postoperative acute renal failure is increased when ketorolac is used for more than 5 days. Similarly, their use may result in the attenuation of antihypertensive therapy, particularly with diuretics or ACE inhibitors. Many haematological disorders and bleeding tendencies are an absolute contraindication to their use, and significant haemorrhage during and after surgery has resulted when NSAIDs have been used concomitantly with low-dose heparin regimes. Even short-term administration may result in gastric erosions and ulceration (particularly with ketorolac), and NSAIDs should not be used postoperatively for more than 5–7 days.

Paracetamol

Although paracetamol was synthesized more than 100 years ago, it has only been widely used as an analgesic since 1949. Paracetamol has analgesic and antipyretic effects that are similar to aspirin, but little or no anti-inflammatory activity. It is generally accepted that it has little effect on extracerebral COX-1 or COX-2, although it inhibits central COX-3. Consequently, it prevents the enhanced synthesis of prostaglandin E$_2$ in the hypothalamus during pyrexia, and thus reduces elevated body temperature. It has similar effects to aspirin on non-specific pain.

Pharmacokinetics

Paracetamol is well absorbed from the gastrointestinal tract and does not cause gastric irritation or bleeding. After absorption, paracetamol is not significantly bound to plasma proteins, and has a short terminal half-life (1.9–2.5 h) and rapid clearance (5.0–7.5 mL min^{-1} kg^{-1}). It is almost completely metabolized by the liver, and approximately 60% is eliminated as a glucuronide conjugate, with the remainder as sulphate and cysteine conjugates. Only trace amounts are eliminated unchanged in urine.

Clinical use

Paracetamol is widely used in the treatment of pain of moderate intensity such as headache, toothache, dysmenorrhoea and pains of musculoskeletal origin. Similarly, it is incorporated into many compound preparations containing aspirin, caffeine, dextropropoxyphene, codeine or dihydrocodeine.

In anaesthetic practice, paracetamol is often used as a premedicant or analgesic, particularly in paediatric patients. In adults, doses of 1–2 g can be given orally or by intravenous infusion, which provides more consistent plasma concentrations and analgesia during the perioperative period. Intravenous paracetamol may be a valuable component of multimodal regimes, and its analgesic effects are probably due to the modulation of descending 5-hydroxytryptaminergic pathways and inhibition of central cyclooxygenases, particularly COX-3.

Paracetamol toxicity

Paracetamol overdosage can lead to potentially fatal hepatocellular necrosis, and less commonly causes renal tubular necrosis. In the UK, it is involved in approximately 15% of all hospital admissions for drug poisoning. Although liver damage has been reported after oral ingestion of 5 g, it is more commonly produced by more than 10–15 g (i.e. 20–30 tablets) of the drug. The initial features of poisoning such as nausea, vomiting and abdominal pain are often slight and may regress, thus engendering a false sense of security. Hepatocellular jaundice and other signs of liver damage are only be apparent after a latent period of 3–6 days, and may be rapidly followed by haemorrhage, hypoglycaemia, encephalopathy and death.

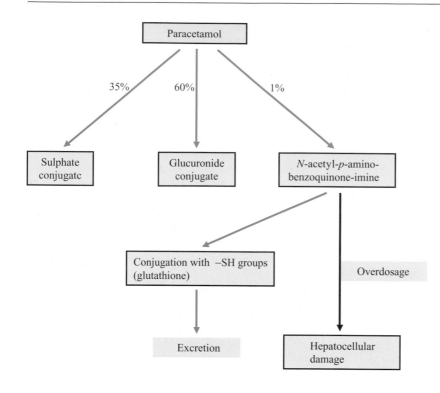

Fig. 11.6 The metabolism of paracetamol. In normal conditions, approximately 95–99% is eliminated as sulphate and glucuronide conjugates. In drug overdosage, excessive amounts of a toxic metabolite are formed, and may produce hepatocellular damage unless conjugated with –SH groups.

Paracetamol is normally metabolized to glucuronide, sulphate and cysteine conjugates. However, small amounts of paracetamol are converted to *N*-acetyl-*p*-amino-benzoquinone-imine, which has a high affinity for sulphydryl groups. This minor metabolite is usually innocuous, since it is inactivated by conjugation with hepatic glutathione. After an overdose of paracetamol, hepatic reserves of glutathione and methionine are conjugated and depleted, and the toxic metabolite combines covalently with sulphydryl groups in liver macromolecules, producing subacute hepatic necrosis (Fig. 11.6). If patients are on enzyme-inducing drugs, the risk of significant hepatic damage is considerably greater. Unless specific therapy is given, some degree of centrilobular hepatic necrosis will occur in 10–20% of patients, and 2–3% will die in hepatic failure. Immediate treatment is essential, since sulphydryl donors such as *N*-acetylcysteine, methionine and cysteamine can conjugate the toxic metabolite and prevent liver damage if given rapidly. Treatment includes gastric lavage, intravenous fluids and the cautious use of antiemetics if there is persistent nausea and vomiting. The sulphydryl donor *N*-acetylcysteine is the treatment of choice, but must be given intravenously within 10–12 hours of ingestion of paracetamol, since it is ineffective

and may be dangerous if given at a later stage. Plasma paracetamol levels are invaluable in assessment, and provide a guide to the likely effectiveness of *N*-acetylcysteine. Vitamin K and other clotting factors may be necessary for the management of coagulation defects.

Paracetamol is usually free from other toxic effects. Occasionally, skin rashes, methaemoglobinaemia and haemolytic anaemia occur, which may be related to erythrocyte glucose 6-phosphate dehydrogenase deficiency.

Other agents

In some circumstances, many drugs that are not primarily analgesics may be used in the management of pain. Thus, antimuscarinic drugs such as hyoscine butylbromide are of value in the treatment of smooth muscle spasms. Pain due to hypertonicity of striated muscle, for instance in upper motor neuron lesions, spasmodic torticollis and muscle tension headaches, may be relieved by dantrolene or centrally acting muscle relaxants, including benzodiazepines and the $GABA_B$ receptor agonist baclofen. Drugs that affect the calibre of blood vessels are also important, and vasodilators often provide symptomatic relief when pain is due to ischaemia of somatic or visceral structures.

Some of the chemical excitants of pain may be inactivated or antagonized by specific agents. Examples include antacid therapy for peptic ulcer, and the use of histamine and 5-HT antagonists in the prophylaxis of migraine. The thyroid hormone calcitonin produces symptomatic relief in Paget's disease and occasionally in other forms of bone pain, possibly due to the translocation of phosphate ions.

Psychotropic drugs are often used as adjuncts in pain therapy. In addition to their action on the reactive components of pain such as anxiety and misery they may have more specific effects. Phenothiazines augment the effects of opioid analgesics and may produce analgesia as part of a generalized deafferentation. Tricyclic antidepressants are thought to facilitate transmission in descending fibres that release 5-HT, and may modify inhibitory input in the substantia gelatinosa (Fig. 11.1).

Nefopam

Although nefopam is chemically related to diphenhydramine, its mode of action is uncertain and it is not classified as an opioid or a simple analgesic. It is normally free from the adverse effects of opioids, such as respiratory depression and drug dependence. Nefopam blocks the uptake of noradrenaline by sympathetic nerve endings, and can also produce antimuscarinic effects. It may also induce excessive sweating, and its atropine-like effects may be mediated within the CNS rather than peripherally. Nefopam has been successfully used in musculoskeletal and cancer pain.

Migraine

Acute attacks of migraine are probably caused by the initial release of 5-HT, which triggers the cerebral vasoconstriction and the associated prodromal symptoms. Further release of 5-HT subsequently occurs, due to platelet aggregation. The typical migraine headache corresponds to the phase of dilatation of extracranial vessels, and may be mediated by the increased production of histamine and plasma kinins, while plasma 5-HT levels are decreasing. The triggering of neurogenic inflammation may result in plasma extravasation in the dura, with resultant nociceptive responses relayed to the most caudal part of the trigeminal nucleus and the dorsal horn of C1 and C2 segments of the spinal cord.

Acute attacks of migraine are usually managed with paracetamol, aspirin or other NSAIDs, and their inhibitory effects on platelet aggregation may impede 5-HT release and be an added advantage. Nausea and vomiting are common in severe attacks, and antiemetic drugs may be valuable.

In current practice 5-HT$_1$ receptor agonists, that act at receptor subtypes B and D ('triptans'), are often used to terminate an acute attack, since they reduce vasodilatation in the carotid circulation without compromising cerebral blood flow. Sumatriptan, which is also used in the treatment of cluster headaches, is available as tablets, a subcutaneous injection, and as a nasal spray, and other triptans are also widely used. Although ergotamine is still available, it is now mainly of historical interest.

For continuous prophylaxis, drugs which antagonize the peripheral effects of 5-HT, histamine and the kinins have been used, including methysergide, cyproheptadine and pizotifen. Some anticonvulsant drugs (e.g. valproate, topiramate) and ß-adrenoceptor antagonists that cross the blood–brain barrier (e.g. propranolol) are also used in the management of migrainous neuralgia and atypical facial pain. Their mode of action in this context is unclear, but it may be related to antagonism of ß$_2$-adrenoceptors in the extracranial vessels, or possibly to inhibitory effects on the synthesis and release of 5-HT from the pineal body.

Trigeminal neuralgia

In trigeminal neuralgia, the sudden attacks of severe lancinating pain are inadequately managed by conventional analgesic therapy. The aetiology of the condition is unknown, but the paroxysmal nature of the pain suggests that it is a type of focal sensory epilepsy. It is therefore not surprising that several drugs that were originally introduced into clinical practice for the treatment of epilepsy are effective, and their membrane-stabilizing activity on the spinal trigeminal nucleus may be of considerable importance. Their mechanism of action may involve the reduction of ectopic responses and Na$^+$ entry at concentrations that do not block nerve conduction.

Carbamazepine is the drug of choice. When taken regularly, it is highly effective in controlling the attacks of pain, and 70% of patients gain relief. The development of drug tolerance may be due to an alteration in its pharmacokinetics, since carbamazepine is an enzyme-inducing agent that can accelerate its own metabolism. Side effects such as drowsiness and ataxia are common although these may disappear with continued dosage, and gastrointestinal intolerance may occur. Blood dyscrasias are an occasional but more serious problem. Other anticonvulsant agents, such as phenytoin and valproate, are logical alternatives when unacceptable side effects are present, although they are not quite as effective. If the symptoms of trigeminal neuralgia are abolished by a surgical procedure, or by a radiofrequency lesion to the Gasserian ganglion or its appropriate branches, anticonvulsant therapy should be gradually withdrawn, since sudden cessation may induce epileptiform attacks.

Suggested reading

Corbett, A.D., Henderson, G., McKnight, A.T. & Paterson, S.J. (2006) 75 years of opioid research: the exciting but vain quest for the Holy Grail. *British Journal of Pharmacology* **147**, S153–S162.

Darland, T. & Grandy, D.K. (1998) The orphanin FQ system: an emerging target for the management of pain? *British Journal of Anaesthesia* **81**, 29–37.

Dray, A., Urban, L. & Dickenson, A. (1994) Pharmacology of chronic pain. *Trends in Pharmacological Sciences* **15**, 190–197.

Duthie, D.J.R. (1998) Remifentanil and tramadol. *British Journal of Anaesthesia* **81**, 51–57.

Finck, A.D. (1989) Opiate receptors and endogenous opioid peptides. *Current Opinion in Anaesthesiology* **2**, 428–433.

Glass, P.S.A., Hardman, D. & Kamiyama, Y., *et al.* (1993) Preliminary pharmacokinetics and pharmacodynamics of an ultra-short acting opioid remifentanil (G187084B). *Anesthesia and Analgesia* **77**, 1031–1040.

Henderson, G. & McKnight, A.T. (1997) The orphan opioid receptor and its endogenous ligand-nociceptin/orphanin FQ. *Trends in Pharmacological Sciences* **18**, 293–300.

Hoskin, P.J. & Hanks, G.W. (1991) Opioid agonist–antagonist drugs in acute and chronic pain states. *Drugs* **41**, 326–344.

Keeble, J.E. & Moore, P.K. (2002) Pharmacology and potential therapeutic applications of nitric oxide-releasing non-steroidal anti-inflammatory and related nitric oxide-donating drugs. *British Journal of Pharmacology* **137**, 295–310.

Martin, W.R., Eades, C.G. & Thompson, J.A., *et al.* (1976) The effects of morphine- and nalorphine-like drugs in the non-dependent chronic spinal dog. *Journal of Pharmacology and Experimental Therapeutics* **97**, 517–532.

Melzack, R. & Wall, P.D. (1965) Pain mechanisms: a new theory. *Science* **150**, 971–979.

Mitchell, R.W.D. & Smith, G. (1989) The control of acute postoperative pain. *British Journal of Anaesthesia* **63**, 147–158.

Morgan, M. (1989) Use of intrathecal and extradural opioids. *British Journal of Anaesthesia* **63**, 165–188.

Pasternak, G.W. (1993) Pharmacological mechanisms of opioid receptors. *Clinical Neuropharmacology* **16**, 1–18.

Pasternak, G.W. (2005) Molecular biology of opioid analgesia. *Journal of Pain Symptom Management* **29**, S2–S9.

Pert, C.B. & Snyder, S.H. (1973) Opiate receptor; demonstration in nervous tissue. *Science* **179**, 1011–1014.

Pleuvry, B.J. (1993) Opioid receptors and their relevance to anaesthesia. *British Journal of Anaesthesia* **71**, 119–126.

Power, I. (2005) Recent advances in postoperative pain therapy. *British Journal of Anaesthesia* **95**, 43–51.

Rathmell, J.P., Lair, T.R. & Naumann, B. (2006) The role of intrathecal drugs in the treatment of acute pain. *Anesthesia and Analgesia* **101**(Suppl 5), S30–S43.

Richmond, C.E., Bromley, L.M. & Woolf, C.J. (1993) Preoperative morphine pre-empts postoperative pain. *Lancet* **342**, 73–75.

Sear, J.W. (1998) Recent advances and developments in the clinical use of i.v. opioids during the preoperative period. *British Journal of Anaesthesia* **81**, 38–50.

Shetty, P.S. & Picard, J. (2006) Adjuvant agents in regional anaesthesia. *Anaesthesia and Intensive Care Medicine* **7**, 407–410.

Vane, J.R. & Botting, R.M. (1995) New insights into the mode of action of anti-inflammatory drugs. *Inflammation Research* **44**, 1–10.

Waldhoer, M., Bartlett, S.E. & Whistler, J.L. (2004) Opioid receptors. *Annual Review of Biochemistry* **73**, 953–990.

Wall, P.D. & Melzack, R. (eds) (1999) *Textbook of Pain*, 4th edn. Edinburgh: Churchill Livingstone.

Watkins, P.B., Kaplowitz, N. & Slattery, J.T., *et al.* (2006) Aminotransferase elevations in healthy adults receiving 4 grams of acetaminophen daily: a randomized controlled trial. *Journal of the American Medical Association* **296**, 87–93.

12 Drugs Used in Premedication and Antiemetic Agents

Many drugs are prescribed or used by anaesthetists before the administration of general or regional anaesthesia. In general, the aims of premedication are

- The relief of fear and anxiety
- A reduction in anaesthetic requirement
- The suppression of unwanted sympathetic or parasympathetic activity, including haemodynamic responses to intubation
- The prevention or diminution of pain, nausea and vomiting in the postoperative period
- The minimization of risks associated with the aspiration of gastric contents, particularly in obstetric anaesthesia.

The development of premedication

For many years opioid analgesics were routinely used as premedicant drugs. Their sedative and analgesic effects had considerable advantages in facilitating the induction and maintenance of anaesthesia in the era prior to the introduction of barbiturates, neuromuscular blocking agents and potent inhalational anaesthetics. However, there are many disadvantages associated with opioid premedication. Dysphoria may occur in the absence of preoperative pain, gastric emptying is prolonged and nausea and vomiting may occur. In addition, interaction with other CNS depressants may be undesirable, and parenteral administration is usually essential. Nevertheless, until 1960 intramuscular morphine or pethidine was commonly used with atropine or hyoscine 30–45 minutes prior to surgery. Some anaesthetists considered that the 'twilight sleep' induced by the combination of papaveretum (Omnopon) and hyoscine (scopolamine) had marked advantages. In recent years, the use of these regimes has greatly declined.

Other forms of premedication were also widely used, but are now only of historical interest. At one time, pre-anaesthetic sedation or basal narcosis was induced by the rectal administration of powerful CNS depressants during the preoperative period. These agents included tribromethyl alcohol (bromethol; Avertin), paraldehyde and thiopentone sodium suspension. This method was considered to be particularly useful in uncooperative children, or in patients with uncontrolled thyrotoxicosis ('stealing the thyroid'). Orally administered barbiturates were sometimes used as hypnotics or preoperative sedatives. All of these techniques are now obsolete.

In current practice, benzodiazepines are widely used for premedication in adult patients. Diazepam, temazepam and midazolam are the main drugs that are used for this purpose. In children, oral midazolam is also widely used or analgesics (e.g. paracetamol suspension, ibuprofen) are given prior to induction. Oral phenothiazines (alimemazine, promethazine) are also sometimes used in children. Antimuscarinic drugs (atropine or hyoscine) are occasionally given by mouth, but are also used intravenously immediately before the induction of anaesthesia. In children undergoing day-case surgery sedative premedication may be unnecessary. Occasionally, oral midazolam or ketamine is used.

In this chapter, premedicant agents are considered in five groups:
- Benzodiazepines
- Phenothiazines
- Antimuscarinic drugs
- α_2-Adrenoceptor antagonists
- Other drugs

Benzodiazepines

Benzodiazepines are probably the most commonly prescribed drugs in the Western World. They are either used as night hypnotics, or administered during the day to produce sedation and anxiolysis. They are the hypnotics and sedatives of choice for short-term oral administration, and are particularly useful in the treatment of insomnia associated with anxiety. Side effects (apart from drowsiness and related central phenomena) are rare, although they occasionally cause nightmares, nausea, skin rashes or an increase in body weight. They do not induce hepatic microsomal enzymes, and do not usually interact with other drugs, apart from other hypnotics and sedatives, including ethyl alcohol. In most subjects, they are relatively safe in overdosage, and patients have recovered from as much as 80 times the normal hypnotic dose. Although most benzodiazepines are suitable hypnotics, a drug with a short half-life (e.g. temazepam) may be preferred when hangover effects impair performance.

Disadvantages

All benzodiazepines impair judgement and increase reaction time, and even short-acting drugs impair psychomotor performance and may produce hangover effects on the day after their administration. Ambulant patients should not drive, work at heights or operate dangerous machinery for at least 24 hours after their administration. Although conventional doses of benzodiazepines do not usually affect respiration, they may depress ventilation in elderly patients with poor pulmonary function. In general, they are poorly tolerated by the elderly, and drowsiness, disorientation and unsteadiness can result in slurred speech, falls and fractures, poor memory and acute confusional states. The increased susceptibility of the elderly is partly due to impaired drug metabolism, and partly to enhanced CNS sensitivity.

Effect on sleep

Benzodiazepines also alter the pattern of physiological sleep. During their administration, the duration of stage 2 sleep is increased, while stages 3, 4 and REM sleep ('dreaming sleep') is reduced. When the hypnotic is stopped, a rebound phenomenon occurs and there is subsequent compensation for the earlier loss of REM sleep. This is sometimes associated with unpleasant dreams and nightmares due to more intense REM mentation. The significance of these changes is unknown.

Tolerance and dependence

In subacute or chronic use (i.e. for more than 2–3 weeks), benzodiazepines are associated with a significant risk of tolerance and drug dependence. Consequently, their use as hypnotics and sedatives should be restricted to less than 1 month. Tolerance to their hypnotic effects may occur after 3–14 days continual administration, and during their chronic use physical dependence is said to occur in 15%

of patients. In recent years, some benzodiazepines (e.g. temazepam, lorazepam) have become notorious drugs of abuse.

At present 13 benzodiazepines are available in the UK as hypnotics, tranquillizers or anticonvulsants (Table 12.1).

Mode of action

Benzodiazepines produce their effects by the enhancement of GABA-mediated inhibitory transmission at GABA$_A$ receptors, which are widely distributed at postsynaptic sites in the CNS. Although they are most numerous in the cerebral cortex, the cerebellar cortex, the corpus striatum and the limbic system,[1] they are also present in the brainstem and the spinal cord.

Structure of GABA$_A$ receptors

GABA$_A$ receptors are integral transmembrane proteins with five distinct subunits surrounding an intrinsic ion pore that is selectively permeable to chloride ions. The five subunits are derived from seven families, and 18 different types have been identified in the mammalian CNS (α_{1-6}, β_{1-3}, γ_{1-3}, δ, ϵ, θ, ρ_{1-3}). Consequently, GABA$_A$ receptors should be considered to be a heterogeneous group of related receptors rather than a single entity. Nevertheless, more than 60% of receptors in the brain contain three different subunits (in the combination α_1, α_1, β_2, β_2 and γ_2). Most GABA$_A$ receptors contain binding sites for both GABA and benzodiazepines, which interact with each other (Fig. 12.1). In addition, the macromolecular complex contains binding sites for barbiturates, steroids and some proconvulsive drugs (e.g. picrotoxin). Both the α- and β-subunits are believed to contribute to the GABA binding site, which is closely related to the chloride channel. In contrast, the benzodiazepine binding site is at the interface between the α- and γ-subunits, close to a histidine residue (histidine 101). The replacement of histidine 101 by arginine results in a 1000-fold decrease in the binding affinity of benzodiazepines for the GABA$_A$ receptor.

GABA and benzodiazepines

GABA is the most important inhibitory neurotransmitter in the CNS and is believed to mediate postsynaptic inhibition at more than 50% of all synapses. It is normally synthesized in presynaptic nerve endings from glutamate

---

[1] The limbic system consists of the hippocampus, the amygdaloid nuclei, the nucleus accumbens, and part of the cerebral cortex and is believed to be mainly concerned with the integration of emotional responses.

Table 12.1 Relative potencies, terminal half-lives and active metabolites of benzodiazepines.

	Approximate hypnotic, sedative or anticonvulsant dose (mg)	Approximate potency	Terminal half-life of parent drug (h)	Active metabolites	Half-lives of significant metabolites (h)
Flurazepam	15	2	2–3	Yes	50–100
Lormetazepam	1	30	8–12	No	
Loprazolam	1	30	6–8	Yes	6–8
Nitrazepam	10	3	18–34	Doubtful	
Temazepam	20	1.5	4–10	Yes	6–25
Midazolam	10	3	1–3	Yes	12–24
Alprazolam	0.5	60	10–12	Yes*	
Chlordiazepoxide	10	3	5–30	Yes	6–25 50–120
Clobazam	20	1.5	10–30	Yes	35–45
Clonazepam	6	5	20–60	No	
Diazepam	10	3	24–48	Yes	4–10 6–25 50–120
Lorazepam	2	15	10–20	No	
Oxazepam	30	1	6–25	No	

*Active metabolites of alprazolam are of no clinical significance.

by the enzyme glutamate decarboxylase and is rapidly broken down by GABA transaminase (Fig. 7.3). In the presence of GABA, chloride channels in GABA$_A$ receptors open, resulting in neuronal hyperpolarization and inhibition. Benzodiazepines act by increasing the affinity of GABA for the receptor, and thus enhance and facilitate the effects of GABA. Consequently, they increase the frequency of chloride channel opening in response to a given stimulus (Fig. 12.1), although channel opening times are unchanged or only slightly increased. In these conditions, more receptors are recruited for activation by GABA, and the amplitude of the peak inhibitory postsynaptic potential is enhanced. There is no evidence that benzodiazepines affect the synthesis or the breakdown of GABA, or influence its action in any other way.

Benzodiazepines may indirectly affect other neurotransmitters in the CNS. For example, they decrease dopamine and 5-HT turnover in specific brain regions, and prevent the increase in noradrenaline turnover induced by stress. These changes are believed to represent secondary effects on brain metabolism.

GABA$_B$ receptors

Other types of GABA receptor are also present in the CNS (particularly in the brainstem and the spinal cord).

GABA$_B$ receptors are metabotropic receptors that are coupled to G$_i$ and adenylate cyclase (Chapter 3), and receptor activation decreases cAMP and has secondary effects on Ca^{2+} and K$^+$ channels. GABA$_B$ receptors do not possess high affinity binding sites for benzodiazepines, and they are mainly present at presynaptic sites in the CNS and peripheral autonomic nerve terminals. They are also present in high concentrations in the dorsal horn and dorsal columns of the spinal cord. GABA$_B$ receptors decrease the release of amines, neuropeptides and excitatory neurotransmitters, and inhibit the release of GABA at presynaptic sites. The GABA analogue baclofen is a specific agonist at GABA$_B$ receptors, and is used to reduce spasticity and prevent flexor spasms in a variety of neurological disorders.

Inverse agonists

Benzodiazepines differ greatly in potency (Table 12.1). The variations in potency appear to be related to the different affinity of benzodiazepines for GABA$_A$ receptors in the CNS, and there is usually a close relation between receptor occupancy and potency. Nevertheless, not all drugs that are bound by benzodiazepine receptors have hypnotic effects. Some extensively bound drugs (e.g. β-carboline esters) may even have proconvulsant effects, which are

(a)

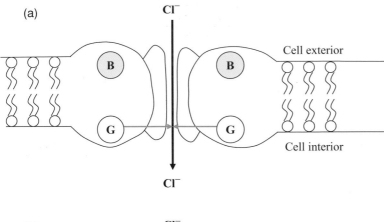

(b)

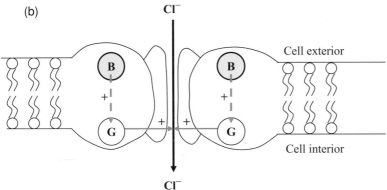

Fig. 12.1 Relationship between benzodiazepine binding sites, GABA binding sites and chloride channels in GABA$_A$ receptors. The receptors shown in (a) and (b) contain binding sites for both GABA (G) and benzodiazepines (B). (a) Binding of GABA at site G (○) opens the chloride channel, resulting in the entry of Cl$^-$; (b) Binding of benzodiazepines at site B (●) increases the binding affinity of GABA at site G and thus increases the frequency of chloride channel opening in response to a given GABA stimulus. In both instances, the enhanced entry of Cl$^-$ results in hyperpolarization of the postsynaptic cell and inhibition of neuronal transmission. (+) represents amplification.

probably due to antagonism of the spontaneous ('constitutive') activity of benzodiazepine receptors (Chapter 3). Similar effects are occasionally produced by the benzodiazepine antagonist flumazenil in man. In recent years, a peptide ('diazepam-binding inhibitor') has been isolated from rat brain, which has similar effects to inverse agonists at GABA$_A$ receptors.

General effects of benzodiazepines

Benzodiazepines are considered to produce sedation, hypnosis, anxiolysis and anterograde amnesia by enhancing inhibitory transmission in the CNS (particularly in the limbic system). Consequently, benzodiazepines produce the following general effects:

• Modification of emotional responsiveness and behaviour due to suppression of neuronal activity between the limbic system and the hypothalamus.

• Decrease in alertness and arousal reactions due to the depression of activity between the limbic system and the reticular system.

• Anticonvulsant effects (probably due to inhibition of amygdaloid nuclei).

• Reduction in voluntary muscle tone due to the suppression of polysynaptic reflexes in the spinal cord.

Pharmacokinetics

Benzodiazepines are nonpolar and highly lipid-soluble drugs. Consequently, they are well absorbed after oral administration, have a high bioavailability and a large apparent volume of distribution. Most of them are extensively bound to plasma proteins (95–99%), but only the unbound fraction can cross the blood–brain barrier and affect the CNS. Although displacement reactions occur in *in vitro* conditions, they are of little significance in practice. Many benzodiazepines have a variable duration of action due to their different half-lives (Table 12.1). These differences have been used to divide them into hypnotics (with a relatively short terminal half-life) and sedatives/tranquillizers (with a relatively long half-life). Although this distinction is rather

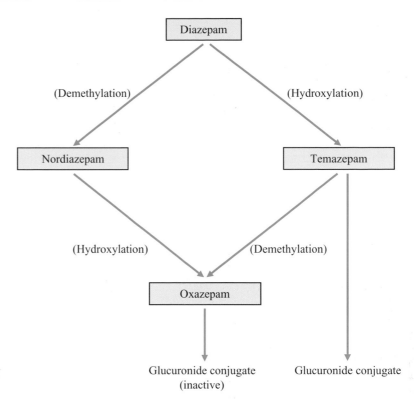

Fig. 12.2 The metabolism of diazepam and its relationship to the metabolism of temazepam and oxazepam.

arbitrary, it may be valuable in practice. Benzodiazepines with short terminal half-lives (and whose active metabolites have short half-lives) are less likely to cause impaired psychomotor performance and hangover effects on the day after their administration.

Metabolism

Benzodiazepines are almost entirely metabolized and only small amounts are excreted unchanged. Many of them (e.g. diazepam) are oxidized by cytochrome P450 isoforms (particularly CYP 2D6 and CYP 3A4) to active metabolites, while others (e.g. temazepam, oxazepam) are directly converted to glucuronide conjugates and subsequently eliminated in urine. Almost all benzodiazepines (with the exception of midazolam) have a low intrinsic hepatic clearance, which is not influenced or dependent on liver blood flow.

Diazepam

Diazepam is metabolized to several active metabolites, including temazepam and desmethyldiazepam (nordiazepam). Both compounds are then partly converted to oxazepam, which is finally eliminated as a glucuronide conjugate (Fig. 12.2). Temazepam is also directly eliminated as a glucuronide conjugate. Nordiazepam is almost as potent as diazepam and is only eliminated slowly, with a terminal half-life of 50–120 hours. Consequently, it tends to accumulate during chronic administration of diazepam, and can prolong the action of the parent compound. Nordiazepam can cross the placenta and accumulate in fetal tissues, causing neonatal depression, hypotonia and hypothermia (page 232). Elderly patients may be extremely sensitive to diazepam, mainly due to the age-dependent decrease in oxidative metabolism by the liver.

Temazepam

Temazepam is predominantly (90%) conjugated by the liver to an inactive 3-oxy-glucuronide, which is subsequently eliminated in urine. Minor amounts of temazepam (2–10%) are demethylated by cytochrome P450 3A4 to oxazepam, which is also eliminated as a glucuronide conjugate.

Midazolam

Midazolam is rapidly metabolized by cytochrome P450 to two active hydroxylated metabolites (1-hydroxymidazolam and 4-hydroxymidazolam), as well as several inactive metabolites. One of these metabolites (1-hydroxymidazolam) has considerable pharmacological activity and may accumulate during prolonged infusions, but is normally converted to an inactive glucuronide, which is eliminated in urine. Drugs that inhibit cytochrome P450 (Chapter 4) reduce the hepatic clearance of midazolam and may prolong its activity.

Lorazepam

Lorazepam is mainly eliminated by metabolism to an inactive phenolic glucuronide conjugate (lorazepam 3-oxyglucuronide), which undergoes enterohepatic circulation and is then slowly eliminated in urine.

Clinical use

Benzodiazepines produce temporary anterograde amnesia, especially after intravenous administration. Consequently, they are particularly useful as premedicant agents, since anxiety and apprehension are reduced and patients may have no recollection of unpleasant events or procedures. Benzodiazepines have a low toxicity and do not affect the pain threshold. Serious drug interactions are uncommon and they do not usually potentiate the effects of other anaesthetic agents.

In the UK, the main benzodiazepines used in anaesthetic practice are

• Diazepam
• Temazepam
• Midazolam
• Lorazepam

Diazepam

Diazepam is widely used as a premedicant agent in adult patients prior to elective surgery, and many regimes have been designed to provide sedation and hypnosis during the preoperative period. Diazepam (usually 5 mg t.d.s.) is normally started on admission to hospital, and continued until the morning of operation. It is not commonly used in day-case surgery since it may have prolonged effects due to its relatively long half-life, and active metabolites can be detected for at least 24–48 hours.

Diazepam (usually 10–15 mg, by slow intravenous injection) has also been widely used to produce sedation and anterograde amnesia during unpleasant or painful procedures such as endoscopy, dentistry or minor surgery under local anaesthesia. It usually acts within 2–3 minutes, producing sedation (for up to 60 min) and amnesia (for 10–30 min).

Aqueous preparations of diazepam can produce local complications after intravenous injection. Solutions of diazepam are acidic and viscous, and often contain various organic solubilizing agents (e.g. propylene glycol, ethanol, benzoic acid). Pain on injection, thrombophlebitis and venous thrombosis are not uncommon, particularly when the drug is injected into small diameter veins on the dorsum of the hand. The incidence of these local complications can be reduced by appropriate techniques, in particular the use of large veins in the antecubital fossa, the injection of the drug into a fast-running infusion, or by 'barbotage'. Some preparations of diazepam contain the drug in a soybean oil-in-water emulsion ('Diazemuls'), and only rarely cause pain and thrombophlebitis after injection, but in other respects are similar to aqueous diazepam. Although diazepam can also be given intramuscularly, this route is generally less satisfactory than oral or intravenous administration, since it is often painful and associated with reduced systemic bioavailability.

Although diazepam is extensively bound to plasma proteins (98–99%), the unbound drug readily crosses the placenta and may affect the foetus. When diazepam is used in late pregnancy or labour (e.g. in the treatment of preeclampsia and eclampsia), it diffuses across the placenta and may be metabolized by foetal tissues. Some of its active metabolites (particularly nordiazepam) may accumulate in the foetus, and can cause neonatal depression, hypotonia and hypothermia. In addition, chronic exposure of the foetus to benzodiazepines during pregnancy can result in hyperreflexia after birth, although there is no evidence that they cause foetal abnormalities. Similarly, the perioperative use of diazepam in children may have unpredictable effects and cause irritability and hyperactivity, and its use should be avoided if possible.

In addition to its use as a hypnotic and sedative, diazepam has been widely used as an anticonvulsant. It is normally the drug of choice in status epilepticus, whether idiopathic or drug-induced (except, perhaps, when thiopental and facilities for artificial ventilation are immediately available). An initial intravenous dose of 10–30 mg is usually given, but repeated administration or continuous infusion may be necessary. A total dose of 200 mg in 24 hours should not be exceeded, unless controlled ventilation has been instituted.

Although diazepam has also been used as an intravenous induction agent, it has a relatively slow onset of action, and produces unpredictable effects on the level of consciousness. It is generally less satisfactory than thiopental or propofol, but is occasionally of value in patients known to be hypersensitive to other agents.

Temazepam

Temazepam (10–30 mg, at night) is often used as an oral premedicant either in tablet form or as a solution, particularly in adult patients prior to elective surgery. It is probably the commonest premedicant drug that is used in current practice. It has an onset within 1 hour, but a relatively short duration of action (usually 6–8 h), due to its rapid metabolism to a glucuronide conjugate (95%) and oxazepam (which is also eliminated as a glucuronide). It is particularly useful as a hypnotic drug in day-case surgery, when it is usually given 1–2 hours before surgery or other procedures, and it normally produces anterograde amnesia for several hours.

Midazolam

Oral midazolam (usually 0.5 mg kg^{-1}) is commonly used for premedication, particularly in children. Although a specific oral preparation is not available in the UK, intravenous midazolam is usually given diluted as a fruit drink or syrup, due to its bitter taste. Unfortunately, oral administration can result in variable plasma concentrations and effects due to its unpredictable first-pass metabolism, and it occasionally causes delirium in young children. Midazolam is also commonly used intravenously (normal adult dose $= 50 - 100 \, \mu g \, kg^{-1}$) prior to regional anaesthesia, therapeutic nerve blocks, uncomfortable diagnostic procedures, conservative dentistry and sometimes as a prelude to general anaesthetic techniques. It has a relatively rapid onset of action, and tends to cause more profound anterograde amnesia than diazepam. There is a wide individual variation in response, and the drug should be injected slowly (i.e. over 4–5 min) until an adequate response is obtained. Drooping of the eyelids is commonly used as an endpoint, but may be an unreliable sign. Elderly patients may be extremely sensitive to midazolam, and the maximum recommended dose is usually 50 $\mu g \, kg^{-1}$. Respiratory depression is a real possibility and facilities for artificial ventilation should always be available. Midazolam is also frequently used to provide sedation in patients requiring controlled or assisted ventilation during intensive care. Although midazolam can be given intramuscularly, this method of administration is only used occasionally.

Midazolam has two main advantages when compared with diazepam:
• Midazolam is injected intravenously in aqueous solution as an ionized drug, but is rapidly converted to a non-ionized and lipid-soluble form in the circulation. Since the drug is given in a water-soluble form (pH <4) pain on injection, thrombophlebitis and venous thrombosis are extremely rare complications. After intravenous injection, the chemical structure of the drug is modified by the

increase to pH 7.4, and 'ring-closure' occurs, increasing its lipid-solubility and entry into the CNS (Fig. 12.3).

• Midazolam has a relatively short terminal half-life (1–3 h), which is associated with a rapid recovery and the absence of any hangover effects. The drug is almost entirely metabolized by the liver, and its clearance (unlike that of other benzodiazepines) is partly dependent on liver blood flow. Its principal metabolite (1-hydroxymidazolam) has some hypnotic activity, and can accumulate during continuous intravenous infusion.

Lorazepam

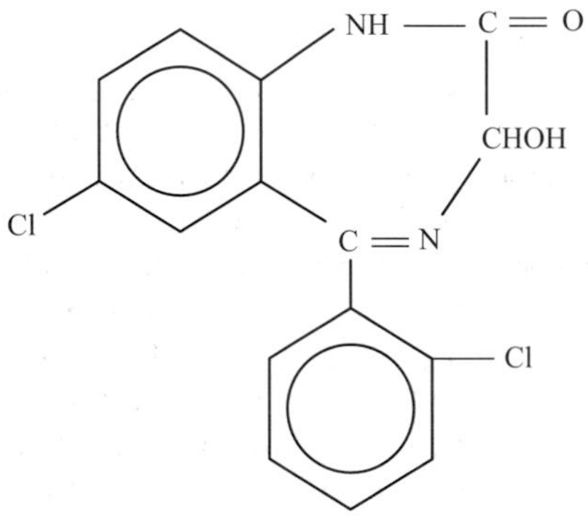

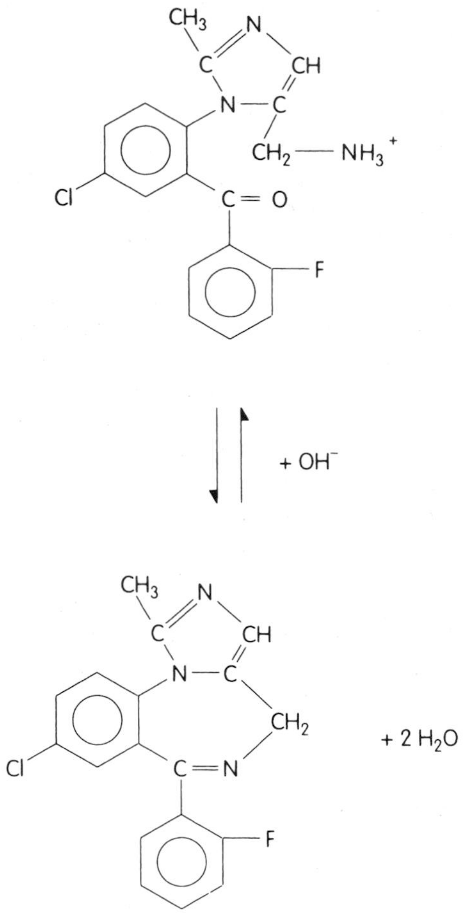

Although lorazepam is sometimes used as an oral premedicant, it is more commonly given intravenously (usual dose = $50\,\mu g\,kg^{-1}$). It has a relatively slow onset of action (usually within 10–20 min) and a prolonged duration of action (up to 6 h) due to its slow distribution to and redistribution from the CNS. It usually produces intense and prolonged anterograde amnesia within 30 minutes, which usually lasts for up to 4 hours. It is less likely to cause local complications than aqueous diazepam. Despite its slow onset of action, it may be of value in prolonged procedures under local anaesthesia, for sedation in intensive care or to diminish the psychotomimetic effects of other drugs.

Other benzodiazepines

Other benzodiazepines are effective in the prophylaxis of many forms of epilepsy (particularly those associated with a generalized EEG discharge), although the doses required often cause an unacceptable degree of sedation and drowsiness. Some benzodiazepines may be useful for short-term prophylaxis, or used as 'add-on therapy' to other anticonvulsant regimes.

Clonazepam and clobazam are benzodiazepine derivatives that have been most widely used in the management of epilepsy. Clonazepam is particularly effective in

Fig. 12.3 The structure of midazolam at pH 4 and pH 7.4. At pH 4, midazolam is water-soluble due to its ionized NH_3^+ group. At pH 7.4, the ionized amine group is incorporated in a non-ionized benzodiazepine nucleus (ring-closure), which significantly increases its lipid solubility.

the long-term control of myoclonic disorders, although problems with oversedation can occur. Like some other anticonvulsant drugs (e.g. carbamazepine, phenytoin), it may be of value in the treatment of trigeminal neuralgia and other painful conditions. Clobazam causes less psychomotor disturbance than clonazepam.

Benzodiazepines are also useful in the management of muscle hypertonicity or spasticity, due to their effects on GABA receptors and the production of central muscle relaxant effects. They may be of value in painful spasms associated with spinal cord injury or demyelinating disorders, 'muscle contraction' headaches and in the management of tetanus. In addition, they are used in the treatment of alcohol withdrawal and the control of night terrors and sleepwalking.

Benzodiazepine antagonists

Flumazenil is a competitive, reversible antagonist of most other benzodiazepines. It may also stimulate benzodiazepine receptors, and some of its actions appear to be unrelated to benzodiazepine antagonism. Flumazenil is mainly metabolized in the liver, and has a rapid onset but relatively brief duration of action due to its short half-life ($\approx$1 h). Consequently, it may need to be given by repeated injection or continuous infusion in order to antagonize the sedation and respiratory depression that are produced by longer acting benzodiazepines. Initially, 0.2 mg is given followed by further 0.1 mg increments at minute intervals until recovery is complete. Flumazenil can be used to reverse the effects of benzodiazepines after anaesthesia or after short diagnostic procedures, although careful supervision is required until recovery is complete. It sometimes causes anxiety, and can precipitate convulsions in epileptic patients and these effects may reflect its inverse agonist effects at GABA$_A$ receptors (Chapter 3). The duration of anterograde amnesia produced by benzodiazepines is usually reduced by flumazenil.

Phenothiazines

Promethazine and alimemazine are sometimes used as sedative premedicant drugs in children, although their use in recent years has declined. Both these drugs have antimuscarinic effects, and indirect evidence suggests that their sedative activity is partly related to antagonism of acetylcholine at central synapses, although antagonism of histamine at central H$_1$-receptors may also be involved. There are numerous cholinergic neurons in the brain and the spinal cord, and acetylcholine is an important excitatory transmitter at many sites in the CNS, including the reticular system and the cerebral cortex. Many other drugs with antimuscarinic activity also produce sedation, including antidepressants, antipsychotics, H$_1$-histamine antagonists and hyoscine.

Promethazine

Promethazine is an H$_1$-histamine antagonist with a prolonged duration of action (up to 24 h). After oral administration it is well absorbed and widely distributed, and usually acts within 30–60 minutes. It is relatively safe in overdosage, and therapeutic doses have little effect on the cardiovascular or respiratory system. Promet-hazine may produce dizziness and disorientation, particularly in elderly patients. In addition to sedative effects, it has antiemetic and antisecretory properties, which contribute to its usefulness as a premedicant drug in children. Promethazine is sometimes used in asthmatic patients since the drug has bronchodilator effects, and may also prevent responses due to histamine release by anaesthetic agents. It may also be useful in the symptomatic relief of various hypersensitivity reactions, although hypnotic and antimuscarinic side effects are common. Promethazine may be valuable in the prophylaxis of motion sickness, and can be used as an antiemetic drug in early pregnancy.

Alimemazine

Alimemazine is an H$_1$-histamine antagonist with more powerful sedative and hypnotic effects than promethazine. It is occasionally used as a premedicant agent in children, and is given as an elixir (1–2 mg kg^{-1}) 1–2 hours prior to surgery. Alimemazine may cause postoperative restlessness, and some delay in recovery from anaesthesia may occur. It can antagonize the effects of 5-HT, dopamine and noradrenaline, and high doses may produce extrapyramidal effects, hypothermia and hypotension. Other central side effects, such as disturbing dreams and possibly hallucinations, have also been reported.

Antimuscarinic drugs

Premedication with antimuscarinic drugs (in particular, atropine and hyoscine) was an established clinical practice for many years. The main advantages were a reduction in the amount of bronchial and salivary secretions, a diminution in the cardiac responses to inhalational anaesthetics with significant vagomimetic activity and a decrease in reflex stimulation during endotracheal intubation and visceral traction.

In current practice, the routine use of these agents is no longer considered to be necessary. Anaesthetic agents that induced pronounced salivation and respiratory secretions (diethyl ether) or vagomimetic activity (cyclopropane) are rarely administered, and neuromuscular blocking agents are used to provide optimal conditions for laryngoscopy and intubation. In addition, the subjective discomforts of antimuscarinic drugs (dry mouth, palpitations and blurring of vision) are obviously undesirable.

Current indications for the use of antimuscarinic drugs as premedicant agents are not well defined. In many instances they are omitted, or are given intravenously at the time of induction of anaesthesia. However, they may have advantages in some situations:

- In small children, when the presence of copious secretions in the airway may be a particular embarrassment.
- When effects mediated through the cardiac vagus may be enhanced. This may occur
  (1) in patients receiving treatment with β-adrenoceptor antagonists or cardiac glycosides;
  (2) during ophthalmic surgery, in order to prevent oculocardiac reflexes;
  (3) when techniques involving intermittent suxamethonium are used.
- In patients with obstructive airways disease, in order to prevent reflex or drug-induced bronchospasm.

The action of antimuscarinic drugs in preventing the regurgitation of stomach contents is not clearly understood. Although antimuscarinic drugs do not significantly affect gastric pH, the volume of secretion is reduced, and treatment with antacids is more effective. In theory, the tone of the cardiac sphincter is increased by antimuscarinic drugs, and this should impede the entry of gastric contents into the oesophagus. However, current concepts suggest that a cardiac 'valve' is produced by the apposition of folds of gastric mucosa at the acutely angled cardiooesophageal junction. Thus, antimuscarinic drugs that produce relaxation of smooth muscle can facilitate regurgitation by lowering the barrier pressure. In spite of other beneficial effects, atropine and related drugs should not be used prior to induction of anaesthesia for obstetric procedures.

Atropine

Systemic administration of a standard adult dose of atropine (0.6 mg) may produce a transient decrease in heart rate prior to the development of tachycardia. Moderate antisialagogue effects and some mydriasis may be observed, although significant elevation of intraocular pressure does not occur in normal conditions. Bronchodilatation results in an increase in the physiological dead space, which is associated with slight stimulation of the cerebral cortex and the medullary centres, and can lead to an increase in the rate and the depth of respiration.

Atropine has a relatively short duration of action (1–1.5 h) since it is extensively metabolized by esterases, and only small amounts of the unchanged drug are normally identified in urine. After oral administration, atropine is extensively (60–70%) absorbed from the small intestine. In children, it is sometimes administered orally with alimemazine as premedication for elective surgical procedures. The recommended dose is 0.05 mg kg^{-1}, up to a maximum dose of 1.2 mg.

Hyoscine

Hyoscine (scopolamine) may also be used as a premedicant drug. In the doses used in adults (0.4 mg), it has a shorter duration of action than atropine and produces less tachycardia. It is a more powerful antisialagogue than atropine, and has more pronounced effects on the eye.

In contrast, it has less bronchodilator activity. In therapeutic doses, it causes depression of the CNS, and drowsiness, amnesia and confusion (particularly in elderly patients) may occur. It also has a short duration of action (1–1.5 h), and is extensively metabolized by esterases, so only trace amounts of hyoscine (approximately 1% of the dose) are eliminated unchanged in urine. Although hyoscine may be given orally, it is less extensively absorbed from the small intestine than atropine.

Glycopyrronium

Glycopyrronium is a synthetic antimuscarinic agent, which is also used as a premedicant drug. Unlike atropine and hyoscine, glycopyrronium is an ionized quaternary amine and does not readily cross cell membranes. Consequently, it does not produce central effects, and placental transfer of the drug is insignificant.

Glycopyrronium is an effective antisialagogue with a prolonged duration of action (approximately 6 h), and sweat gland activity is affected for a similar period of time. However, moderate doses do not tend to cause other antimuscarinic effects. Heart rate may not increase, and a slight but insignificant bradycardia sometimes occurs. Cardiac arrhythmias are rare, and changes in pupillary size are minimal. Nevertheless, larger doses will cause typical antimuscarinic effects.

Glycopyrronium may be given intramuscularly or intravenously, in doses ranging from 0.1 to 0.4 mg in adults. It is usually considered that 0.2 mg intramuscularly produces optimal premedicant effects. Larger doses (2–8 mg) may be given orally, but there is a predictable delay in the onset of action.

α$_2$-Adrenoceptor agonists

Agonists at α$_2$-receptors decrease noradrenaline release in both central and peripheral sympathetic nerves (Chapter 13). In the CNS, their main sites of action include the tractus solitarius (leading to hypotension and bradycardia), the locus coeruleus (causing sedation) and certain vagal nuclei. In addition, they have profound analgesic effects. These may involve actions at spinal and supraspinal sites, including enhancement of descending inhibitory pathways to the dorsal horn, as well as the depression of thalamocortical pathways. Their peripheral effects decrease heart rate and reduce vascular smooth muscle tone. Their use may be associated with oversedation or excessive hypotension, and respiratory depression can occur with high dosage.

In recent years, the partial agonist clonidine has been occasionally used as a premedicant and anaesthetic adjunct. Clonidine was introduced as a nasal decongestant, but was subsequently used in the treatment of migraine and hypertension, and in the management of withdrawal syndromes in opioid-dependent patients. Clonidine inhibits catecholamine release in both central and peripheral neurons, and there is a decrease in the anaesthetic requirement for both intravenous and inhalational agents (Table 8.1). The sympathoadrenal responses associated with anaesthesia and surgery are also attenuated. Clonidine also produces marked analgesia, and can enhance the effects of opioid analgesics and local anaesthetic agents. It has been given prior to surgery to produce perioperative analgesia (100–300 μg, orally), and has also been used extradurally and intrathecally for postoperative and chronic pain.

Other α_2-adrenoceptor agonists have also been used as anaesthetic adjuncts in man, particularly dexmedetomidine and azepexole. Dexmedetomidine is a more highly selective and potent α_2-agonist than clonidine, and has been used in veterinary practice for its sedative, hypnotic and analgesic properties. In man, high doses can reduce the MAC of inhalational anaesthetics by approximately 90%.

Miscellaneous drugs

The popularity of NSAIDs as anaesthetic adjuvants has led to their frequent use as premedicant drugs, particularly for minor surgery. Diclofenac and ketorolac are commonly used for this purpose. Both drugs can be given orally and by intramuscular and intravenous injection, and diclofenac can also be administered as suppositories. Paracetamol suspension and ibuprofen are also commonly used for oral premedication in children. These drugs are considered in detail in Chapter 11. Very occasionally, ketamine is used in children for premedication.

Premedication and obstetric anaesthesia

The main aim of drug therapy before the administration of general anaesthesia for Caesarian section, or other op-erative procedures during late pregnancy and labour, is to minimize the risks associated with the aspiration of gastric contents, as well as any depressant effects on the foetus.

Opioids should never be used in these circumstances. In addition to their undesirable effects on the foetus, opioids delay gastric emptying and increase the likelihood of regurgitation. Benzodiazepines should also be avoided, as cumulation leading to oversedation, hypotonia and hypothermia in the baby may occur (page 232).

Although apomorphine has been used to produce vomiting before anaesthesia, the procedure is unpleasant for the patient and cannot be relied upon to empty the stomach efficiently. Apomorphine acts by stimulation of dopaminergic receptors in the chemoreceptor trigger zone, and produces a combination of excitatory and depressant effects on the CNS. It is rarely used for this purpose in current practice.

More specific methods are used to reduce the acidity of the stomach contents, since a gastric pH above 2.5–3 is known to alleviate the severity of pulmonary complications in the event of aspiration. For many years, an oral suspension of magnesium trisilicate was given, but is no longer used due to its slow onset of action and the risks of particulate matter being deposited in the lungs following aspiration.

H_2-histamine antagonists are now commonly used in preoperative preparation. They reduce the volume of gastric juice and pepsin secreted, and increase its pH. Ranitidine is the drug of choice and is usually administered orally (150 mg) at 6 hours intervals throughout labour, with a further intravenous dose (50 mg) following a decision to operate. Hypersensitivity responses are extremely rare, although bradyarrhythmias occasionally occur. H_2-histamine antagonists will not neutralize acid already present in the stomach, so a soluble antacid (sodium citrate; 30 mL of 0.3 mol L^{-1}) is given prior to induction. Metoclopramide, which increases the tone of the oesophageal sphincter and promotes gastric emptying, may also be given intravenously before induction, but atropine should be avoided.

Antiemetic drugs

Physiological and pharmacological factors
Nausea and vomiting can be induced by many physiological and pathological factors. These include:
• Pregnancy
• Acute pain

- Raised intracranial pressure
- Ionizing radiation
- Psychogenic factors
- Labyrinthine or vestibular disturbances
- Metabolic disorders
- Inflammation or irritation of the gastrointestinal tract
- Many drugs and ingested toxins

Drugs and ingested toxins

Drugs such as ipecacuanha, squill, NSAIDs, chloral hydrate and ammonium chloride act immediately after oral administration, and have a local irritant effect on the stomach, or activate visceral afferent nerves in the intestinal mucosa or the portal vein. Afferent stimuli are then conducted by the vagus nerve to the brain.

Other drugs with significant emetic effects (e.g. opioids, digitalis glycosides) predominantly affect central pathways concerned with the control of nausea and vomiting. Cytotoxic drugs with pronounced emetic properties (e.g. cisplatin, dacarbazine) act by both peripheral and central mechanisms.

Vomiting centre

For many years, it was generally accepted that nausea and vomiting were primarily controlled and coordinated by the vomiting centre in the lateral reticular formation of the medulla. Recent evidence suggests that the existence of a discrete vomiting centre may be questionable, but that it is best considered as the area in the brain stem that integrates emetic responses. Its functions are probably dependent on complex interactions between the reticular formation, the nucleus tractus solitarius (NTS) and the dorsal vagal nucleus. The neurochemistry of these interactions is extremely complex, since more than 40 different neurotransmitters have been identified in this region. Efferent impulses from the vomiting centre influence vasomotor, respiratory and salivary nuclei, and then pass in the vagus, phrenic and spinal nerves to the gastrointestinal tract, to initiate the vomiting reflex.

Chemoreceptor trigger zone

The vomiting centre is influenced by the afferent input from many centres but is primarily affected by the chemoreceptor trigger zone (CTZ), which is situated close to the area postrema in the floor of the fourth ventricle. It is physiologically outside the blood–brain and CSF–brain barriers, and is extremely sensitive to emetic stimuli in the circulation. It may also be concerned with the control of

blood pressure, sleep and the regulation of food intake. Many emetic drugs stimulate the CTZ and thus indirectly affect the vomiting centre (Fig. 12.4). Several neurotransmitters are known to influence the activity of the CTZ, including:

- Dopamine
- 5-Hydroxytryptamine
- Acetylcholine, acting on M_1-receptors
- Histamine, acting on H_1-receptors
- Enkephalins, acting on δ-opioid receptors

Dopamine

In physiological conditions, dopamine is released from the peripheral processes of astrocytes that synapse with the CTZ, and acts directly on D_2-receptors in the CTZ, the area postrema and the nucleus tractus solitarius (NTS). D_2-receptors in the CTZ are also sensitive to apomorphine, opioids, bromocriptine, cardiac glycosides and cytotoxic drugs, and are antagonized by metoclopramide and sulpiride. D_2-receptors are also present in the gastrointestinal tract and may inhibit intestinal motility and mediate emetic stimuli.

5-Hydroxytryptamine

5-Hydroxytryptamine, acting via $5-HT_3$ receptors, is also an important neurotransmitter in the CTZ. $5-HT_3$ receptors in the CTZ play an important part in drug-induced emesis (particularly with cytotoxic agents), and they are also present in the stomach and the small intestine. $5-HT_3$-receptor antagonists are highly effective antiemetic drugs.

Acetylcholine

The vomiting centre has an afferent input from several other sites in the CNS (Fig. 12.4). Stimuli from the labyrinths in the inner ear that are mediated by vestibular and cerebellar nuclei affect the vomiting centre and may cause nausea and vomiting. At least one of the synaptic connections in this pathway is cholinergic, and is antagonized by centrally acting antimuscarinic drugs, acting on M_1-receptors.

Histamine

Histamine is physiologically released from the axons of neurons that originate in the hypothalamus, and acts on H_1-postsynaptic excitatory receptors in the CTZ. Histamine release follows a circadian pattern, and is increased

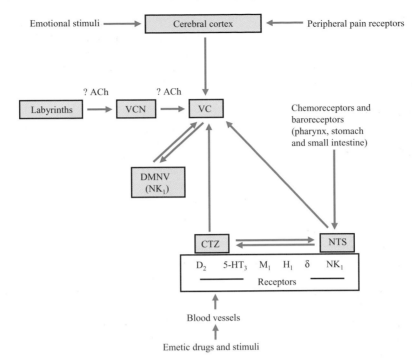

Fig. 12.4 Central and peripheral pathways affecting the activity of the chemoreceptor trigger zone (CTZ) and the vomiting centre (VC). Emotional stimuli and peripheral pain are projected to the cerebral cortex, and efferent cortical pathways then directly affect the VC. Similarly, stimuli from the labyrinths in the inner ear are projected via vestibular and cerebellar nuclei (VCN) to the VC. This pathway probably depends on central muscarinic receptors and is mediated by acetylcholine (ACh). Afferent pathways from chemoreceptors and baroreceptors in the pharynx, stomach and small intestine directly affect the activity of the nucleus tractus solitarius (NTS). The CTZ is connected to the NTS, and both have efferent connections with the VC and contain numerous receptors for dopamine (D_2), 5-hydroxytryptamine ($5\text{-}HT_3$), acetylcholine (M_1), histamine (H_1), opioids (δ) and neurokinins (NK_1). Since the CTZ (but not the NTS) is outside the blood–brain barrier, it can be directly affected by emetic drugs and stimuli in the blood vessels and circulation. The main efferent pathway from the vomiting centre is projected to the dorsal motor nucleus of the vagus, which initiates nausea and vomiting. This efferent pathway is mediated centrally by neurokinins (mainly substance P) via NK_1-receptors.

during daytime. It is not as powerful an emetic stimulus as other neurotransmitters.

Enkephalins

Enkephalins are also believed to influence the activity of the CTZ, and the vomiting centre is affected by afferent stimuli from chemoreceptors in the gut and the CNS, as well as peripheral pain receptors (Fig. 12.4).

Efferent pathways

Until recently, little was known of the neurotransmitter involved in the chemical efferent pathway from the vomiting centre to the gastrointestinal tract. There is some experimental evidence that this pathway is partly controlled by substance P via tachykinin NK_1-receptors, which are

Table 12.2 Drugs that are used in the prevention or control of postoperative nausea and vomiting.

Dopamine D_2-receptor antagonists
  Prochlorperazine
  Metoclopramide
$5\text{-}HT_3$-receptor antagonists
  Ondansetron
  Granisetron
  Tropisetron
  Dolasetron
Histamine H_1-receptor antagonists
  Cyclizine
  Promethazine
Corticosteroids
  Dexamethasone

present in the NTS and the dorsal motor nucleus of the vagus nerve. Antagonists at NK_1-receptors (e.g. septide, aprepitant) inhibit responses to a wide range of emetic stimuli, suggesting that they are acting on the final efferent pathway from the vomiting centre.

Summary

Current evidence suggests that the neurotransmitters dopamine (via D_2-receptors in the CTZ and NTS), 5-hydroxytryptamine (via 5-HT_3 receptors in the area postrema, the CTZ and the NTS) acetylcholine (via central cholinergic pathways and vestibular nuclei), histamine (via postsynaptic excitatory H_1-receptors), and substance P (via tachykinin NK_1-receptors in the NTS and dorsal motor nucleus of the vagus nerve) may play an important part in the central control of nausea and vomiting. Consequently, most antiemetic drugs, including those that are used to control postoperative nausea and vomiting, are antagonists of one or more than one of these neurotransmitters (Table 12.2). In addition, they may affect the peripheral pathways concerned with nausea and vomiting.

Antiemetic drugs can be classified pharmacologically as
- Dopamine antagonists
- 5-HT_3 antagonists
- Acetylcholine antagonists (antimuscarinic drugs)
- Histamine antagonists
- Miscellaneous agents

Dopamine antagonists

Dopamine has an important physiological role and acts on D_2-receptors in the CTZ and the NTS, and may also have a peripheral inhibitory effect on gastrointestinal motility. Consequently, all drugs that antagonize D_2-receptors in the CNS have antiemetic properties. Nevertheless, only prochlorperazine and metoclopramide are now used to prevent or treat perioperative nausea and vomiting.

Prochlorperazine

Prochlorperazine, like most other phenothiazines, has many pharmacological effects and can modify the effects of many central and peripheral neurotransmitters. It is an antagonist of dopamine (at D_1- and D_2-receptors), acetylcholine (at M_1- and M_3-receptors), noradrenaline (at α_1- and α_2-receptors) and histamine (at H_1-receptors). In addition, it has membrane stabilizing activity and prevents the uptake of noradrenaline at sympathetic nerve endings ($Uptake_1$).

Like other phenothiazines, it may produce extrapyramidal side effects, particularly acute dystonic reactions such as facial and skeletal muscle spasms, which may present with or develop into oculogyric crises. These reactions are not infrequent (particularly in the young), and the use of prochlorperazine should be avoided in children. It may also cause postural hypotension, and its dosage should be reduced in elderly subjects.

The antiemetic effects of prochlorperazine are mainly due to D_2-receptor antagonism (centrally and peripherally), although antagonism of H_1-receptors and M_1-receptors may be contributory factors. Consequently, it is extremely effective in the control of nausea and vomiting, whether induced by drugs or other causes (e.g. uraemia, neoplastic disease). Prochlorperazine has been widely used as an antiemetic during the postoperative period. The usual dose is 12.5 mg intramuscularly, although a buccal preparation (3 mg) and a suppository preparation (5 mg) are sometimes used. After oral administration, prochlorperazine is well absorbed but has a large and variable first-pass effect, and is extensively metabolized to a sulphoxide. It has an extremely large volume of distribution, and a terminal half-life of about 6 hours.

Metoclopramide

Although the antiemetic properties of metoclopramide are mainly due to dopamine antagonism, high doses also antagonize 5-HT_3 receptors in the CTZ and the NTS. Metoclopramide produces widespread antagonism at D_2-receptors in the corpus striatum, and may produce dose-related extrapyramidal effects, particularly in children, young women and the elderly. These effects can be prevented or treated by centrally acting drugs with antimuscarinic properties (e.g. procyclidine, benzatropine), or by benzodiazepines. Other acute reactions, apart from restlessness and drowsiness, are relatively rare.

Metoclopramide also has peripheral effects on the gastrointestinal tract. It increases the rate of gastric emptying by enhancing fundal and antral contractility, relaxes the pyloric sphincter, stimulates peristalsis and increases lower oesophageal sphincter pressure ('barrier pressure'). These effects may be related to the peripheral antagonism of dopamine at D_2-receptors in the gastrointestinal tract.

Metoclopramide is sometimes used as a prokinetic and antiemetic agent and in the prophylaxis of Mendelson's syndrome. In anaesthetic practice, 10 mg (intramuscularly or intravenously) is sometimes used postoperatively in adults, but is often of limited efficacy. Although higher doses antagonize both D_2- and HT_3-receptors, their use is often associated with acute dystonic reactions, particularly in children and adolescents.

In recent years, metoclopramide has been superseded by more effective agents and is less commonly used in the prophylaxis and treatment of postoperative nausea and vomiting.

Domperidone

Domperidone is a chemically related antiemetic drug with both central and peripheral effects, which are mainly due to dopamine antagonism. Like metoclopramide, it increases the rate of gastric emptying and increases the lower oesophageal sphincter pressure. Domperidone also antagonizes D_2-receptors in the CTZ and the NTS, but is less likely to produce acute dystonic reactions than metoclopramide, since it does not readily cross the blood–brain barrier and affect the corpus striatum. In large doses, domperidone may cause cardiac arrhythmias, which are sometimes fatal. It has been mainly used as an antiemetic drug during chemotherapy with cytotoxic drugs, and is not usually recommended for postoperative nausea and vomiting.

5-HT$_3$-receptor antagonists

5-Hydroxytryptamine has an important role in the peripheral and central control of nausea and vomiting. In the stomach and small intestine, 5-HT_3 receptors are present on vagal afferent fibres in the myenteric plexus. Opioids, cytotoxic agents, radiotherapy and surgical stress release 5-HT which acts on peripheral 5-HT_3 receptors and causes nausea and vomiting. In the CNS, the neurotransmitter is focally released from vagal afferent neurons in the medulla and area postrema, and combines with 5-HT_3 receptors in the CTZ and the NTS, thus increasing the excitability of the vomiting centre. All 5-HT_3 receptors are ionotropic and are only present on neurons. They consist of five subunits (two 5-HT_{3A} subunits and three 5-HT_{3B} units) in the order A-B-A-B-B, which surround an intrinsic cation channel. Both the 5-HT_{3A} subunits contains a single binding site for 5-HT.

In recent years, 5-HT_3-receptor antagonists have been widely used in the prevention and treatment of emesis associated with chemotherapy and radiotherapy, and in the control of postoperative nausea and vomiting. They are extremely effective agents for the prevention or treatment of postoperative emesis and have largely replaced other drugs in the management of this condition, although they are rather expensive. Occasionally, they are used with other antiemetic agents in resistant postoperative nausea and vomiting.

Ondansetron

Ondansetron is a potent and selective 5-HT_3-receptor antagonist. It is well absorbed after oral administration, is moderately bound to plasma proteins, and has a large volume of distribution (160 L), and a short terminal half-life (3 h). Approximately 95% of the drug is metabolized by the liver to inactive products, and the dose should be reduced in patients with significant hepatic impairment.

Ondansetron increases bowel transit time, and constipation is common. Other side effects include headaches, sensations of warmth or flushing, transient visual disturbances and occasionally chest pain and cardiac arrhythmias (which may be related to the antagonism of other 5-HT-receptor subtypes). Hypersensitivity reactions have also been reported.

Ondansetron may be given orally or parenterally. A prophylactic dose (8 mg) is given by mouth 1 hour before anaesthesia, followed by two further oral doses (8 mg) at 8-hourly intervals (if necessary). Alternatively, a single oral dose (16 mg) is given preoperatively, or the drug (4 mg) is given by intramuscular or intravenous injection at induction of anaesthesia. In the treatment of established nausea and vomiting, a similar dose is given parenterally and may be repeated at intervals according to the severity of the symptoms.

Granisetron

Granisetron is a similar specific 5-HT_3-receptor antagonist. Although it is well absorbed after oral administration, its bioavailability is reduced due to first-pass metabolism, and it is moderately (65%) bound to plasma proteins. Granisetron has a large volume of distribution (210 L), and a variable terminal half-life (9 h). Approximately 85% of the drug is metabolized by the liver (mainly by N-demethylation, oxidation and conjugation).

Granisetron decreases bowel motility, and constipation is not uncommon. Other side effects include headaches, minor skin reactions and occasional hypersensitivity and anaphylactic responses.

In the prevention of postoperative nausea and vomiting, a prophylactic dose (1 mg diluted in 5 mL saline, intravenously) is usually given before the induction of anaesthesia. A similar regime is used in established postoperative nausea and vomiting, and may be repeated. The total dosage should not exceed 2 mg in 24 hours. Its use in children is not recommended.

Tropisetron

Tropisetron is also a specific 5-HT$_3$-receptor antagonist. It is well absorbed after oral administration, although its bioavailability is reduced by first-pass metabolism. Tropisetron is extensively (70–80%) bound to plasma proteins (particularly α_1-acid glycoprotein), and has a large volume of distribution (400–600 L). It is metabolized in the liver by CYP 2D6, an enzyme isoform, which is subject to genetic polymorphism (Chapter 1). In extensive metabolizers the terminal half-life is 8 hours, but is 4–5 times longer in poor metabolizers. Approximately 80–90% of the drug is metabolized, mainly by hydroxylation and glucuronide conjugation. Its metabolism is increased by enzyme-inducing agents (e.g. phenobarbital, rifampicin).

Tropisetron decreases bowel motility, and may cause constipation and other common side effects include headaches, dizziness and fatigue. Hypersensitivity responses (including anaphylaxis) have also been reported, but are relatively rare.

In anaesthetic practice, a prophylactic dose (2 mg, intravenously) is usually given shortly before the induction of anaesthesia. A similar regime may be used in established postoperative nausea and vomiting, and should be given within 2 hours of recovery from anaesthesia. The total dosage should not exceed 6 mg in any 24 hour period.

Dolasetron

Dolasetron is a specific 5-HT$_3$-receptor antagonist. After oral administration it is well absorbed from the gut and has a significant first-pass effect. It is rapidly metabolized in the liver to an active metabolite (hydrodolasetron), which has a terminal half-life of approximately 8 hours, and is mainly responsible for its antiemetic activity. In common with other 5-HT$_3$ antagonists, it may cause constipation, headaches, fatigue and dizziness. Dolasetron can be given orally (50 mg) or intravenously (12.5 mg) before the induction of anaesthesia, or a similar dose (12.5 mg, intravenously) can be used to treat postoperative nausea and vomiting. Its use in children is not recommended.

Palonosetron

Palonosetron is an alternative 5-HT$_3$ antagonist that is used in the prevention of nausea and vomiting during chemotherapy for malignant disease. It is not currently licensed for use in postoperative nausea and vomiting in the UK.

Acetylcholine antagonists (antimuscarinic drugs)

All drugs that antagonize the muscarinic effects of acetylcholine and cross the blood–brain barrier may have antiemetic properties, particularly in motion sickness, labyrinthine disease, or vestibular disorders. They mainly act by inhibiting one or more cholinergic synapses from the labyrinths to the vomiting centre, via the vestibular and cerebellar nuclei.

Although the antiemetic activity of antimuscarinic agents is mainly due to their central effects, they also decrease muscle tone and intestinal secretions in the gut. In general, atropine is a less potent and less effective antiemetic agent than hyoscine (although its activity on intestinal motility and secretions is greater). Both drugs decrease the opening pressure of the lower oesophageal sphincter ('barrier pressure') and thus predispose to gastrooesophageal regurgitation. They also produce characteristic autonomic side effects due to peripheral parasympathetic blockade and hyoscine may cause profound sedation. Both atropine and hyoscine suppress the emetic effects of therapeutic doses of opioid analgesics.

Histamine antagonists

Many classical antihistamine drugs that act by competitive antagonism at H$_1$-receptors have antiemetic properties, although their precise mode of action is uncertain. Histamine is physiologically released from the axons of neurons that originate in the hypothalamus, and antihistamines may act by antagonism of H$_1$-postsynaptic excitatory receptors in the CTZ and the NTS. However, many of them also have some antimuscarinic activity, which may contribute to their antiemetic properties by their action on vestibular and cerebellar nuclei.

In the UK, cinnarizine, cyclizine and promethazine have been frequently used as antiemetic drugs. Promethazine (a phenothiazine) has a longer duration of action than other H$_1$-antihistamines. They are of most value in the prevention and treatment of motion sickness, and in the management of labyrinthine disorders (e.g. Meniere's disease), but are sometimes used in postoperative nausea and vomiting. All these drugs have antimuscarinic properties, which may cause characteristic side effects, including sedation, dryness of the mouth, urinary retention and drowsiness. These effects are usually less marked with cyclizine and cinnarizine than with promethazine.

Antihistamines can suppress the emetic effects of opioid analgesics. Promethazine can be used for premedication in children (page 235), while cyclizine is available as a compound preparation with morphine ('Cyclimorph'), which is sometimes used in the perioperative period. It is also present with dipipanone in 'Diconal' (Chapter 11), which is used in pain therapy.

H_1-antagonists that do not cross the blood–brain barrier (e.g. acrivastine, cetirizine) or H_2-antagonists are of no value as antiemetic drugs.

Miscellaneous agents

Nabilone

Nabilone is a synthetic cannabinoid with antiemetic properties and is chemically related to tetrahydrocannabinol. Specific $G_{i/o}$-protein coupled cannabinoid receptors (CB_1 and CB_2) are present in the CNS as well as at peripheral sites, and an endogenous agonist anandamide (*N*-arachidonoyl-ethanolamine) has been identified. Nabilone may also act on opioid receptors in the area postrema and the CTZ, and its antiemetic effects may be partially antagonized by naloxone.

Nabilone (usually 1–4 mg daily) is only used as an antiemetic drug during cancer chemotherapy due to the possibility of drug dependence and misuse. Unwanted effects, particularly drowsiness, dizziness and dry mouth, and psychotic reactions including dysphoria, depression, nightmares and hallucinations are relatively common.

Lorazepam

Lorazepam is a potent benzodiazepine with profound sedative and amnesic properties, which has also been used as an antiemetic drug during cancer chemotherapy. Its mode of action is obscure; it may modify central pathways concerned with the control of nausea and vomiting. In addition, its powerful amnesic action prevents anticipatory vomiting which occurs in approximately 20% of patients during repeated courses of chemotherapy.

Dexamethasone

Dexamethasone (0.5–10 mg daily), as well as other glucocorticoids, has been used as an antiemetic drug during cancer chemotherapy and to control postoperative nausea and vomiting. In these conditions, dexamethasone is well tolerated and is as effective as prochlorperazine or metoclopramide. Its mode of action is uncertain, although it has been suggested that its action depends on the decreased release of arachidonic acid, reduced turnover of 5-HT or decreased permeability of the blood–brain bar-

rier. It is often used in combination with other antiemetic drugs.

Aprepitant

Aprepitant is a tachykinin NK_1 (neurokinin-1) receptor antagonist, which produces blockade of emetic pathways controlled by substance P and other neurokinins in the NTS and the dorsal motor nucleus of the vagus nerve. Aprepitant and other antagonists at NK_1-receptors (e.g. septide) inhibit responses to a wide range of emetic stimuli, suggesting that they are acting on the final efferent pathway from the vomiting centre. It is only used with other antiemetic drugs (e.g. 5-HT$_3$ antagonists, dexamethasone) to prevent nausea and vomiting induced by cancer chemotherapy.

Postoperative nausea and vomiting in anaesthetic practice

Many patients who undergo anaesthesia and surgery experience nausea and vomiting in the early postoperative period. The incidence is variable, but causal factors that may be involved include:
- Patient susceptibility, in particular, previous experiences of nausea and vomiting in association with anaesthesia, or a history of motion sickness. Patients with delayed gastric emptying due to gastrointestinal hypomotility, or who have had recent food or fluid intake, also have an increased risk of postoperative nausea and vomiting. The incidence is also increased in non-smokers, for unknown reasons.
- Specific surgical procedures, especially abdominal, gynaecological and ear, nose and throat surgery. The risk is particularly high in middle-aged women undergoing laparoscopic procedures, and is also increased after prolonged surgery (> 1 h).
- Anaesthetic agents that are used during surgical procedures. Classically, a high incidence of postoperative nausea and vomiting (approximately 80%) was associated with the use of diethylether and cyclopropane. In current practice, opioids are now widely used as anaesthetic adjuvants and are potent emetic drugs. The use of anticholinesterase drugs to reverse neuromuscular blockade is also associated with an increased incidence of nausea and vomiting. There is considerable evidence that 'stormy' induction of anaesthesia, hypoxic episodes, insufflation of anaesthetic gases into the oesophagus and inadequate suppression of reflex autonomic activity are other contributory factors.

In contrast, the use of propofol (particularly in TIVA) is undoubtedly associated with antiemetic effects that are believed to be due to the enhancement of inhibitory transmission at $GABA_A$ receptors, and the decreased release of 5-HT in the CTZ and the NTS.

Antiemetic drugs may be given for the prophylaxis and treatment of postoperative nausea and vomiting. Although anticholinergic drugs may confer some protective effect, their side effects can be a disadvantage. Dopamine antagonists are sometimes used, and both prochlorperazine and metoclopramide inhibit the emetic effects of opioids, but their duration of action is relatively short. In addition, there is a significant incidence of extrapyramidal reactions even after single doses, particularly in adolescent females. In recent years, the 5-HT_3 antagonists (ondansetron, granisetron, tropisetron and dolasetron) have been extensively used in the prophylaxis of postoperative nausea and vomiting, and can be given during the induction of anaesthesia or at the end of surgery. Alternatively, they can be used postoperatively for the treatment of established vomiting. In general, they are extremely effective and do not produce extrapyramidal problems, but their high cost (approximately 10–20 times that of prochlorperazine or metoclopramide) has tended to limit their use in anaesthetic practice.

Dexamethasone (0.5–10 mg, intravenously) during the induction of anaesthesia may reduce the incidence of postoperative nausea and vomiting, particularly when combined with other antiemetic drugs.

Suggested reading

Bormann, J. (2000) The 'ABC' of GABA receptors. *Trends in Pharmacological Sciences* **21**, 16–19.

Diemunsch, P., Schoeffler, P., Bryssine, B., *et al.* (1999) Antiemetic activity of the NK_1 receptor antagonist GR205171 in the treatment of established postoperative nausea and vomiting after major gynaecological surgery. *British Journal of Anaesthesia* **82**, 274–276.

Fisher, D.M. (1997) The 'big little problem' of postoperative nausea and vomiting: do we know the answer yet? *Anesthesiology* **87**, 1271–1273.

Gesztesi, Z.S., Song, D. & White, P.F. (1998) Comparison of a new NK_1 receptor antagonist (CP122,721) to ondansetron in the prevention of postoperative nausea and vomiting. *Anesthesia and Analgesia* **86**(Suppl 2), S32.

Hayashi, Y. & Maze, M. (1993) Alpha$_2$ adrenoceptor agonists and anaesthesia. *British Journal of Anaesthesia* **71**, 108–118.

Heffernan, A.M. & Rowbotham, D.J. (2000) Postoperative nausea and vomiting – time for balanced antiemesis? *British Journal of Anaesthesia* **85**, 675–677.

Henzi, I., Walder, B. & Tramer, M.R. (1999) Metoclopramide in the prevention of postoperative nusea and vomiting: a quantitative systematic review of randomized, placebo-controlled studies. *British Journal of Anaesthesia* **83**, 761–771.

Johnston, G.A.R. (1996) $GABA_A$ receptor pharmacology. *Pharmacology and Therapeutics* **69**, 173–198.

Lee, C.R., Plosker, G.L. & McTavish, D. (1993) Tropisetron: a review of its pharmacodynamic and pharmacokinetic properties, and therapeutic potential as an antiemetic. *Drugs* **46**, 925–943.

Markham, A. & Sorkin, E.M. (1993) Ondansetron: an update of its therapeutic use in chemotherapy-induced and postoperative nausea and vomiting. *Drugs* **45**, 931–952.

McDonald, R.L. & Olsen, R.W. (1994) $GABA_A$ receptor channels. *Annual Review of Neuroscience* **17**, 569–602.

Mitchelson, F. (1992) Pharmacological agents affecting emesis: a review (Part I). *Drugs* **43**, 295–315.

Mitchelson, F. (1992) Pharmacological agents affecting emesis: a review (Part II). *Drugs* **43**, 443–463.

Pleuvry, B. (2001) Anxiolytics and hypnotics. *Anaesthesia and Intensive Care Medicine* **2**, 233–236.

Pleuvry, B. (2001) Premedication. *Anaesthesia and Intensive Care Medicine* **2**, 245–249.

Plosker, G.L. & Goa, K.L. (1991) Granisetron: a review of its pharmacological properties and therapeutic use as an antiemetic. *Drugs* **42**, 805–824.

Reynolds, J.M. & Blogg, C.E. (1995) Prevention and treatment of postoperative nausea and vomiting. *Prescribers Journal* **35**, 111–116.

Rose, J.B. & Watcha, M.F. (1999) Postoperative nausea and vomiting in paediatric patients. *British Journal of Anaesthesia* **83**, 104–117.

Rosen, M. & Camu, F. (1994) Postoperative nausea and vomiting. *Anesthesia* **49**, 1–11.

Rowbotham, D.J. (1992) Current management of postoperative nausea and vomiting. *British Journal of Anaesthesia* **69**, 46S–59S.

Rust, M. (1995) Intravenous administration of ondansetron vs. metoclopramide for the prophylaxis of postoperative nausea and vomiting. *Anaesthetist* **44**, 288–290.

Sieghart, W. (1995) Structure and pharmacology of γ-aminobutyric acid$_A$ receptor subtypes. *Pharmacological Reviews* **47**, 182–234.

Sigel, E. & Buhr, A. (1997) The benzodiazepine binding site of $GABA_A$ receptors. *Trends in Pharmacological Sciences* **18**, 425–429.

Sinclair, D.R., Chung, F. & Mezei, G. (1999) Can postoperative nausea and vomiting be predicted? *Anesthesiology* **91**, 109–118.

Tanelian, D.L., Kosek, P., Mody, I. & MacIver, M.B. (1993) The role of the $GABA_A$ receptor/chloride channel complex in anesthesia. *Anesthesiology* **78**, 757–776.

Tramer, M.L. (2001) A rational approach to the control of PONV: evidence from systematic reviews. Part I. Efficacy and harm of antiemetic interventions, and methodological issues. *Acta Anaesthesiologica Scandinavica* **45**, 4–14.

Tramer, M.L. (2001) A rational approach to the control of PONV: evidence from systematic reviews. Part II. Recommendations for prevention and treatment, and research agenda. *Acta Anaesthesiologica Scandinavica* **45**, 14–20.

Watcha, M.F. & White, P.F. (1992) Postoperative nausea and vomiting. Its etiology, treatment, and prevention. *Anesthesiology* **77**, 162–184.

Watcha, M.F. & White, P.F. (1999) Postoperative nausea and vomiting. Prophylaxis versus treatment. *Anesthesia and Analgesia* **89**, 1337–1339.

White, P.F. (1995) Management of postoperative pain and emesis. *Canadian Journal of Anaesthesia* **42**, 1053–1055.

13 Drugs and the Autonomic Nervous System

Anatomy and physiology of the autonomic nervous system

The autonomic nervous system consists of all efferent fibres which leave the CNS, apart from those which innervate skeletal muscles. Consequently, the system is widely distributed throughout the body. In all cases, the autonomic outflow from the brain stem and spinal cord makes synaptic connections with peripheral neurons, and these synapses normally occur in autonomic ganglia. The postganglionic fibres that originate from ganglion cells are usually unmyelinated, and are responsible for the innervation of effector organs.

The activity of the autonomic nervous system is involuntary and cannot be influenced by individual will or volition. Nevertheless, cellular function in many organs is influenced by autonomic activity, including contraction of smooth muscle in the heart and the uterus, secretion in the salivary, mucous and sweat glands, and endocrine secretion by the adrenal medulla.

Afferent fibres from visceral structures are usually carried to the CNS by major autonomic nerves, such as the vagus and splanchnic nerves or the pelvic plexus. These pathways are concerned with the mediation of visceral sensation and the regulation of vasomotor and respiratory reflexes. In addition, specialized afferent autonomic fibres arise from the baroreceptors and chemoreceptors in the carotid sinus and the aortic arch, and play an important part in the reflex control of heart rate, blood pressure and respiratory activity. Autonomic afferent fibres from blood vessels, which are concerned with the transmission of painful impulses, are usually carried by somatic nerves.

Reflex activity in the autonomic nervous system may occur at a spinal level, and can be demonstrated in humans after spinal cord transection. Vital functions such as respiration and the control of blood pressure are locally mediated via nuclei in the medulla oblongata. However, the central integration of autonomic function mainly occurs in the hypothalamus, which is regulated by the cerebral cortex and has important connections with the limbic system and the pituitary gland.

The autonomic nervous system is divided on anatomical and physiological grounds into two divisions, the parasympathetic and the sympathetic nervous system.

Parasympathetic division

The preganglionic fibres of the parasympathetic nervous system emerge from the CNS in two separate regions. The cranial outflow originates in the midbrain and the medulla, and its axons are carried by the 3rd (oculomotor), 7th (facial), 9th (glossopharyngeal) and the 10th (vagus) cranial nerves. The oculomotor, facial and glossopharyngeal nerves convey fibres that affect ocular accommodation and salivary gland secretion, while the vagus nerve carries fibres to the heart, lungs, bronchi, stomach and the upper small intestine. The sacral outflow occurs from the 2nd, 3rd and 4th sacral segments of the spinal cord and its efferent nerves form pelvic plexuses, which innervate the distal colon and rectum, the bladder and reproductive organs. In both the cranial and the sacral regions, parasympathetic ganglia are usually closely related to their target organs, and postganglionic parasympathetic fibres are very short.

The parasympathetic nervous system is concerned with the conservation and restoration of energy, and increased parasympathetic tone slows the heart rate, reduces blood pressure and facilitates the digestion and absorption of nutrients as well as the excretion of waste material.

Sympathetic division

The cells of origin of the sympathetic nervous system are in the lateral horns of the thoracic and upper lumbar segments of the spinal cord. Their axons travel a short distance in the mixed spinal nerves, and then branch off as white

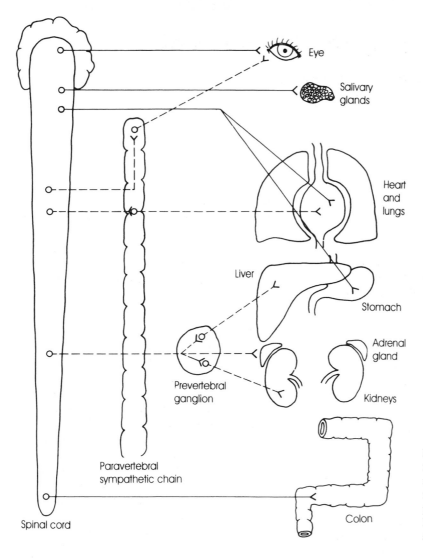

Fig. 13.1 Diagrammatic representation of the autonomic nervous system, showing the main neuronal pathways in the parasympathetic nervous system (solid line) and the sympathetic nervous system (broken line).

rami to enter the sympathetic ganglia. These consist of bilateral chains lying anterolateral to the vertebral bodies and extending from the cervical to the sacral region. The preganglionic fibres or white rami that enter the sympathetic chain may have three different terminations:

• They may make a synaptic connection with a cell body at the same dermatomal level, and the postganglionic fibres may then return to the spinal nerve (via grey rami).

• They may pass in the sympathetic chain to a ganglion at a higher or a lower level before forming a synapse, so that postganglionic fibres subsequently rejoin adjacent spinal nerves.

• They may entirely traverse the sympathetic chain and synapse with prevertebral ganglia and plexuses in the abdominal cavity. Some preganglionic fibres, which emerge from the lower thoracic segments of the sympathetic chain travel in the greater splanchnic nerve, and directly synapse with chromaffin cells in the adrenal medulla (Fig. 13.1). Experimental studies suggest that an intact sympathetic nervous system, although not essential for life, enables the body to be prepared for 'fear, fight or flight'. Sympathetic responses include an increased heart rate and blood pressure, diversion of blood flow from skin and splanchnic vessels to skeletal muscle, an increase in the availability of glucose due to liver glycogenolysis, pupillary and bronchiolar dilatation and the contraction of sphincters.

Cholinergic nervous system

Acetylcholine

Although acetylcholine was first synthesized by Baeyer in 1867, definite evidence for its role in neurohumoral transmission was first provided by the classical experiments of Otto Loewi in the early 1920s. Stimulation of the vagus nerve of an isolated and perfused frog's heart, and the subsequent transfer of the perfusion fluid to a second frog's heart, slowed its rate of contraction. Loewi originally called the released substance 'Vagusstoff', but a few years later it was chemically identified as acetylcholine.

Subsequent investigations established that acetylcholine had a widespread role as a neurotransmitter, and was physiologically released at the following sites:

• All postganglionic parasympathetic nerve endings.
• Postganglionic sympathetic nerve endings supplying the sweat glands ('sympathetic cholinergic fibres').[1]
• All preganglionic nerve endings that synapse in sympathetic and parasympathetic ganglia, including preganglionic sympathetic fibres that synapse with chromaffin cells in the adrenal medulla.
• Motor nerve terminals at the neuromuscular junction.
• Some excitatory nerve endings in the CNS (Chapter 12).

All nerve fibres that release acetylcholine are referred to as cholinergic fibres, and the synthesis, storage, release and subsequent fate of acetylcholine is similar at most cholinergic nerve endings (see Chapter 10).

Muscarinic and nicotinic effects of acetylcholine

Some of the effects of acetylcholine are mimicked by muscarine, an alkaloid derived from the poisonous red mushroom, Amanita muscaria. These responses, which include vasodilatation, hypotension and bradycardia, are similar to those produced by parasympathetic nerve stimulation and are described as the muscarinic (M) effects of acetylcholine. They are due to the action of released acetylcholine at postganglionic nerve endings, and can be competitively antagonized by small doses of atropine.

However, larger doses of acetylcholine produce different effects after its muscarinic actions are blocked. Blood pressure is increased due to stimulation of sympathetic ganglia, enhanced vasoconstrictor tone and the secretion of adrenaline from the adrenal medulla. Stimulation and fasciculation of skeletal muscle also occurs. These effects are described as the nicotinic (N) effects of acetylcholine since they resemble those produced by nicotine, and reflect the effects of acetylcholine at autonomic ganglia and chromaffin cells in the adrenal medulla, as well as the neuromuscular junction.

All the effects of acetylcholine are mediated by cholinergic receptors (cholinoceptors), which are usually classified as muscarinic (M) or nicotinic (N) receptors.

Muscarinic receptors

The effects of acetylcholine at postganglionic nerve endings are mediated by five different types of muscarinic receptor (Table 13.1). Their identification is based on molecular cloning, autoradiographic and radioligand binding studies, and the selectivity of some muscarinic antagonists. M_1-, M_2- and M_4-receptors all contain 460–480 amino acids, while M_3- and M_5-receptors are slightly larger.

All five types of muscarinic receptors have seven transmembrane segments and are coupled to GTP-binding proteins (Chapter 3). They all appear to produce excitatory or inhibitory effects by changes in K^+ conductance, although secondary effects on Ca^{2+} channels may also occur (Table 13.1).

M_1-, M_3- and M_5-receptors produce excitatory responses, and are coupled to the G_q family of GTP-binding proteins. They act by activation of phospholipase C and the inositol trisphosphate (IP_3) pathway. Excitatory responses are usually produced by a decrease in K^+ conductance, resulting in membrane depolarization. In contrast, M_2- and M_4-receptors mediate inhibitory responses and are coupled to G_i and adenylate cyclase. Consequently, their activation decreases cAMP synthesis and increases K^+ conductance, resulting in membrane hyperpolarization.

M₁-receptors

M_1-receptors (neuronal receptors) produce excitatory effects, and have been identified in the CNS, peripheral neurons and gastric parietal cells, where they mediate the increased gastric secretion induced by vagal stimulation. They are also present in all autonomic ganglia, and produce slow depolarization of ganglion cells during synaptic transmission. They have a relatively high affinity

---

[1] In some species, vascular smooth muscle is supplied by sympathetic cholinergic vasodilator nerves. In humans, local or circulating acetylcholine can cause vasodilatation by releasing nitric oxide from vascular endothelium, resulting in the increased synthesis of cGMP by vascular smooth muscle (Chapter 3).

Table 13.1 The distribution and pharmacological effects produced by activation of muscarinic and nicotinic receptors.

Type of receptor	Location	Principal effects	Cellular mechanism	Antagonists
Muscarinic receptors				
M_1 (neuronal)	CNS		activation of PLC	pirenzepine
	peripheral neurons		$\uparrow IP_3 \uparrow DAG$	mamba toxin MT7
	gastric parietal cells	$\uparrow$gastric secretion	$\downarrow K^+$ conductance	
	autonomic ganglia	slow depolarization	$\uparrow[Ca^{2+}]_i$	
M_2 (cardiac)	presynaptic sites	$\downarrow$NA release	inhibition of AC	gallamine
	(nerve terminals)	$\uparrow$ACh release	$\downarrow$cAMP	himbacine
	myocardium	bradycardia	$\uparrow K^+$ conductance	tripitramine
	cerebellum		$\downarrow[Ca^{2+}]_i$	
M_3 (glandular-smooth muscle)	postsynaptic sites		activation of PLC	atropine
	salivary glands	$\uparrow$salivary secretion	$\uparrow IP_3 \uparrow DAG$	hyoscine
	mucous glands	$\uparrow$mucous secretion	$\downarrow K^+$ conductance	glycopyrronium
	smooth muscle	NO release from endothelium	$\uparrow[Ca^{2+}]_i$	darifenacin
M_4	CNS	? bradycardia	inhibition of AC	himbacine
	cardiac muscle		$\downarrow$cAMP	mamba toxin MT3
	bronchial muscle		$\uparrow K^+$ conductance	
			$\downarrow[Ca^{2+}]_i$	
M_5	? CNS	? central cholinergic transmission	activation of PLC	darifenacin
			$\uparrow IP_3 \uparrow DAG$	guanylpirenzepine
			$\downarrow K^+$ conductance	tripitramine
			$\uparrow[Ca^{2+}]_i$	
Nicotinic receptors				
N_1 (muscle receptors)	motor endplate	neuromuscular transmission	ion channel	non-depolarizing
			$\uparrow Na^+ \uparrow Ca^{2+}$ entry	muscle relaxants
N_2 (neuronal receptors)	autonomic ganglia	ganglionic transmission	ion channel	mecamylamine
			$\uparrow Na^+ \uparrow Ca^{2+}$ entry	trimetaphan
	presynaptic nerve terminals	ACh release		

PLC, phospholipase C; IP_3, inositol trisphosphate; DAG, diacylglycerol; cAMP, cyclic adenosine monophosphate; NO, nitric oxide; AC, adenylate cyclase; NA, noradrenaline; ACh, acetylcholine; $[Ca^{2+}]_i$, intracellular calcium ions.

for some muscarinic antagonists (e.g. pirenzepine, green mamba toxin MT7).

M₂-receptors

M₂-receptors (cardiac receptors) produce presynaptic inhibition at some central and peripheral nerve endings. For instance, they inhibit the release of noradrenaline from adrenergic nerve terminals, and increase the release of acetylcholine from vagal nerve endings. They are present in the myocardium, the cerebellum and nerve terminals supplying visceral smooth muscle. M₂-receptors are antagonized by gallamine (allosterically) as well as some experimental drugs (e.g. himbacine, tripitramine). In addition, the receptors may be involved in the autonomic effects of certain agents such as the initial bradycardia sometimes seen after the administration of atropine, and the bronchoconstriction induced by low doses of ipratropium.

M₃-receptors

M$_3$-receptors (glandular secretion/smooth muscle receptors) are found at classical postsynaptic sites in mucous and salivary glands and visceral smooth muscle. They mediate excitatory effects, and their activation increases glandular secretions and causes smooth muscle contraction. They may mediate the release of nitric oxide from endothelial cells, resulting in activation of guanylate cyclase, accumulation of cGMP and vasodilatation (Chapter 3). They are antagonized by some experimental drugs (e.g. darifenacin) as well as classical antimuscarinic drugs, which produce blockade at all muscarinic receptors. When therapeutic doses of atropine are administered, antagonism at M$_3$-receptors overshadows any effects at M$_2$-receptors.

M₄-receptors

M$_4$-receptors have been identified in the CNS, cardiac muscle and bronchial smooth muscle. They are antagonized by himbacine and green mamba toxin MT3.

M₅-receptors

Although M$_5$-receptors are probably present in the CNS, little is known of their function, and their existence has been questioned. They are non-selectively antagonized by many drugs with relatively low affinity (e.g. darifenacin, tripitramine).

In some instances, the clinical significance of the various types of muscarinic receptors is obscure, although they have been implicated in the differential effects of atropine and hyoscine at central and peripheral sites, and the additive effects of atropine and gallamine on cardiac rate.

Nicotinic receptors

Nicotinic receptors are present at the neuromuscular junction, at autonomic ganglia and in the CNS (Table 13.l). They have a pentameric structure, and contain a non-selective cation channel that opens when the receptor is bound by acetylcholine or similar agonists (Chapter 3). Nicotinic receptors invariably mediate excitatory responses, and are divided into two types (muscle and neuronal receptors), which have different subunit structures. Muscle receptors are present at the motor endplate and are invariably sensitive to certain snake toxins (α-bungarotoxin and α-cobratoxin), while neuronal receptors are present in autonomic ganglia and the CNS. Acetylcholine receptors at the neuromuscular junction are considered in detail in Chapter 10.

Adrenergic nervous system

Adrenaline and noradrenaline

During the early years of the twentieth century, it was established that the vascular responses produced by adrenal gland extracts were similar to the effects of sympathetic nerve stimulation. Although it was originally considered that adrenaline might be the sympathetic neurotransmitter, it became clear that the effects of adrenaline and sympathetic nerve stimulation were not identical. For many years, the nature of the substance released at postganglionic sympathetic nerve endings was controversial, but in 1946, von Euler established that noradrenaline[2] was the main transmitter involved. Although small amounts of adrenaline and dopamine are also released by sympathetic nerves, the fibres are most correctly described as noradrenergic.

All three adrenergic neurotransmitters, dopamine, adrenaline and noradrenaline, are chemically related and are commonly referred to as catecholamines, since they are derivatives of catechol (dihydroxybenzene), and have an amine side-chain.

Adrenergic receptors (adrenoceptors)

In 1948, Ahlquist compared the relative potencies of six different sympathomimetic agents, including noradrenaline, adrenaline and isoprenaline, on various tissues. Contraction of smooth muscle was most marked with adrenaline and noradrenaline, but cardiac stimulation and relaxation of smooth muscle were greatest with isoprenaline and least with noradrenaline. On the basis of these studies Ahlquist proposed that two types of adrenergic receptors were present in tissues (α- and β-adrenoceptors). At α-receptors, the potency of the three catecholamines was ranked in the order noradrenaline > adrenaline > isoprenaline. In contrast, at β-receptors their potency was ranked as isoprenaline > adrenaline > noradrenaline. In general, α-adrenoceptors mediated vasoconstriction in most vascular beds as well as smooth muscle contraction, while β-adrenoceptors produced an increase in the force, rate and conduction velocity of the heart, as well as arteriolar vasodilatation and smooth muscle relaxation (Table 13.2).

---

[2] Noradrenaline is the demethylated analogue of adrenaline, and 'nor' is reputed to be an acronym for 'Nitrogen ohne radikal'. The prefix was apparently first used some 100 years ago, when German was the main language for scientific communication.

Table 13.2 Location and pharmacological responses mediated by adrenergic receptors.

Type of receptor	Location	Response	Cellular mechanism	Selective antagonists
α_1	smooth muscle		activation of PLC	doxazosin
	blood vessels	vasoconstriction	$\uparrow IP_3 \uparrow DAG$	prazosin
	bronchi	constriction	$\uparrow Ca^{2+}$ entry	terazosin
	bladder	contraction	$\uparrow[Ca^{2+}]_i$	
	intestine	relaxation		
	uterus	contraction		
	iris (radial muscle)	contraction		
	cardiac muscle	contraction		
	liver/skeletal muscle	glycogenolysis		
α_2	platelets	aggregation	inhibition of AC	yohimbine
	pancreatic β-cells	$\downarrow$insulin secretion	$\downarrow$cAMP	rauwolscine
	blood vessels	vasoconstriction	$\downarrow[Ca^{2+}]_i$	
	sympathetic nerve endings	$\downarrow$NA release		
β_1	heart	$\uparrow$rate	activation of AC	atenolol
		$\uparrow$force of contraction	$\uparrow$cAMP	bisoprolol
		$\uparrow$excitability	$\uparrow[Ca^{2+}]_i$	metoprolol
	sympathetic nerve endings	$\uparrow$NA release		nebivolol
	renal juxtamedullary cells	$\uparrow$renin secretion		
	salivary glands	$\uparrow$amylase secretion		
β_2	smooth muscle		activation of AC	butoxamine
	blood vessels	vasodilatation	$\uparrow$cAMP	α—methylpropanol
	bronchi	dilatation	PKA activation	
	bladder	relaxation	MLCK inactivation	
	uterus	relaxation		
	heart	$\uparrow$rate	activation of AC	
		$\uparrow$force of contraction	$\uparrow$cAMP	
	sympathetic nerve endings	$\uparrow$NA release	$\uparrow[Ca^{2+}]_i$	
	pancreatic β-cells	$\uparrow$insulin secretion		
	liver	glycogenolysis	$\uparrow$phosphorylase	
	skeletal muscle	tremor		
		hypokalaemia	$\uparrow Na^+/K^+$ ATPase	
β_3	fat	thermogenesis	activation of AC	bupranolol
	subcutaneous tissues	lipolysis	$\uparrow$cAMP	cyanopindolol
	? skeletal muscle	glucose uptake	$\uparrow[Ca^{2+}]_i$	

PLC, phospholipase C; IP_3, inositol trisphosphate; DAG, diacylglycerol; AC, adenylate cyclase; cAMP, cyclic adenosine monophosphate; NA, noradrenaline; PKA, protein kinase A; MLCK, myosin light chain kinase; $[Ca^{2+}]_i$, intracellular calcium ions.

Both α- and β-receptors were subsequently divided into several subgroups. α-Receptors are currently classified as α_1- and α_2-receptors, while β-receptors are divided into β_1-, β_2-, and β_3-receptors.

α-Adrenergic receptors

α_1-Receptors

α_1-Adrenoceptors are primarily present at postsynaptic sites in vascular smooth muscle, but are also present in bronchi, bladder, intestine, uterus, iris, liver and heart. They mediate a wide variety of autonomic effects, including

- vasoconstriction in most blood vessels
- bronchoconstriction
- contraction of the bladder and uterus
- relaxation of intestinal muscle
- mydriasis
- glycogenolysis
- cardiac inotropic effects

Some α_1-receptors are more sensitive to noradrenaline than adrenaline, although both catecholamines are equipotent at some sites. They are all selectively antagonized by doxazosin, prazosin and terazosin. All α_1-adrenoceptors are coupled to the GTP-binding protein G_q, and act by activation of phospholipase C and the phosphatidyl-inositol pathway. Consequently, receptor activation increases IP_3 synthesis and the release of intracellular Ca^{2+} (Table 13.2).

α_2-Receptors

α_2-Adrenoceptors are present in platelets, in pancreatic β-cells, in vascular smooth muscle and at sympathetic nerve endings. They mediate a number of physiological effects, including

• inhibition of noradrenaline release from sympathetic postganglionic neurons. Noradrenaline normally inhibits its own release by its action on presynaptic α_2-receptors (an example of an autoinhibitory feedback system)
• platelet aggregation
• inhibition of insulin release
• vasoconstriction (in some vascular smooth muscle beds)
All α_2-adrenoceptors are more sensitive to adrenaline than noradrenaline, and are selectively antagonized by yohimbine and rauwolscine. Other drugs, including clonidine, dexmedetomidine and azepexole, are agonists or partial agonists at α_2-receptors. All α_2-receptors are coupled to the GTP-binding protein G_i, and their activation results in the inhibition of adenylate cyclase and a reduction in intracellular cAMP (Table 13.2).

β-Adrenergic receptors

The subdivision of β-adrenoceptors into β_1 and β_2 groups was originally based on the relative potency of adrenaline and noradrenaline in different tissues. β_3-Receptors were subsequently identified on the basis of their atypical metabolic effects. All β-adrenoceptors are coupled to the GTP-binding protein G_s, and agonists at β-receptors activate adenylate cyclase and increase intracellular cAMP synthesis, with resultant effects on protein phosphorylation and Ca^{2+} mobilization (Table 13.2).

β_1-Adrenoceptors

At most β_1-receptors, noradrenaline is equipotent with adrenaline (although both are less potent than isoprenaline). β_1-Adrenoceptors have been identified at postsynaptic sites in the heart, at adrenergic nerve terminals, in the juxtaglomerular cells in the kidney and in salivary glands. At these sites, activation of β_1-receptors

• increases the rate and force of cardiac contraction
• facilitates the release of noradrenaline
• increases the secretion of renin from juxtaglomerular cells
• increases amylase secretion in salivary glands

β_2-Adrenoceptors

β_2-Adrenoceptors are 10–50 times more sensitive to adrenaline than noradrenaline, and are primarily involved in mediating physiological responses to circulating catecholamines. They are widely present in vascular, bronchial, vesical and uterine smooth muscle, and at presynaptic sites on adrenergic neurons. In some tissues (lymphocytes, liver, skeletal muscle) they are not associated with a sympathetic nerve supply.

Activation of β_2-receptors produces
• vasodilatation
• bronchodilatation
• vesical smooth muscle relaxation
• uterine relaxation
• increased noradrenaline release from sympathetic nerves
• glycogenolysis
• increased insulin secretion
• muscle tremor and hypokalaemia

Myocardial β_1- and β_2-receptors

In humans, normal myocardium contains both β_1- and β_2-adrenoceptors in the approximate ratio of 3:1. β_1-Receptors are predominantly present at postsynaptic sites in the immediate vicinity of sympathetic nerves, and respond to locally released noradrenaline (as well as adrenaline). In contrast, β_2-receptors are present at extrajunctional as well as postsynaptic sites, and partly mediate responses to circulating adrenaline. Changes in the proportion of myocardial β_1- and β_2-receptors are known to occur in various pathological conditions, including heart failure. In these circumstances, excessive sympathetic drive and increased noradrenaline release leads to the down-regulation of β_1-adrenoceptors, resulting in the relative overexpression of extrajunctional β_2-adrenoceptors, and an enhanced response to circulating adrenaline. In severe heart failure, the ratio of β_1- to β_2-adrenoceptors may change from 3:1 to 3:2.

β_3-Adrenoceptors

β_3-Adrenoceptors are usually equally sensitive to noradrenaline and adrenaline, and have been identified in omental and subcutaneous tissues, brown fat and the gall-bladder and colon. They mediate atypical metabolic responses, including

- thermogenesis (in skeletal muscle and adipose tissue)
- lipolysis (in adipose tissue)
- glucose uptake (by skeletal muscle)

They are antagonized by bupranolol and cyanopindolol, but are relatively resistant to many standard β_1- and β_2-antagonists, which may sometimes act as partial agonists or agonists.

β_4-Adrenoceptors

β_4-Adrenoceptors are not novel or true receptors, but represent alternative sites of action of some β_1-partial agonists.

Dopaminergic receptors

Dopamine is the immediate metabolic precursor of noradrenaline and small concentrations are released from sympathetic nerve terminals. Although its peripheral role is limited, it is an important central neurotransmitter, and five different types of dopamine receptor have been identified in the CNS.

All dopamine receptors are coupled to GTP-binding proteins, and their activation affects the synthesis of cAMP by adenylate cyclase. D_1-like receptors (D_1 and D_5) are coupled to G_s, and their activation increases intracellular cAMP synthesis. In contrast, D_2-like receptors (D_2, D_3 and D_4) are coupled to G_i, and their activation decreases cAMP synthesis. Some D_2- and D_4-receptors have alternative transduction mechanisms (G_q coupling) that use the inositol trisphosphate pathway (Chapter 3).

In humans, the D_2-receptor has splice variants (D_{2S} and D_{2L}) and the D_4-receptor is subject to genetic polymorphism, which does not appear to affect its function.

Central dopamine receptors

In the CNS, dopamine receptors are expressed at both presynaptic and postsynaptic sites. D_1-receptors are present in the basal ganglia, the nigrostriatal pathway, the hypothalamus and the limbic system. D_2-receptors are also present at all these sites, as well as in the anterior and intermediate lobes of the pituitary gland. D_3- and D_4-receptors have been primarily identified in the limbic system, but are not present in the nigrostriatal pathway or the corpus striatum.

In general, D_2-receptors have an important functional role in the CNS. Activation of D_2-receptors

- decreases the secretion of prolactin
- produces emesis (via receptors in the CTZ and NTS; Chapter 12)
- influences the local release of acetylcholine and endorphins

Activation of D_1-receptors is also involved in hormonal and neurosecretory activity, and modulates extrapyramidal activity. In the corpus striatum, there appears to be functional interaction between D_1- and D_2-receptors. In parkinsonism, changes in the receptor population may account for the 'on-off' therapeutic response and the development of tardive dyskinesia after administration of non-selective dopamine agonists.

Peripheral dopamine receptors

D_1- and D_2-receptors have also been identified at peripheral sites, where they may have a limited functional role. D_1-receptors are present in the renal and mesenteric blood vessels, and their activation causes vasodilatation and increased Na^+ excretion (Table 13.3). In autonomic ganglia, specific SIF[3] cells release dopamine, which then acts on ganglionic D_1-receptors, producing hyperpolarization and decreasing the release of noradrenaline from sympathetic neurons.

Synthesis of noradrenaline and adrenaline
Synthesis of noradrenaline in sympathetic nerve endings

Postganglionic sympathetic nerve endings are the terminal axons of neurons that originate in sympathetic autonomic ganglia, and they synthesize dopamine and noradrenaline from the simple amino acid precursors phenylalanine and tyrosine. Initially, phenylalanine is hydroxylated to tyrosine, which is then actively transported into sympathetic nerve endings. Tyrosine is subsequently hydroxylated to dihydroxyphenylalanine (DOPA) by tyrosine hydroxylase, which is a relatively selective enzyme and the main rate-controlling step in noradrenaline synthesis. Tyrosine hydroxylase is inhibited by noradrenaline, which thus exerts negative feedback control on the rate of neurotransmitter synthesis. Subsequently, DOPA is decarboxylated to dopamine by DOPA decarboxylase, a relatively non-specific enzyme, which is also present in many extraneuronal tissues. Dopamine is then transported into synaptic vesicles from the axoplasm, and noradrenaline is

---

[3] Small intensely fluorescent cells due to their high dopamine content.

Table 13.3 Adrenergic receptors that are involved in different sympathetic responses.

Organ or tissue	Response	Receptor
Heart		
	↑rate	$\beta_1 (? \beta_2)$
	↑force of contraction	$\beta_1 (? \beta_2) \alpha_1$
	↑automaticity	$\beta_1 (? \beta_2)$
Vascular smooth muscle		
skin	vasoconstriction	$\alpha_1 (? \alpha_2)$
skeletal muscle	vasoconstriction	$\alpha_1 (? \alpha_2)$
	vasodilatation	β_2
splanchnic area	vasoconstriction	$\alpha_1 (? \alpha_2)$
	vasodilatation	$\beta_2 D_1$
renal vessels	vasoconstriction	$\alpha_1 (? \alpha_2)$
	vasodilatation	$\beta_2 D_1$
Non-vascular smooth muscle		
bronchi	constriction	α_1
	dilatation	β_2
intestine	contraction	α_1
	relaxation	$\alpha_1 \beta_2$
uterus	contraction	α_1
	relaxation	β_2
Other effects		
renin secretion	increased	β_1
	decreased	α_1
glycogenolysis	increased	$\alpha_1 \beta_2$
lipolysis	increased	β_3
insulin secretion	increased	β_2
	decreased	α_2

synthesized from dopamine by dopamine-β-hydroxylase. This membrane-bound enzyme is present in some vesicular proteins (chromogranins) and mediates the final step in the synthesis of noradrenaline (Fig. 13.2). The neurotransmitter is stored in the synaptic vesicles, where it forms a complex with ATP and is bound by chromogranins. Any extravesicular noradrenaline in the axoplasm is subsequently metabolized by monoamine oxidase (MAO), which is present on the surface membrane of mitochondria.

Synthesis of adrenaline in the adrenal medulla

In the adrenal medulla, noradrenaline is synthesized by this pathway and in some medullary cells it is converted to adrenaline by an *N*-methyltransferase (phenylethanolamine *N*-methyltransferase). This enzyme is mainly located in specific juxtamedullary cells close to the adrenal cortex, and its activity is induced by the adjacent cortical hormones. In adults, adrenaline is the main hormone synthesized by the adrenal medulla, and in physiological conditions forms 80–85% of the catecholamines released into the circulation. Different proportions are present in foetal life, early childhood and in patients with phaeochromocytomata.

Noradrenaline release

When a nerve impulse arrives at a noradrenergic nerve terminal, its action potential causes depolarization and opens Ca^{2+} channels in the axonal membrane. The entry of extracellular Ca^{2+} results in the fusion of synaptic vesicles with the terminal membrane, and the release of their contents (noradrenaline, ATP, chromogranin and small amounts of dopamine and dopamine-β-hydroxylase) into the synaptic gap. Other mediators (e.g. neuropeptide Y) may also be released simultaneously. Normally, the contents of 200–300 vesicles are released over a relatively wide area from the terminal varicosities of adrenergic nerves.

Indirectly acting sympathomimetic amines, such as tyramine, ephedrine and amphetamine cause the release of noradrenaline from synaptic vesicles into extracellular fluid. In addition, many physiological agents, including acetylcholine, angiotensin II, prostaglandins, purines and neuropeptides, as well as α_2- and β_2-adrenergic agonists, can combine with receptors on the presynaptic nerve terminal and modulate the release of noradrenaline from synaptic vesicles.

Noradrenaline uptake

When noradrenaline is released from the nerve terminal, it diffuses into the synaptic gap, but only 10–20% combines with α- and β-receptors in blood vessels and other postsynaptic sites. Some of the noradrenaline combines with α_2-receptors on the presynaptic nerve terminal, resulting in decreased cAMP synthesis and the inhibition of further release of the neurotransmitter (an autoinhibitory or negative feedback mechanism). Other agonists at α_2-receptors (e.g. clonidine, dexmedetomidine) also decrease the release of noradrenaline from sympathetic neurons, while α_2-antagonists (e.g. phenoxybenzamine, yohimbine) increase its release. Most of the noradrenaline in the synaptic gap is removed by two different active transport systems (Fig. 13.3).

Uptake₁

Uptake₁ (neuronal uptake) is a neuronal membrane transport process with a high affinity but a low capacity for

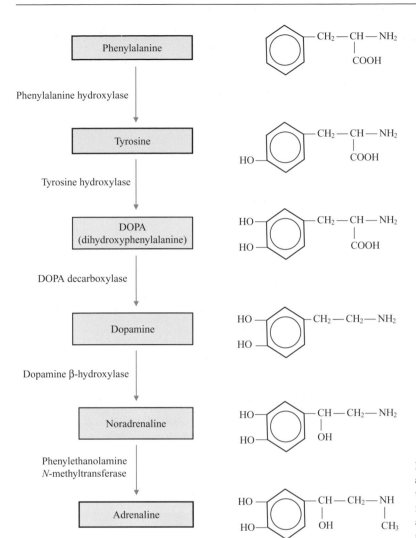

Fig. 13.2 The synthesis of noradrenaline and adrenaline from phenylalanine and tyrosine. In sympathetic nerve endings, noradrenaline is the final product. In the adrenal medulla, noradrenaline is subsequently methylated to adrenaline.

noradrenaline. Uptake$_1$ is relatively specific, although it can also transport other amines (including adrenaline), but with a much lower affinity. After transport by Uptake$_1$, noradrenaline is either metabolized by mitochondrial MAO or stored by synaptic vesicles. Uptake$_1$ can be blocked by various drugs, including cocaine, some tricyclic antidepressants and phenothiazines, amphetamines and phenoxybenzamine.

Uptake$_2$

Uptake$_2$ (extraneuronal uptake) mainly occurs in extraneuronal tissues such as cardiac and smooth muscle cells and vascular endothelium. It has a low affinity for noradrenaline, but a higher affinity for adrenaline, and is probably mainly responsible for the removal of the hormone from plasma. Uptake$_2$ has a higher capacity and maximum rate of transport than Uptake$_1$, and is inhibited by phenoxybenzamine and many glucocorticoids. After their transport by Uptake$_2$, catecholamines are metabolized intracellularly (probably by mitochondrial MAO).

Metabolism of noradrenaline

Noradrenaline is metabolized by two enzyme systems, monoamine oxidase (MAO) and catechol-O-methyl

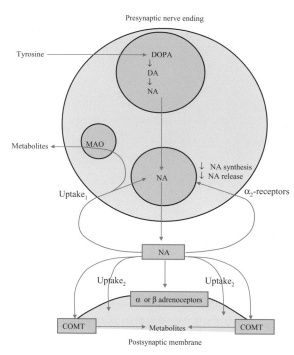

Fig. 13.3 The adrenergic nerve terminal, showing the synthesis, release and uptake of noradrenaline. DOPA, dihydroxyphenylalanine; DA, dopamine; NA, noradrenaline; MAO, monoamine oxidase; COMT, catechol-*O*-methyltransferase.

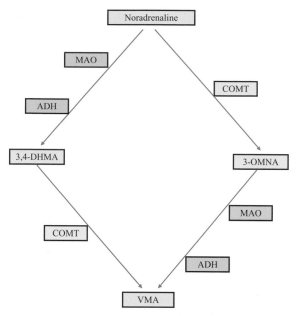

Fig. 13.4 The metabolism of noradrenaline in the peripheral nervous system. MAO, monoamine oxidase; ADH, aldehyde dehydrogenase. COMT, catechol-*O*-methyltransferase; 3,4-DHMA, 3,4-dihydroxymandelic acid; 3-OMNA, 3-oxymethylnoradrenaline; VMA, vanillylmandelic acid (3-methoxy-4-hydroxymandelic acid). In the CNS, a reductive pathway is predominant, resulting in the formation of 3-methoxy-4-hydroxy-phenylethylene glycol.

transferase (COMT). In many tissues, the two systems complement each other and metabolize catecholamines in a sequential manner. In most neurons (and some extraneuronal tissues), noradrenaline is initially metabolized by mitochondrial MAO and aldehyde dehydrogenase (ADH) to dihydroxymandelic acid (DHMA), which is then converted by COMT to vanillylmandelic acid (VMA). In many extraneuronal tissues, noradrenaline is initially converted by COMT to *O*-methylnoradrenaline, and is subsequently oxidized by MAO (and ADH) to VMA (Fig. 13.4). In the CNS, noradrenaline metabolism is slightly different, and a reductive pathway is predominant, resulting in the formation of 3-methoxy-4-hydroxy-phenylethylene glycol (MHPEG). Consequently, changes in urinary MHPEG levels have been used to reflect noradrenergic activity in the CNS.

Other autonomic neurotransmitters

In addition to acetylcholine and noradrenaline, many other endogenous compounds can mimic or enhance autonomic activity, including histamine, 5-HT, ATP, adenosine, endothelins, vasoactive intestinal peptide, neuropeptide Y, substances P and K, and nitric oxide. These agents are generally considered to be local neurotransmitters (local hormones), and this type of transmission is called non-adrenergic non-cholinergic (NANC) transmission. The effects produced by these neurotransmitters may be mediated by other known or putative receptors, or may involve modulation of the synthesis, release or activation produced by classical neurotransmitters.

Parasympathomimetic agents

All agonists at muscarinic receptors have parasympathomimetic properties, and produce effects that are similar to stimulation of the parasympathetic nervous system. They usually produce characteristic effects on the eye, the heart, non-vascular smooth muscle and glandular secretions, due to their non-selective effects on muscarinic receptors at these sites.

Acetylcholine

$$CH_3 - CO - O - CH_2 - CH_2 - \overset{\overset{\displaystyle CH_3}{|}}{\underset{\underset{\displaystyle CH_3}{|}}{\overset{+}{N}}} - CH_3$$

Acetylcholine has widespread effects at all muscarinic and nicotinic receptors, but an evanescent action due to its rapid destruction by cholinesterase. In the past, it has been used to induce convulsions in schizophrenia. It is still occasionally used in ophthalmic practice to produce rapid and complete miosis immediately prior to anterior segment ophthalmic surgery.

Other drugs with parasympathomimetic properties are usually classified as
• choline esters
• naturally occurring parasympathomimetic amines
• anticholinesterase agents

Choline esters

Synthetic choline esters (e.g. carbachol, bethanechol) are more stable than acetylcholine due to their slow hydrolysis or resistance to cholinesterases. They are only rarely used in current practice.

Bethanechol is resistant to enzymatic destruction, increases detrusor muscle contraction, and is occasionally used in the treatment of urinary retention and postoperative atony of the bladder.

Natural parasympathomimetic amines

Some parasympathomimetic agents occur naturally, including muscarine (from the poisonous red mushroom, *Amanita muscaria*), arecoline (from the betel nut palm, *Areca catechu*) and pilocarpine (from a South American shrub, *Pilocarpus jaborandi*). Pilocarpine is still used as a miotic in patients with raised intraocular pressure or angle-closure glaucoma (either as eye drops or as an ophthalmic gel). It is also used systemically (10–30 mg daily, by mouth) to treat xerostomia after head and neck irradiation, or in patients with Sjögren's syndrome. In order to be effective in the treatment of xerostomia, patients must have some residual salivary function.

Anticholinesterase agents

Anticholinesterase agents inhibit acetylcholinesterase (AChE) and/or butyrylcholinesterase (BChE), and thus prevent the enzymic destruction of acetylcholine. Consequently, they allow the neurotransmitter to accumulate at all its peripheral sites of release, resulting in widespread muscarinic and nicotinic effects. Some anticholinesterase drugs (physostigmine and organophosphorus agents) are non-polar and lipid-soluble, and can readily cross the blood–brain barrier and produce central effects (Chapter 10).

Anticholinesterase drugs that are used clinically include:
• Edrophonium
• Neostigmine
• Pyridostigmine
• Physostigmine
• Distigmine

Edrophonium

$$C_2H_5 - \overset{\overset{\displaystyle CH_3}{|}}{\underset{\underset{\displaystyle CH_3}{|}}{\overset{+}{N}}} - \bigcirc - OH$$

At one time the quaternary amine edrophonium was widely used as a diagnostic test in myasthenia gravis. Although it is still occasionally used for this purpose, it has been largely superseded by other methods of diagnosis (e.g. electromyography). Edrophonium has also been used to reverse non-depolarizing blockade (particularly with short-acting muscle relaxants). Large doses of the drug may be required (e.g. 500–700 μg kg^{-1}), and should be given with atropine in order to prevent muscarinic side effects.

Neostigmine

$$CH_3 - \overset{\overset{\displaystyle CH_3}{|}}{\underset{\underset{\displaystyle CH_3}{|}}{\overset{+}{N}}} - \bigcirc - O - \overset{\overset{\displaystyle O}{\|}}{C} - N \overset{\displaystyle CH_3}{\underset{\displaystyle CH_3}{}}$$

In anaesthetic practice, neostigmine is primarily used to reverse nonpolarizing neuromuscular blockade (Chapter 10). It is also used orally or intramuscularly to improve neuromuscular function in myasthenia gravis and related conditions. Overdosage in myasthenia can cause muscular weakness or even paralysis ('cholinergic crisis').

Pyridostigmine

Pyridostigmine is also used orally in the treatment of myasthenia gravis. It has a longer duration of action than neostigmine due to its slower metabolism.

Physostigmine

Physostigmine (eserine) is a naturally occurring tertiary amine that crosses the blood–brain barrier. It is derived from the Calabar bean, and was once widely used as a miotic drug. It has sometimes been used in the treatment of atropine poisoning.

Distigmine

Distigmine is a combination of two molecules of pyridostigmine and has a relatively long duration of action. It is sometimes used in the treatment of postoperative urinary retention, and in upper motor neuron lesions that result in a neurogenic bladder.

Antimuscarinic drugs

Some naturally occurring and synthetic agents can competitively antagonize the muscarinic effects of acetylcholine and other parasympathomimetic drugs. They principally affect organs innervated by postganglionic parasympathetic fibres (M_3-receptors), and have characteristic effects on the eye, the heart, non-vascular smooth muscle and glandular secretions. Some of them also inhibit ganglionic transmission or have significant CNS activity, but they have little or no effect at nicotinic sites (e.g. the neuromuscular junction). Transient bradycardia is some-

times observed following the administration of antimuscarinic drugs (particularly atropine). This was formerly believed to be due to an effect on the CNS, but is now considered to represent an initial response by cardiac M_2-receptors.

Antimuscarinic drugs ('anticholinergic drugs') can be classified as
- Naturally occurring agents (atropine and hyoscine)
- Synthetic compounds

Naturally occurring antimuscarinic drugs

Atropine and hyoscine are organic esters that are derived from solanaceous plants and are chemically related to cocaine. Both drugs are esters of tropic acid and a tertiary base (either tropine or scopine).

Atropine

Atropine has been used in anaesthetic practice for many years, both for premedication and to antagonize the muscarinic effects produced by anticholinesterase drugs (Chapter 10). It is also used in the management of intraoperative bradycardia during general anaesthesia, or in the treatment of local anaesthetic overdosage. Although it is now only rarely used for premedication (Chapter 12), it is still widely used for other purposes.

Atropine is used in myocardial infarction when bradycardia is associated with hypotension, or when prolonged atrioventricular conduction results in ventricular 'escape' and multiple extrasystoles. It is also administered topically as a mydriatic in the treatment of iritis and choroiditis, although its effects may last up to 2 weeks and produce profound cycloplegia. Atropine is also used in the treatment of poisoning with organophosphorus insecticides, and is a specific antidote in the treatment of muscarine poisoning, whether induced by poisonous mushrooms (*Amanita muscaria*) or other fungi. In these conditions, large and repeated doses of atropine (e.g. 2 mg every 5–10 min) may be required until pupillary dilatation and tachycardia occur.

Atropine poisoning

Although therapeutic doses of atropine only produce slight stimulation of the CNS, larger doses can cause excitement, hallucinations and hyperpyrexia. In untreated cases, respiratory depression and coma will eventually occur. Children are most frequently affected by atropine poisoning due to the accidental consumption of deadly nightshade berries (*Atropa belladonna*). Treatment includes gastric lavage, the reduction of body temperature, administration of physostigmine and the use of controlled ventilation.

Hyoscine (scopolamine)

In contrast to atropine, therapeutic doses of hyoscine hydrobromide produce depressant effects on the CNS, suggesting that the two drugs may have different affinities for central muscarinic receptors. Its sedative and amnesic effects may be of value, and it has been used as a premedicant drug (particularly in children). In elderly subjects, its use may lead to undue excitation with confusion and ataxia, behavioural abnormalities and excessive drowsiness ('the central anticholinergic syndrome').

Hyoscine hydrobromide induces less tachycardia than equivalent doses of atropine, has greater antisecretory activity and produces more pronounced ocular effects. It is often used prophylactically in the management of motion sickness, and can also be employed to prevent nausea and vertigo in Meniere's disease, or after middle-ear surgery. Its mechanism of action involves inhibition of cholinergic

pathways from the labyrinths to cerebellar and vestibular nuclei and the medullary centres (Chapter 12).

Synthetic antimuscarinic drugs

Many synthetic and semisynthetic antimuscarinic agents produce fewer peripheral side effects than atropine or hyoscine. Consequently, they have been developed and used in many different conditions, including
- Drug-induced extrapyramidal syndromes
- Gastrointestinal disorders
- Urinary incontinence
- Obstructive pulmonary disease
- Mydriasis and cycloplegia

Drug-induced extrapyramidal disorders

Many synthetic antimuscarinic drugs (e.g. benzatropine, procyclidine) are commonly used to control tremor and rigidity in drug-induced parkinsonism and extrapyramidal syndromes. They are not used as frequently in classical idiopathic parkinsonism, since they are less effective than dopamine agonists and often cause cognitive impairment. Benzatropine and procyclidine are also used to reverse acute dystonia induced by phenothiazines, metoclopramide and similar drugs.

Gastrointestinal disorders

Synthetic antimuscarinic drugs are used as antispasmodics in various gastrointestinal conditions, particularly irritable bowel syndrome and diverticular disease. They are also used prior to endoscopy or radiological examination.

Dicycloverine produces fewer peripheral side effects than atropine, and is a tertiary amine that directly affects intestinal smooth muscle. Other antimuscarinic drugs (including hyoscine butylbromide and propantheline) are quaternary amines that are poorly absorbed from the gut and do not significantly cross the blood–brain barrier. They also have more affinity for M_1 (ganglionic) receptors and may abolish the effects of sympathetic nerve activity on muscle tone, particularly in the sphincters. Glycopyrronium is a similar quaternary amine that is used in premedication prior to anaesthesia, and during the reversal of neuromuscular blockade (Chapter 10).

Urinary incontinence

Antimuscarinic drugs are frequently used to reduce contractions of the detrusor muscle and to control incontinence, frequency and nocturia. Some of these drugs also have direct relaxant effects on vesical smooth muscle.

Drugs that are used for this purpose include flavoxate, oxybutynin and tolterodine.

Obstructive pulmonary disease

Ipratropium and tiotropium are muscarinic M_3-receptor antagonists that are used in the treatment of acute bronchospasm and chronic obstructive pulmonary disease.

Ipratropium is a quaternary analogue of *N*-isopropylatropine, which is not significantly absorbed from the respiratory tract, so that its effects are localized to the bronchi. It is a non-selective antagonist at all types of muscarinic receptors, and prevents bronchoconstrictor effects that are produced by parasympathetic stimulation. It is only given by inhalation as a powder, an aerosol or as a nebulized solution, and usually acts within 30 minutes. It normally acts for 3–6 hours and can be used with other antiasthmatic drugs.

Mydriasis and cycloplegia

Some synthetic or semisynthetic antimuscarinic drugs are used to produce pupillary dilatation and paralysis of accommodation prior to ophthalmological examination. When locally applied to the eye, homatropine has a shorter duration of action than atropine and has been used as a mydriatic for diagnostic procedures. Tropicamide and cyclopentolate are related synthetic compounds with a weak and evanescent action, which are currently used to facilitate examination of the optic fundus.

Sympathomimetic agents

Many sympathomimetic agents have inotropic properties, and their administration increases the force of cardiac contraction. These effects are due to a rise in intracellular Ca^{2+} in myocardial cells, which enhances the release of Ca^{2+} from the sarcoplasmic reticulum, and thus increases the force of cardiac contraction. The concentration of Ca^{2+} in myocardial cells is often extremely low (≈ 100 nanomolar) but may be increased by a variety of mechanisms, including

• inhibition of myocardial Na^+/K^+ ATPase (e.g. digoxin)
• increased formation of intracellular cAMP (e.g. adrenaline, noradrenaline, dopamine)
• reduced metabolism of intracellular cAMP (e.g. enoximone, milrinone)
• infusions of calcium chloride or calcium gluconate
A rise in intracellular cAMP increases myocardial Ca^{2+} by enhancing its entry through voltage-dependent (L-type) Ca^{2+} channels during myocardial depolarization. Consequently, Ca^{2+} is released from the sarcoplasmic reticulum. The effects of inotropic agents on cardiac rate vary with individual drugs.

Inotropic agents

Adrenaline

Infusions of adrenaline produce characteristic physiological responses, which are mediated by both α- and β-adrenoceptors in the heart and the circulation. Heart rate, force of contraction and conduction velocity are invariably increased, and arrhythmias are not uncommon. Systolic pressure is increased, but diastolic pressure may fall due to vasodilatation, which is mediated by $β_2$-adrenoceptors in splanchnic and skeletal muscle blood vessels. At higher doses or rates of infusion, effects on $α_1$-adrenoceptors in the peripheral vasculature are predominant, and peripheral resistance is increased. Cutaneous blood flow is invariably reduced, but coronary arterioles are dilated, due to the metabolic changes produced by the increased work of the heart. Coronary vasodilatation overshadows the vasoconstrictor responses that are mediated through α-adrenoceptors in the myocardial circulation.

Anaphylaxis

The prompt use of adrenaline is of fundamental importance in the treatment of anaphylaxis. It is currently recommended that 500 μg (0.5 mL of 1 in 1000 adrenaline) should be given intramuscularly, and repeated if necessary at 5-minute intervals depending on the blood pressure, pulse and respiration. Alternatively, 500 μg adrenaline may be given by slow intravenous injection (5 mL of 1 in 10,000 adrenaline) at a rate of 100 μg min^{-1}, when the peripheral circulation is compromised and absorption is uncertain. The use of 1 in 10,000 adrenaline intravenously is also recommended for the first line treatment of severe hypersensitivity responses occurring during anaesthesia (Chapter 7).

Cardiac arrest

In cardiac arrest, intravenous adrenaline (5–10 mL of 1 in 10,000 adrenaline) should be given (preferably via a central vein) when there is ECG evidence of asystole, or when fine fibrillation (high-frequency, low-amplitude waves) needs to be coarsened prior to DC cardioversion.

Cardiac surgery and hypotension

Adrenaline is sometimes used as a primary inotropic drug in patients with ventricular dysfunction after cardiopulmonary bypass surgery. It has also been used to increase cardiac output when hypotension and sepsis are unresponsive to dopamine. Its use in these circumstances may be limited by its propensity to induce cardiac arrhythmias.

Local anaesthesia

Adrenaline is commonly incorporated into local anaesthetic solutions, in order to reduce bleeding and decrease systemic absorption. The addition of adrenaline prolongs local anaesthetic activity and reduces its systemic toxicity (Chapter 9). Concentrations of 1 in 200,000 ($5\ \mu g\ mL^{-1}$) or 1 in 300,000 ($3.3\ \mu g\ mL^{-1}$) are commonly used (though concentrations of 1 in 80,000 are used in dental surgery).

Other uses

Nebulized solutions of 1 in 1000 adrenaline ($1\ mg\ mL^{-1}$) are sometimes useful in the treatment of severe croup in children, and adrenaline eye drops may be of value in the treatment of primary open angle glaucoma. The vasoconstrictor effect will reduce the secretion of aqueous humour, as well as increasing its reabsorption through the trabecular network.

Noradrenaline

The effects of infused noradrenaline are almost entirely mediated by α-adrenoceptors. Peripheral resistance and systolic and diastolic pressures are invariably raised due to generalized vasoconstriction. Although noradrenaline has direct effects on the heart, these are often obscured by the reflex baroreceptor responses to increased blood pressure, which usually results in slight bradycardia. Other effects on the heart are usually minimal.

Acute hypotension

Noradrenaline infusions are sometimes used in the treatment of acute hypotension, particularly when this is due to sepsis or neurogenic shock following spinal cord injury. Nevertheless, blood pressure may be maintained at the expense of reduced tissue perfusion, and extravasation of the infusion into tissues can produce severe necrosis. Noradrenaline infusions are sometimes used in hypotensive patients with cardiogenic shock who are unresponsive to plasma expansion and dopamine alone. The effects of noradrenaline on α- and β_1-adrenoceptors in the myocardium may complement the positive inotropic effects of other drugs, and when relatively low doses are used (e.g. 0.05–$0.5\ \mu g\ kg^{-1}\ min^{-1}$), excessive vasoconstriction is not usually a problem. Nevertheless, the effects of combinations of vasoactive drugs are variable and unpredictable, and the monitoring of cardiovascular parameters is essential.

Isoprenaline

Isoprenaline is a synthetic catecholamine with powerful effects on β_1- and β_2-adrenoceptors. After infusion of isoprenaline, both heart rate and cardiac output are increased, and arrhythmias are not uncommon. Peripheral resistance falls, and coronary perfusion may be reduced due to tachycardia and a reduction in diastolic pressure.

At one time, isoprenaline infusions were used in the management of cardiovascular shock, various bradyarrhythmias and bronchospasm. Its use is now obsolete and it is only available on special order.

Dopamine

Dopamine is an endogenous catecholamine that is formed as an intermediate compound during noradrenaline and adrenaline synthesis, and is also used as an inotropic agent. It has complex pharmacological actions, since it differentially affects D_1- and D_2-dopamine receptors (as well as α- and β-adrenoceptors). Dopamine is usually given by intravenous infusion, and when low doses (1–$2\ \mu g\ kg^{-1}\ min^{-1}$) are used, renal blood flow is enhanced and urinary output increased due to its direct effects on D_1-receptors in the renal and mesenteric vasculature. Dopamine D_2-receptors in autonomic ganglia and sympathetic nerves are also activated, resulting in decreased noradrenaline release. At higher rates of infusion (2–10 $\mu g\,kg^{-1}\,min^{-1}$), the effects of dopamine are primarily mediated by β_1-adrenoceptors, resulting in an increase in cardiac output. In these circumstances, dopamine has inotropic effects that primarily increase cardiac contractility rather than heart rate. However, tachycardia can sometimes be a problem, particularly in underhydrated patients. At still higher rates of infusion (10–15 $\mu g\,kg^{-1}\,min^{-1}$), α_1-adrenoceptor effects are predominant, leading to profound vasoconstriction and decreased renal blood flow. Cardiac arrhythmias may also occur.

In practice, the effects of dopamine on the circulation are not always consistent with this dose-dependent gradation of pharmacological effects, and a wide range of vascular responses to infused dopamine may occur. Dopamine is widely used for its inotropic effects after cardiac surgery, when renal insufficiency is associated with a low cardiac output, in endotoxic and cardiogenic shock, and in refractory congestive cardiac failure.

Dopamine and parkinsonism

In most cases of parkinsonism, dopamine stores in the corpus striatum are depleted, and their replenishment is an effective method of treatment. Although dopamine does not readily cross the blood–brain barrier, its immediate precursor levodopa can be used for this purpose. In parkinsonism, levodopa is usually given with a dopa-decarboxylase inhibitor, either benserazide (in co-beneldopa) or carbidopa (in co-careldopa), to minimize side effects such as nausea, vomiting and cardiac arrhythmias, which are mainly due to the formation of extracerebral dopamine. Other drugs, which may be used to increase dopaminergic activity within the CNS are dopamine D_2-receptor agonists (e.g. apomorphine, bromocriptine), selective inhibitors of monoamine oxidase B (selegiline, rasagiline),[4] and amantidine, which increases the presynaptic release of dopamine.

Dobutamine

Dobutamine is a synthetic catecholamine that resembles dopamine, and is used clinically as a mixture of two stereoisomers. It directly increases cardiac contractility and output by activating β_1-adrenoceptors, and produces moderate vasodilatation by its effects on β_2-receptors. Dobutamine has little or no effect on α-adrenoceptors. Unlike dopamine, it has no effect on the renal vasculature and does not directly increase urinary output.

Dobutamine has a very short plasma half-life (2–3 min) due to its rapid metabolism in the liver to inactive conjugates. The drug is therefore given by continuous intravenous infusion (normal dose range = 2.5–10 $\mu g\,kg^{-1}\,min^{-1}$, although doses up to 40 $\mu g\,kg^{-1}\,min^{-1}$ have been used). It is sometimes used in combination with renal doses of dopamine in the treatment of shock states with a low cardiac output (e.g. septic or cardiogenic shock). In these conditions, it may have a more selective inotropic action than dopamine, and cause a lesser increase in myocardial oxygen requirements.

Dobutamine is readily oxidized and is unstable in alkaline solutions (e.g. 8.4% sodium bicarbonate), and should not normally be mixed with other drugs.

Dopexamine

Dopexamine hydrochloride (an analogue of dopamine) is a potent β_2-adrenoceptor agonist and also acts on peripheral dopaminergic receptors (both D_1 and D_2). In contrast to dopamine, it has no α- and β_1-agonist activity, although it inhibits the neuronal uptake of noradrenaline (Uptake$_1$). Dopexamine has positive inotropic effects, due to its effects on cardiac β_2-adrenoceptors and the inhibition of Uptake$_1$ (which increases the effects of released noradrenaline at β_1-adrenoceptors). In addition, it produces vasodilatation by its effects on peripheral β_2-receptors. It is normally infused at rates of 0.5–6.0 $\mu g\,kg^{-1}\,min^{-1}$, and sometimes induces tachycardia or tachyarrhythmias.

Aminophylline

Dobutamine

---

[4] Monoamine oxidase type B is the main enzyme that breaks down dopamine in the CNS.

Aminophylline is a stable combination of theophylline and ethylenediamine, which is 20 times more water-soluble than the parent drug. Theophylline (a methylxanthine derivative) is a potent but non-specific inhibitor of all the isoforms of phosphodiesterase (Chapter 3), and many of its pharmacological effects are due to the accumulation of intracellular cAMP (and possibly cGMP). These changes affect Ca^{2+} translocation in smooth muscle and in the myocardium, producing smooth muscle relaxation and positive inotropic and chronotropic effects on the heart. Other less plausible but possible modes of action include blockade of adenosine receptors, or effects on the release and availability of endogenous catecholamines.

Aminophylline is a highly effective bronchodilator, and was widely used in the treatment of bronchospasm before the advent of β_2-selective agonists. It is now infrequently used in the treatment of acute asthmatic attacks. In anaesthetic practice, it is occasionally used to control bronchospasm induced by other drugs or procedures, or as a prophylactic measure in patients with a history of bronchospasm.

Aminophylline should be given by extremely slow intravenous injection (250–500 mg over 20 min) or as an infusion (500 μg kg^{-1} h^{-1}). Tachyarrhythmias and gastrointestinal disturbances are sometimes encountered. At high dose levels convulsions may occur, and plasma levels should be monitored if patients have been given oral theophylline.

Enoximone

Mode of action

Enoximone, a derivative of imidazoline, is a selective inhibitor of type III phosphodiesterase (PDE-III), which is principally present in the myocardium, smooth muscle and platelets. PDE-III ('cardiac PDE') is also inhibited by the accumulation of cGMP (Chapter 3), and normally breaks down both cAMP and cGMP. Conse-

quently, inhibition of the enzyme results in the accumulation of cAMP and cGMP in cardiac and smooth muscle cells, resulting in translocation of Ca^{2+}, positive inotropic effects and vasodilatation. In cardiac muscle, cAMP phosphorylates L-type calcium channels and phospholamban, resulting in increased Ca^+ entry during depolarization, and its enhanced release from the sarcoplasmic reticulum. In vascular smooth muscle cAMP phosphorylates protein kinase and myosin-light-chain kinase, resulting in vasodilatation. Since it acts on both cardiac and vascular smooth muscle, enoximone and other PDE-III inhibitors are sometimes known as 'inodilators'. Enoximone also increases platelet cAMP (by inhibition of platelet PDE) and prevents platelet aggregation.

Pharmacological effects

Enoximone increases cardiac output and contractility, and reduces ventricular filling pressure as well as systemic and pulmonary vascular resistance. The decrease in systemic vascular resistance can cause a fall in blood pressure, and the drug should be used with caution in hypotensive patients. Although tachycardia, ectopic beats and ventricular arrhythmias may occur, these are less marked than with catecholamines, and myocardial oxygen requirements are not significantly increased. Enoximone inhibits platelet aggregation (due to an increase in platelet cAMP), as well as suppressing intimal hyperplasia after endothelial injury and decreasing the formation of proinflammatory cytokines after cardiac surgery.

Clinical use

Enoximone is used in the treatment of congestive cardiac failure, particularly when ventricular filling pressure is increased, or when heart failure has proved refractory to treatment with other drugs (e.g. ACE inhibitors). Sustained haemodynamic and clinical benefits have been observed in patients treated for up to 48 hours, but there is no conclusive evidence of any reduction in mortality (indeed, in some circumstances increases in mortality have occurred). The use of enoximone may be associated with significant side effects, including tachyarrhythmias, hypotension, thrombocytopenia, nausea and vomiting, fever, oliguria and limb pain.

Enoximone is usually administered by slow intravenous infusion (initially 90 μg kg^{-1} min^{-1} for 10–30 min, followed by 5–20 μg kg^{-1} min^{-1}). The solution in ampoules is extremely alkaline (pH 12.0) and must be diluted before-hand and mixed in plastic syringes or infusion containers, as crystal formation has been observed when glass apparatus is used. The drug is mainly eliminated by the kidney as a sulphoxide metabolite, which has some inotropic activity. The elimination half-life of the parent drug is 4–7 hours in healthy volunteers, but is longer in patients with congestive cardiac failure.

Milrinone

Milrinone is a dipyridone derivative with similar actions and properties to enoximone that has been extensively used as an inodilator during and after cardiac surgery. It is also used for the short-term treatment of congestive cardiac failure in patients who fail to respond to standard therapy (e.g. with ACE inhibitors). Milrinone improves left ventricular function and causes widespread vasodilatation, in a similar manner to enoximone. It is usually given as a loading dose ($50 \ \mu g \ kg^{-1}$) followed by an intravenous infusion ($0.5 \ \mu g \ kg^{-1} \ min^{-1}$), which usually increases cardiac output.

Digoxin

Although they are not classified as autonomic drugs, digoxin and related cardiac glycosides have inotropic effects, and increase the force of myocardial contraction as well as reducing atrioventricular conduction. They have been used in the treatment of cardiac failure for over 250 years. Their inotropic action is dependent on the inhibition of membrane Na^+/K^+ ATPase in myocardial cells (Chapter 15). In these conditions, intracellular Na^+ is increased, and Na^+ entry during depolarization is reduced. Consequently, the activity of the Na^+/Ca^{2+} pump in the sarcolemmal membrane, which normally couples Na^+ entry to the active extrusion of Ca^{2+}, is reduced. In these conditions, the extrusion of Ca^{2+} by the Na^+/Ca^{2+} pump is limited and intracellular Ca^{2+} increases, thus increasing the force of myocardial contraction.

Ephedrine

Ephedrine is the active principle of a traditional Chinese drug (Ma Huang). Although it occurs naturally in *Ephedra vulgaris* (a member of the seascape genus), it is now usually synthesized. Although it has two chiral centres, only l-ephedrine and the racemic mixture have been used clinically.

Pharmacological effects

Ephedrine has α-, β_1- and β_2-effects on adrenergic receptors due to its direct and indirect sympathomimetic activity. It directly stimulates α_1- and β_2-receptors, but is also actively taken up by sympathetic nerve endings (Uptake$_1$) and displaces noradrenaline from its storage granules into the synapse, thus producing indirect α- and β_1-sympathomimetic effects. In addition, ephedrine also inhibits the intraneuronal metabolism of noradrenaline by mitochondrial MAO.

Ephedrine has similar effects to adrenaline, and usually increases heart rate, cardiac output, blood pressure and systemic vascular resistance. In addition, it occasionally causes attacks of supraventricular tachycardia. Although ephedrine relaxes bronchial smooth muscle, it increases the tone of the vesical sphincter, and may precipitate acute urinary retention. Its continuous use results in tachyphylaxis (rapid tolerance) to its effects, due to the depletion of noradrenaline stores in the synaptic vesicles of postganglionic sympathetic neurons. Ephedrine readily crosses the blood–brain barrier, and produces CNS stimulation.

Clinical use

Ephedrine (3–6 mg every 3–4 min, intravenously) is widely used in the treatment of hypotension produced by sympathetic blockade during spinal anaesthesia. Single intravenous doses last for several minutes, although the drug has a relatively long half-life (3–6 h). Although some tachycardia may occur, the combined α and β_2 effects do not usually affect uterine blood flow during obstetric anaesthesia, and are unlikely to compromise placental perfusion and foetal oxygenation. Nevertheless, ephedrine crosses the placenta, increasing foetal heart rate and catecholamine levels, and commonly causes slight foetal acidosis.

Ephedrine is also widely used as a nasal decongestant, and is sometimes of value in neuropathic postural hypotension (e.g. in autonomic diabetic neuropathy). Although it is still occasionally used in the treatment of bronchospasm, it may cause cardiac arrhythmias and is less suitable than many other drugs (e.g. selective β_2-receptor agonists). It has been used in the management of narcolepsy and nocturnal enuresis.

Amphetamines and related compounds (e.g. methylphenidate, phentermine) have peripheral actions, which are similar to ephedrine. Chronic administration of all indirectly acting sympathomimetic agents tends to produce tachyphylaxis, since they all cause the rapid depletion of noradrenaline from sympathetic nerve endings. In addition, they may produce hazardous drug interactions in patients who are receiving monoamine oxidase inhibitors.

Metaraminol

Metaraminol is a vasopressor drug with direct and indirect sympathomimetic effects. It directly stimulates α_1-adrenergic receptors, and also releases noradrenaline from synaptic vesicles in postganglionic sympathetic nerves. Metaraminol (15–100 mg, intravenously) is sometimes used in the treatment of untoward hypotension during anaesthesia, particularly after subarachnoid or extradural blockade or when ganglion-blocking drugs have been employed. It has a longer duration of action than ephedrine, and excessive vasopressor responses may cause a prolonged rise in blood pressure.

In the UK, it is not available as a proprietary preparation, but can be obtained on special order from regional hospital manufacturing units.

Phenylephrine

Phenylephrine is a close structural analogue of adrenaline and noradrenaline. It is a selective α_1-adrenoceptor agonist, but has little or no indirect sympathomimetic action. Consequently, its pharmacological effects are similar to noradrenaline, although its duration of action is longer. Phenylephrine is sometimes used as a vasopressor agent in acute hypotension after spinal anaesthesia (0.1–0.5 mg intravenously), although it may cause reflex bradycardia. It is also used as a mydriatic agent or a decongestant, and is sometimes incorporated into local anaesthetic solutions for topical use in ENT surgery (lidocaine with phenylephrine solution).

Ergotamine

Ergotamine has more than 300 times the affinity of noradrenaline for α-adrenoceptors. It acts as a partial agonist, and initially causes direct stimulation of smooth muscle. These agonist effects are usually followed by α-adrenoceptor antagonism. Ergotamine may also act on some 5-HT receptors.

In the past, ergotamine was widely used in the treatment of acute attacks of migraine. However, it is unpredictably absorbed after oral administration, and may cause nausea, vomiting and abdominal pain. It is sometimes used in combinations with other drugs (e.g. caffeine, cyclizine). In acute migraine, it has been largely superseded by 5-HT$_{1D}$ agonists (the 'triptans').

Prolonged administration of ergot alkaloids may produce symptoms of vascular insufficiency, and result in gangrene of the extremities. Marked effects on the CNS, including headache, loss of consciousness and convulsions, can also occur. Historically, endemic episodes of ergotism ('St Anthony's fire') have occurred after the ingestion of rye bread manufactured from grain contaminated with ergot fungus.

Ergometrine has powerful oxytocic activity, and is used in obstetrics to control postpartum bleeding. It has considerably less effect on vascular smooth muscle than ergotamine (either as a partial agonist or as an antagonist). Ergometrine should be administered with special care to hypertensive patients or those with pre-existing cardiac disease.

Selective β_2-adrenoceptor agonists

Selective β_2-adrenoceptor agonists are used in the treatment of bronchospasm. They have relatively specific effects on β_2-adrenoceptors in bronchial smooth muscle, but little or no direct effect on the heart. Tachycardia and palpitations occasionally occur (particularly after systemic administration), and probably reflect direct effects on cardiac β_2-receptors, rather than a reflex response to vasodilatation. These effects may be enhanced in cardiac failure, when there is a relative preponderance of β_2-adrenoceptors.

All β_2-adrenoceptor agonists, including adrenaline and isoprenaline, may cause hypokalaemia, due to stimulation of membrane bound Na^+/K^+ ATPase and increased K^+ uptake by skeletal muscle. There is some evidence that hypokalaemia may be a contributory factor in the occurrence of cardiac arrhythmias induced by sympathomimetic amines.

Salbutamol

```
                             ,--- Chiral centre
                            /
HO — CH₂              CH — CH₂ — NH
              ⬡                    |
HO                   OH    CH₃ — C — CH₃
                                  |
                                 CH₃
```

Salbutamol can be given orally, by injection, by inhalation or as a nebulized solution. Salbutamol may be given as a bolus dose (250 μg, intravenously) or by continuous infusion (3–20 μg min^{-1}) in the treatment of severe bronchospasm. Alternatively, salbutamol may be administered in severe asthmatic states as a respirator solution through a suitably driven nebulizer.

Terbutaline

Terbutaline is a β_2-receptor agonist with similar effects to salbutamol. It is sometimes used as a prodrug (bambuterol).

Long-acting β_2-receptor agonists

Salmeterol and formoterol are longer acting β_2-receptor agonists that are normally given twice daily with inhaled corticosteroids. They are used in the long-term management of chronic asthma and obstructive airway disease.

Myometrial relaxants

β_2-Adrenoceptor agonists relax uterine smooth muscle, and some of them, particularly ritodrine, salbutamol and terbutaline, are given by continuous infusion to inhibit premature labour between 24 and 33 weeks gestation. These drugs cause tremor and nervous tension, although it is not clear whether these are central or peripheral side effects.

Antagonists of sympathetic activity

The activity of the sympathetic nervous system can be inhibited or modified by various drugs, including
• centrally acting agents
• drugs that block autonomic ganglia
• drugs that block adrenergic neurons
• α-adrenoceptor antagonists
• β-adrenoceptor antagonists
Most of these drugs reduce peripheral resistance or decrease cardiac output, and have been used in the treatment of essential hypertension (Chapter 14).

Centrally acting agents

The activity of noradrenergic pathways in the CNS can modify peripheral sympathetic responses. Central pathways in the hypothalamus, the nucleus tractus solitarius, and the cardioaccelerator and vasomotor centres in the medulla are under the modulatory control of α_2-adrenoceptors (an example of an autoinhibitory negative feedback system). Both clonidine and methyldopa reduce blood pressure by their agonist or partial agonist effects on central noradrenergic neurons. Similarly moxonidine decreases blood pressure by its agonist effects on central imidazoline receptors, which reduces central noradrenergic tone (Chapter 14).

Drugs that block autonomic ganglia

Drugs in this group (e.g. pempidine, mecamylamine) occlude ion channels in nicotinic acetylcholine receptors on the postsynaptic membrane of ganglion cells. These agents produce indiscriminate blockade of both sympathetic and parasympathetic ganglia, and at one time were widely used in the treatment of hypertension. However, due to their many disadvantages, the clinical use of these agents is now obsolete.

In the past, the ganglion-blocking drug trimetaphan was sometimes used to produce controlled hypotension in operative surgery, but is not currently available in the UK.

Drugs that block adrenergic neurons

Drugs acting in this manner are transported into adrenergic neurons by Uptake$_1$ (page 254), and then interfere with the intraneuronal storage of catecholamines. At the present time, only guanethidine is available in the UK. It is only occasionally used as an antihypertensive agent.

Guanethidine

Guanethidine is transported into sympathetic nerve endings by Uptake$_1$, and then taken up by synaptic vesicles, where it prevents the storage and release of noradrenaline by competing for granular binding sites. Since guanethidine is actively transported by the adrenergic neuron, its uptake is antagonized by other drugs that are transported by Uptake$_1$ (e.g. tricyclic antidepressants, phenothiazines, cocaine, ephedrine). Guanethidine lowers blood pressure by depleting the store of noradrenaline in synaptic vesicles, and thus reduces the amount that is available for release by nerve impulses. Paradoxically, after rapid intravenous injection it may cause hypertension and acute sympathomimetic effects, due to the displacement of stored noradrenaline. At one time, guanethidine was extensively used in the treatment of hypertension, although it is now only occasionally used for this purpose (Chapter 14).

α-Adrenoceptor antagonists

α-Adrenoceptor antagonists combine with α-adrenoceptors, and prevent or inhibit the sympathetic responses that are mediated by them. They can be divided into three groups:
- Non-selective α-adrenoceptor antagonists
- Selective α_1 adrenoceptor antagonists
- Selective α_2-adrenoceptor antagonists

Non-selective α-adrenoceptor antagonists

Drugs in this group block both α_1- and α_2-receptors, and may also inhibit pharmacological responses to other transmitters (e.g. histamine, 5-HT). Since they produce blockade of presynaptic α_2-adrenoceptors, they increase the physiological release of noradrenaline from sympathetic neurons (page 254). Although postsynaptic α_1-

adrenoceptors are also blocked, β_1- and β_2-receptors are unaffected. This results in an enhanced response to the β-effects of released noradrenaline, producing tachycardia and postural hypotension. Consequently, non-selective α-adrenoceptor antagonists are of little value in patients with essential hypertension. Nevertheless, they may control blood pressure in patients with secondary hypertension that is associated with high levels of circulating catecholamines.

Phentolamine

Phentolamine is a reversible antagonist at α-adrenoceptors, and has a short duration of action (usually 5–10 min). It may be used in the management of hypertensive episodes during the surgical removal of phaeochromocytomata. It may also be used to ablate sympathetic responses to anaesthesia and surgery in uncontrolled hypertensive patients.

Phenoxybenzamine

Phenoxybenzamine is an irreversible antagonist that forms covalent bonds with α-adrenoceptors, so that the effects of single doses can last for at least several days. The restoration of normal responsiveness to α-adrenoceptor agonists is dependent on the synthesis of new receptors. Phenoxybenzamine is used in the preoperative preparation of patients with phaeochromocytoma, and in their long-term management when surgery is precluded. In the past, it has been used to improve peripheral perfusion in shocked states, particularly when combined with an inotropic agent. Dopamine antagonists (e.g. phenothiazines, butyrophenones) are also α_1-adrenoceptor antagonists and have been used for similar purposes.

Labetalol

Labetalol is a non-selective α-adrenoceptor antagonist that also produces β-adrenoceptor blockade (Table 13.4). It is sometimes used in the treatment of hypertension (Chapter 14).

Carvedilol is a β-adrenoreceptor antagonist that also blocks α-receptors in a non-selective manner.

Selective α_1-adrenoceptor antagonists

Selective α_1-adrenoceptor antagonists (e.g. doxazosin, prazosin) are sometimes used with other drugs in the treatment of essential hypertension (Chapter 14). In addition to blocking postsynaptic α_1-adrenoceptors, they also have vasodilator properties. In addition, they have been used in the treatment of urinary outflow obstruction in benign

Table 13.4 Properties of β-adrenoceptor antagonists.

Drug	β_1/β_2 selectivity	Partial agonist activity (intrinsic sympathomimetic activity)	Na$^+$ channel blockade (local anaesthetic activity)
Acebutolol	<20	+	+
Atenolol	75	−	−
Bisoprolol	119	−	−
Carvedilol*	<10	−	−
Celiprolol†	<10	+	+/−
Esmolol	70	−	−
Labetalol*	<10	+/−	+
Metoprolol	74	−	+/−
Nadolol	<10	−	−
Nebivolol	293	−	−
Oxprenolol	<10	+	+
Pindolol	<10	++	+/−
Propranolol	<10	−	++
Sotalol	<10	−	−
Timolol	none	+/−	−

* Carvedilol and labetalol are also α-adrenoceptor antagonists.

† Celiprolol also has partial β₂-agonist activity.

(−), no effect; (+/−), minimal effect; (+), moderate effect; (++), marked effect.

prostatic hyperplasia. Tamsulosin is an α_1-adrenoceptor antagonist that may have selective effects on α_1-receptors in vesical muscles.

Selective α_2-adrenoceptor antagonists

Yohimbine and idazoxan are selective α_2-adrenoceptor antagonists that block hypotensive responses to the α_2-agonist clonidine.

β-Adrenoceptor antagonists

β-Adrenoceptor antagonists inhibit the β-effects of adrenaline and noradrenaline on the heart and smooth muscle, as well as some of their metabolic effects. Their effects depend on the degree of sympathetic tone, and in resting conditions they may have little or no effect (particularly in the young). In contrast, when sympathetic tone is raised they often cause

• bradycardia
• prolonged AV conduction
• decreased cardiac contractility
• decreased cardiac output
• decreased coronary blood flow
• reduced myocardial oxygen consumption

In susceptible patients, they may induce heart block and cardiac failure.

Many β-adrenoceptor antagonists are used in clinical practice for the treatment of various cardiovascular disorders, particularly hypertension, angina and cardiac arrhythmias. Propranolol was the first β-adrenoceptor antagonist that was used, although at least 15 of these drugs are now used clinically (Table 13.4).

Non-selective β-adrenoceptor antagonists

The majority of β-adrenoceptor antagonists have non-selective effects at both β₁- and β₂-receptors. β₂-Adrenoceptor blockade may be responsible for some of the unwanted effects of these drugs, such as the occurrence of bronchospasm and symptoms of peripheral vascular insufficiency. Non-selective antagonists may also reduce blood glucose and potentiate the effects of other hypoglycaemic drugs.

Selective β_1-adrenoceptor antagonists

Other β-adrenoceptor antagonists are relatively selective and only block β₁-adrenoceptors in the heart and certain other tissues, e.g. juxtaglomerular cells in the kidney. Cardioselective β₁-adrenoceptor antagonists are usually preferred when therapy is required in patients with bronchial asthma, insulin-dependent diabetes and peripheral vascular disease. Nevertheless, the β₁-selectivity of antagonists

Table 13.5 The pharmacokinetics and elimination of some β-adrenoceptor antagonists.

Drug	Lipid solubility	Absorption (%)	Bioavailability (%)	Protein binding (%)	Terminal half-life (h)	Elimination
Acebutolol*	moderate	100	40	80	3	M
Atenolol	low	50	45	3	6	R
Bisoprolol	low	100	90	50	18	M & R
Carvedilol	high	100	25	98	8	M
Celiprolol	low	100	50	50	12	M & R
Esmolol	high	N/A	N/A	N/A	0.13	M
Labetalol	high	100	50	50	4	M & R
Metoprolol	high	90	50	98	10	M
Nadolol	low	30	30	30	22	R
Nebivolol	moderate	90	50	80	12	M
Oxprenolol	high	80	50	80	2	M
Pindolol	moderate	90	90	40	4	M & R
Propranolol*	high	100	20	90	5	M
Sotalol	low	100	90	0	15	R
Timolol	high	90	70	10	4	M

*Drugs with active metabolites: M, mainly eliminated by metabolism; R, mainly eliminated by renal excretion of unchanged drug; M & R, eliminated by both metabolism and renal excretion; N/A, not applicable.

is relative rather than absolute, and these drugs can cause bronchospasm or peripheral vascular insufficiency in susceptible patients.

Partial agonist activity

Some β-adrenoceptor antagonists have partial agonist activity or 'intrinsic sympathomimetic activity' (Table 13.4). They may cause less bradycardia, or even a mild tachycardia (due to their agonist effects), but also protect the heart from excessive sympathetic activity (due to their antagonist effects). They may be less likely than other β-adrenoceptor antagonists to induce severe bradyarrhythmias or cardiac failure. Nevertheless, their advantages in clinical practice are unclear.

Local anaesthetic activity

β-Adrenergic antagonists may also block Na^+ channels in myocardial cells ('local anaesthetic' or 'membrane-stabilizing' effects, Table 13.4). These drugs decrease the rate of depolarization and increase the refractory period of cardiac muscle. Experimental studies suggest that these effects are only produced by extremely high doses of β-antagonists, and are of little clinical significance.

Lipid solubility

The pharmacokinetic properties of β-adrenoceptor antagonists are mainly determined by their lipid solubility. Highly lipid-soluble agents are well absorbed after oral administration but are subject to significant first pass effects due to hepatic metabolism (Table 13.5). Consequently, their bioavailability is susceptible to numerous factors, including pharmacogenetic influences, liver disease and concomitant therapy with other drugs. Lipid-soluble β-adrenoceptor antagonists usually have a short terminal half-life and are extensively bound by plasma proteins. They also readily cross the blood–brain barrier, and may produce central side effects such as sedation, sleep disturbances and bizarre dreams. They may also cross the placenta, and cause foetal bradycardia and hypoglycaemia.

In contrast, water-soluble β-adrenoceptor antagonists are less absorbed from the gut, but are susceptible to first-pass metabolism. They have longer terminal half-lives, are predominantly eliminated by the kidney, and may cumulate in renal failure. In addition, they do not readily cross the blood–brain or placental barriers, so that effects on the CNS or the foetus are unlikely.

Clinical uses

β-Adrenoceptor antagonists are widely used in the treatment of hypertension (Chapter 14). They are also used in angina pectoris and certain tachyarrhythmias that are related to abnormal catecholamine activity, such as those induced by exercise, emotion or thyrotoxicosis (Chapter 15). In almost all cases, their beneficial effects are due to β_1-adrenoceptor blockade.

Other less common uses of β-adrenoceptor antagonists include the control of the peripheral responses to stress, the management of pathological anxiety states, the prophylaxis of migraine and the treatment of schizophrenia. Some drugs in this group (e.g. timolol, betaxolol) are also used as topical preparations in the treatment of chronic simple glaucoma. Intraocular pressure is reduced by a mechanism which is not entirely clear but probably involves a reduction in the rate of production of aqueous humour.

Drugs have been developed which exhibit selective antagonism at β_2-adrenoceptors (e.g. butoxamine, α-methylpropranol), although they are unlikely to achieve a clinical role.

Suggested reading

Ahlquist, R.R. (1948) A study of the adrenergic receptors. *American Journal of Physiology* **153**, 586–600.

Barnett, D.B. (1948) Myocardial β-adrenoceptor function and regulation in heart failure: implications for therapy. *British Journal of Clinical Pharmacology* **27**, 527–538.

Boldt, J., Knothe, C., Zickmann, B., *et al.* (1992) The role of enoximone in cardiac surgery. *British Journal of Anaesthesia* **69**, 45–50.

Craven, J. (2005) The autonomic nervous system, sympathetic chain and stellate ganglion. *Anaesthesia and Intensive Care Medicine* **6**, 37–38.

Goldberg, L.I. (1974) Dopamine – clinical uses of an endogenous catecholamine. *New England Journal of Medicine* **291**, 707–710.

Goyal, R.K. (1989) Muscarinic receptor subtypes: physiology and clinical implications. *New England Journal of Medicine* **321**, 1022–1029.

Guinmaraes, S. & Moura, D. (2001) Vascular adrenoceptors: an update. *Pharmacological Reviews* **53**, 319–356.

Handy, J.M. & Cordingley, J. (2003) Postoperative cardiac intensive care. *Anaesthesia and Intensive Care Medicine* **4**, 258–261.

Hayashi, Y. & Maze, M. (1993) Alpha$_2$ adrenoceptor agonists and anaesthesia. *British Journal of Anaesthesia* **71**, 108–118.

Hieble, I.P., Bondinell, W.E. & Ruffolo, R.R. (1995) α- and β-adrenoceptors; from the gene to the clinic. 1. Molecular biology and adrenoceptor subclassification. *Journal of Medicinal Chemistry* **38**, 3415–3444.

Hulme, E.C., Birdsall, N.J.M. & Buckley, N.J. (1990) Muscarinic receptor subtypes. *Annual Review of Pharmacology and Toxicology* **30**, 633–673.

Insel, P.A. (1996) Adrenergic receptors – evolving concepts and clinical implications. *New England Journal of Medicine* **334**, 580–585.

Kilbinger, H. (1984) Presynaptic muscarinic receptors modulating acetylcholine release. *Trends in Pharmacological Sciences* **5**, 103–105.

Langer, S.Z. & Hicks, P.E. (1984) Physiology of the sympathetic nerve ending. *British Journal of Anaesthesia* **56**, 689–700.

Liu, Y. & Edwards, R.H. (1997) The role of vesicular transport proteins in synaptic transmission and neural degeneration. *Annual Review of Neurosciences* **20**, 125–156.

Pleuvry, B.J. (2005) Drugs affecting the autonomic nervous system. *Anaesthesia and Intensive Care Medicine* **6**, 34–36.

Ruffolo, R.R. (1987) The pharmacology of dobutamine. *American Journal of Medical Sciences* **294**, 244–248.

Ruffolo, R.R., Bondinell, W. & Hieble, J.P. (1995) α- and β-adrenoceptors; from the gene to the clinic. 2. Structure–activity relationships and therapeutic applications. *Journal of Medicinal Chemistry* **38**, 3681–3716.

Saravanan, S., Kocarev, M., Wilson, R.C., Watkins, E., Columb, M.O. & Lyons, G. (2006) Equivalent dose of ephedrine and phenylephrine in the prevention of post-spinal hypotension in Caesarean section. *British Journal of Anaesthesia* **96**, 95–99.

Small, R. (2001) Pharmacological modulation of myocardial function, vascular resistance and blood pressure: drugs used during cardiopulmonary resuscitation. *Anaesthesia and Intensive Care Medicine* **2**, 34–39.

Starke, K., Gothert, M. & Kilbinger, H. (1989) Modulation of neurotransmitter release by presynaptic autoreceptors. *Physiological Reviews* **69**, 864–989.

Stephan, H., Sonntag, H., Henning, H. & Yoshimine, K. (1990) Cardiovascular and renal haemodynamic effects of dopexamine: comparison with dopamine. *British Journal of Anaesthesia* **65**, 380–387.

Summers, R.J. & McMartin, L.R. (1993) Adrenoceptors and their second messenger systems. *Journal of Neurochemistry* **60**, 10–23.

Zaugg, M., Schaub, M.C., Pasch, T. & Spahn, D.R. (2002) Modulation of β-adrenergic receptor subtype activities in perioperative medicine: mechanisms and sites of action. *British Journal of Anaesthesia* **88**, 101–123.

14 Antihypertensive Agents: Drugs that Are Used to Induce Hypotension

Although hypertension has been recognized as a disease for more than a century, effective treatment has only been generally available during the past five decades. Before this time, treatment was mainly directed to patients with the most severe forms of the disease. The remedies that were used included prolonged bed rest, the use of sedative drugs and surgical attempts to extirpate the sympathetic nervous system.

Treatment of hypertension

Blood pressure is a continuously distributed physiological variable, and there is no individual value that marks the transition between normal and hypertensive states. In current practice, treatment is usually considered when values are consistently greater than 140/90 (particularly in diabetic patients). It is generally accepted that specific therapy aimed at reducing systolic and diastolic levels will decrease the morbidity and mortality that results from the disease. In particular, large-scale studies have demonstrated that the incidence of renal complications, haemorrhagic stroke and cardiac failure is diminished, and that myocardial infarction is less likely. Before specific antihypertensive therapy is initiated, the use of non-specific measures should be encouraged, including the cessation of smoking and excessive alcohol consumption, the reduction of weight and salt intake, and regular appropriate exercise. The existence of related diseases should also be excluded (particularly diabetes mellitus and hypercholesterolaemia), since their effective treatment may significantly improve the control of hypertension. It is now accepted that elderly subjects with hypertension should be treated as well as the young, and that the benefits of treatment can be demonstrated up to the age of 85.

The immediate treatment of hypertension is essential when blood pressure levels greater than 200 mm Hg systolic and 110 mm Hg diastolic are consistently present. With lesser degrees of hypertension, the decision when to commence therapy is usually determined by the presence of cardiovascular complications or of end-organ damage (e.g. renal impairment, retinal changes). However, drug treatment is always indicated if the mean systolic pressures is above 160 mm Hg and diastolic pressure is above 100 mm Hg over a period of 3–6 months. Isolated systolic hypertension is common in elderly patients, and its treatment results in a significant reduction in the incidence of cardiac and cerebrovascular complications.

In all patients with hypertension, the regular assessment of blood pressure is essential, and the use of 24-hour ambulatory monitoring devices is an invaluable adjunct in milder forms of hypertension. 'White-coat hypertension' occurs in approximately 20% of patients, and may be an important factor in preoperative assessment.

Causes of hypertension

In a minority of cases (5–10%), hypertension is secondary to an identifiable and sometimes curable cause. Secondary hypertension is commoner in younger patients, and may be due to

- renal disease (e.g. renal artery stenosis)
- endocrine disease (e.g. acromegaly, phaeochromocytomata, carcinoid tumours, Cushing's disease and hyperaldosteronism)
- congenital abnormalities (e.g. coarctation of the aorta)
- drug abuse (e.g. cocaine dependence)

In contrast, in most hypertensive patients the precise cause is unknown (essential hypertension), although excessive alcohol consumption and obesity may be contributory factors. It is believed that physiological or biochemical

271

factors may lead to morphological changes in the arteriolar wall, resulting in increased peripheral resistance and a subsequent rise in blood pressure.

Role of electrolytic changes

It has been suggested that imprecisely defined changes in Na^+, K^+ or Ca^{2+} balance in arteriolar walls may have a causal relationship with essential hypertension. Increased salt intake may lead to plasma volume expansion and hypertension, although normal Na^+ balance is usually maintained by an intact renin–angiotensin–aldosterone system. Consequently, therapeutic regimes involving drastic reductions in salt intake have been widely used in the past, but usually produce little or no long-term benefit. Nevertheless, in some individuals a substantial reduction in sodium intake produces a modest fall in blood pressure, and patients who modify their diet while taking antihypertensive therapy often achieve sustained periods of normotension. In some instances, unidentified genetic mutations in the renin–angiotensin–aldosterone system may lead to increased Na^+ reabsorption, or the presence of an endogenous ouabain-like compound may inhibit the Na^+ pump (Na^+/K^+-ATPase).

There is also some evidence that increased K^+ intake and Ca^{2+} supplementation may produce beneficial effects in hypertensive patients, and that the dietary intake of Mg^{2+} may be an important factor.

Role of endogenous transmitters

Endogenous transmitters may have an important role in the control of peripheral resistance. Endothelin-1 (ET-1) promotes vasoconstrictor tone via ET_A-receptors on vascular smooth muscle. Endothelin receptors (ET_A and ET_B) are activated by endogenous peptides (ET-1, ET-2 and ET-3), and these may play an important part in the control of vascular resistance and are linked to the synthesis of prostaglandins and nitric oxide. Experimental studies with ET_A-receptor antagonists produce effective hypotensive responses in animal models of hypertension, and increase peripheral blood flow in human volunteers. The presence of nitric oxide ('endothelium-derived relaxant factor'), which has both vasodilator and antiproliferative effects in the vascular bed, may be significant.

Physiological and pharmacological factors

Arterial blood pressure is determined by the cardiac output and the impedance of the resistance vessels (mainly arterioles), and is maintained by the efficiency of both the sympathetic nervous system and the renin–angiotensin–

Table 14.1 Site and mode of action of antihypertensive agents in current use.
Inhibitors of sympathetic nervous system activity
• Centrally acting drugs
• Adrenergic neuron-blocking agents
• α-Adrenoceptor antagonists
• β-Adrenoceptor antagonists
Inhibitors of the renin–angiotensin–aldosterone system
• $β_1$-Adrenoceptor antagonists (inhibitors of renin secretion)
• Angiotensin-converting-enzyme inhibitors
• Angiotensin II receptor antagonists
• Aldosterone antagonists
Peripheral vasodilators
• Dihydropyridine calcium antagonists
• Hydralazine
• Thiazide diuretics

aldosterone system. Pharmacological methods of reducing blood pressure may involve the modification of these physiological pathways at various sites. Drugs that directly relax vascular smooth muscle or alter vessel wall compliance by effects on extracellular fluid volume are effective antihypertensive agents. In some instances, drugs also affect capacitance vessels and reduce venous return and cardiac output, or have negative inotropic or chronotropic effects on the heart. The sites of action of the various drugs employed in the treatment of hypertension are shown in Table 14.1, although it must be emphasized that this physiological classification is not related to their practical importance. In this chapter, drugs used in the treatment of hypertension are discussed in the sequence:

(1) Diuretics

(2) β-Adrenoceptor antagonists

(3) Drugs affecting the renin–angiotensin–aldosterone system

(4) Vasodilators

(5) α-Adrenoceptor antagonists

(6) Centrally acting drugs

(7) Other antihypertensive drugs

Diuretics

Thiazide diuretics

Thiazide diuretics are acidic compounds that are structurally related to the sulphonamides, and are commonly used in the long-term management of oedema associated with congestive cardiac failure, hepatic cirrhosis and the nephrotic syndrome.

Mechanism of diuretic action

Although thiazides are actively secreted in the proximal tubule, their principal site of action is the distal renal tubule, where they inhibit the reabsorption of Na^+ and Cl^- by combining with the Cl^- cotransporter. Thiazide diuretics increase K^+ loss, since they cause excessive Na^+/K^+ exchange at the aldosterone sensitive site in the collecting tubule, and increase the intracellular–luminal K^+ gradient. The elimination of Mg^{2+} is also increased, while Ca^{2+} and urate excretion is reduced. Supplementation with potassium salts is sometimes necessary during continuous thiazide therapy. In addition, long-term use of thiazide diuretics may impair insulin secretion and cause hyperglycaemia, resulting in diabetes mellitus.

Antihypertensive effects

Thiazide diuretics initially reduce blood pressure by decreasing plasma volume due to the enhanced renal elimination of water and electrolytes. However, their antihypertensive effects are attained at doses far lower than those required to produce significant loss of free water, Na^+ or K^+. It is now recognized that thiazide diuretics activate K_{ATP} channels, resulting in the hyperpolarization of vascular smooth muscle. In addition, they may affect intracellular Na^+/K^+ balance. Consequently, the thiazides are peripheral vasodilators, and increase vascular compliance in hypertension.

Bendrofluazide

Bendrofluazide (bendroflumethiazide) is the most important and widely used thiazide in the control of mild and moderate hypertension. Other thiazide diuretics and their related analogues are less commonly used, and have no significant clinical advantages. After oral administration, bendrofluazide acts within 1–2 hours and lasts for 18–24 hours, and conventional doses (2.5 mg, daily) cause little or no electrolyte or metabolic disturbance. The use of low-dose regimes is safe and effective, and many of the classical side effects of thiazides, such as hypokalaemia, urate retention, hyperglycaemia and dyslipidaemia, are extremely uncommon. Bendrofluazide enhances the effects of other antihypertensive drugs, and is commonly combined with other agents that have different mechanisms of action.

Most non-steroidal anti-inflammatory drugs decrease the synthesis of vasodilator prostaglandins by afferent arterioles, and may interfere with the diuretic and antihypertensive effects of bendrofluazide and other thiazides.

Other diuretics

Loop diuretics

Loop diuretics (e.g. furosemide, bumetanide) are extremely potent diuretics with a relatively short duration of action. They are highly protein-bound drugs and are secreted by the proximal renal tubule, but act on the $Na^+/K^+/2Cl^-$ cotransporter in the ascending limb of the loop of Henle. Loop diuretics usually increase renal blood flow and the glomerular filtration fraction, and are often used to produce rapid diuresis in severe cardiac failure, as well as pulmonary and cerebral oedema. They are also valuable when administered with blood transfusions in severe anaemia, particularly when cardiac failure due to fluid overloading is anticipated. Loop diuretics are not normally used in the treatment of hypertension.

Potassium-sparing diuretics

Potassium-sparing diuretics have a mild diuretic action, but are frequently used to prevent hypokalaemia associated with thiazide or loop diuretic therapy. They either act directly on the collecting tubule (e.g. triamterene, amiloride), or competitively inhibit the action of aldosterone on distal tubular cells (e.g. spironolactone, eplerenone). Aldosterone normally acts in the distal renal tubule, promoting Na^+ reabsorption in exchange for K^+ (and H^+) excretion.

Carbonic anhydrase inhibitors

Carbonic anhydrase inhibitors are now rarely used as diuretic agents. However, they reduce bicarbonate production and the secretion of aqueous humour, and are sometimes used to reduce intraocular pressure in glaucoma.

Osmotic diuretics

Mannitol

$$CH_2OH$$
$$|$$
$$(HCOH)_4$$
$$|$$
$$CH_2OH$$

Mannitol is the only osmotic diuretic in current use, and in contrast to other agents it commonly produces a moderate increase in blood pressure after administration. It is a poly-hydric alcohol with a molecular weight of about 200, and is usually synthesized by reduction of the monosaccharide mannose. After intravenous administration, mannitol is widely distributed throughout the vascular bed and interstitial tissues, and its volume of distribution (200 mL kg^{-1}) usually reflects extracellular fluid volume. Mannitol is pharmacologically inert, but is freely filtered by the renal glomerulus and is not significantly reabsorbed. When administered as a hypertonic infusion (usually 50 g as a 10% or 20% solution, given over 20 min) it produces a rapid diuresis due to its osmotic effects, since it reduces water and electrolyte reabsorption in the renal tubule. Mannitol is used in the prophylaxis of renal failure, during aortic aneurysm surgery, or during operations in the presence of severe jaundice, in the treatment of cerebral oedema and glaucoma, and to promote forced diuresis in cases of drug overdose.

β-Adrenoceptor antagonists

Although β-adrenoceptor antagonists have been used in the treatment of hypertension for over 40 years, their mode of action is unclear. A number of possible explanations have been advanced, for example:
- Reduction in cardiac output due to β-adrenoceptor blockade.
- Resetting of carotid and aortic baroreceptors.
- Inhibition of renin secretion and the renin–angiotensin–aldosterone system (particularly in patients with high plasma renin activity).
- Presynaptic inhibition of noradrenaline release from sympathetic nerve terminals.
- Effects on the CNS. In experimental conditions, hypotensive responses are produced after the intraventricular injection of β-adrenoceptor antagonists.

It seems probable that the antihypertensive effects of β-adrenoceptor antagonists are due to their actions on the CNS and to their effects on the renin–angiotensin system. The release of renin from the juxtaglomerular apparatus is controlled by β$_1$-adrenoceptors, and is inhibited by most antagonists. Hypertensive patients with high plasma renin activity are usually controlled with low doses of β-adrenoceptor antagonists.

Most currently available β-adrenoceptor antagonists (Table 13.4) have been used in the treatment of hypertension. Although propranolol was the first drug that was widely employed for this purpose, it is now used less frequently.

Propranolol

Propranolol is a non-selective β-adrenoceptor antagonist with no partial agonist activity (intrinsic sympathomimetic activity). It is now considered to be less suitable than atenolol as an antihypertensive agent.

Some of the undesirable effects of propranolol are due to blockade at β$_2$-receptors, for example bronchospasm, peripheral vasoconstriction, and hypoglycaemia. Consequently, selective antagonists (e.g. atenolol) are usually preferred.

Propranolol is a highly lipid-soluble and extensively protein-bound drug. Because of its lipid-solubility, it readily crosses the blood–brain barrier and may cause central side effects, including sedation, sleep disturbances and bizarre dreams. Propranolol also crosses the placenta and may cause foetal bradycardia and hypoglycaemia.

Atenolol

Atenolol is a selective β$_1$-adrenoceptor antagonist, with no partial agonist activity or intrinsic sympathomimetic activity. Consequently, it is unlikely to produce problems due to β$_2$-adrenoceptor blockade. Atenolol is a relatively polar (water-soluble) drug that is only partly absorbed from the intestine (50%), but is poorly metabolized and has little or no first-pass effect. Although it has a relatively short half-life (about 6 h), single doses act for up to 24 hours, and it is mainly eliminated unchanged in urine. Because of its poor lipid-solubility, it does not cross the blood–brain barrier or the placenta readily, and only rarely causes central side effects.

Atenolol has been used in the treatment of hypertension. Bisoprolol, celiprolol and nebivolol are related drugs that have similar advantages.

β-Adrenoceptor antagonists are also discussed in Chapters 13 and 15.

Drugs affecting the renin–angiotensin–aldosterone system

The renin–angiotensin system plays an important part in the regulation of vascular tone. It also controls the secretion of aldosterone, which has a modulatory effect on sodium balance and fluid retention.

Renin secretion

Renin is a proteolytic enzyme that is synthesized by cells in the juxtaglomerular apparatus of afferent arterioles in the renal cortex. It is secreted in response to three physiological stimuli (Fig. 14.1):

• Arteriolar pressure: a decrease in renal perfusion pressure reduces the tension in the wall of the afferent arteriole, and causes the release of renin.
• Sodium concentration: a decrease in Na^+ concentration in the macula densa in the distal tubule increases renin secretion from the adjacent juxtaglomerular apparatus.
• Neurogenic factors: stimulation of nerves in the renal plexus causes the secretion of renin. This secretomotor effect is mediated by efferent sympathetic nerves, resulting in the release of noradrenaline and activation of β_1-adrenoceptors.

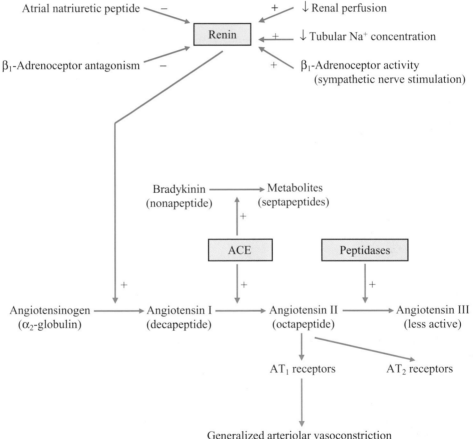

Fig. 14.1 The physiological regulation of the renin–angiotensin–aldosterone system. ACE, angiotensin-converting enzyme; AT_1, angiotensin-1 receptors; AT_2, angiotensin-2 receptors; + facilitatory pathways; − inhibitory pathways. The boxes correspond to enzymes.

Formation of angiotensin II

After its release, renin acts on a plasma α_2-globulin (angiotensinogen) and splits off a terminal decapeptide (angiotensin I), which has little or no activity. However, the decapeptide angiotensin I is rapidly converted to the octapeptide angiotensin II by angiotensin-converting-enzyme (ACE or kininase II), which also inactivates bradykinin and various other biologically active peptides. ACE is mainly present in vascular endothelium (particularly in the lung, but also in most other tissues). Angiotensin II has an extremely short half-life, and is rapidly broken down by various aminopeptidases to other peptides (angiotensin III and angiotensin IV).

Angiotensin receptors

The actions of angiotensin II, which is a highly potent pressor amine, are mediated by two distinct types of receptors (Fig. 14.1). AT_1-receptors are more numerous than AT_2-receptors, and have a higher affinity for angiotensin II. They mediate most of the effects of angiotensin II, and are linked to GTP-binding proteins (G_q) and phosphoinositide metabolism (Chapter 3). In contrast, effects at AT_2-receptors are mediated by tyrosine phosphorylation in proteins, and may have an important role in physiological processes such as cell growth and differentiation.

The effects of angiotensin II that are mediated by AT_1-receptors include:
• generalized arteriolar vasoconstriction
• release of catecholamines from the adrenal medulla
• release of noradrenaline from sympathetic nerve endings
• facilitation of transmission in autonomic ganglia
• secretion of aldosterone by the zona glomerulosa cells in the adrenal cortex

Inhibition of the renin–angiotensin–aldosterone system

The renin–angiotensin–aldosterone system can be inhibited at several sites and by different mechanisms (Fig. 14.2). The four main types of physiological or pharmacological inhibitors are
• Inhibitors of renin secretion
• Angiotensin-converting-enzyme inhibitors (ACE inhibitors)
• Angiotensin receptor antagonists
• Aldosterone antagonists

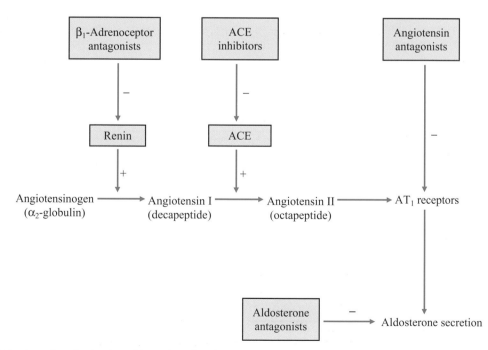

Fig. 14.2 The site and mode of action of drugs that affect the renin–angiotensin–aldosterone system. ACE, angiotensin-converting enzyme; AT_1, angiotensin-1 receptors; + facilitatory pathways; − inhibitory pathways.

Inhibitors of renin secretion

The secretion of renin is inhibited by atrial natriuretic peptide (ANP), a hormone that is stored in an inactivated form by atrial myocytes (Fig. 14.1). ANP decreases the formation or release of angiotensin II and aldosterone, as well as other hormones (endothelin, antidiuretic hormone). The rate of secretion of ANP is dependent on atrial wall tension, and levels are raised after blood volume expansion, and in congestive cardiac failure and renal impairment. ANP increases both the glomerular filtration rate and the fractional excretion of Na^+, and experimental evidence suggests that it is a vasodilator with selective effects on arterioles.

The antihypertensive effects of β-adrenoceptor antagonists may be partly due to inhibition of renin secretion, which is mediated by $β_1$-receptors in the juxtaglomerular apparatus. Other orally active inhibitors of renin have also been developed (e.g. enalkiren, remikiren), but are not in current clinical use.

Angiotensin-converting-enzyme inhibitors

Angiotensin-converting-enzyme can be inhibited by many drugs that are commonly known as ACE inhibitors (Table 14.2). Various snake venoms were found to contain peptides that inhibit kininase II (which is identical with ACE), the enzyme that inactivates bradykinin. Orally effective inhibitors of ACE with a similar steric configuration were then synthesized and used in the treatment of hypertension and congestive cardiac failure.

ACE inhibitors decrease blood pressure by inhibiting the conversion of angiotensin I to angiotensin II and thus reducing peripheral resistance (mainly by an effect on arteriolar tone). The compliance of large arteries is also increased, and may contribute to the hypotensive effect. Heart rate is unchanged or slightly increased, and postural hypotension is infrequent. Renal blood flow is usually increased, and aldosterone secretion is inhibited, thus promoting Na^+ excretion. However, ACE inhibitors occasionally cause significant renal impairment, particularly in patients with pre-existing kidney disease or renal artery stenosis, and in elderly patients or those receiving NSAIDs. Hyperkalaemia sometimes occurs, and renal function and electrolytes should be measured prior to treatment and subsequently monitored.

Common adverse effects that may be induced by ACE inhibitors include a persistent dry cough, loss of taste sensation, gastrointestinal disturbances, proteinuria and occasionally bone marrow depression. In diabetic patients, the use of ACE inhibitors has been associated with increased insulin sensitivity. A symptom complex including fever, myalgia, eosinophilia, photosensitivity and other skin reactions has also been reported. A number of these undesirable effects may be related to the accumulation of bradykinin (since its degradation is prevented by ACE inhibitors).

ACE inhibitors are used in the treatment of mild to moderate hypertension, usually as an adjunct to diuretic therapy. They can produce vasodilatation in patients with low levels of plasma renin, possibly due to potentiation

Table 14.2 Pharmacokinetic properties of ACE inhibitors.*

	Bioavailability (%)	Protein binding (%)	Terminal half-life (h)	Elimination by metabolism (M) or excretion (E)
Captopril	65	30	2.2	ME
Cilazapril	60	70	9	E
Enalapril	40	<50	11	E
Fosinopril	35	>95	11.5	ME
Imidapril	40	70	8	ME
Lisinopril	25	0	12	E
Moexipril	13	90	2–9	ME
Perindopril	70	<30	1	ME
Quinapril	55	97	2.2	E
Ramipril	45	55	14	ME
Trandolapril	50	80	21	ME

*With the exception of captopril and lisinopril all ACE inhibitors in current use are prodrugs. In these instances, the pharmacokinetic data relates to the active metabolite (which has the suffix 'at', e.g. enalaprilat).

Table 14.3 Angiotensin II receptor antagonists (AT$_1$ antagonists) in current clinical use.

Candesartan
Eprosartan
Irbesartan
Losartan
Olmesartan
Telmisartan
Valsartan

of the effects of bradykinin and other relaxant factors on vascular smooth muscle. ACE inhibitors are particularly useful in hypertensive patients with insulin-dependent diabetic nephropathy. Since they reduce both preload and afterload, they also have an important role in the treatment of congestive cardiac failure.

At least 11 ACE inhibitors are now available in the UK, and have variable pharmacokinetic properties (Table 14.2). The majority of these compounds are prodrug esters and are hydrolysed in the body to pharmacologically active derivatives (usually the related dicarboxylic acids).

Angiotensin receptor antagonists

Angiotensin receptor antagonists (Table 14.3) have a high affinity and selectivity for angiotensin AT$_1$-receptors, and thus antagonize the effects of angiotensin II. Thus, many of their properties and effects are similar to those of ACE inhibitors, although they do not inhibit the breakdown of bradykinin and related kinins. Consequently, they can be used instead of ACE inhibitors in patients with adverse effects that are due to bradykinin. They are a particularly useful alternative to ACE inhibitors in patients who develop a dry and troublesome cough. However, hyperkalaemia may occur and monitoring of electrolyte levels is recommended, especially in the elderly.

Aldosterone antagonists

Aldosterone antagonists are selectively bound by aldosterone receptors in the distal tubule and inhibit their mineralocorticoid effects. At present two aldosterone antagonists, spironolactone and eplerenone, are available in the UK. At one time, spironolactone was extensively used in the management of essential hypertension. It is now only used in the treatment of primary hyperaldosteronism (Conn's syndrome) and in refractory oedema associated with cirrhosis of the liver, congestive cardiac failure or the nephrotic syndrome. Adverse effects, such as gastrointestinal disturbances, gynaecomastia and hyperkalaemia, are not uncommon. Eplerenone is a newer but extremely expensive alternative, which is sometimes used in patients who cannot tolerate the hormonal side effects of spironolactone.

Vasodilators

Vasodilators that are used in the treatment of hypertension include:
• Calcium channel-blocking drugs (calcium antagonists)
• Hydralazine
• Minoxidil

Calcium channel-blocking drugs

Calcium ions play an important part in the contraction of vascular smooth muscle. During depolarization, Ca^{2+} ions enter through voltage-dependent or ligand-dependent channels, or are released from the endoplasmic reticulum. They subsequently combine with calmodulin, and the Ca^{2+}-calmodulin complex activates myosin light chain kinase, causing the phosphorylation of light chain myosin and its separation from actin filaments, resulting in muscle contraction. Calcium channel-blocking drugs block voltage-dependent Ca^{2+} channels (L-type channels) and prevent Ca^{2+} entry, causing relaxation of vascular smooth muscle. Some of these drugs (e.g. verapamil, diltiazem) also affect cardiac conduction and contractility, and are sometimes used as antiarrhythmic agents (Chapter 15). In contrast, dihydropyridine calcium antagonists only affect vascular smooth muscle, and are extensively used in the treatment of angina and hypertension (Table 14.4). They produce arteriolar vasodilatation at concentrations which have little or no effect on cardiac conduction. Nevertheless, they have indirect effects on the

Table 14.4 Dihydropyridine calcium antagonists that are currently used in the treatment of hypertension.

Amlodipine
Felodipine
Isradipine
Lacidipine
Lercanidipine
Nicardipine
Nifedipine
Nimodipine
Nisoldipine

heart, since coronary blood flow and subendocardial perfusion are improved and there is a reduction in the work of the left ventricle.

Although many dihydropyridine calcium antagonists have been used in the treatment of essential hypertension, in current practice amlodipine (5–10 mg) and felodipine (5–10 mg) are probably more commonly used than other agents. They have a long duration of action and their most frequent adverse effects, such as ankle oedema, headache, flushing, dizziness and postural hypotension, are related to peripheral vasodilatation. Experimental evidence indicates that calcium antagonists also antagonize the effects of ET-1 and may inhibit the progress of atherosclerosis.

Hydralazine

Hydralazine produces relaxation of vascular smooth muscle by the inhibition of Ca^{2+} release from the sarcoplasmic reticulum by inositol trisphosphate. Since it mainly acts on the arterial circulation and selectively inhibits arteriolar tone, postural hypotension does not usually occur. Reflex tachycardia and fluid retention are relatively frequent, but can be modified by the addition of a β-adrenoceptor antagonist and a diuretic. Hydralazine is sometimes used intravenously in the treatment of hypertensive emergencies, and in the management of severe hypertension associated with pregnancy. Chronic therapy, particularly with high doses, may produce an immune response that is similar to systemic lupus erythematosis. The metabolism of hydralazine is subject to genetic polymorphism, and 'slow acetylators' of the drug are more prone to develop this complication.

Minoxidil

Minoxidil is a potent vasodilator, mainly due to activation and opening of K_{ATP} channels in vascular smooth muscle. It causes salt and water retention and peripheral oedema, and is only occasionally used in severe hypertension. It also causes hirsutism and hypertrichosis and has been used topically in the treatment of baldness.

α-Adrenoceptor antagonists

α-Adrenoceptor antagonists that are used in the treatment of hypertension are
- Phenoxybenzamine
- Phentolamine
- Indoramin
- Prazosin
- Other agents

In the past, α-adrenoceptor antagonists have been predominantly used in the treatment of hypertension secondary to an increase in circulating catecholamines, rather than for the management of essential hypertension. They were also used to improve organ blood flow in the treatment of shock, and occasionally as peripheral vasodilators.

Phenoxybenzamine and phentolamine are non-selective antagonists at both α_1- and α_2-receptors, so they facilitate the release of noradrenaline (Chapter 13). As only α-adrenoceptors are antagonized, there will be an enhanced response to the β-effects of noradrenaline that are mediated by β_1-adrenoceptors. Consequently, tachycardias, cardiac dysrhythmias and postural hypotension are relatively common.

In recent years, α-adrenoceptor antagonists have been developed which have selective effects on postsynaptic α_1-adrenoceptors (e.g. indoramin, prazosin). These drugs do not increase noradrenaline release from sympathetic nerve endings or cause tachycardia and postural hypotension, and have been used in essential hypertension and the symptomatic treatment of prostatic hyperplasia.

Phenoxybenzamine

Phenoxybenzamine is bound covalently by α-adrenoceptors, resulting in irreversible α-adrenoceptor blockade, and the effects of a single dose may last for several days after its total elimination from the body. It is used in the preoperative management of patients with phaeochromocytoma, or in their long-term treatment when surgery is precluded. Phenoxybenzamine has also been used to improve splanchnic and renal perfusion in shock states, and in these circumstances monitoring of the central venous pressure is essential. The drug may be administered orally (initial dose 10 mg daily), or by infusion (1 mg kg^{-1} in 200 mL normal saline over 2 h) when intensive care facilities are available.

Phentolamine

Phentolamine was occasionally used as a diagnostic agent in the diagnosis of phaeochromocytoma. However, false-positive responses were common, and a dangerous degree of hypotension sometimes occurred, probably due to its direct relaxant effects on vascular smooth muscle. Identification and measurement of urinary metabolites of catecholamines and localization of the tumour by radiological techniques are more rational methods of diagnosis. Nevertheless, phentolamine infusions (0.1–2 mg min^{-1}) are sometimes useful in the management of hypertensive crises that occur during surgical removal of a phaeochromocytoma, especially during manipulation of the tumour.

Indoramin

Indoramin is an α_1-adrenoceptor antagonist that has local anaesthetic properties and some antihistamine activity. It is sometimes used in the treatment of hypertension, usually in combination with a thiazide diuretic or a β-adrenoceptor antagonist. It has also been used in the management of prostatic hyperplasia and to reduce the frequency of attacks of migraine. Indoramin interacts with ethyl alcohol, and can cause drowsiness. It may also cause extrapyramidal side effects.

Prazosin

Prazosin has a highly selective action on α_1-adrenoceptors, and is approximately 10 times more potent than phentolamine in controlling vasoconstrictor responses to noradrenaline. Since it does not increase transmitter output, it rarely produces tachycardia or dysrhythmias. Prazosin is available as an oral preparation for the treatment of essential hypertension. A number of incidents of fainting with loss of consciousness have occurred when a course of treatment is initiated (first-dose phenomenon). It is unclear whether this effect is due to severe postural hypotension from peripheral adrenoceptor blockade, or whether central mechanisms are involved. This untoward response can be minimized by commencing treatment with a low dose taken on retiring to bed.

Other α-adrenoceptor antagonists

Terazosin and doxazosin have similar properties but a longer duration of action than prazosin.

Doxazosin has also been used in the preparation of patients prior to surgery for phaeochromocytoma, since it is unlikely to cause preoperative tachycardia or arrhythmias.

Other selective α_1-adrenoceptor antagonists (e.g. alfuzosin, tamsulosin) are also used in the symptomatic treatment of benign prostatic hyperplasia. Alternative agents exhibiting α-adrenoceptor antagonist activity include the neuroleptic phenothiazines and some ergot alkaloids (Chapter 13).

Centrally acting drugs
Methyldopa

Methyldopa readily traverses the blood–brain barrier and is converted into α-methylnoradrenaline in the CNS. This metabolite subsequently inhibits cardioregulatory centres in the tractus solitarius in the medulla oblongata, through effects that are mediated by α_2-adrenoceptors. Adverse effects of methyldopa include drowsiness and depression, oedema, drug rashes and hepatotoxicity. With prolonged therapy, 10–20% of patients show a positive direct Coombs test and haemolytic anaemia occurs in a small proportion. Methyldopa only rarely causes postural hypotension, and the drug is safe to use in pregnancy, and in patients with asthma and heart failure. Nevertheless, its use in recent years has significantly declined.

Clonidine

Clonidine was originally introduced as a topical vasoconstrictor, and its potent antihypertensive effects were discovered by accident. Intravenous administration of clonidine produces a transient rise in blood pressure associated with peripheral vasoconstriction, an effect which is mediated by α_1-adrenoceptors. However, the secondary responses of bradycardia and hypotension are mainly due to agonist effects on α_2-adrenoceptors in the CNS. Clonidine commonly causes sedation and a dry mouth.

Its use as an antihypertensive drug has been considerably restricted by severe rebound phenomena that may occur following sudden withdrawal of the drug. Clonidine has also been used in low dosage in the prophylaxis of migraine, and in the management of Gilles de la Tourette syndrome. Clonidine has also been shown to reduce the MAC value of anaesthetic agents and to exhibit an antinociceptive effect (Chapters 8 and 11).

Moxonidine

Moxonidine is a centrally acting agent that exerts its principal antihypertensive effects via imidazoline I_1-receptors in the medulla oblongata. The drug has a low affinity for

α_2-receptors, and sedation is unlikely to occur. Moxonidine is well absorbed orally, is not subject to first-pass elimination and is not extensively metabolized, although two of its breakdown products have some hypotensive effects. The parent drug and its metabolites are excreted in urine, and its terminal half-life is relatively short (2–3 h). There are a number of contraindications to its use including heart failure, significant arrhythmias and peripheral vascular disorders.

Other antihypertensive drugs
Guanethidine

Guanethidine lowers blood pressure by acting at postganglionic sympathetic nerve endings, where it affects the transport, storage and subsequent release of noradrenaline. It primarily acts on storage vesicles in sympathetic nerve terminals by displacing noradrenaline from its binding sites and preventing its further uptake from the axoplasm. The drug has a long duration of action, and the effects of a single dose can persist for up to 4 days and cumulation is likely. Adverse effects include postural hypotension, diarrhoea and failure of ejaculation, although effects on the CNS are uncommon as guanethidine does not readily cross the blood–brain barrier. The effects of guanethidine are antagonized by drugs that inhibit Uptake$_1$ (e.g. tricyclic antidepressants, cocaine, amphetamines). Conversely, those patients receiving long-term treatment with guanethidine exhibit a marked 'supersensitivity' to pressor amines.

Guanethidine has also been used to produce intravenous regional sympathetic blockade in the treatment of intractable limb pain when there is evidence of autonomic dysfunction. The drug also has significant local anaesthetic activity. In current practice, it is rarely used in the treatment of hypertension.

Metirosine

Metirosine (α-methyl-p-tyrosine) is a competitive inhibitor of tyrosine hydroxylase, and thus prevents the conversion of tyrosine to DOPA in central and peripheral sympathetic neurons (including the adrenal medulla). Metirosine has been used in the preoperative preparation of patients prior to the removal of a phaeochromocytoma, or in the long-term management of those unsuitable for surgery. Adverse effects include moderate or severe sedation, diarrhoea and extrapyramidal effects. Metirosine is not used in the treatment of essential hypertension, and in the UK it is only available on a 'named-patient' basis.

Treatment of hypertension

In many patients with moderate or severe essential hypertension, blood pressure can be slowly and gradually controlled by oral therapy. In most instances, more than one drug is required, and many patients are stabilized on 2–4 different antihypertensive drugs. The use of drug combinations usually increases the efficacy of treatment and the control of blood pressure, but minimizes the prevalence of adverse effects.

Until recently, thiazide diuretics or β-adrenoceptor antagonists were commonly recommended as first-line therapy. The choice of these drugs was influenced by the presence of certain coexisting disorders, particularly angina pectoris, obstructive airway disease, peripheral vascular insufficiency, diabetes and gout. Peripheral vasodilators (e.g. hydralazine), centrally acting drugs (e.g. methyldopa) or adrenergic neuron-blocking drugs (e.g. guanethidine) were added to this regime in resistant cases.

In recent years, the rationale and effectiveness of these regimes has been reassessed. Thiazides are still considered a drug of first choice, particularly in the elderly, although they have many disadvantages. They are relatively non-potent drugs, may induce hypokalaemia and have adverse effects on plasma lipids. In addition, in chronic use they can cause hyperglycaemia and diabetes and precipitate gout. Similarly, the extensive use of β-adrenergic antagonists has recently been re-evaluated. Many of the lipid-soluble drugs produce undesirable central effects, and may interact with other antianginal drugs (e.g. diltiazem, verapamil). In addition, all β-blockers have adverse effects on plasma lipids. They may be less effective than other drugs in reducing cerebrovascular complications, possibly because they preferentially reduce brachial rather than carotid arterial pressure.

In current practice, dihydropyridine calcium antagonists, ACE inhibitors or angiotensin II receptor antagonists, and α_1-adrenoceptor antagonists are more commonly used in the treatment of hypertension. Although minor side effects are relatively common, their use in long-term management is now well established, and they all have neutral or beneficial effects on plasma lipids. They may be specifically indicated in the treatment of associated diseases. For example, ACE inhibitors are used in incipient heart failure, calcium channel blockers are used in patients with angina and peripheral vascular insufficiency, and α_1-adrenoceptor antagonists are useful in prostatism.

Most patients with essential hypertension are also treated with statins (hydroxymethyl-glutaryl-coenzyme A reductase inhibitors) and aspirin.

Hypertensive emergencies

In certain hypertensive emergencies, the blood pressure should be lowered immediately. These situations include hypertensive encephalopathy, intracranial haemorrhage, dissecting aortic aneurysm, acute congestive cardiac failure and severe hypertension associated with toxaemia of pregnancy. Parenteral therapy may be indicated in these instances, although a precipitous fall in blood pressure must be avoided to minimize further complications from a reduction in cerebral, myocardial or renal blood flow. Drugs that are used for this purpose include diazoxide, hydralazine, labetalol and sodium nitroprusside. The latter three drugs are discussed elsewhere in this chapter.

Diazoxide

Diazoxide has a close structural resemblance to the thiazide diuretics, although it (paradoxically) causes Na^+ retention. Diazoxide (like thiazide diuretics) produces antihypertensive effects by the activation of K_{ATP} channels in vascular smooth muscle, resulting in enhanced K^+ loss and hyperpolarization. These changes cause the relaxation of arteriolar smooth muscle, although there appears to be little or no effect on capacitance vessels. The baroreceptor response produced by the fall in blood pressure may lead to an increased heart rate and stroke volume, and the secretion of renin is enhanced. When used in a hypertensive crisis, diazoxide is administered by rapid intravenous injection ($1-3$ mg kg^{-1}, with a maximal single dose of 150 mg). An optimal response occurs within a few minutes and if further treatment is not instituted, blood pressure returns to its original level within 4–24 hours. The concomitant use of a rapidly acting diuretic such as furosemide may be necessary if the hypertensive emergency is associated with pulmonary oedema or renal failure. Diazoxide and thiazide diuretics decrease insulin secretion by the activation of K$_{ATP}$ channels in the islets of Langerhans. Consequently, it has diabetogenic properties and can antagonize the effects of oral hypoglycaemic agents. Since it decreases endogenous insulin secretion, diazoxide is sometimes used orally in the management of chronic hypoglycaemia associated with hyperplasia or islet cell tumours of the pancreas. It is of no value in the treatment of acute insulin-induced hypoglycaemia.

Hypertension in pregnancy

The presence of hypertension during pregnancy is one of the leading causes of maternal death and of foetal mortality and morbidity. Even moderate increases in diastolic or mean arterial pressure in the middle trimester are often associated with an increased incidence of stillbirths and intrauterine growth retardation. Rises in blood pressure during the third trimester are frequently correlated with an increased maternal risk. Consequently, it is important to control elevated blood pressure during pregnancy, whether this due to pre-existing essential or secondary hypertension, or to pre-eclampsia. Non-pharmacological methods (e.g. strict bed rest) are sometimes of value, but drug treatment is often required. However, the choice of an appropriate antihypertensive agent needs careful consideration.

Thiazide diuretics, ACE inhibitors, lipid-soluble β-adrenoceptor antagonists and clonidine should all be avoided during pregnancy. Thiazide diuretics do not prevent the development of toxaemia, and may cause hypovolaemia and decrease placental perfusion. In addition, neonatal thrombocytopenia, jaundice, hyponatraemia and an increased probability of hypertension at maturity have been reported. ACE inhibitors may adversely affect foetal and neonatal blood pressure control and renal function, and may cause skull defects and oligohydramnios. Lipid-soluble β-adrenoceptor antagonists (e.g. propranolol) can cross the placenta and may restrict intrauterine growth and cause foetal bradycardia, respiratory depression and severe neonatal hypoglycaemia. Clonidine can lower the foetal heart rate, and experimental studies suggest that it may be teratogenic in pregnancy. Although calcium antagonists are apparently safe, they can

potentially inhibit the progress of labour. Nevertheless, prolonged release preparations of nifedipine are sometimes used to lower blood pressure during pregnancy.

Methyldopa and non-lipophilic β-adrenoceptor antagonists (e.g. atenolol) are safe to administer during pregnancy and oral hydralazine is a useful alternative. Intravenous hydralazine may be necessary to control hypertensive crises associated with eclampsia.

Antihypertensive drugs and anaesthesia

Historical perspective

Many of the agents used in anaesthetic practice can exert significant activity on the autonomic nervous system and can theoretically augment the effects of established antihypertensive therapy. At one time it was considered desirable to withdraw antihypertensive drugs for up to 14 days prior to anaesthesia and surgery. Various tests were used to assess the magnitude of residual sympathetic activity, including the measurement of responses to the Valsalva manoeuvre or to postural changes, or the administration of indirectly acting sympathomimetic amines such as ephedrine or tyrosine.

This view is no longer tenable. The attendant dangers of a rising blood pressure are an obvious disadvantage, and the enhanced pressor responses, which are observed during laryngoscopy and intubation in uncontrolled hypertensive patients may be particularly hazardous. Furthermore, the sudden withdrawal of clonidine, β-adrenoceptor antagonists and possibly other agents may lead to dangerous rebound phenomena.

Antihypertensive drugs and surgery

It is now standard practice to continue antihypertensive therapy until a few hours prior to surgery. However, special vigilance is still necessary to prevent the excessive hypertension and tachycardia that may result from airway manipulation or surgical stimulation. In this context, the depth of anaesthesia is of considerable importance. The concentrations of volatile agents required to suppress these haemodynamic responses are considerably greater than their MAC values, and may lead to depression of an already compromised myocardium.

In this situation, the use of rapidly acting opioid analgesics (e.g. fentanyl, alfentanil) during induction may be especially valuable. Topical lidocaine applied to the larynx before intubation and, on occasions, the prior administration of glyceryl trinitrate, would also appear to be beneficial.

Perioperative β-adrenoceptor blockade

Recent studies suggest that aggressive perioperative β_1-receptor blockade may be particularly beneficial in hypertensive patients with coronary artery disease, and is associated with a reduction in morbidity and mortality. In these circumstances, the ultra short-acting β-adrenoceptor antagonist esmolol may also prove to be of immediate value. Esmolol is a cardioselective agent with no intrinsic sympathomimetic or membrane-stabilizing activity. It has a rapid onset of action after intravenous infusion ($50–200\ \mu g\ kg^{-1}\ min^{-1}$), and no significant activity is detected after 20 minutes. The short half-life (approximately 9 min) is due to rapid biotransformation by esterases to an inactive acidic metabolite and methyl alcohol. These properties suggest that the drug is particularly suitable for the management of hypertensive responses that occur during the induction or recovery phases of anaesthesia. Esmolol has also been used in the treatment of supraventricular tachycardias, and may be effective in the management of acute myocardial ischaemia and unstable angina.

Other drugs

Adenosine has negative inotropic and chronotropic effects on the heart and a transient duration of action, and may also be useful during the perioperative period. α_2-Adrenoceptor agonists (e.g. dexmedetomidine, azepexole) reduce anaesthetic requirements, and also decrease adrenergic activity by both central and peripheral mechanisms. They may develop a role in the modification of cardiovascular reflex responses during anaesthesia (Chapter 13).

Other measures

In both treated and untreated hypertensive patients, untoward changes in cardiovascular parameters are more prone to occur during anaesthesia than in normotensive subjects. Special attention must thus be paid to the maintenance of blood volume, ventilatory parameters and positioning the patient on the operating table.

Induced hypotension

Historical perspective

Deliberate hypotension was employed for many years to reduce bleeding during surgical procedures. The techniques originally used included controlled arteriotomy, the application of negative pressures to the lower limbs and the production of high spinal or extradural blockade with local anaesthetic agents. More recently volatile inhalational agents, which produce dose-dependent effects on blood pressure, were employed to produce moderate and predictable hypotension during anaesthesia. Controlled ventilation was mandatory and at one time the muscle relaxant tubocurarine was extensively used in this technique. Similarly, the ganglion-blocking drug trimetaphan was frequently used in hypotensive techniques, but is not now available in the UK. The use of controlled hypotension during surgery has undoubtedly declined during the past two decades. At the present time, sodium nitroprusside and glyceryl trinitrate are sometimes used to produce controlled hypotension during surgery (particularly ENT and neurosurgery).

Sodium nitroprusside

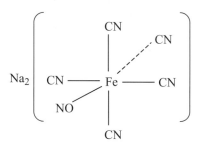

Although sodium nitroprusside was first shown to reduce blood pressure in 1929, another 30 years elapsed before it was used in anaesthetic practice to produce controlled hypotension.

Mode of action

The nitroso group ($-N = O-$) in sodium nitroprusside reacts with sulphydryl groups (–SH) in vascular smooth muscle, forming nitric oxide and nitrosothiol derivatives. Both these metabolites stimulate guanylate cyclase, increasing cGMP levels and producing generalized relaxation of vascular smooth muscle. Consequently, sodium nitroprusside produces both arterial and venular dilatation. These effects result in increased venous capacitance and pooling, leading to a reduction in peripheral resistance and cardiac output. Since sodium nitroprusside has little or no direct effect on cardiac function, reflex tachycardia may occur and sometimes requires β_1-adrenergic blockade.

Renal blood flow and glomerular filtration rate are usually unaltered, and plasma renin is increased. Sodium nitroprusside may increase cerebral blood flow and intracranial pressure, and its effects on the autoregulation of the cerebral circulation are controversial. A fall in arterial oxygen tension may also occur.

Administration

Sodium nitroprusside must be given by intravenous infusion, and is normally administered as a solution (50–200 $\mu g\,mL^{-1}$) in 5% dextrose. Solutions of the drug should be freshly prepared, and have a faint orange-brownish tint. When exposed to light, sodium nitroprusside is broken down to cyanide ions (–CN) and other derivatives. Solutions subsequently become dark brown or blue and must then be discarded. The infusion solution should be protected by wrapping the container in aluminium foil or other opaque material.

Sodium nitroprusside has a rapid onset (within 1 min) and a short duration of action (2–4 min), and is an extremely potent and toxic drug. It is normally infused until a mean arterial pressure of 50–60 mm Hg (6.7–8.0 kPa) is achieved. It is suggested that the dose used to provide controlled hypotension during anaesthesia should not normally exceed 1.5 $\mu g\,kg^{-1}min^{-1}$.

The evanescent action of sodium nitroprusside is due to its rapid breakdown to cyanide ions, which are then converted into thiocyanate and excreted by the kidney. This reaction is dependent on the presence of thiosulphate (which provides –SH groups) and the enzyme rhodanase. Alternatively, cyanide ions are eliminated by combination with hydroxocobalamin (forming cyanocobalamin).

Cyanide ions can accumulate with high rates of infusion, or when their elimination is impaired. Cellular oxidative processes that depend on cytochrome oxidase are inhibited by cyanide ions, and the resultant metabolic acidosis may present as sweating, hyperventilation, cardiac arrhythmias and an accentuated fall in blood pressure. The appearance of toxic effects is sometimes delayed until 1–3 hours after the administration of sodium nitroprusside.

When cyanide toxicity occurs, sodium nitroprusside infusions should be stopped immediately and an antidote, either sodium thiosulphate to promote conversion to thiocyanate, or dicobalt edetate that chelates cyanide ions, given intravenously. The administration of intravenous sodium nitrite or inhaled amyl nitrite is also valuable, since they induce the formation of methaemoglobin, which has a greater affinity for cyanide than cytochrome oxidase. Calcium salts may help to restore blood pressure. Hydroxocobalamin is sometimes used to provide an alternative route for the elimination of cyanide.

The use of sodium nitroprusside should be avoided in patients with disorders of Vitamin B_{12} metabolism. It is also contraindicated in hypothyroid states, since thiocyanate inhibits the uptake of iodide by the thyroid gland. Nitroprusside is also contraindicated in renal failure, since thiocyanate can accumulate.

Glyceryl trinitrate

$$CH_2 — O — NO_2$$
$$CH — O — NO_2$$
$$CH_2 — O — NO_2$$

Glyceryl trinitrate (nitroglycerine) can be used to enhance or induce controlled hypotension.

Mode of action

Glyceryl trinitrate is metabolized by blood vessels, forming nitric oxide and various nitrosothiol derivatives. Both metabolites stimulate guanylate cyclase, increasing cGMP levels and producing generalized relaxation of vascular smooth muscle. Consequently, glyceryl trinitrate causes peripheral vasodilatation by the action of its metabolites on peripheral blood vessels. In contrast to nitroprusside, there appears to be a more selective effect on capacitance vessels. Thus venular tone (and 'preload') is decreased to a greater extent than arterial tone (and 'afterload'). Consequently, the hypotensive action of glyceryl trinitrate is highly susceptible to positional changes, and is less likely to induce direct effects on cerebral blood flow than nitroprusside.

Administration

Glyceryl trinitrate is normally diluted prior to use with normal saline or isotonic dextrose, to produce an intravenous solution (0.01% or 100 $\mu g\,mL^{-1}$). The drug should be prepared in glass or polyethylene containers, since loss of activity occurs in packs or bags of polyvinyl chloride (Viaflex or Steriflex). The resulting solution is normally infused at a dose range of 10–200 $\mu g\,min^{-1}$ until the desired level of blood pressure is achieved. Its rapid onset of action (2–3 min) is due to the formation of nitric oxide, and tolerance to the effects of the drug is not usually a problem with short-term use.

Glyceryl trinitrate is also given by infusion in the treatment of unstable angina, the management of congestive cardiac failure following myocardial infarction, or to control myocardial ischaemia during and after cardiovascular surgery. It is also administered by different routes (sublingual, buccal or percutaneous) in the management of anginal attacks. In these conditions, left ventricular end-diastolic pressure and myocardial wall tension are reduced and there is a resultant decrease in myocardial oxygen demand.

Magnesium sulphate and labetalol (an α- and β-adrenoceptor antagonist) have also been used to facilitate controlled hypotension during surgery (Chapter 13).

Suggested reading

Aitken, D. (1977) Cyanide toxicity following nitroprusside induced hypotension. *Canadian Anaesthetists Society Journal* **24**, 651–660.

Antonaccio, M.J. (1982) Angiotensin-converting-enzyme (ACE) inhibitors. *Annual Review of Pharmacology and Toxicology* **27**, 57–87.

Bearner, J.E.R. & Warwick, J. (2001) Critical incidents: the cardiovascular system. *Anaesthesia and Intensive Care Medicine* **2**, 412–417.

Burnier, M. & Brunner, H.R. (2000) Angiotensin II receptor antagonists. *Lancet* **355**, 637–645.

Elsharnouby, N.M. & Elsharnouby, M.M. (2006) Magnesium sulphate as a technique of hypotensive anaesthesia. *British Journal of Anaesthesia* **96**, 727–731.

Goldman, L. & Caldera, D.L. (1979) Risks of general anaesthesia and elective operation in the hypertensive patient. *Anaesthesiology* **50**, 285–292.

Howell, S.J., Sear, J.W. & Foëx, P. (2001) Peri-operative β-blockade: a useful treatment that should be greeted with cautious enthusiasm. *British Journal of Anaesthesia* **86**, 161–164.

Howell, S.J., Sear, J.W. & Foëx, P. (2004) Hypertension, hypertensive heart disease and perioperative cardiac risk. *British Journal of Anaesthesia* **92**, 570–583.

Jacobi, K.E., Bohmo, B.E., Rickauer, A.J., Jacobi, C. & Hemmerling, T.M. (2000) Moderate controlled hypotension with sodium nitroprusside does not improve surgical conditions or decrease blood loss in endoscopic sinus surgery. *Journal of Clinical Anesthesia* **12**, 202–207.

Johnston, C.I. (1995) Angiotensin receptor antagonists: focus on losartan. *Lancet* **346**, 1403–1407.

Jones, K.G. & Powell, J.T. (2000) Slowing the heart saves lives: advantages of perioperative of perioperative β-blockade. *British Journal of Surgery* **87**, 689–690.

Kaplan, N.M. & Opie, L.H. (2006) Controversies in Cardiology 2. Controversies in hypertension. *Lancet* **367**, 168–176.

Leigh, J.M. (1975) The history of controlled hypotension. *British Journal of Anaesthesia* **47**, 745–749.

Lenders, J.W.M., Eisenhofer, G., Mannelli, M. & Pacak, K. (2005) Phaechromocytoma. *Lancet* **366**, 665–675.

Lindholm, L.H., Carlberg, B. & Samuelsson, O. (2005) Should β blockers remain first choice in the treatment of primary hypertension? A meta-analysis. *Lancet* **366**, 1545–1553.

MacIndoe, A.K. (2002) Recognition and management of phaeochromocytoma. *Anaesthesia and Intensive Care Medicine* **3**, 319–324.

Moss, E. (1994) Cerebral blood flow during induced hypotension. *British Journal of Anaesthesia* **74**, 635–637.

Nicolson, D.J., Dickinson, H.O., Campbell, F. & Mason, J.M. (2004) Lifestyle interventions or drugs for patients with essential hypertension: a systematic review. *Journal of Hypertension* **22**, 2043–2048.

Prys-Roberts, C., Meloche, R. & Foëx, P. (1971) Studies of anaesthesia in relation to hypertension. I. Cardiovascular responses of treated and untreated patients. *British Journal of Anaesthesia* **43**, 122–137.

Sambrook, A. & Small, R. (2003) Antiarrhythmic drugs: antihypertensive drugs in pregnancy. *Anaesthesia and Intensive Care Medicine* **4**, 266–272.

Small, R. (2001) Pharmacological modulation of myocardial function, vascular resistance and blood pressure. *Anaesthesia and Intensive Care Medicine* **2**, 34–39.

Spahn, D.R. & Priebe, H.-J. (2004) Preoperative hypertension: remain wary? 'Yes' – cancel surgery? 'No'. *British Journal of Anaesthesia* **92**, 461–464.

15 Antiarrhythmic and Antianginal Drugs

Antiarrhythmic drugs

Cardiac arrhythmias may be defined as irregular or abnormal heart rhythms. By convention, they also include bradycardias or tachycardias outside the physiological range (55–90 beats per minute in adults). Arrhythmias may present before surgery and are commonly seen in patients admitted to intensive care units. During anaesthesia, they may be precipitated by surgical stimuli, or by physiological and pharmacological factors. In all these circumstances, the use of antiarrhythmic drugs may be necessary to control cardiac irregularities or maintain cardiac output.

Electrophysiology of normal cardiac muscle

The understanding of the mode of action of antiarrhythmic drugs depends on an appreciation of cardiac physiology, and the manner in which this is modified by disease. Microelectrode studies on single muscle fibres in the heart have clarified these concepts. The heart contains
• Pacemaker cells in the sinoatrial (SA) and atrioventricular (AV) nodes. Normally, the SA node initiates the cardiac impulse, although in abnormal conditions the AV node can take over and control the rhythm and rate of the heart.
• Conducting pathways (bundle of His and Purkinje network), which preferentially conduct cardiac impulses to ventricular muscle.
• Contractile cells (atrial and ventricular muscle fibres), which respond to cardiac impulses by depolarization, resulting in muscle contraction.

Structural differences

There are important structural differences between pacemaker cells, conducting pathways and contractile muscle fibres. In the SA and AV nodes, small round pacemaker cells are interspersed with larger, slender and more elongated cellular elements. The conducting pathways in Purkinje tissues consist of similar elongated, delicate, fusiform cells that contain relatively few myofibrils and are faintly striated, and are embedded in dense connective tissue. In contrast, typical cardiac contractile muscle cells contain numerous myofibrils, which are responsible for the prominent striations seen on light microscopy. The myofibrils consist of filaments of myosin and actin, which interact when the intracellular Ca^{2+} concentration increases above the resting level (excitation–contraction coupling). Each muscle cell is partly divided at multiple sites by the transverse (T) tubular system, and their limiting sarcolemmal membranes contain numerous ion channels that control the electrical gradient across the membrane. Cardiac muscle fibres form a syncytium (there are no clear cellular boundaries), and branch frequently. They are separated from each other by intercalated discs.

Electrophysiological differences

These structural differences are paralleled by electrophysiological differences that are responsible for the sequential conduction of the cardiac impulse. In the diastolic phase of the cardiac cycle, the inside of all conducting tissues and muscle fibres is electrically negative compared to the outside (the resting membrane potential). As in other tissues, this 'potassium diffusion potential' mainly reflects the balance between the tendency of K^+ to diffuse from cells along ion-specific channels, and the attraction of K^+ for negatively charged intracellular phosphate groups.

SA node

In the SA and AV nodes, the changes in electrical potential during the cardiac cycle differ from those in atrial and

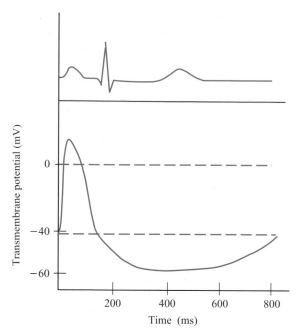

Fig. 15.1 The transmembrane potential in the SA node during the cardiac cycle. The bell-shaped action potential in the SA node lasts for 150–200 milliseconds, and is mainly produced by the entry of Ca^{2+} through L-type channels. Repolarization is mainly due to Ca^{2+} channel closure and the outward diffusion of K^+. After repolarization, the resting membrane potential is only constant for a short time, and then decreases from −60 mV to −40 mV during the latter part of atrial diastole (the prepotential or pacemaker potential). When the resting potential reaches −40 mV, depolarization occurs. Simultaneous changes in the electrocardiogram are shown for comparison.

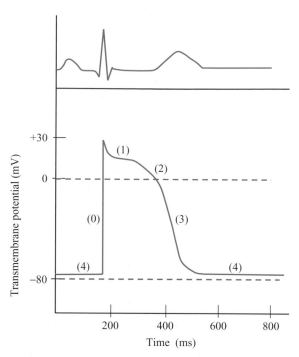

Fig. 15.2 Transmembrane potential of a ventricular muscle fibre during the cardiac cycle. The resting membrane potential is stable and constant during diastole (approximately −80 mV), and the ventricular action potential lasts for 200–300 milliseconds. Transmembrane potential changes during the cardiac cycle are divided into five phases (0–4), corresponding to rapid depolarization (phase 0), partial repolarization (phase 1), the plateau potential (phase 2), repolarization (phase 3), and the resting potential (phase 4). Simultaneous changes in the electrocardiogram are shown for comparison. The QRS complex represents ventricular depolarization, and the Q-T interval corresponds to the duration of the ventricular action potential.

ventricular muscle. In the SA node, the resting membrane potential is unstable, and decreases from approximately −60 mV to −40 mV during atrial diastole. This change in potential (the pacemaker potential or prepotential) is mainly related to a decrease in K^+ permeability and the opening of rapidly inactivated Ca^{2+} channels (T or transient channels) in the SA node. When the resting potential reaches −40 mV, a further group of voltage-dependent Ca^{2+} channels opens (L or long-lasting channels), resulting in a rapid increase in Ca^{2+} permeability and depolarization. The resultant action potential in the SA node is usually bell-shaped and lasts for 150–200 milliseconds (Fig. 15.1). Repolarization is due to closure of the slowly inactivating L-channels and the unopposed diffusion of K^+, which re-establishes the normal resting potential. β_1-Adrenoceptor stimulation increases the slope of the pace-

maker potential, since it increases intracellular cAMP and Ca^{2+} entry into SA nodal cells. Similar ionic changes occur during depolarization in the AV node.

Atrial and ventricular muscle

In contrast, in atrial and ventricular muscle the resting potential is stable ($\approx$ −80 mV), and the changes in electrical potential during the cardiac cycle are usually divided into five phases (Fig. 15.2). During phase 0, the myocardial cell depolarizes from approximately −80 mV to +30 mV, due to the rapid influx of Na^+ along voltage-dependent channels (and to a lesser extent, of Ca^{2+}), which usually lasts for less than 1 millisecond. In phase 1 (partial repolarization), the amplitude of the action potential slightly decreases as the fast Na^+ channels are inactivated, and transiently outward channels (K^+_{TO}) allow a brief efflux of K^+. During phase 2 (the plateau phase), there is a slow influx of Ca^{2+} along voltage-dependent L-channels, balanced by an efflux of K^+, and the action potential is maintained between 0 and −20 mV for a period of 100–150 milliseconds. In phase 3 (the repolarization phase), the action potential rapidly returns to its resting value of −80 mV, due to the inactivation of Ca^{2+} L-channels, and the continued efflux of K^+. Between depolarization and the middle of phase 3, cardiac muscle will not respond to any further stimulus (the absolute refractory period), although after this period it will respond to high intensity stimulation (the relative refractory period). In phase 4, the potential is maintained at a value of approximately −80 mV, since normal atrial and ventricular muscle fibres are effectively impermeable to Na^+ and Ca^{2+} during diastole. During this phase, the ionic movements across the myocardial membrane are reversed due to the activity of the ion pump (Na^+/K^+ ATPase), which exchanges 3 Na^+ for 2 K^+, resulting in a negative intracellular potential. Since the total duration of the atrial or ventricular action potential (200–300 ms) is greater than the time required to produce muscle contraction, cardiac muscle cannot be tetanized and can only contract intermittently.

AV node and the His–Purkinje system

These differences in electrical behaviour between the SA node, and atrial and ventricular muscle, are reflected in other conducting tissues. Thus, the shape of the action potential in the AV node is similar to the SA node, while the His–Purkinje system has characteristics that are similar to normal ventricular muscle. The duration of the cardiac action potential (i.e. the beginning of phase 1 to the end of phase 3) is shorter in the bundle of His and ventricular muscle (150–200 ms) than in the terminal Purkinje fibres (250–300 ms) and is approximately equal in duration to the refractory period. In the electrocardiogram, the QRS duration corresponds to ventricular depolarization, while the Q-T interval reflects the duration of the myocardial action potential.

Origin and propagation of the cardiac impulse

The origin and propagation of the cardiac impulse can be interpreted in terms of the differences in electrical behaviour between pacemaker cells, conduction pathways, and contractile myocardial cells. In normal conditions, the

diastolic membrane potential reaches its threshold value in the SA node earlier than in other cardiac tissues (Fig. 15.1). Consequently, the SA node is depolarized sooner than other cells, and therefore initiates the cardiac impulse. Excitation is propagated over the right atrium by means of local currents between atrial muscle cells that are in longitudinal contact with each other (and have a low electrical resistance to current flow). Similarly, the AV node and the His–Purkinje system are depolarized before ventricular muscle, and their depolarization results in action potentials that rapidly spread over the entire subendocardial surface of the ventricles.

The physiology of cardiac arrhythmias

Bradycardia and bradyarrhythmias

Bradycardia will occur due to defects in impulse initiation in the SA node. Other bradyarrhythmias are associated with delays in propagation of impulses via the AV node and the His–Purkinje system. These arrhythmias are frequently induced by drugs (e.g. digoxin, verapamil), or may result from reflex stimulation leading to vagal overactivity. When there is marked bradycardia or SA block, the cardiac impulse can be initiated by other junctional tissues (AV node, bundle of His or the His–Purkinje system). These 'escape beats' may be induced by excessive vagal tone, and are responsible for the phenomenon of 'vagal escape'. Bradyarrhythmias may also be induced by underlying structural heart disease, when permanent cardiac pacing may be required.

Tachycardia and tachyarrhythmias

Tachycardia and some tachyarrhythmias may result from
• Ectopic foci that result in enhanced automaticity
• Re-entry or reciprocating mechanisms
• Spontaneous after-depolarization potentials
These phenomena are believed to be concerned in the production of many tachyarrhythmias such as atrial flutter, atrial fibrillation, ventricular extrasystoles, ventricular tachycardia and many supraventricular tachycardias (including the Wolff–Parkinson–White syndrome).

Ectopic foci that result in enhanced automaticity

In normal conditions, the pacemaker potential in the SA node (Fig. 15.1) reaches the threshold value for depolarization earlier than in other conducting pathways, or in atrial or ventricular muscle. Consequently, the SA node is depolarized earlier than other cardiac tissues, and therefore acts as the pacemaker. In some physiological and patho-logical conditions, the resting potential of other cells may decrease and become less electronegative earlier than the SA node. In these conditions, the ectopic focus acts as the pacemaker, and the normal activity of the SA node is sup-pressed. If myocardial cells reach their excitation threshold before the SA node, they may act as an ectopic focus and thus induce cardiac arrhythmias. Ectopic rhythms may also originate in junctional tissues that can undergo spon-taneous depolarization (AV node and His–Purkinje sys-tem). In pathological conditions, ischaemia may produce abnormal changes in myocardial muscle cells, and allow them to assume the electrical characteristics of pacemaker cells. Consequently, they may become more permeable to Na^+, resulting in an unstable resting potential and spon-taneous depolarization during diastole. Similar changes may be produced by hypokalaemia, which tends to cause an unstable resting membrane potential (phase 4) in my-ocardial cells. These conditions will favour the develop-ment of an ectopic focus in atrial or ventricular muscle (as well as in conducting tissues).

Re-entry and reciprocating mechanisms

Re-entry and reciprocating mechanisms usually arise in anatomical sites that possess the opportunity for differen-tial rates of conduction along alternative pathways. They are particularly common when impulses can pass down al-ternative pathways with different conduction times and re-fractory periods, and when these impulses can be blocked. These pathways may be present in the AV node and in ter-minal Purkinje fibres, as well as in damaged atrial and ventricular muscle. Terminal Purkinje fibres frequently branch as they approach the myocardium, so that a sin-gle cardiac muscle fibre can be innervated by more than one terminal (Fig. 15.3). If there is no delay in conduc-tion, impulses can pass down both terminal arborizations and are extinguished or neutralized in the muscle fibre. By contrast, if one of these terminals has a relatively longer refractory period (due to physiological or pathological causes), conduction may only occur down one branch, since the other may still be refractory. In these conditions, the impulse is not extinguished in the muscle fibre, and can approach the previously refractory arborization in a ret-rograde manner. If this branch has recovered, retrograde conduction of the impulse occurs, followed by antero-grade conduction in the contralateral limb, and a recipro-cal rhythm is set up due to re-entry of the impulse. This phenomenon may occur in a fixed anatomical pathway, as in some supraventricular tachycardias (ordered re-entry),

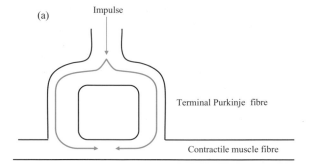

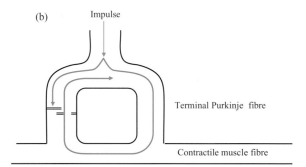

Fig. 15.3 The probable mechanism for the establishment of re-entrant arrhythmias. (a) The impulse is conducted along two alternative pathways with normal conduction times in the terminal arborization of the Purkinje system. Normal conduction occurs down both pathways and the impulse is extinguished in the contractile muscle fibre. (b) One of the terminal branches has a prolonged conduction time and refractory period. If this branch is refractory (════) on the arrival of the impulse, conduction only occurs down the opposite terminal. The impulse is not extinguished in the muscle fibre, and can approach the previously refractory arborization in a retrograde manner. If this branch has recovered (= = =), retrograde conduction of the impulse continues, followed by anterograde conduction in the opposite branch. In this manner, an ectopic focus is set up.

or may constantly change in an incoordinated manner (random re-entry, as in atrial fibrillation). In the Wolff–Parkinson–White syndrome, an accessory, fast responsive pathway between the atria and the ventricles (the bundle of Kent) competes with slower conducting fibres across the AV node. Conduction along the conventional pathway al-lows the impulse to gain retrograde re-entry to the atria via the bundle of Kent, producing a reciprocating supraven-tricular tachycardia. Although this arrhythmia responds to calcium antagonists and β-adrenoceptor antagonists, it is more commonly treated by surgical ablation.

Spontaneous after-depolarization potentials

Spontaneous after-depolarization potentials (triggered activity) refer to the occurrence of one or more spontaneous after-potentials after a normal action potential. They are usually associated with pathological changes in ischaemic myocardium, and are divided into two types:

- Early after-depolarization
- Delayed after-depolarization

Early after-depolarization

Early after-depolarization (EAD) refers to an additional phase of depolarization occurring at the end of phase 2 or at the middle of phase 3 (Fig. 15.4). They are usually associated with the activation or reactivation of calcium channels, resulting in enhanced Ca^{2+} entry through L-channels (phase 2 EAD) or T-channels (phase 3 EAD). The early after-potentials are often associated with bradycardia, and are more likely to occur when the myocardial action potential (Q-T interval) is prolonged by hypokalaemia, hypercalcaemia, or anti-arrhythmic drugs, or when inherited abnormalities in Na^+ or K^+ channels results in congenital long Q-T syndromes (Romano–Ward syndrome, Jervell and Lange–Nielsen syndrome). In these conditions, Q-T prolongation may precipitate polymorphic ventricular tachycardia or 'torsade de pointes'.

Delayed after-depolarization

Delayed after-depolarization (DAD) is an additional phase of depolarization that occurs when repolarization is complete at the beginning of phase 4 (Fig. 15.4). The occurrence of delayed after-potentials may result in the generation of single or multiple repetitive action potentials, resulting in an ectopic focus. It is often associated with rapid heart rates and the accumulation of intracellular Ca^{2+}, and may occur during myocardial ischaemia, heart failure, and in digoxin toxicity. It may also be induced by catecholamine secretion or administration, which produces β_1-adrenoceptor stimulation, accumulation of cyclic AMP, and Ca^{2+} entry.

Early after-depolarization potential

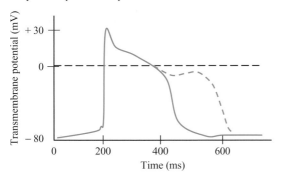

Delayed after-depolarization potential

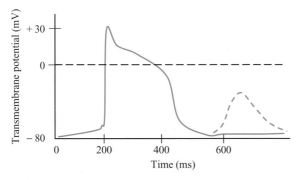

Fig. 15.4 After-depolarization potentials (- - -) occur after ventricular action potentials. Early after-depolarization potentials occur at the end of phase 2 or the middle of phase 3. In contrast, delayed after-depolarization potentials occur at the beginning of phase 4, when repolarization is complete. Both early and delayed after-depolarization potentials may give rise to a second ventricular action potential, particularly at high rates of stimulation or during tachycardia.

Classification of antiarrhythmic drugs

In atrial flutter and atrial fibrillation, treatment is usually directed towards a reduction in the rate of ventricular response by the suppression of AV conduction. In most other arrhythmias, the aim of treatment is the restoration of sinus rhythm, either by decreasing the enhanced automaticity of ectopic foci or by interruption (dissociation) of the process of re-entry. Drugs that produce these effects are usually divided into four groups, depending on their effects on the ionic and electrical characteristics of cardiac muscle (Table 15.1).

Sodium channel blockade (class 1 activity)

Sodium channel blockade reduces the entry of Na^+ into cardiac muscle fibres during depolarization, and thus decreases the maximum rate of rise of phase 0 of the action potential (Fig. 15.2). Drugs that block Na^+ channels often affect other excitable tissues, and may have local anaesthetic and membrane stabilizing activity.

Table 15.1 The mode of action of some common antiarrhythmic drugs.

	Sodium channel blockade	β-Adrenoceptor blockade	Potassium channel blockade	Calcium channel blockade	Other modes of action
Adenosine	−	−	−	−	+
Atenolol	−	+	−	−	−
Propranol	+	+	−	−	−
Sotalol	−	+	+	−	−
Verapamil	−	−	−	+	−
Digoxin	−	−	−	−	+
Disopyramide	+	−	+	−	−
Amiodarone	−	−	+	−	−
Propafenone	+	−	+	−	−
Flecainide	+	−	−	−	−
Lidocaine	+	−	−	−	−
Mexiletine	+	−	−	−	−

+, presence of activity; −, absence of activity.

They can be divided into three groups, depending on their effect on the duration of the action potential:

• Class 1a drugs increase the duration of the action potential (e.g. quinidine, procainamide)
• Class 1b drugs reduce the duration of the action potential (e.g. lidocaine, mexilitine)
• Class 1c drugs do not affect the duration of the action potential (e.g. flecainide)

Most class 1 drugs show the property of use–dependence, where the degree of blockade is dependent on the activation of Na^+ channels. Class 1a and 1c drugs associate and dissociate from Na^+ channels slowly, and channel blockade is constant throughout the cardiac cycle. In contrast, class 1b drugs associate and dissociate rapidly during each cardiac cycle, so that they suppress premature beats without interference with the subsequent action potential.

Most class 1 drugs modify arrhythmias that are due to enhanced automaticity or to re-entry. When cardiac arrhythmias are due to enhanced automaticity, they reduce Na^+ entry, and may thus reduce the rate of diastolic depolarization in abnormal ectopic foci. In these conditions, the diastolic potential in the ectopic focus reaches the threshold for depolarization less rapidly, and this may allow the SA node to resume its normal role as a pacemaker. Some drugs with class 1 activity may also raise the threshold for depolarization. When cardiac arrhythmias are due to re-entry, drugs with class 1a activity may increase the action potential duration and refractory period of the pathway that is responsible for re-entry. This may prevent retrograde conduction of the impulse

(Fig. 15.3) and produce bidirectional (rather than unidirectional) block in the pathway concerned. Conversely, drugs with class 1b activity reduce the duration of the action potential, and may thus prevent unidirectional blockade and restore normal conduction.

β-Adrenoceptor blockade (class 2 activity)

Drugs that produce β-adrenoceptor blockade antagonize the effects of endogenous catecholamines on the heart. They may also affect terminal postganglionic sympathetic neurons and prevent the release of noradrenaline. Nevertheless, their main action is to produce postsynaptic β-adrenoceptor blockade and protect the heart from circulating adrenaline, as well as the β-effects of locally released noradrenaline. β-Adrenoceptor agonists (e.g. adrenaline) increase the rate of diastolic depolarization (i.e. the slope of phase 4 of the action potential) in the SA node and conducting tissue, and increase Ca^{2+} entry through L-type channels. Consequently, β-adrenoceptor antagonists slow the rate of diastolic depolarization and decrease inward movement of Ca^{2+}. They produce their antiarrhythmic effects by slowing the sinus rate, inhibiting the automaticity of the conducting system during diastolic depolarization, and prolonging the effective refractory period of the AV node. β-Adrenoceptor antagonists are most useful in the management of arrhythmias produced by endogenous or administered catecholamines, although many β-adrenoceptor antagonists also produce Na^+ channel blockade (Table 15.1).

Potassium channel blockade (class 3 activity)

Some antiarrhythmic drugs prolong the duration of the action potential in both conducting tissues and in cardiac muscle fibres. Many of these drugs act by decreasing the rate of K^+ loss through ion channels, or by modifying the rate of Ca^{2+} entry. This effect is most marked in the bundle of His, anomalous AV conduction pathways, and in atrial and ventricular muscle. Some drugs that prolong the action potential also antagonize the effects of catecholamines (e.g. sotalol) or modify the ionic changes responsible for generation of the action potential (e.g. disopyramide). Nevertheless, these drugs primarily increase the duration of the action potential and consequently prolong the refractory period of the His–Purkinje system and cardiac muscle. Ectopic foci due to enhanced automaticity in atrial and ventricular muscle are suppressed, and reciprocal rhythms that are due to re-entry are prevented. Antiarrhythmic agents that prolong the duration of the action potential may be of value in the management of patients with supraventricular tachyarrhythmias, or in arrhythmias associated with anomalous conduction pathways. Nevertheless, all drugs that prolong the ventricular action potential may induce torsade de pointes (prolongation of the Q-T interval followed by episodes of polymorphic tachycardia).

Calcium channel blockade (class 4 activity)

Calcium channel blockers prevent the voltage-dependent entry of Ca^{2+} into cardiac muscle cells during depolarization. Pacemaker cells in the SA and the AV node are almost entirely dependent on inward Ca^{2+} currents for depolarization. Drugs that block Ca^{2+} channels prevent this process, and are particularly effective in preventing reentrant arrhythmias in the AV node and including nodal tachycardia. Ca^{2+} also plays an important part in the excitation of vascular smooth muscle (Chapter 14), so Ca^{2+} channel blockade decreases vascular tone and induces vasodilatation.

Other antiarrhythmic drugs

Although the classification of antiarrhythmic drugs by their electrophysiological effects emphasizes the differences between their mode of action, it is of limited clinical significance. It does not reflect the clinical use of drugs in cardiac arrhythmias, and does not include certain drugs with valuable antiarrhythmic properties (e.g. adenosine, digoxin). In addition, many drugs possess more than one type of antiarrhythmic activity (Table 15.1). Commonly used antiarrhythmic drugs may act on the SA and AV nodes, the atria, or the ventricles (Table 15.2), and for practical purposes can be divided into three groups:
• Agents that are used in supraventricular arrhythmias
• Agents that are used in supraventricular and ventricular arrhythmias
• Agents that are used in ventricular arrhythmias

Table 15.2 The principal site or sites of action of common antiarrhythmic drugs.

SA and AV node	Atrium	Ventricle
Adenosine	Disopyramide	Disopyramide
β-Adrenoceptor antagonists	Amiodarone	Amiodarone
Verapamil	Propafenone	Propafenone
Digoxin		Flecainide
		Lidocaine
		Mexiletine

Drugs that are used in supraventricular arrhythmias

Adenosine

Physiology

Adenosine is an endogenous nucleoside and chemical mediator, and consists of a purine base (adenine) linked to a pentose sugar (D-ribose). It is produced during normal metabolic activity by the action of various intracellular enzymes on high energy phosphates, and is also formed from S-adenosylhomocysteine. Experimental studies indicate that extracellular levels of adenosine are significantly increased during hypoxic and ischaemic episodes. Adenosine receptors mediate several physiological effects concerned with cellular conservation, including vasodilatation, inhibition of Ca^{2+} transport and glutamate release, as well as K^+ channel activation and glucose mobilization.

Pharmacological effects

Adenosine has negative inotropic effects on the heart, and particularly affects SA automaticity, AV nodal excitation and conduction in anomalous pathways. These effects are mediated by adenosine A_1-receptors, which are coupled to G-proteins (G_i). Consequently, receptor activation produces a decrease in intracellular cAMP, opening of K^+_{Ach} channels and hyperpolarization, and adenosine slows the rate of rise of the pacemaker potential.

Administration

Adenosine is frequently the drug of choice in the treatment of supraventricular arrhythmias, particularly paroxysmal supraventricular tachycardia, and arrhythmias associated with anomalous pathways. It is given by rapid intravenous injection as three incremental bolus doses (3 mg, 6 mg and 12 mg) until the desired effect is attained. The effects of adenosine are transient, as its plasma half-life is only 8–10 seconds, due to its rapid uptake by erythrocytes and subsequent metabolism. Adenosine may also be used as a diagnostic aid in the management of tachyarrhythmias, and as a coronary vasodilator during radionuclide myocardial perfusion imaging.

Adverse effects

Adenosine has several adverse effects (some of which are not mediated by adenosine A_1-receptors), including facial flushing, bronchospasm and chest pain. It also decreases the atrial refractory period and may induce atrial fibrillation or flutter. Severe bradycardia has been reported, and its half-life may be prolonged and its activity enhanced by the concurrent administration of dipyridamole, which decreases the uptake of adenosine by erythrocytes. Adenosine triphosphate has also been used during anaesthesia to attenuate the sympathetic responses to laryngoscopy and endotracheal intubation.

β-Adrenoceptor antagonists

β-Adrenoceptor antagonists are sometimes used in the treatment of paroxysmal supraventricular tachycardia and sinus tachycardia associated with thyrotoxicosis, and when arrhythmias are due to increased sympathetic activity or increased concentrations of catecholamines. In atrial fibrillation, they can be used with digoxin to suppress a rapid ventricular response. They are also commonly used after myocardial infarction, in order to control arrhythmias and decrease the possibility of recurrent attacks. They decrease cardiac output and may precipitate or exacerbate cardiac failure, and should be avoided in patients with heart block, since they increase the refractory period of the SA node and the bundle of His. Their antiarrhythmic activity is mainly due to β-adrenoceptor blockade.

β-Adrenoceptor antagonists are also considered in Chapters 13 and 14.

Verapamil

Pharmacological effects

Depolarization in pacemaker cells is almost entirely dependent on the entry of Ca^{2+} from extracellular fluid through T- and L-channels. Verapamil is a calcium channel-blocking drug that prevents Ca^{2+} transport through L-channels in SA and AV nodal cells, and has similar (but less marked) effects on myocardial contractile

Table 15.3 The effect of calcium channel blocking drugs on the heart and circulation.

	Heart rate	AV conduction	Myocardial contractility	Coronary and peripheral blood vessels
Verapamil	Decreased	Prolonged	Decreased	Slight dilatation
Diltiazem	Decreased	Prolonged	Slightly decreased	Moderate dilatation
Dihydropyridines	Increased	Enhanced*	Increased*	Marked dilatation

*Mainly due to reflex effects induced by hypotension.

tissue and vascular smooth muscle (Table 15.3). Consequently, the conduction velocity of cardiac impulses in nodal cells is decreased, and their refractory period is increased. Verapamil can precipitate AV block in patients on other drugs that depress AV conduction, such as cholinergic agents or β-adrenoceptor antagonists. In addition, verapamil may cause bradycardia and precipitate or intensify cardiac failure. Although the drug has only limited effects on vascular smooth muscle, it may cause vasodilatation and hypotension.

Administration

Verapamil can be given intravenously or orally (usually 120–360 mg daily, given in divided doses) and there may be considerable individual variability in the response. Although verapamil is well absorbed after oral administration, it is subject to extensive presystemic metabolism, and its bioavailability is only 20–30%. It is extensively bound to plasma proteins (80–90%) and is mainly metabolized by the liver to inactive metabolites, which are eliminated in urine. The terminal half-life of verapamil is usually 3–7 hours.

Verapamil has been mainly used in the treatment of acute and chronic supraventricular tachycardias. In atrial fibrillation and flutter, it slows the ventricular rate and may restore sinus rhythm. In addition to its use as an antiarrhythmic drug, verapamil has also been used in the treatment of angina and hypertension. Unfortunately, it may cause bradycardia, hypotension and congestive cardiac failure, particularly in patients on β-adrenoceptor antagonists and other drugs that depress AV conduction.

Digoxin

Digoxin is a glycoside derived from the dried leaves of the foxglove (*Digitalis lanata*). Its parent glycoside (lanatoside C) has also been used as an antiarrhythmic drug. Digoxin consists of a sugar (digitoxose) combined with an aglycone (digitoxigenin), and its effectiveness is mainly dependent on digitoxigenin. Digoxin has little effect on the normal heart, and its actions are most evident in patients with atrial flutter or fibrillation.

Indirect effects that are mediated by the vagus nerve

Indirect effects of digoxin cause
• bradycardia (by slowing the rate of rise of the pacemaker prepotential in the SA node)
• reduced refractory period in atrial muscle
• increased refractory period in AV node and bundle of His

All of the indirect effects of digoxin are antagonized by atropine and other antimuscarinic drugs.

Direct effects on cardiac muscle and conducting tissue

Direct effects of digoxin result in
• increased inotropic effects (although the rate of ventricular contraction and relaxation are unaffected)
• increased refractory period in AV node and bundle of His
• reduced refractory period in ventricles
• increased ventricular excitability

The direct effects of digoxin are due to inhibition of Na^+/K^+ ATPase, which mainly governs the ionic balance in cardiac cells. Inhibition of this enzyme increases intracellular Na^+, which decreases Na^+ entry during depolarization and Na^+/Ca^{2+} exchange, and thus enhances intracellular Ca^{2+}, ventricular excitability and the force of myocardial contraction.

Clinical use

Digoxin is most commonly used in the treatment of atrial flutter and fibrillation. In these conditions, numerous impulses impinge on the AV node, and a significant proportion are conducted to the His–Purkinje system, resulting in a rapid and irregular ventricular rate. Digoxin (by both its indirect and direct actions) increases the refractory period of the AV node and the bundle of His. Consequently, the rate of ventricular contraction is decreased, allowing more time for ventricular filling to occur. Nevertheless, the pulse rate should not be allowed to fall below 60 beats per minute. Digoxin may increase atrial arrhythmias, since it reduces the duration of the atrial refractory period.

Digoxin is also used in the treatment of chronic heart failure in patients with sinus rhythm (although its use for this purpose has declined). Although it initially increases myocardial contractility and cardiac output, its positive inotropic effects may not be maintained during chronic treatment. In mild and moderate heart failure, diuretics and ACE inhibitors are usually more effective.

Although digoxin has also been used in the treatment of paroxysmal atrial tachycardia, it is now rarely used for this purpose, since adenosine, β-adrenergic antagonists or verapamil are usually preferred.

Digoxin should never be given to patients with ventricular extrasystoles or tachycardia, since it increases cardiac excitability and may precipitate ventricular fibrillation.

Administration

Patients are usually digitalized by the oral administration of 0.75–1.0 mg digoxin daily, until an optimum effect is obtained. Maintenance doses are usually 0.25–0.5 mg in 24 hours. Digoxin is completely absorbed from the small intestine (as long as drug dissolution is complete). Maximum plasma concentrations are present within 30–60 minutes, although therapeutic effects are not observed for several hours. Digoxin is almost entirely eliminated by glomerular filtration, and cumulation may occur in elderly subjects or patients with renal failure. It has a long terminal half-life (24–36 h), an extremely large volume of distribution (approximately 10 L kg^{-1}), and its concentration in skeletal or cardiac muscle is often 20–30 times greater than the plasma level.

Adverse effects

Digoxin has a low therapeutic ratio, and the relation between the toxic and therapeutic doses is close. The initial effects of toxicity are often anorexia, nausea, vomiting and abdominal discomfort. Neurological side effects (headache, fatigue and visual disturbances) are not infrequent, and skin rashes and gynaecomastia are occasionally seen.

In addition, digoxin has serious toxic effects on the heart, and almost any arrhythmia may be produced and can simulate cardiac disease. The commonest arrhythmias induced are ventricular extrasystoles (including coupled beats), ventricular tachycardia, and various types of AV block. Digoxin toxicity may be precipitated by electrolyte abnormalities such as hypokalaemia or hypercalcaemia, and by acid–base changes. It is particularly common in elderly subjects and in patients with poor renal function. Digoxin therapy should be controlled (when possible) by the measurement of its serum concentration by radioimmunoassay. Serum concentrations of less than 1 ng mL^{-1} are usually ineffective, while concentrations greater than 2.5 ng mL^{-1} are commonly associated with toxic effects.

Digoxin-specific antibody

Digoxin overdosage can be treated with digoxin-specific antibody fragments (Digibind). This preparation consists of the F (ab) fragments of immunoglobulin G (IgG) antibodies raised in sheep. The affinity of digoxin for the antibody fragments is more than 10 times greater than its affinity for Na$^+$/K$^+$ ATPase, so that the drug is removed from the enzyme and other digoxin receptors and eliminated in urine as a protein-bound complex. Treatment with digoxin-specific antibody fragments is potentially hazardous, and should be restricted to severe and life-threatening cases of drug overdose.

Antimuscarinic agents

Antimuscarinic drugs (e.g. atropine, glycopyrronium) are widely used to prevent or antagonize bradycardia during general anaesthesia. They are considered in detail in Chapter 13.

Drugs that are used in supraventricular and ventricular arrhythmias

Disopyramide

Disopyramide produces blockade of Na$^+$ channels, and consequently prolongs the rise time of phase 0 of the cardiac action potential (Fig. 15.2) in atrial and ventricular muscle. The threshold potential that is required to initiate phase 0 may also be increased. In addition, disopyramide increases the duration of the action potential by delaying repolarization, and thus prolongs the effective refractory period of atrial and ventricular muscle. Disopyramide

has considerable anticholinergic activity, and may produce atropine-like effects in tissues that are innervated by the parasympathetic nervous system. Excessive doses may cause depression of myocardial contractility, AV block, increased ventricular excitability and cardiac arrest.

Disopyramide is mainly used in the prevention and treatment of ventricular arrhythmias, particularly those induced by myocardial infarction, surgical procedures or digoxin overdose. It is sometimes useful in arrhythmias that do not respond to lidocaine or mexiletine. Disopyramide is occasionally used in supraventricular tachycardia, atrial arrhythmias or in arrhythmias associated with anomalous conducting pathways.

Disopyramide can be given intravenously or orally (usual dose range = 300–800 mg daily), and is mainly eliminated unchanged. Its terminal half-life is 4–6 hours, but is considerably prolonged in patients with cardiac or renal failure. In these conditions, the dosage of the drug should be modified.

Amiodarone

Amiodarone produces blockade of K$^+$ channels, and thus increases the duration of the action potential by approximately 20–30%. The maximum rate of repolarization is decreased, phase 3 is prolonged, and the onset of phase 4 is delayed (Fig. 15.2). The refractory period of the myocardium and the entire conducting system is increased.

Amiodarone is mainly used in arrhythmias associated with anomalous conducting pathways (particularly the Wolff–Parkinson–White syndrome), but is sometimes used in other supraventricular and ventricular arrhythmias when other drugs are ineffective. It commonly causes mild sinus bradycardia, and when used with other drugs that slow the heart (e.g. digoxin, β-adrenoceptor antagonists), marked bradycardia and a reduction in cardiac output may occur. Amiodarone is an iodinated drug that affects thyroid function, and occasionally causes hypothyroidism. It commonly causes the formation of microdeposits of lipofuscin in the cornea, and photosensitivity and pigmentation of the skin may also occur. Pulmonary fibrosis, peripheral neuropathy and hepatotoxicity are other long-term adverse effects. Amiodarone is extensively bound to plasma protein, and has a relatively long terminal half-life (approximately 28 days). It may be given intravenously or orally (usual dose = 200–600 mg daily), and an antiarrhythmic response usually occurs within 1 week, and may persist for 4–6 weeks after administration ceases. Amiodarone is mainly eliminated by metabolism to desethylamiodarone.

Since amiodarone prolongs the ventricular action potential and Q-T interval, it may precipitate polymorphic ventricular tachycardia (torsade de pointes) in susceptible patients.

Propafenone

Propafenone is an antiarrhythmic agent that decreases the rate of depolarization of phase 0 of the action potential and slows conduction, particularly in the His–Purkinje system. The duration of the action potential is prolonged in atrial and ventricular muscle, as well as in anomalous pathways. Thus, propafenone may be useful in both supraventricular and ventricular arrhythmias.

Propafenone is used as a racemic mixture, and its S(+)-enantiomer is a non-selective antagonist at β-adrenoceptors in addition to its membrane-stabilizing activity. It has a number of adverse effects, including minor gastrointestinal disorders, antimuscarinic effects, drug rashes and occasional hypersensitivity responses. Undesirable effects due to β_2-adrenoceptor receptor antagonism (e.g. bronchospasm) have also been reported. Propafenone is metabolized by an isoform of cytochrome P450, which shows genetic polymorphism (CYP 2D6), and is more slowly metabolized in patients with enzyme deficiency. It may also increase the bioavailability of other antiarrhythmic agents, particularly digoxin.

Flecainide

Flecainide is a fluorinated derivative of procainamide. It decreases Na^+ entry into myocardial cells, and prolongs the rise time of phase 0 but does not affect the duration of the action potential. Flecainide also reduces automaticity and prolongs atrial, nodal and ventricular conduction. In addition, it has negative inotropic effects, and may precipitate cardiac failure in susceptible patients.

Flecainide is used in the prophylaxis and treatment of paroxysmal atrial fibrillation, and is also sometimes used in ventricular arrhythmias. Unfortunately, it occasionally precipitates arrhythmias and sudden death in patients after myocardial infarction. Flecainide causes minor adverse effects (e.g. nausea, dizziness, tremor) in approximately 25% of patients. It has a long terminal half-life (12–27 h), which may be further prolonged in the elderly and in renal failure. Flecainide is eliminated equally by metabolism and excretion, and has significant pharmacokinetic interactions with many other drugs, including digoxin, propranolol and amiodarone.

β-Adrenoceptor antagonists

β-Adrenoceptor antagonists are also widely used in the prevention and treatment of various atrial and ventricular arrhythmias (Chapters 13 and 14). Sotalol is a non-selective β_1 and β_2 antagonist that prolongs the duration of the ventricular action potential (Q-T interval) and may induce torsade de pointes in susceptible patients. Consequently, in current practice its clinical use is usually restricted to the treatment of paroxysmal atrial tachycardia and various ventricular arrhythmias.

Drugs that are used in ventricular arrhythmias

Lidocaine

Lidocaine blocks Na^+ channels in cardiac muscle cells, as well as in motor and sensory nerve fibres (Chapter 9). It decreases automaticity in conducting pathways and ventricular ectopic foci by reducing the slope of phase 4, and may also alter the threshold for excitability. In addition, lidocaine decreases the duration of the action potential of cardiac muscle, particularly in the preterminal Purkinje fibres, and suppresses arrhythmias that are due to re-entry or established reciprocal rhythms.

Lidocaine is primarily used in the management of ventricular arrhythmias, particularly those induced by myocardial infarction or cardiac surgery. It is of no value in the treatment of atrial arrhythmias, and therapeutic concentrations do not significantly affect AV conduction. Rarely, lidocaine may precipitate or exacerbate intraventricular conduction blockade. Moderate doses have no significant effect on heart rate, blood pressure or myocardial contractility.

Lidocaine may produce toxic effects on the CNS, which are associated with high plasma concentrations of the drug (Chapter 9), and its safe and effective use depends on accurate administration. Optimal antiarrhythmic effects are present at plasma concentrations of 2–4 $\mu g\,mL^{-1}$. These concentrations can be produced by a bolus injection of 75–100 mg, followed by a constant infusion of 4 mg min^{-1} for 30 minutes, 2 mg min^{-1} for 2 hours, and then 1 mg min^{-1}. The terminal half-life of lidocaine in patients with normal hepatic and cardiac function ranges from 100 to 120 minutes. Consequently, when the drug is infused at a constant rate, cumulation may occur for at least 7 hours before a steady state is reached. In the presence of liver disease, cardiac failure or drugs that impair hepatic blood flow, this period may be prolonged.

Mexiletine

Mexiletine is chemically related to lidocaine, and has similar effects on ventricular arrhythmias. It slows the rise time of phase 0 of the cardiac action potential (i.e. it reduces the maximum rate of depolarization) without significantly affecting the resting membrane potential. The duration of the action potential is slightly reduced, due to the shortening of repolarization (phase 3). Mexiletine is mainly used as an alternative to lidocaine in the prevention and treatment of ventricular arrhythmias induced by coronary artery disease and myocardial infarction. It is effective when given orally or intravenously (usual intravenous dose = 100–250 mg).

Mexiletine is used cautiously in patients with cardiac conduction defects. Its therapeutic ratio is low and the drug commonly causes side effects, which may affect the CNS or the cardiovascular system. Mexiletine is mainly eliminated by hepatic metabolism, and its terminal half-life is usually 10–15 hours. Small amounts of the drug (approximately 10% of the dose) are excreted unchanged in urine.

Other antiarrhythmic drugs

Quinidine

Quinidine is an isomer of quinine with more powerful antiarrhythmic effects. It increases the threshold for depolarization by Na^+ channel blockade, and prolongs the duration of the action potential by blockade of K^+ and Ca^{2+} channels. It also has antimuscarinic effects on the heart, and antagonizes the effects of increased vagal tone.

Quinidine is highly protein-bound drug and a potent inhibitor of CYP 2D6, and may be involved in significant drug interactions. In addition, the antiarrhythmic dose of the drug (1–3 g in 24 h) is close to its toxic dose. It may induce various bradyarrhythmias and conduction defects, prolongs the Q-T interval and may be associated with torsade de pointes. Quinidine commonly affects the CNS and may produce various hypersensitivity responses.

In the past, quinidine has been used in the management of atrial and ventricular arrhythmias. Because of its many disadvantages, it is rarely used in current practice.

Procainamide

The actions of procainamide are similar to quinidine, although it has no antimuscarinic activity and has fewer cardiac depressant effects. In the past, it was commonly used in the management of ventricular arrhythmias.

Procainamide has a short plasma half-life (3–4 h), and is mainly eliminated unchanged in urine. It is also partly hydrolysed by amidases, and is acetylated to an active metabolite with anti-arrhythmic properties (N-acetylprocainamide). The acetylation of procainamide is controlled by genetic polymorphism, and patients can be divided into slow and fast acetylators. A long-term hazard of chronic oral treatment is the development of antinuclear antibodies and a syndrome resembling systemic lupus erythematosus (SLE). Slow acetylators of procainamide are more liable to develop signs of drug toxicity, including SLE. Procainamide has been superseded by other agents, and is rarely used in current practice.

Magnesium salts

Magnesium is the fourth most common cation in the body (after Na$^+$, K$^+$ and Ca^{2+}), and approximately 35–40% is present in cardiac and skeletal muscle. It has an established or putative role in many physiological systems, including the inhibition of acetylcholine and noradrenaline release, and antagonism of NMDA receptors in the CNS. Magnesium ions are bound to cellular ATP, and act as a cofactor for Na$^+$/K$^+$ ATPase, so that intracellular concentrations of Mg^{2+} may affect Na$^+$ and K$^+$ transfer.

Decreased Mg^{2+} concentrations may be associated with a variety of cardiac arrhythmias, and the effects observed are similar to hypokalaemia. Magnesium deficiency may facilitate Ca^{2+} influx, which has a central role in cellular death during myocardial ischaemia.

Clinical use

Magnesium salts have been used in the treatment of supraventricular arrhythmias for at least 75 years. Magnesium sulphate [20 mmol (2.5 g), given as 5 mL 50% over 20–30 min] is commonly used in ventricular tachycardia and torsade de pointes induced by antiarrhythmic agents, or to reverse arrhythmias associated with digitalis toxicity. In shock and refractory ventricular fibrillation, magnesium sulphate (8–16 mmol, i.e. 1–2 g) is sometimes given via a peripheral vein. After myocardial infarction, a bolus dose followed by an infusion of 65–72 mmol in 24 hours has been recommended. Mortality appears to be reduced, and there may be a prophylactic effect on the development of arrhythmias. However, an improvement in coronary blood flow (due to the vasodilating properties of magnesium) and a reduction in platelet aggregation may be contributory factors.

Antiarrhythmic drugs and general anaesthesia

General anaesthesia presents special risks in patients receiving antiarrhythmic drugs. These hazards may be related to the existence of cardiovascular disease, or to concurrent drug therapy. Verapamil and β-adrenoceptor antagonists reduce cardiac output, and the use of anaesthetic agents that produce similar effects may be hazardous. Similarly, many antiarrhythmic drugs increase the refractory period of junctional tissues and delay AV conduction. These effects may be potentiated by anaesthetic agents that depress AV conduction, such as suxametho-

nium, neostigmine and some inhalational anaesthetics, and partial or complete heart block may be precipitated.

Cardiac arrhythmias are not uncommon during general anaesthesia, although they are often relatively benign and may require little or no intervention or treatment. Occasionally, they are life threatening and require the immediate administration of antiarrhythmic drugs. Although they may have no identifiable cause, they are often precipitated by physiological or pharmacological factors associated with general anaesthesia. Thus, arrhythmias may be due to

- electrolyte abnormalities (particularly in K$^+$, Mg^{2+} or Ca^{2+} levels)
- hypoxia and hypercarbia
- increased secretion of catecholamines (which may be induced by hypoxia or hypercarbia)
- hypovolaemia
- extremes of body temperature
- surgical stimulation under light anaesthesia
- operative manipulations that alter vagal or sympathetic tone
- drugs used during anaesthesia

Operative manipulations that alter vagal or sympathetic tone

Stimulation of the upper airways is associated with a reflex increase in sympathetic activity and increased catecholamine secretion. Consequently, arrhythmias may occur during laryngoscopy, bronchoscopy, endotracheal intubation and extubation, and dental surgery. Traction or stimulation of the heart, the lungs and many intra-abdominal viscera may also cause reflex effects, including arrhythmias. Similarly, neurosurgical procedures in the posterior fossa, ocular surgery, and stimulation of the carotid sinus may cause bradycardia or cardiac arrhythmias.

Drugs used during anaesthesia

Drugs used during anaesthesia (e.g. adrenaline, suxamethonium) may precipitate cardiac arrhythmias. Some inhalational anaesthetics sensitize the heart to the effects of administered or endogenous adrenaline, and may cause abnormalities in cardiac rhythm. Arrhythmias associated with catecholamines or increased catecholamine sensitivity can be treated with atenolol (2.5 mg over 3 min), which may be repeated at 2 minutes intervals until a response is observed, or a maximum dose of 10 mg has been given. Alternatively, the short-acting β$_1$-adrenoceptor antagonist esmolol may be used. Non-selective β-adrenoceptor antagonists are less suitable, particularly in patients with obstructive pulmonary disease, diabetes or peripheral vascular disease. Arrhythmias produced by suxamethonium invariably respond to atropine (0.3–0.6 mg). Although atropine itself may produce arrhythmias, these are usually benign and of little importance.

Patients with pre-existing cardiovascular disease or with certain endocrine disorders may develop arrhythmias during surgery. Arrhythmias associated with thyrotoxicosis, thyroid surgery or phaeochromocytomas usually respond to β_1-adrenoceptor antagonists.

Drugs used in the treatment of angina

Anginal pain occurs when coronary blood flow cannot meet the metabolic demands of the myocardium. Myocardial hypoxia leads to the accumulation of local metabolites, such as potassium ions, adenosine, prostaglandins and bradykinin, resulting in precordial pain. Drugs are mainly useful for the prophylaxis of anginal attacks rather than their treatment, since the precordial pain usually responds rapidly to termination of the precipitating stimulus. Occasionally, anginal attacks are prolonged, and drug treatment is necessary.

Several groups of drugs are commonly used to prevent attacks of anginal pain:
• Nitrates
• Calcium channel blockers (calcium antagonists)
• β-Adrenoceptor antagonists
• Potassium channel activators

Nitrates
Pharmacological effects
Nitrates selectively dilate small veins, resulting in the pooling of blood in capacitance vessels. Ventricular filling pressure (ventricular end-diastolic pressure) is reduced, and both ventricular size and myocardial wall tension is decreased. Consequently, there is increased perfusion of subendocardial blood vessels (which are normally subjected to the greatest pressure during ventricular systole). Myocardial work and oxygen requirements are reduced, and blood is redistributed to ischaemic regions.

Nitrates also act on the resistance vessels, and some arteriolar dilatation occurs so that peripheral resistance is reduced. Consequently, cardiac work is reduced, although compensatory tachycardia sometimes causes a fall in coronary perfusion pressure. Nitrates directly dilate coronary blood vessels and atherosclerotic stenoses, so that collat-

eral flow is increased and the oxygenation of ischaemic myocardium is enhanced.

Since nitrates primarily affect capacitance vessels, they may produce postural hypotension. In supine patients they have only minor effects on blood pressure, although profound hypotension occurs on standing (particularly in younger subjects). The effect of nitrates on pulse rate is variable, but in small doses they cause bradycardia. Higher doses commonly produce tachycardia due to a compensatory increase in sympathetic tone.

Mode of action
The vasodilator effects of all nitrates (including sodium nitroprusside) are mainly due to their intracellular metabolism to nitric oxide (NO), which is identical to endothelium-derived relaxant factor (EDRF). All organic nitrates are lipid-soluble compounds that readily penetrate many cells, including smooth muscle and vascular endothelial cells. They are metabolized intracellularly by glutathione-S-transferases and cytochrome P450 enzymes to nitrite ions and NO, which diffuses into vascular smooth muscle and reacts with sulphydryl groups to form reactive intermediates (S-nitrosothiols). NO and nitrosothiols activate soluble guanylate cyclase, increasing the conversion of GTP to cGMP. This intermediate messenger subsequently activates protein kinase, resulting in the phosphorylation of membrane proteins, reduced sequestration of Ca^{2+} and relaxation of vascular smooth muscle (Fig. 3.7).

All nitrates may rapidly induce the development of tolerance to their vasodilator effects, unless there is a daily drug-free period of 6–8 hours. Tolerance is probably due to the depletion of sulphydryl (–SH) groups from vascular smooth muscle cells (Chapter 5).

Glyceryl trinitrate

$$CH_2 - O - NO_2$$
$$|$$
$$CH - O - NO_2$$
$$|$$
$$CH_2 - O - NO_2$$

Glyceryl trinitrate (GTN) tablets (0.3–1 mg) are used to provide rapid symptomatic relief of angina. They are also of value in providing short-term extension of exercise tolerance, and should be taken approximately 1–2 minutes before any activity that is liable to provoke angina. After sublingual administration, their action is almost immediate, and usually lasts for 20–30 minutes. Oral administration has little or no effect, due to extensive presystemic metabolism of the drug by the gut wall and the liver. Glyceryl trinitrate is volatile and slowly evaporates from the tablets at ambient temperatures, so they often deteriorate within 2–6 months of preparation. Although controlled release tablets are also available, they are of less value in the prophylaxis of angina.

Other preparations of glyceryl trinitrate have been extensively used to prevent or control anginal pain. Sustained release sublingual or buccal tablets have an equally rapid onset but a longer duration of action than conventional preparations. Metered aerosol sprays are often used for sublingual administration, and since they are relatively stable, they may be useful in patients who require infrequent prophylaxis.

Transdermal preparations are also widely used. Glyceryl trinitrate is an extremely potent and lipid-soluble drug, which is readily absorbed through the skin. Transdermal patches containing a slow release formulation of GTN can be applied to any area of hairless skin in the body (e.g. the chest wall, the shoulder, the thigh or the abdomen). The rate of drug delivery is controlled by a semipermeable membrane between the drug and the skin, and usually releases 5–10 mg of GTN over a 24-hour period. This preparation may be particularly useful for patients who suffer from nocturnal anginal attacks. GTN ointment is also used as a transdermal preparation, which is covered by an occlusive dressing. This preparation provides prophylaxis for 2–3 hours, but is inconvenient to apply and is unsuitable for long-term use.

All of these preparations are associated with the rapid and sustained systemic absorption of GTN, and avoid extensive presystemic metabolism by the liver. Intravenous infusions of glyceryl trinitrate have occasionally been used in the prophylaxis of angina, and have also been used to provide controlled hypotension during surgical procedures (Chapter 14).

Other nitrates

Oral preparations of other nitrates have also been widely used in the prophylaxis of angina. In general, these preparations decrease the frequency of attacks and may extend exercise tolerance, but they are of no value in the immediate treatment of anginal pain.

In current practice, oral preparations of isosorbide dinitrate and isosorbide mononitrate are most commonly used. Isosorbide dinitrate is metabolized by the gut and the liver into isosorbide mononitrate, which has a longer terminal half-life than the parent drug. The metabolite isosorbide mononitrate, which has a systemic bioavailability of 100%, is also used in the management of angina. Although it is also absorbed after sublingual administration, its duration of action is usually no greater than sublingual GTN.

Calcium channel blockers (calcium antagonists)
Calcium ions and physiological processes

Calcium ions are involved in many cellular processes, including glandular secretion, neuronal excitability, neurotransmitter release, excitation–contraction coupling and blood coagulation. In addition, they play an important role in the excitation and depolarization of cardiac muscle and vascular smooth muscle. During excitation, Ca^{2+} pass from extracellular fluid into junctional and myocardial cells through specific voltage-sensitive ion channels, resulting in depolarization. Similar changes occur during excitation in vascular smooth muscle.

Calcium channel blockers

Drugs that prevent Ca^{2+} entry during depolarization are usually known as calcium channel blockers or calcium antagonists, and may interfere with cardiac excitation or conduction, decrease the force of myocardial contraction or cause relaxation of vascular smooth muscle. All calcium channel blockers that are currently available selectively prevent Ca^{2+} ion entry through L- (long lasting) channels, but do not have significant effects on other ion channels. In angina, they usually increase coronary and peripheral blood flow, reduce blood pressure, decrease the work of the heart, and improve the efficiency of myocardial contraction, so that the imbalance between oxygen supply and demand is corrected. In addition, calcium channel blockers relax vascular spasm, and are usually effective in vasospastic angina (Prinzmetal's angina), as well as classical exertional angina.

Low voltage dependent T- (transient) channels are also present in vascular smooth muscle as well as the conducting tissues of the heart.

Commonly used calcium channel blockers are
- Verapamil
- Diltiazem
- Dihydropyridine derivatives

The clinical effects of individual calcium antagonists are often different, possibly due to variability in their affinity for L-channels in junctional tissues, cardiac muscle and vascular smooth muscle.

A number of other drugs have non-selective effects on calcium channels, including lidoflazine, prenylamine, perhexiline and fluorinated anaesthetic agents.

Verapamil

In the SA node and the AV node, depolarization is dependent on the influx of Ca^{2+} from extracellular fluid. Verapamil prevents Ca^{2+} entry into nodal cells, but has less marked effects on myocardial contractile tissue and vascular smooth muscle. Consequently, verapamil has been primarily used in the treatment of supraventricular arrhythmias (page 294), but may also be of value in angina. It has significant negative inotropic effects and may cause bradycardia and cardiac failure, particularly in patients on β-adrenoceptor antagonists and other drugs, which depress AV conduction. Although verapamil has only limited effects on vascular smooth muscle, it may reduce peripheral resistance and cause hypotension. The usual oral dose ranges from 120 to 360 mg daily, given in divided doses.

Diltiazem

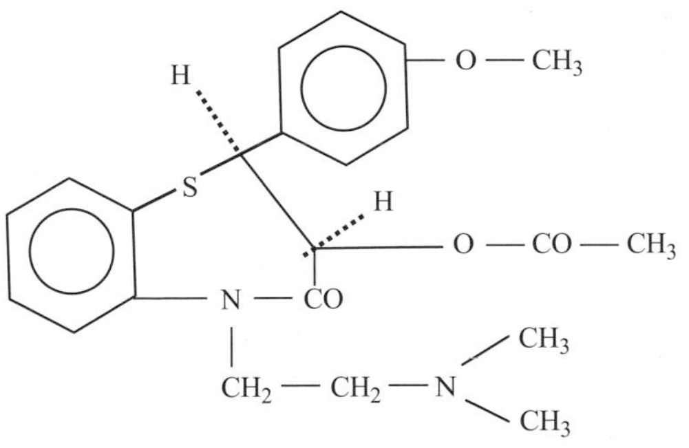

Diltiazem is a calcium channel blocker that affects the heart and in the peripheral circulation. Thus, it impairs cardiac conduction and contractility, and also causes vasodilatation in coronary and peripheral blood vessels (Table 15.3). Diltiazem reduces the automaticity of the SA node, and impairs conduction of the cardiac impulses through the AV node. Consequently, the P-R interval is usually prolonged, and heart rate is reduced. Diltiazem also affects Ca^{2+} channels in vascular smooth muscle and the coronary circulation, and peripheral resistance is decreased. Systolic and diastolic pressures

fall, due to the decrease in cardiac output and the reduction in peripheral resistance, although reflex tachycardia does not usually occur. After oral administration, diltiazem is almost completely absorbed from the small intestine, but is subject to considerable presystemic metabolism. Approximately 60% is metabolized by the liver, while the remainder is eliminated unchanged by the kidney. Although diltiazem has antiarrhythmic effects, it is mainly used in the treatment of angina, hypertension and peripheral vascular disease (including Raynaud's disease).

Dihydropyridine derivatives

Dihydropyridine derivatives that are commonly used clinically are

- Nifedipine
- Nicardipine
- Amlodipine
- Felodipine
- Nisoldipine
- Nimodipine

Nifedipine

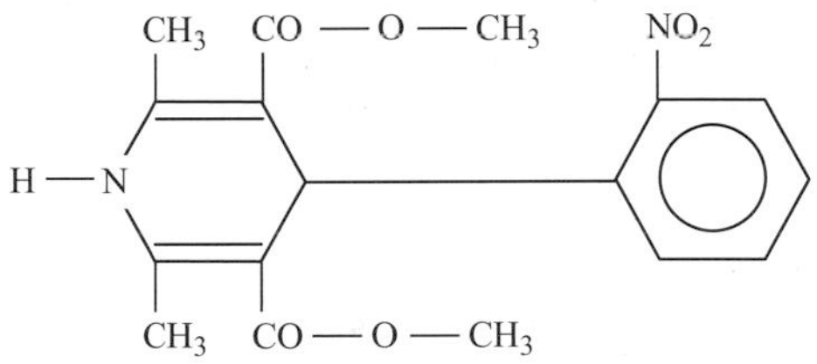

Nifedipine primarily affects the peripheral vasculature and the coronary circulation. It has little or no direct effect on myocardial contractility or AV conduction. It is unclear whether this is related to the preferential localization of the drug in vascular smooth muscle, or to its differential effects on Ca^{2+} channels in the peripheral circulation and cardiac muscle. Current evidence suggests that nifedipine may reduce the duration of L-type calcium channel opening, and thus inhibit the entry of Ca^{2+} into vascular smooth muscle during depolarization.

Nifedipine is a powerful vasodilator, and is approximately 30–50 times more potent than verapamil on vascular smooth muscle. It mainly affects Ca^{2+} channels in arterioles, and has little or no effect on capacitance vessels. Consequently, nifedipine decreases systemic resistance and blood pressure and increases peripheral and coronary blood flow (Table 15.3). In the isolated heart, nifedipine has direct depressant effects and decreases myocardial contractility and AV conduction. In *in vivo* conditions, these effects are overshadowed by reflex tachycardia and increased stroke volume, resulting in a rise in cardiac output. Most of the side effects of nifedipine are due to peripheral vasodilatation and the subsequent reduction in blood pressure (e.g. headache, dizziness, palpitations). Occasionally, nifedipine (and other dihydropyridines) increase the frequency of anginal attacks and prolong ischaemic pain, due to decreased peripheral resistance and the associated reflex tachycardia.

After oral administration, nifedipine is well absorbed although approximately 50% is eliminated by presystemic metabolism. The terminal half-life is approximately 5–6 hours, and its clearance is 20–30% of liver blood flow. Since nifedipine has a short duration of action, it is normally used as a modified release preparation in the treatment of angina and hypertension.

Nicardipine

Nicardipine is closely related to nifedipine. It was originally introduced in Japan as a cerebral vasodilator, and was subsequently used in the treatment of essential hypertension. Nicardipine is a potent vasodilator, decreases systemic vascular resistance and diastolic blood pressure, and increases peripheral and coronary blood flow. It has less direct depressant effects on the heart than nifedipine, and often causes reflex tachycardia and an increase in cardiac output. After oral administration, nicardipine is rapidly absorbed and extensively metabolized by the liver. Its systemic bioavailability is only 30–35%, due to extensive presystemic metabolism, and only small amounts of the unchanged drug are eliminated in urine. The terminal half-life of nicardipine is 7–9 hours, and its clearance is approximately 30–50% of liver blood flow.

Nicardipine is used as a modified release preparation in the treatment of hypertension and angina.

Amlodipine

Amlodipine has similar effects to nicardipine but has a longer duration of action and is usually given once daily. It has selective effects on calcium channels in vascular smooth muscle, but has little or no effect on the heart. It is widely used in the treatment of hypertension and angina.

Nimodipine

Nimodipine has preferential effects on cerebral arterioles, and is used in the prevention and treatment of ischaemic neurological deficits following subarachnoid haemorrhage.

β-Adrenoceptor antagonists

β-Adrenoceptor blockade reduces the work of the heart, decreases oxygen consumption and reduces systemic arterial pressure. In addition, the associated bradycardia improves coronary and myocardial perfusion. Thus, β-adrenoceptor antagonists restore the balance between myocardial oxygen supply and demand, and decrease cardiac activity to a level that does not induce attacks of angina. They also modify sympathetic drive and the effects of circulating catecholamines, and thus reduce chronotropic and inotropic responses during exercise or stress. Consequently, β-adrenoceptor antagonists are widely used to decrease the frequency and severity of attacks of exertional angina. Unlike calcium channel blockers, they are not used in vasospastic (Prinzmetal) angina, since they may exacerbate this condition by promoting coronary vasoconstriction via α-adrenoceptors. They may also precipitate cardiac failure in patients with a poor cardiac reserve.

Although non-selective β_1- and β_2-adrenoceptor antagonists are sometimes used in angina, they may produce β_2-receptor blockade, resulting in bronchospasm, decreased peripheral blood flow, hypoglycaemia, and an increase in uterine tone. These effects are less common with selective β_1-antagonists and 'cardioselective' drugs are often preferred for patients with obstructive airways disease, peripheral vascular disease, and diabetes. The less lipid-soluble agents are not significantly metabolized and have a relatively long half-life, so that once-daily oral administration may produce adequate β-adrenoceptor blockade for up to 24 hours. In addition, they do not readily cross the placenta or the blood–brain barrier.

Potassium channel activators
Potassium channels

The resting potential in vascular smooth muscle is approximately −50 mV, and reflects the distribution of K^+ across the cell membrane. In normal conditions, K^+ diffuse from vascular smooth muscle cells to extracellular fluid through potassium channels, and thus produces the negative resting potential (a 'potassium diffusion potential'). Potassium channels in cell membranes have been divided into at least 21 subfamilies. One of these subfamilies (the $K_{IR}6.x$ subfamily) consists of ATP-sensitive K^+ channels, that are inhibited by ATP and many sulphonylureas. In physiological conditions, K_{ATP} channels close in the presence of excessive ATP, but open when ATP stores are depleted, and this negative feedback process plays an important part in the regulation of intracellular ATP and cellular metabolism. There is considerable evidence that K_{ATP} channels have an important influence on smooth muscle tone during ischaemia and other pathophysiological states. Drugs that activate K_{ATP} channels (e.g. diazoxide, thiazide diuretics) increase K^+ loss from smooth muscle cells, producing hyperpolarization and vasodilatation.

Nicorandil

Nicorandil is a nitrated derivative of nicotinamide that causes relaxation of vascular smooth muscle by two independent mechanisms.

Nicorandil activates K_{ATP} channels, causing hyperpolarization and relaxation of vascular smooth muscle. Experimental patch-clamp studies with glibenclamide (a K_{ATP} channel inhibitor) suggest that nicorandil specifically activates these channels, resulting in arteriolar vasodilatation (particularly in peripheral and coronary blood vessels).

Nicorandil also releases nitrate ions, which are metabolized to nitric oxide and combine with –SH groups in tissues to form nitrosothiol derivatives. These metabolites stimulate soluble guanylate cyclase, and thus increase the synthesis of cGMP and the activation of protein kinase, resulting in vasodilatation. These changes particularly affect small veins and venules, resulting in venous pooling in capacitance vessels. Consequently, nicorandil accelerates recovery from myocardial contraction and may prolong the time for diastolic filling. In experimental studies, it reduces infarct size, and has a cardioprotective effect in ischaemic conditions.

Although other drugs activate K_{ATP} channels and produce vasodilatation (e.g. aprokalim, cromakalim and pinacidil), none of these agents are in current clinical use.

Clinical use

Nicorandil (20–60 mg day^{-1}) is used orally in the prophylaxis of angina, particularly in patients who are resistant or unresponsive to nitrates, β-adrenergic antagonists or calcium channel blockers. Many of its adverse effects including headache, facial flushing, dizziness, postural hypotension and reflex tachycardia, appear to be related to the activation of guanylate cyclase or nitric oxide production.

Drug combinations in angina

Nitrates, calcium channel blockers, β-adrenoceptor antagonists and potassium channel activators have different modes and sites of action on the heart and the circulation, and their use in combination may therefore be beneficial. Nitrates primarily dilate the venous system, and thus reduce venous return and end-diastolic pressure; calcium channel blockers mainly affect the heart and peripheral arterioles, decreasing arterial pressure; while β-adrenoceptor antagonists reduce the work and the oxygen demand of the myocardium. Combinations of nitrates and β-adrenoceptor antagonists are often used together in the treatment of angina. Indeed, their disadvantages may be diminished by combined therapy, since β-receptor antagonists decrease tachycardia due to nitrates, while nitrates limit the alterations in ventricular size produced by β-adrenoceptor antagonists. Similarly, combinations of peripherally acting dihydropyridines, β-adrenoceptor antagonists and nitrates are sometimes used in the control of anginal pain. The potassium channel activator nicorandil can also be used with other drugs. However, combinations of verapamil with other antianginal drugs are potentially dangerous due to its effects on cardiac conduction and myocardial contractility. This may precipitate heart failure in susceptible patients.

Angina and general anaesthesia

Classical angina is usually indicative of the presence of coronary artery disease. Consequently, patients with angina usually have pre-existing cardiovascular pathology, and general anaesthesia may present special hazards. In particular, tachycardia and significant changes in blood pressure should be avoided. Preoperative drug therapy with nitrates, β-adrenoceptor antagonists, calcium channel blockers or potassium channel activators should be maintained until surgery, and resumed as soon as possible after surgery. Patients on low doses of β-adrenoceptor antagonists may require the dose to be slightly increased. In addition, patients who have a high risk of myocardial ischaemia should continue to receive β-blockade (e.g. metoprolol 5 mg or atenolol 5–10 mg). Premedication should be sufficient to allay the undesirable haemodynamic effects of preoperative anxiety, and intravenous opioids (alfentanil, remifentanil) may be useful in decreasing the dose requirements of induction agents and in suppressing the undesirable haemodynamic responses to laryngoscopy and intubation. Muscle relaxants that produce tachycardia should be avoided, while the choice of inhalational anaesthetics is controversial, since isoflurane may cause the redistribution of coronary blood flow away from ischaemic areas (Chapter 8). Intravenous anaesthetics, inhalational agents, and other drugs may affect the cardiovascular response to antianginal drug therapy, and haemodynamic changes that are of little significance in healthy patients may result in serious morbidity or death.

Suggested reading

Aggarwal, A. & Wartlier, D.C. (1994) Adenosine: present uses, future indications. *Current Opinion in Anaesthesiology* **7**, 109–123.

Barnett, D.B. (1988) Myocardial ischaemia: progress in drug therapy. *British Journal of Anaesthesia* **61**, 11–23.

Booker, P.D., Whyte, S.D. & Ladusans, E.J. (2003) Long QT syndrome and anaesthesia. *British Journal of Anaesthesia* **90**, 349–366.

Ertel, S.I. & Ertel, E.A. (1999) Low-voltage-activated T-type Ca^{2+} channels. *Trends in Pharmacological Sciences* **18**, 37–42.

Fawcett, W.J., Haxby, E.J. & Male, D.A. (1999) Magnesium: physiology and pharmacology. *British Journal of Anaesthesia* **83**, 302–309.

Godfraind, T. & Govani, S. (1995) Recent advances in the pharmacology of Ca^{2+} and K^+ channels. *Trends in Pharmacological Sciences* **16**, 1–4.

Hammil, S. & Hubmayr, R. (2000) The rapidly changing management of cardiac arrhythmias. *American Journal of Respiratory and Critical Care Medicine* **161**, 1070–1073.

Ijzerman, A.P. & Soudijn, W. (1989) The antiarrhythmic properties of β-adrenoceptor antagonists. *Trends in Pharmacological Sciences* **10**, 31–36.

Kaplinsky, E. (1992) Management of angina pectoris. Modern concepts. *Drugs* **43**(Suppl 1), 9–14.

Kirkman, E. (2006) Initiation and regulation of the heartbeat. *Anaesthesia and Intensive Care Medicine* **7**, 255–258.

Kirkman, E. (2006) Myocardial action potential. *Anaesthesia and Intensive Care Medicine* **7**, 259–263.

Kirkman, E. (2006) The electrocardiogram. *Anaesthesia and Intensive Care Medicine* **7**, 264–266.

Nestico, P.F., Morganroth, J. & Horowitz, L.N. (1988) New antiarrhythmic drugs. *Drugs* **35**, 286–319.

Reiz, S. (1988) Myocardial ischaemia associated with general anaesthesia. *British Journal of Anaesthesia* **61**, 68–84.

Richards, K.J.C. & Cohen, A.T. (2001) Cardiac arrhythmias in the critically ill. *Anaesthesia and Intensive Care Medicine* **2**, 384–389.

Roden, D.M. (1994) Risks and benefits of antiarrhythmic drug therapy. *New England Journal of Medicine* **331**, 785–791.

Rutherford, J.D. (1993) Pharmacologic management of angina and acute myocardial infarction. *American Journal of Cardiology* **72**, 16C–20C.

Sambrook, A. & Small, R. (2003) Antiarrhythmic drugs; antihypertensive drugs in pregnancy. *Anaesthesia and Intensive Care Medicine* **4**, 266–272.

Silvestry, F.E. & Kimmel, S.E. (1996) Calcium-channel blockers in ischaemic heart disease. *Current Opinion in Cardiology* **11**, 434–439.

Thadani, U. (1992) Role of nitrates in angina pectoris. *American Journal of Cardiology* **70**, 43B–53B.

Van Zweiten, P.A. (1996) Clinical pharmacology of calcium antagonists as antihypertensive and anti-anginal drugs. *Journal of Hypertension* **14**(Suppl), S3–S9.

Vaughan Williams, E.M. (1992) Classifying antiarrhythmic actions: by facts or speculation. *Journal of Clinical Pharmacology* **32**, 964–977.

16 Antiplatelet Drugs, Anticoagulants and Fibrinolytic Agents

Haemostasis and blood coagulation

Haemostasis

Haemostasis is a complex biological process that is designed to prevent blood loss after vascular injury. Following trauma or tissue damage, the arrest of haemorrhage depends on:

- arteriolar contraction
- platelet adhesion and aggregation
- blood coagulation, resulting in a fibrin clot

Platelet adhesion and aggregation

Many of the physiological and biochemical steps involved in platelet adhesion and aggregation are now well established (Fig. 16.1).

1 After vascular damage, platelets adhere to collagen in the vessel wall by means of von Willebrand factor[1] and similar adhesive proteins.

2 Platelet adhesion results in the synthesis and release of adenosine diphosphate (ADP), 5-HT and other mediators from damaged endothelial cells and intracellular granules. ADP then combines with specific P2Y receptors on the platelet membrane and mediates changes in shape and the formation of pseudopodia during activation.

3 Platelet-activating factor (PAF) and thromboxane A_2 (TXA_2) are synthesised from phospholipids in the platelet membrane. PAF is synthesised by the lysosomal enzyme phospholipase A_2, and thromboxane (TXA_2) is formed from arachidonic acid and the cyclic endoperoxides PGG_2 and PGH_2 by cyclooxygenase-1 (COX-1).

---

[1] von Willebrand factor is an elongated protein synthesised by the Weibel–Palade bodies in the vascular endothelium and by the alpha granules of platelets. In addition to its role in haemostasis, it acts as a protective carrier for circulating factor VIII.

4 The synthesis of PAF and TXA_2 is associated with a decrease in platelet cyclic AMP, which may be mediated by inhibition of prostaglandin receptors.

5 The decrease in cyclic AMP and the generation of ADP, PAF and TXA_2 results in the exposure and expression of glycoprotein IIb/IIIa receptors by the platelet membrane. Their generation is the 'final common pathway' in platelet activation and results in the cross-linking of receptor sites in adjacent platelets by fibrinogen, von Willebrand factor and other adhesive proteins, and thus produces aggregation.

Platelet glycoprotein IIb/IIIa receptors are usually classified as integrins (i.e. transmembrane proteins that provide a link between cells and the extracellular matrix). They consist of an α_{IIb}- and a β_3-subunit, and many ligands that combine with them contain a characteristic tripeptide adhesion sequence (arginine–glycine–aspartate).

Antiplatelet drugs

Platelets play an important role in the production of arterial thrombi in patients with pre-existing vascular damage due to atheroma, and may also be involved in the process of atherogenesis. The role of platelets in the production of venous thrombi is less clearly defined. Consequently, antiplatelet agents are mainly used in the prevention or treatment of thromboembolism on the arterial side of the circulation. This includes the prophylaxis of thromboembolism after cardiac surgery, arterial surgery or angioplasty, the prevention and treatment of cerebral ischaemia or myocardial infarction and the inhibition of thrombus formation in haemodialysis equipment or in pump oxygenators. Drugs that affect platelet function may also prevent accelerated atherosclerosis in coronary arteries after heart transplantation and

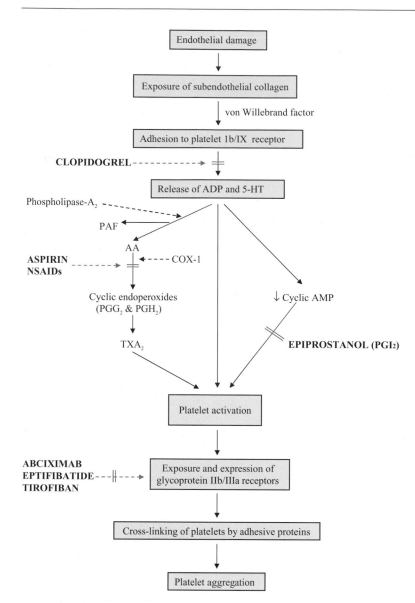

Fig. 16.1 Platelet adhesion, activation and aggregation, and its modification by antiplatelet drugs. AA, arachidonic acid; PAF, platelet-activating factor; TXA$_2$, thromboxane A$_2$; COX-1, cyclooxygenase-1. ---||----▶ Pathways inhibited by drugs (in boldface).

small-vessel occlusion in transplanted kidneys, which have been attributed to immune-mediated endothelial injury.

Mode of action of antiplatelet drugs

Antiplatelet drugs interfere with one or more of the physiological or biochemical processes involved in platelet adhesion and aggregation. Consequently, they act by:

- ADP antagonism
- COX-1 inhibition
- prostaglandin receptor agonism
- phosphodiesterase inhibition
- glycoprotein IIb/IIIa receptor antagonism

ADP antagonism

ADP plays an important part in platelet activation, and drugs that are antagonists at ADP receptors interfere with platelet aggregation.

Clopidogrel

Clopidogrel is a thienopyridine derivative that produces irreversible antagonism of most ADP receptors and inhibits platelet function for the duration of their lifespan (7–9 days). The antiplatelet activity of clopidogrel is dependent on its conversion to an active metabolite by hepatic cytochrome P450 1A1. Current evidence suggests that it is as effective as aspirin in preventing the complications or recurrence of myocardial infarction or ischaemic stroke. It is also widely used with aspirin as antiplatelet therapy for 3–12 months after percutaneous coronary intervention. Unfortunately, its use is associated with increased blood loss and significant blood product replacement, particularly after cardiac surgery. At present it is unclear whether treatment with clopidogrel should be stopped or modified prior to elective surgery, as its cessation after recent coronary intervention may lead to major postoperative thrombotic complications.

Ticlopidine

Ticlopidine is chemically related to clopidogrel and also acts by irreversible antagonism of platelet ADP receptors. Platelet function is affected only after several days, and its maximum effects are delayed for 5–8 days. In the past, ticlopidine was used to prevent the occurrence or recurrence of stroke in cerebrovascular and coronary artery disease and to reduce the risk of complications after coronary angioplasty and stenting. Unfortunately, ticlopidine was associated with neutropenia, agranulocytosis and thrombocytopenia, and regular blood counts were required at frequent intervals. Ticlopidine is not currently available in the UK.

COX-1 inhibition

The integrity of vascular endothelium is partly dependent on the balanced synthesis of prostacyclin (in the endothelium) and thromboxane (in platelets) by cyclooxygenase enzymes (Fig. 16.2). Both mediators are derived from the inactive precursor arachidonic acid, which is present in the phospholipid membrane of most cells, and from which it is released by a lysosomal enzyme (phospholipase A_2). In platelets, the conversion of arachidonic acid to the cyclic endoperoxides PGG_2 and PGH_2 depends on the constitutive enzyme COX-1, and the resultant endoperoxides are subsequently converted to thromboxanes (TXA_2), which induce platelet aggregation and vasoconstriction. In vas-

cular endothelium, the conversion of arachidonic acid to cyclic endoperoxides is partly dependent on COX-1, although inducible COX-2 may also have an important role, particularly after vascular damage or local arterial inflammation. In the endothelium, the resultant endoperoxides are subsequently converted to prostacyclin (PGI_2), which inhibits platelet aggregation and produces vasodilatation. It is believed that the balance between the formation of thromboxanes (by the platelets) and prostacyclin (by the vascular endothelium) plays an important part in maintaining the integrity of platelets in circulating blood. When the balance between their mutually opposing cardiovascular effects is disturbed, thrombosis may occur. Clearly, drugs that are selective inhibitors of COX-1 but have no effect on COX-2 will have antiplatelet effects and protect against thromboembolism, since they will entirely prevent platelet thromboxane synthesis but may have relatively little effect on endothelial prostacyclin (particularly in pathological conditions).

Aspirin

In physiological conditions, aspirin produces selective inhibition of COX-1 and thus prevents platelet aggregation. Aspirin acetylates and irreversibly inhibits a serine residue (serine 530) in the active centre of platelet COX-1, and thus decreases the synthesis of TXA_2. Platelets that are exposed to aspirin cannot synthesise new COX-1 during their limited lifespan (7–9 days). In contrast, the synthesis of PGI_2 by the vascular endothelium is less impaired, since it is exposed to lower concentrations of aspirin and is partly dependent on COX-2.

It is believed that as little as 160 mg aspirin daily will completely inhibit platelet COX-1. Doses of 75–325 mg daily are commonly used in the primary and secondary prevention of myocardial infarction and are also used to reduce the prevalence of myocardial infarction in patients with unstable angina. In cerebral ischaemia, it is generally accepted that aspirin reduces the frequency of transient ischaemic attacks and the prevalence of cerebrovascular strokes.

There is some evidence that aspirin can also reduce the incidence of postoperative thromboembolic phenomena. Nevertheless, its use may also predispose patients to significant postoperative haemorrhage. In general, aspirin is not discontinued prior to dental or minor surgery, but is usually withdrawn within 48 hours of higher risk surgery (e.g. prostatic, orthopaedic or neurosurgery). In emergency situations, aprotinin or desmopressin is sometimes used to inhibit the effects of aspirin.

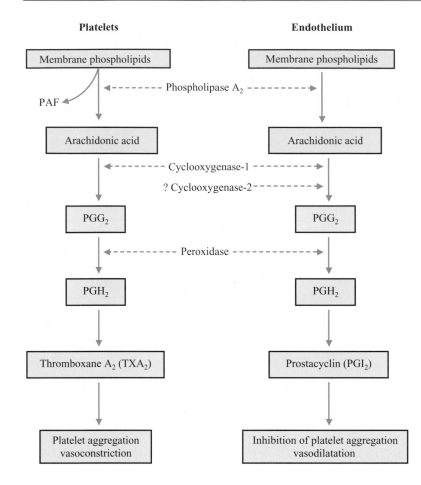

Fig. 16.2 The parallel synthesis of thromboxane A_2 (by platelets) and prostacyclin (by the vascular endothelium) and their opposing pharmacological effects. PAF, platelet-activating factor.

Other NSAIDs

Other non-selective NSAIDs usually produce reversible inhibition of COX-1 and COX-2, and their effects on platelet aggregation are therefore less marked and transient. In addition, their concurrent administration may interfere with the antiplatelet effects of aspirin. Consequently, they are not normally used as antiplatelet drugs. Nevertheless, the use of all NSAIDs during the perioperative period occasionally results in severe bleeding during or after the surgical procedure and can be difficult to control. In general, all non-selective NSAIDs are discontinued prior to transurethral prostatectomy and retinal surgery, due to the increased risk of perioperative haemorrhage.

Although selective COX-2 inhibitors have no significant effects on platelet aggregation, they may produce adverse effects on the cardiovascular system and they are not generally used in ischaemic heart disease or cerebrovascular disease (Chapter 11).

Prostaglandin receptor agonism

A decrease in cyclic AMP occurs during platelet activation and is associated with the expression of glycoprotein IIb/IIIa receptors by the platelet membrane. Drugs that are agonists at prostaglandin IP receptors increase cAMP and thus inhibit platelet aggregation.

Epoprostenol

Epoprostenol (prostacyclin, PGI_2) is a naturally occurring prostaglandin which is synthesised in the vascular endothelium from arachidonic acid. It combines with prostanoid IP receptors in platelets, activates adenylate cyclase and thus increases intracellular cAMP. Consequently, it is an extremely potent vasodilator and inhibitor of platelet aggregation. In the circulation, the half-life of epoprostenol is only 2–3 minutes, and it must be given by intravenous infusion due to its rapid spontaneous hydrolysis to 6-keto prostaglandin F. Epoprostenol is sometimes used to inhibit platelet aggregation during renal dialysis (either alone or with heparin) and is occasionally used in primary pulmonary hypertension. It commonly causes flushing, headache and hypotension, and bradycardia, pallor and sweating may occur with higher doses or rates of infusion.

Phosphodiesterase inhibition

Cyclic AMP is synthesised by platelets and is then rapidly degraded by one of the phosphodiesterase isoenzymes (usually Type V). Consequently, drugs that inhibit platelet phosphodiesterase may increase the local concentration of cAMP and thus inhibit platelet aggregation.

Dipyridamole

Dipyridamole inhibits platelet aggregation in two different ways:
• It inhibits platelet phosphodiesterase (isoenzyme V) and thus increases cyclic AMP. Ca^{2+} release is inhibited, and the synthesis of 5-HT and ADP is decreased.
• It prevents the uptake of adenosine by blood cells and increases its local concentration. Adenosine stimulates platelet adenylate cyclase and increases intracellular cAMP.

Dipyridamole is a vasodilator which was originally used in the treatment of angina. It has been used (with oral anticoagulants) to prevent thrombus formation on prosthetic heart valves and for prophylaxis against transient ischaemic attacks and cerebrovascular strokes. Dipyridamole may produce postural hypotension and a throbbing headache (particularly in patients with migraine), which is probably due to inhibition of phosphodiesterase in the cerebral circulation. In current practice, it is not commonly used as an antiplatelet drug.

Glycoprotein IIb/IIIa receptor antagonism

The expression of glycoprotein IIb/IIIa receptors by the platelet membrane is the 'final common pathway' in activation, resulting in the cross-linking of receptor sites in adjacent platelets by fibrinogen, von Willebrand factor and other adhesive proteins. Abciximab, eptifibatide and tirofiban are glycoprotein IIb/IIIa receptor antago-

nists that interfere with the binding of adhesive proteins and thus prevent platelet aggregation (Fig. 16.1).

Abciximab

Abciximab is the F(ab) fragment of a hybrid (mouse–human) monoclonal antibody directed against the glycoprotein IIb/IIIa receptor. Conventional doses produce 80–90% receptor blockade and inhibit platelet aggregation by preventing the binding of fibrinogen, von Willebrand factor and other adhesive molecules to the receptor. Abciximab also binds to vitronectin receptors in platelets and endothelial cells. It is used as an adjunct to heparin and aspirin during percutaneous coronary intervention and decreases the risk of ischaemic complications, including angina and myocardial infarction. It is given intravenously and has an immediate onset of action, which lasts for approximately 12 hours. Abciximab is usually broken down and subsequently eliminated by the kidney. Since it is antigenic and may cause thrombocytopenia in 2–3% of cases, it is used only on a single occasion. A major hazard of abciximab is the occurrence of spontaneous bleeding.

Eptifibatide

Eptifibatide is a synthetic cyclic heptapeptide based on the arginine–glycine–aspartate sequence and is a reversible antagonist of glycoprotein IIb/IIIa receptors. It is used with aspirin and heparin in the management of unstable angina and early myocardial infarction (without S-T segment changes). Eptifibatide is given intravenously and usually acts within 15 minutes. Its maximum effect (6 h) gradually decreases over 6–8 hours, and the drug is mainly (50–60%) eliminated unchanged in urine. Recommended doses produce almost complete blockade of glycoprotein IIb/IIIa receptors, which is associated with a two- to threefold increase in bleeding time.

Tirofiban

Tirofiban is a derivative of the amino acid tyrosine, but is a non-peptide reversible and competitive antagonist of the glycoprotein IIb/IIIa receptor. It is used (with aspirin and heparin) in unstable angina and early myocardial infarction. After intravenous infusion, tirofiban usually acts within 15 minutes, has a circulation half-life of 2–4 hours and acts for about 4–8 hours after its administration is discontinued. Recommended doses produce 90–95% blockade of glycoprotein IIb/IIIa receptors, which is associated with a two- to threefold increase in the bleeding time and activated clotting time. Tirofiban partly blocks the response of platelets to arachidonic acid and thromboxane A_2 and may also cause thrombocytopenia and spontaneous haemorrhage (although probably less commonly than abciximab).

Other agents that affect platelet function

Etamsylate

Etamsylate is a haemostatic agent which probably acts by improving capillary stability and by promoting normal platelet function. It is given orally (2 g daily, in divided doses) and has been used in the treatment of menorrhagia and to reduce capillary bleeding.

After systemic administration, the bleeding time is usually reduced, although platelet levels and clotting factors are unaffected. Adverse effects are relatively rare, although etamsylate may cause headache, nausea and skin rashes.

Dextrans

When added to blood *in vitro*, dextrans appear to have no effect on platelet function. Nevertheless, following the infusion of dextran solutions, bleeding time may be prolonged, polymerisation of fibrin impaired and platelet function reduced. Other colloidal volume expanders such as hydroxyethyl starch and urea-bridged gelatin (Haemaccel) may also impair platelet aggregation. Dextrans are now rarely used in the prophylaxis of thromboembolic disease following surgical procedures.

Blood coagulation

The extrinsic system

After platelet adhesion and aggregation has occurred (page 307), blood coagulation is initiated by platelet phospholipids, which interact with lipoproteins released from the vessel wall (tissue factor) and various precursor proteins that are present in plasma. Platelet phospholipids and tissue factor react with activated factor VII (VIIa) and Ca^{2+} to convert factor X to factor Xa, which plays a central role in blood coagulation (Fig. 16.3). In the presence of phospholipids, Ca^{2+} and activated factor V (Va), factor Xa converts prothrombin (an inactive precursor glycoprotein) into thrombin (an active proteolytic enzyme). Thrombin then acts on fibrinogen to release fibrinopeptides A and B and generate fibrin monomers, which subsequently form cross-links with adjacent molecules to produce an insoluble fibrin clot.

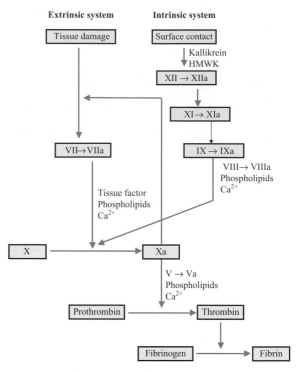

Fig. 16.3 A simplified diagram of the extrinsic and intrinsic systems of coagulation. The activated forms of coagulation factors are designated by the suffix 'a'. HMWK, high-molecular-weight kininogen.

Thrombin affects other coagulation factors and also interacts with thrombomodulin, producing conformational changes that activate a physiological inhibitor of coagulation (protein C). In addition, it affects platelets and leads to further platelet aggregation.

This process of blood coagulation in response to tissue injury is classically described as the extrinsic system, since the process depends on tissue damage, platelet aggregation and factors derived from blood vessels.

The intrinsic system

In the intrinsic system, all the activating factors are present in plasma and a cascading series of proteolytic reactions occurs when blood is allowed to contact a foreign surface. Individual coagulation factors are precursor proteins or proenzymes, which are converted to active enzymes by the product of the immediately preceding proteolytic process. The active enzymes then catalyse the next stage in the reaction. The intrinsic system leads to the formation of factor Xa ('the prothrombin activating complex') and then follows the same pathway as the extrinsic system. In general, both pathways must be intact for adequate haemostasis.

Vitamin K and the synthesis of blood coagulation factors

Most blood coagulation factors are synthesised in the liver from inactive precursor proteins. Vitamin K plays an essential role in the biosynthesis of factors II, VII, IX and X, as well as protein C and protein S.

Vitamin K

Vitamin K was originally discovered during experimental studies when it was shown that deficiency of an ether-soluble substance caused a haemorrhagic disease in chickens. This substance was later isolated and identified as vitamin K, which is present naturally in two different forms. Vitamin K_1 (phytomenadione) is found in green vegetables and salad plants, while vitamin K_2 (menaquinone) consists of one or more compounds that are synthesised in the small intestine by gram-negative microorganisms. Both vitamin K_1 and vitamin K_2 are fat-soluble and their intestinal absorption is dependent on bile salts. Vitamin K deficiency may result from a poor dietary intake, reduced intestinal synthesis, failure of absorption or impaired utilisation by the liver.

Role of vitamin K

The deficiency of vitamin K impairs the hepatic synthesis of prothrombin (factor II), as well as factors VII, IX and X, and proteins C and S. During normal biosynthesis, glutamate residues in their precursor proteins are converted to γ-carboxyglutamate groups, which are essential for the chelation of Ca^{2+} and their subsequent coupling to phospholipids (Fig. 16.4). This process is dependent on the availability of reduced vitamin K, which is simultaneously converted from a hydroquinone to an epoxide (vitamin K 2,3-epoxide). In vitamin K deficiency, γ-carboxylation of blood coagulation factors does not occur. Consequently, the vitamin K-dependent factors are biologi-

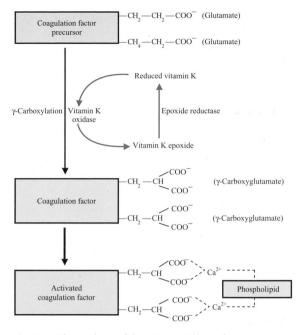

Fig. 16.4 The synthesis of the vitamin K-dependent coagulation factors (II, VII, IX and X, and proteins C and S).

cally inactive, and their defective synthesis may produce bleeding.

Clinical situations in which vitamin K deficiency can occur include haemorrhagic disease of the newborn, various malabsorption syndromes, obstructive jaundice, biliary fistulae and cirrhosis of the liver.

Phytomenadione

Phytomenadione is routinely given to all newborn babies as prophylaxis of haemorrhagic disease of the newborn. It may be given orally, as a mixed micelle preparation (2 mg on two or three occasions) or intramuscularly (1 mg). Larger doses (10–20 mg daily for 3 days preoperatively) usually restore prothrombin levels to normal in jaundiced patients. When jaundice is associated with severe hepatocellular damage, infusion of fresh frozen plasma may be necessary.

Menadione

Menadione (vitamin K_3) is a synthetic compound which can be converted into a water-soluble preparation (menadiol sodium phosphate), which is sometimes administered orally to prevent vitamin K deficiency in malabsorption syndromes. Occasionally, menadiol sodium phosphate causes haemolysis in patients deficient in glucose 6-phosphate dehydrogenase.

Hereditary disorders of blood coagulation
Haemophilia

Haemophilia is transmitted as a sex-linked recessive coagulation defect, although about 40% of cases are due to random mutation. In haemophilia A (classical haemophilia), there is a deficiency of factor VIII (antihaemophilic globulin), while in haemophilia B (Christmas disease), there is a deficiency of factor IX (Christmas factor). When patients require surgery, levels of the coagulation factors can be temporarily raised by desmopressin (DDAVP) or high-purity factor VIII or IX concentrates. In new patients and children under 16, recombinant coagulation factors are often used.

von Willebrand's disease

von Willebrand's disease is the commonest hereditary haemorrhagic disorder and is an autosomal dominant condition which affects both sexes. The deficiency or abnormal production of von Willebrand factor can result in mucosal bleeding, subcutaneous bruising, menorrhagia and epistaxis. There is usually a prolonged bleeding time and a reduction in the activity of factor VIII. When patients require surgery, tranexamic acid or DDAVP often prevent significant haemorrhage, although factor VIII concentrates can be used if required.

Thrombogenesis

Thrombogenesis is an altered state of haemostasis which results in the formation of an intravascular thrombus. The main precipitating factors are changes in the vessel wall, altered blood flow (stasis) and increased coagulability of the blood, as recognised by Rudolph Virchow more than 100 years ago. Thrombi can form in three main sites:

• arteries (white thrombus), which leads to ischaemic changes in vital tissues or organs
• veins (red thrombus), which may lead to pulmonary emboli
• atria or ventricles, where intramural deposits can lead to emboli in the cerebral circulation

Thromboembolic disease is a common cause of morbidity and mortality, and has special implications during the postoperative period. Several preventable and treatable causes of vascular pathology such as obesity, diabetes, cigarette smoking, hypercholesterolaemia and essential hypertension can produce the 'at-risk' patient. Furthermore, the venous stasis induced by prolonged surgery and postoperative immobilisation may be remedied by a number of non-pharmacological measures that include careful positioning during surgery, leg exercises, adequate hydration and the use of elasticated hosiery.

Hypercoagulable states

A hypercoagulable state may be associated with changes that are conducive to thrombosis formation, particularly if additional factors (e.g. vascular stasis) are present. Hypercoagulability may be due to changes in coagulation factors, platelets, the fibrinolytic system or physiological inhibitors of haemostasis. Although increased levels of clotting factors do not enhance the rate of fibrin formation, raised concentrations of factor VIII and fibrinogen are associated with an increased risk of ischaemic heart disease. Diminished fibrinolysis is a risk factor for venous thrombosis and results from insufficient availability or dysfunction of plasminogen activators, plasminogen and fibrin cofactor activity.

Oral contraception

There is also an increased risk of thromboembolism in young women who are taking oestrogen-containing oral contraceptives. Oestrogens have been shown to accelerate blood coagulation and to raise the concentration of some coagulation factors, particularly fibrinogen and factors VII and X, and the levels of antithrombin may fall. This abnormal state of hypercoagulation may not revert to normal until 2–3 months following the cessation of oestrogen therapy. The use of combined oral contraceptives has been associated with an increased risk of thromboembolism. The risk is particularly high in women who have hereditary thrombophilia (e.g. Leiden factor V mutation). However, during the perioperative period the role of other factors promoting platelet adhesion and aggregation may be equally important.

It is usually recommended that oestrogen-containing contraceptives are discontinued for 4–6 weeks prior to major elective surgery and all surgery on the lower limbs, particularly when prolonged immobilisation is necessary. The oestrogen is recommenced at least 2 weeks after full mobilisation. In addition, a thromboprophylactic regime is usually used during the perioperative period. In other types of surgery, subcutaneous heparin and graduated compression hosiery are often used. It should be recognised that the cessation of oral contraception may involve the risk of an undetected pregnancy, and this possibility should be excluded before surgery is undertaken.

Hereditary thrombophilia

In hereditary thrombophilia, the presence of a hypercoagulable state is due to the presence of genetic risk factors. In general, it may be due to:
• inherited deficiency or absence of a physiological inhibitor of coagulation
• inheritance of an abnormal coagulant protein

Inherited deficiency

There are numerous physiological inhibitors of blood coagulation and platelet activation, including heparin, heparan sulphate, antithrombin, protein C, protein S and heparin cofactor II.

Although genetic deficiencies in the synthesis of some of these factors are uncommon, they are characterised by a hypercoagulable state and a predisposition to thrombotic disease.

Inheritance of an abnormal coagulant protein

In the commonest form of inherited thrombophilia, a genetic defect or mutation produces a variant in factor V at the site of its interaction with protein C, which is a physiological inhibitor of coagulation. The variant protein (factor V Leiden) is present in about 5% of the population and is associated with resistance to activated protein C, producing an increased tendency to venous embolism and thromboembolic disease. Similarly, a genetic defect or mutation in prothrombin synthesis may impair its control by physiological inhibitory mechanisms, and an inherited variant in an enzyme (methylene tetrahydrofolate reductase) may increase plasma homocysteine. Both these genetic variants predispose to venous and arterial thrombosis.

Management of hereditary thrombophilia

In most patients with hereditary thrombophilia, the initial episode of venous thrombosis occurs between the ages of 20 and 30, and a precipitating factor is present in approximately 50% of these cases. If surgery is contemplated, the use of short-term anticoagulation should be considered (if long-term therapy is not already being used). Concentrates of antithrombin or fresh frozen plasma administered on the day of surgery may also be useful.

Anticoagulant drugs

Anticoagulant drugs either inhibit the activity or interfere with the synthesis of coagulation factors. They can be divided into five groups:
• heparin
• low molecular weight heparins (LMWHs)
• heparinoids
• hirudins
• oral anticoagulants

Heparin
Physiology

Heparin is a naturally occurring anticoagulant which was originally identified in the liver, but is also present in high concentrations in many other tissues (e.g. lungs, intestinal mucosa). It is usually localised in the secretory granules of mast cells, where it is present with histamine and various proteolytic enzymes. Although its precise physiological role is unclear, heparin and histamine are released from basophil leucocytes and mast cells during anaphylactic shock, and render the blood less coagulable. Heparin and other naturally occurring heparinoids (e.g. heparan sulphate, chondroitin-4-sulphate) appear to have other functions that are independent of anticoagulant activity. Heparin affects the migration of immune cells in inflammatory disorders and metastatic tumours, and also has antiproliferative effects on smooth muscle cells and fibroblasts, which may contribute to pathological changes in atherosclerosis and asthma.

Structure

Natural heparin is a polysaccharide (a glycosaminoglycan) which is synthesised as alternate D-glucuronic acid and sulphated acetyl-D-glucosamine residues:

After further sulphation and isomerisation (epimerisation), it is stored in mast cell granules as a complex mixture of polysaccharides with a mean molecular weight of 15 kDa (range = 3–30 kDa). Due to its numerous ionised sulphate groups, it has a strong electronegative (anionic) charge at physiological pH values. Its anticoagulant activity depends on a specific pentasaccharide sequence:

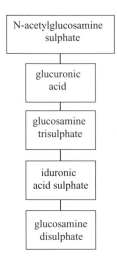

which is present in about 30% of heparin molecules.

Action of heparin on antithrombin

Heparin acts by accelerating the rate of reaction of an endogenous antithrombin in plasma (formerly known as antithrombin III or heparin cofactor) with many activated clotting factors. Antithrombin is a serpin (a *serine protease inhibitor*) which normally combines with many activated proteolytic factors in plasma and neutralises their coagulant activity by forming a stable complex. Heparin significantly increases the rate of binding of antithrombin to thrombin, thus producing immediate anticoagulant effects (both *in vivo* and *in vitro*). Heparin also inhibits factor Xa, but in a rather different manner. Its reaction with antithrombin produces a conformational change that facilitates its binding with factor Xa, and its action does not depend on the simultaneous binding of antithrombin and factor Xa by heparin.

Other actions

Heparin affects blood coagulation in several other ways. In high doses, it inhibits platelet aggregation and prolongs the bleeding time. Heparin also activates lipoprotein lipase in vascular endothelium, hydrolysing plasma triglycerides to glycerol and free fatty acids and reducing plasma turbidity. The resultant increase in free fatty acid levels may interfere with the plasma protein binding of certain drugs (e.g. propranolol, phenytoin) in blood sampled from cannulae which are intermittently flushed with heparin.

Pharmacokinetics

In general, heparin crosses cellular membranes with difficulty due to its polarity and large molecular size. Consequently, it is ineffective when administered orally or sublingually, and does not readily cross the placenta or the blood–brain barrier. When given as a single intravenous injection, its effects usually lasts for 3–4 hours, although its duration of action and half-life is dependent on the dose. After large doses, its terminal half-life progressively increases from 1 to 5 hours, presumably due to saturation of its uptake by the reticuloendothelial system. Heparin is normally metabolised in the liver by the enzyme heparinase, but is also partially excreted unchanged in urine.

The anticoagulant effects of heparin may be prolonged in renal failure or hepatic cirrhosis, but is sometimes reduced in pulmonary embolism.

Heparin preparations

Conventional heparin preparations are referred to as standard, unfractionated heparin in order to distinguish them from LMWHs. Commercial preparations of unfractionated heparin are obtained from bovine lung or porcine intestinal mucosa. Since preparations may differ in potency, they are standardised by biological assay and their activity is measured in units mL^{-1} (100 units ≈ 1 mg). Preparations intended for clinical use contain sodium heparin (1000, 5000, or 25,000 units mL^{-1}) or calcium heparin (25,000 units mL^{-1}).

Heparin monitoring

In clinical practice, the effects of heparin on blood coagulation are most commonly monitored by the activated partial thromboplastin time (APTT). In this test, Ca^{2+}, negatively charged phospholipids and a particulate substance such as kaolin (aluminium silicate) are added to plasma which has previously been treated with citrate or a chelating agent to bind ionic calcium. In these circumstances the clotting time is normally 25–35 seconds, although it varies with the methods and the reagents used.

During cardiopulmonary bypass (CPB), heparin anticoagulation is usually assessed in the operating theatre by the activated clotting time (ACT), which is maintained at 480 seconds or more. Although this provides an indication of heparinisation, it may not be significantly related to actual heparin concentrations and is affected by the concurrent use of antifibrinolytic agents (e.g. aprotinin).

Alternatively, heparin assays are based on chromogenic anti-Xa assays and depend on the inhibitory effect of the heparin–antithrombin complex on factor Xa. The effects of heparin can also be monitored by the thrombin time, i.e. the time required for plasma to clot in the presence of added thrombin. Although high doses of heparin also affect the prothrombin time, this is a relatively insensitive test.

Adverse effects of heparin

The most important adverse effects of heparin are:
- haemorrhage
- thrombocytopenia
- osteoporosis
- hyperkalaemia

Haemorrhage

Haemorrhage is the commonest and most important adverse effect of heparin and is often resolved by stopping its administration. When necessary, haemorrhage can be controlled by protamine, a basic agent derived from salmon sperm that forms an ionic bond with heparin. Protamine is also used routinely to reverse heparinisation after CPB. The action of heparin depends on ionised sulphate groups ($-SO_3^-$) that are attached to its glucosamine residues, and their neutralisation by basic groups ($-NH_3^+$) in protamine rapidly reverses the effects of heparin. After a test dose, protamine sulphate is given intravenously over 10–20 minutes. The dose required depends on the time since heparin was given, but does not usually exceed 1–1.5 mg per 80–100 units of heparin. Automated protamine titration systems can be used to determine the precise dose required to neutralise heparin, and the dose can be monitored by an *in vitro* test. Protamine may produce transient systemic hypotension and an increase in pulmonary vascular resistance. In addition, it may produce anaphylactoid responses (e.g. bronchoconstriction) that are partly mediated by complement activation, although true anaphylaxis is rare. Cross-sensitivity may occur in patients with fish allergy as well as in diabetic pa-

tients on protamine zinc insulin. Protamine has an immediate action and a rapid clearance, and 'heparin rebound' may occur within several hours of its use, due to its release from heparin–protamine complexes in extravascular tissues. Overdosage with protamine may exacerbate any bleeding problems, since protamine itself has antiplatelet activity and is a weak anticoagulant.

Thrombocytopenia

Thrombocytopenia occurs in about 5% of patients during long-term treatment with heparin, and platelet counts should be carried out in all patients who are given heparin for more than 5 days. It is usually considered to be a cytolytic (type II hypersensitivity) response to circulating complexes of heparin and platelet factor 4, which induce the formation of IgG or IgM antibodies. The immunoglobulins bind to platelets resulting in their aggregation in the circulation, and this may cause subsequent venous or arterial thrombosis. It usually occurs 5–10 days after the start of treatment and is commoner with standard heparin than with LMWHs. When thrombocytopenia occurs, heparin should be immediately stopped and replaced with alternative anticoagulants (e.g., danaparoid, lepirudin, or warfarin). Occasionally, thrombocytopenia occurs immediately after the administration of heparin, and is believed to be an anaphylactoid reaction involving the alternate complement pathway.

Other hypersensitivity reactions to heparin are extremely uncommon, but may occur in patients with a history of allergic disorders.

Osteoporosis

Osteoporosis occasionally occurs with long-term (3–6 months) heparin administration and may cause spontaneous vertebral fractures. This may reflect the similarity between the structure of heparin and various heparanoids, which form part of the extracellular matrix of cells. Alopecia may also occur after long-term use.

Hyperkalaemia

Heparin can inhibit aldosterone secretion and cause an increase in serum K^+. This rare complication is commoner in patients with diabetes mellitus, chronic renal failure or acidosis, who may already have some degree of hyperkalaemia.

Heparin resistance

Patients receiving intermittent or continuous heparin are sometimes resistant to its effects, and daily doses of 35,000 units or more may be required to significantly prolong the APTT, although different results may be obtained by other methods, such as anti-Xa assays. Heparin resistance is sometimes related to its increased binding by plasma proteins, including platelet factor 4, factor VIII, fibrinogen and the histidine-rich glycoprotein vitronectin, which inhibits the binding of heparin to antithrombin. A short initial APTT may be due to increased concentrations of factor VIII. In addition, heparin resistance may be due to inherited or acquired antithrombin deficiency, as in cirrhosis, the nephrotic syndrome or inherited intravascular coagulation.

Clinical uses

Unfractionated heparin is used in the prophylaxis and treatment of deep vein thrombosis, pulmonary embolism and myocardial infarction. Therapeutic doses of heparin are also used to prevent thrombosis occurring during cardiac and major vascular surgery and during haemodialysis. Low-dose heparin is frequently used in the prophylaxis of thromboembolic complications in patients who undergo a wide variety of surgical procedures, particularly those who may be considered at special risk. Important considerations include major surgery with prolonged immobilisation, obesity, congestive cardiac failure, venous stasis in the lower limbs and previous thromboembolic episodes. Heparin is usually contraindicated in haemorrhagic states, after recent ophthalmic or neurosurgery, in patients with peptic ulceration or oesophageal varices, in hypertensive patients with a diastolic pressure greater than 110 mm Hg and in cases of known hypersensitivity to heparin.

Deep vein thrombosis and pulmonary embolism

Standard heparin is usually given intravenously, preferably by continuous infusion. A loading dose of 100 units kg^{-1} of heparin sodium is followed by the continuous infusion of 1000–1500 units h^{-1}. The dose should be titrated to maintain the APTT between 1.5 and 2.5 times its control value. In most instances requiring prolonged anticoagulation, oral anticoagulants are started at the same time and heparin can be withdrawn after these have achieved their therapeutic effect (usually after 3–5 days).

An alternative regime is used when intravenous administration is not feasible or oral anticoagulants are contraindicated (e.g. during pregnancy). Standard heparin is given subcutaneously, usually into the anterolateral wall of the abdomen near the iliac crest, using a concentrated preparation (25,000 units mL^{-1}). An initial dose of 10,000–15,000 units is administered 12-hourly, and the dose is adjusted daily by monitoring the APTT. Regular platelet counts should be carried out in all patients receiving heparin for more than 5 days.

Prophylaxis of thrombosis in surgical patients

Standard heparin (5,000 units subcutaneously) may be given 2 hours before operation and repeated at 8–12 hourly intervals for 7 days, or until the patient is mobile. Calcium heparin preparations are often preferred, since they produce fewer haematomata at tissue injection sites. In general, low-dose heparin regimes do not require laboratory monitoring.

It is widely recognised that pulmonary embolism is an important cause of mortality (7% of all deaths) in postoperative surgical patients. There is little doubt that the failure to use prophylactic anticoagulant therapy for patients in whom it is considered appropriate may have important therapeutic and medicolegal consequences. Nevertheless, there are many systemic and surgical contraindications to the use of heparin, and special care must be taken with patients who are concomitantly receiving NSAIDs. All drugs in this group may promote bleeding, and the concomitant use of ketorolac and low-dose heparin regimes in the postoperative period is usually contraindicated. Similar, dose-related effects can be anticipated when other NSAIDs are used. In addition, the timing of spinal and extradural blockade in the presence of anticoagulants must be carefully considered. Present recommendations are that these blocks should be performed before heparin is administered, or at least 4–6 hours after the last dose.

Anticoagulation during cardiac and vascular surgical procedures

Standard heparin is routinely used as an anticoagulant during CPB. In adults, the initial dose is usually 300–500 units kg^{-1}, with a pump-priming dose of 5000–10,000 units. Supplemental doses of heparin (5000–10,000 units) may be required, depending on the ACT. Baseline measurements of the ACT are required, and its prolongation should be confirmed before the institution of bypass. At the end of the procedure, heparin is usually antagonised by protamine (page 317). A similar regime of heparinisation is required prior to aortic clamping in peripheral vascular surgery.

Table 16.1 Differences between standard unfractionated heparin and low molecular weight heparin.

	Unfractionated heparin	Low molecular weight heparin
Molecular weight		
Mean	15 kDa	4.5 kDa
Range	3–30 kDa	2–10 kDa
Coagulant protein bound	Antithrombin and thrombin	Antithrombin
Anti-Xa/Anti IIa activity	1:1	Ranges between 2:1 and 4:1
Platelet aggregation	Inhibited	Unaffected
Pharmacokinetics	Less predictable	More predictable
Bioavailability (subcutaneous injection)	50%	100%
Tissue binding	High affinity	Low affinity
Anticoagulant activity (half-life)	1–2 h	2–4 h
Elimination	Hepatic metabolism (50%) and renal excretion (50%)	Renal excretion
Duration of action (subcutaneous injection)	6–12 h	12–24 h
Frequency of administration (in 24 h)	2–4	1–2
Haemorrhage	More common	Less common
Monitoring	APTT	Unnecessary (usually)
Antagonism by protamine	Predictable	Less predictable
Thrombocytopenia during continuous treatment	3–5%	<1%

Disseminated intravascular coagulation

Heparin may also be used in the treatment of disseminated intravascular coagulation (DIC). This condition can be caused by severe infections, neoplastic conditions, obstetric disorders, major trauma, liver disease and incompatible blood transfusion. The widespread development of thrombi consumes clotting factors and liberates fibrin degradation products, and so the circulating blood becomes incoagulable and a haemorrhagic diathesis occurs. It is important to replace platelets (by leukodepleted platelet concentrate) and fibrinogen (by cryoprecipitate) immediately, followed by other factors (using fresh frozen plasma and red cells). Other agents such as antithrombin concentrate, protein C concentrate or prostacyclin may be of value in some situations. Although the use of heparin is controversial, it may arrest the coagulation process by allowing the accumulation of clotting factors and lead to the cessation of bleeding. Unfortunately, it may also lead to clinical deterioration, and reversal of the effects of heparin by protamine may be required. In these circumstances, inhibitors of fibrinolysis (e.g. aprotinin, tranexamic acid) may also be useful. Even when blood coagulation is controlled by heparin, patients may die from the adult respiratory distress syndrome.

Low molecular weight heparins

- Bemiparin
- Dalteparin
- Enoxaparin
- Reviparin
- Tinzaparin

Standard (unfractionated) heparin can be fractionated by gel filtration chromatography to produce preparations with a lower molecular weight (mean = 4.5 kDa, range = 2–10 kDa). All these preparations have an analogous structure to standard heparin, and all contain the critical pentasaccharide sequence (page 316). LMWHs cannot bind both antithrombin and thrombin (factor IIa) simultaneously, due to their small molecular size. Consequently, they mainly produce their anticoagulant effects by combining with antithrombin and causing a conformational change that facilitates its reaction with factor Xa, but with lesser effects on factors IXa, XIa and XIIa. They only have slight inhibitory effects on thrombin (anti-Xa/anti-IIa activity ranges between 2:1 and 4:1). They are incompletely and unpredictably antagonised by protamine sulphate (Table 16.1).

LMWHs have a more predictable pharmacokinetic profile than unfractionated heparin, since they have a lower binding affinity for platelets, von Willebrand factor and endothelial cells, and they are entirely cleared unchanged by the kidney. In contrast to standard heparin, they do not affect platelet aggregation or prolong the bleeding time. They have a greater bioavailability, a longer terminal half-life (4–6 h) and a longer duration of action (at least 8–12 h) than unfractionated heparin, and are commonly given by subcutaneous administration once daily.

In recent years, LMWHs have largely replaced standard heparin in the prophylaxis and treatment of deep venous thrombosis and pulmonary embolism. They are as safe and effective as standard heparin and reduce the incidence of pulmonary embolism in patients undergoing general surgical or orthopaedic procedures. They are less likely to produce haemorrhagic complications, and monitoring of their activity is not usually required. When necessary, their activity can be assessed by anti-Xa activity in plasma. Different LMWHs do not have identical potencies, and so dose requirements vary with individual drugs and the degree of anticoagulation required.

The timing of spinal and extradural blockade in relation to the administration of LMWHs must be carefully considered. It is generally recommended that blockade is performed before LMWHs are administered or that a relatively long latent period (10–12 h) is observed after their use.

Fondaparinux

Fondaparinux is a synthetic pentasaccharide and contains a similar sequence to the pentasaccharide group in heparin that facilitates the reaction between antithrombin and thrombin (page 316). Consequently, it mainly affects blood coagulation by combining with antithrombin. Due to its small molecular size, it produces conformational changes in antithrombin that inhibit factor Xa. It has a long terminal half-life (21 h) and is usually given by daily subcutaneous injection. It is used in patients undergoing major joint replacement surgery, and in the treatment of deep venous thrombosis and pulmonary embolism.

Heparinoids

Heparinoids are naturally occurring polysaccharides that have a close structural relationship to heparin. They are present on the surface of most cells and are also found in the extracellular matrix.

Danaparoid

Danaparoid is a mixture of three heparinoids: heparan sulphate (84%), dermatan sulphate (12%) and chondroitin sulphate (4%). It has a low molecular weight (5.5–6 kDa) and is obtained from porcine intestinal mucosa. Its anticoagulant effects are primarily due to the binding of antithrombin by heparan sulphate, which increases its anti-Xa activity. It also has some antithrombin activity (which is mainly due to dermatan sulphate). Nevertheless, danaparoid is a more selective inhibitor of factor Xa than other drugs (anti-Xa/anti-IIa activity = 25:1). After subcutaneous injection, its anti-Xa activity is maximal at 5 hours and lasts for 24 hours. It is sometimes used in the prophylaxis of thromboembolism, particularly in patients who have developed heparin-induced thrombocytopenia.

Hirudins

Hirudins are compounds that directly inhibit thrombin, and were originally derived from the salivary glands of the medicinal leech (*Hirudinea medicinalis*). In recent years, a number of recombinant hirudins have synthesised by molecular biological techniques and are now in clinical use.

Bivalirudin

Bivalirudin is a synthetic peptide and an analogue of hirudin that is a direct inhibitor of both free and bound thrombin (factor IIa). It is widely distributed in extracellular fluid and has a relatively short half-life (30 min). Although it is partially metabolised, it is mainly eliminated unchanged in urine. Bivalirudin is given by intravenous infusion, and has been used as an anticoagulant in patients during percutaneous coronary intervention and as an adjunct to aspirin in unstable angina. Its adverse effects include occasional hypersensitivity reactions and anaphylaxis, as well as spontaneous haemorrhages. Since it is partially eliminated by the kidney, bleeding is more likely when it is used in patients with impaired renal function.

Lepirudin

Lepirudin is a recombinant hirudin derived from yeast cells, which directly inhibits the effects of free and bound thrombin. It is distributed in extracellular fluid, has a half-life of 2 hours and is mainly eliminated unchanged in urine. Lepirudin has been used as an alternative to

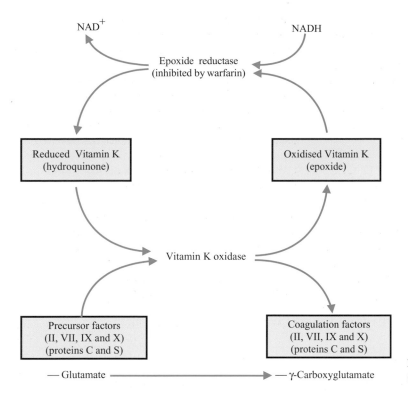

Fig. 16.5 The mode of action of warfarin (and other oral anticoagulants).

heparin when resistance occurs or in heparin-induced thrombocytopenia. Its effects are independent of antithrombin, and it can be used as an anticoagulant for patients with heparin-induced thrombocytopenia. In some patients antihirudin antibodies may develop, but do not appear to be associated with adverse effects. Since it is mainly eliminated by the kidney, lepirudin is usually avoided in renal failure as it may induce spontaneous haemorrhages. Its effects can be monitored by the APPT (when necessary).

Oral anticoagulants

History

Oral anticoagulants were introduced into clinical practice after the accidental discovery that cattle fed on spoiled sweet-clover silage developed a haemorrhagic disorder. The cause was eventually traced to a reduction in plasma prothrombin, and it was subsequently shown that the defect could be prevented by adding alfalfa (a rich source of vitamin K) to the cattle feed. The haemorrhagic agents in silage were identified later as bishydroxycoumarin (di-

coumarol) and its derivatives, and dicoumarol was first used clinically as an anticoagulant in 1941. Warfarin sodium was subsequently developed and patented by the *Wisconsin Alumni Research F*oundation, and is an analogue of bishydroxycoum*arin.* It was originally used as a rat poison and considered to be too toxic for human use, but is now the standard oral anticoagulant. Although acenocoumarol (nicoumalone) and phenindione (an indanedione) are also available in the UK, they have a number of disadvantages and are rarely used.

Mode of action

All oral anticoagulants prevent the synthesis of the vitamin K-dependent coagulation factors (II, VII, IX and X) from their precursor proteins. The carboxylation of 10–15 glutamate groups in the precursor proteins of these factors is essential for their chelation by Ca^{2+} and their binding by platelet phospholipids during blood coagulation. This process is linked to the oxidation of vitamin K, which converts the vitamin from a reduced hydroquinone to an epoxide (Fig. 16.5).

The regeneration of reduced vitamin K is dependent on NADH and a reductase enzyme and is essential for the continual synthesis of coagulation factors. This enzyme is inhibited by oral anticoagulants, causing the accumulation of vitamin K epoxide and the depletion of reduced vitamin K. In these conditions, the synthesis of the vitamin K-dependent factors is impaired, resulting in their depletion and producing anticoagulant effects.

Effects on coagulation factors

Oral anticoagulants have no effect on previously synthesised clotting factors and are therefore ineffective in *in vitro* conditions. After oral administration, their effects are delayed until previously synthesised coagulation factors are consumed and eliminated from plasma. The approximate half-lives of the vitamin K-dependent factors are factor II (prothrombin), 48 hours; factor VII, 6 hours; factor IX, 24 hours; factor X, 36 hours; protein C, 8 hours; protein S, 30 hours. Since the action of oral anticoagulants are mainly dependent on reductions in factors II and X, their effects are delayed for at least 12 hours and the maximum response may take 48–72 hours to develop.

The synthesis of physiological inhibitors of coagulation (protein C and protein S) is also dependent on vitamin K, and their concentrations may rapidly decrease during the introduction of anticoagulant therapy. This may be responsible for transient hypercoagulability and some adverse effects (e.g. 'purple toes' and skin necrosis) which occasionally occur at the onset of oral anticoagulation.

Warfarin sodium

Warfarin sodium is the most commonly used oral anticoagulant and is related in chemical structure to vitamin K_1 (page 313). After oral administration, it is rapidly and completely absorbed from the gastrointestinal tract, and peak plasma concentrations are achieved within 1–2 hours. It is extensively bound (98%) to plasma proteins, particularly albumin. Consequently, its diffusion across cellular membranes is restricted, and the volume of distribution of the drug (140 mL kg^{-1}) is similar to extracellular fluid volume. Nevertheless, warfarin is relatively lipid-soluble and readily crosses the blood–brain barrier and the placenta. Its administration during early pregnancy may cause mental retardation and congenital malformations (chondrodysplasia). During the last trimester, fetal haemorrhage and intrauterine death may occur between 36 and 40 weeks. The clearance of warfarin is independent of liver blood flow, and its elimination half-life is normally about 40 hours. It is almost entirely metabolised, and its breakdown products are eliminated as inactive glucuronide conjugates in urine.

Warfarin is a chiral drug and is normally given as a racemic mixture. There are significant differences in the potency and metabolism of its enantiomers, as well as in their effects on the synthesis of coagulation factors.

Warfarin monitoring

It is essential that the anticoagulant effects of warfarin are monitored and its dosage adjusted accordingly using the prothrombin time and the international normalised ratio (INR). In the measurement of prothrombin time, tissue thromboplastin (a saline extract of brain containing tissue factor and phospholipids) is added to recalcified plasma, and coagulation normally occurs in 12–15 seconds. Unfortunately, tissue thromboplastins differ in potency, and individual results require to be standardised by reference to the INR. This index has a normal value of 1, and is the ratio of the prothrombin time of a patient to that obtained with a standard human thromboplastin. It is commonly used in the regulation of oral anticoagulant therapy and permits the standardisation of results between different laboratories throughout the world.

Variability in response

There is considerable interindividual variability in the response of patients to warfarin due to three main factors:
- the availability of vitamin K
- genetic variability
- drug interactions

Availability of vitamin K

Any factor that reduces the availability of vitamin K will enhance the response to warfarin.

Broad-spectrum antibiotic therapy decreases the synthesis of endogenous vitamin K in the small intestine. Patients with liver disease may also be sensitive to warfarin, due to impaired synthesis of coagulation factors. In contrast, increased vitamin K intake in fats, oils, green vegetables, salads and some fruit juices increases the dose requirement. The breakdown of coagulation factors is affected by the metabolic rate, and so the response to warfarin is decreased in myxoedema but enhanced in fever and hyperthyroidism.

Genetic variability

In some instances, variability in response and inherent resistance to oral anticoagulants is due to hereditary factors. Genetic variations in suppressor proteins may inhibit the synthesis of coagulation factors, or resistant forms of the reducing enzyme (epoxide reductase) may be present. Congenital deficiency or impaired synthesis of antithrombin may also cause severe reactions to warfarin.

Drug interactions

Warfarin is commonly involved in drug interactions that have serious clinical consequences (Table 16.2). Some drugs may impair the absorption of both vitamin K and warfarin (e.g. colestyramine), and aspirin and most NSAIDs will enhance the effects of oral anticoagulants. Even a small dose of aspirin will inhibit platelet aggregation, prolong the bleeding time and impair haemostasis, while larger doses interfere with prothrombin synthesis. In addition, some NSAIDs may potentiate anticoagulant effects by displacing warfarin from plasma proteins or inhibit its metabolism.

A number of other drugs can also prolong and enhance the response to warfarin, and thus increase the likelihood of bleeding. In most instances, competition for protein binding sites and inhibition of hepatic cytochrome P450 is involved. Although chronic, moderate alcohol intake may induce hepatic enzymes, acute consumption can prolong the effects of warfarin and reduce its clearance (particularly in patients with impaired liver function).

In contrast, drugs with significant hepatic enzyme-inducing activity often increases the metabolism of warfarin and its dose requirements. When the administration of the inducing agent is stopped, the activity of warfarin is increased and severe haemorrhage may occur if the dosage is not adjusted.

Clinical use of warfarin

Oral anticoagulants are used in the prophylaxis and treatment of deep venous thrombosis and pulmonary embolism, and in atrial fibrillation. They are also used to prevent the deposition of thrombi on mechanical prosthetic heart valves and vascular grafts. When oral anticoagulant therapy is instituted, the INR should be determined until a stable level is attained. The usual induction dose of warfarin is 10 mg daily for 2 days, but this should be re-duced in small or elderly subjects, in patients with liver disease or cardiac failure or if the baseline prothrombin time is prolonged. The subsequent daily maintenance doses are normally 3–9 mg, which should be taken at the same time each day. In the treatment of deep vein thrombosis, pulmonary embolism, atrial fibrillation, cardioversion, dilated cardiomyopathy, mural thrombus in myocardial infarction and rheumatic mitral valve disease, the INR should be maintained as close to 2.5 as possible. In recurrent deep vein thrombosis or pulmonary embolism, arterial grafts and mechanical prosthetic cardiac valves, a higher level (INR 3.5) is recommended. In general, an INR within 0.5 units of the target value is satisfactory. Since the anticoagulant effects of warfarin are usually delayed for at least 2–3 days, heparin must be administered simultaneously when an immediate anticoagulant effect is required.

Surgery in patients on warfarin

When surgery is required in patients on oral anticoagulants, the INR should be measured. Minor elevations, i.e. 1.5–2.5, are acceptable and may even be desirable as prophylaxis against further thrombotic episodes. In general, minor surgery, including dental extraction and tissue biopsy, can be carried out with levels of up to 2.5, unless there is a risk of serious haemorrhage.

In major procedures, and in patients with prosthetic heart valves and recurrent or recent thrombosis, warfarin can be temporarily discontinued several days before surgery. A regime of standard unfractionated heparin is then substituted, in order to decrease the problems of perioperative control and interactions with other drugs that are administered during anaesthesia. Heparin is normally infused to give an acceptable APTT ratio (1.5–2.5), but is stopped 4–6 hours before surgery. Heparin infusion is recommenced 12 hours after surgery, and warfarin is reintroduced as soon as possible. Heparin is then discontinued when the INR has reached its preoperative level.

When the initial INR is greater than 2.5 and emergency surgery is necessary, management will depend upon the urgency of the surgery and the need for anticoagulant control. If this cannot be achieved sufficiently rapidly, the infusion of prothrombin complex concentrate or fresh frozen plasma (with appropriate haematological monitoring) is a rapidly effective and controllable method of correcting the coagulation defect. Vitamin K_1 should not be used, since it has a relatively slow onset of action and its effects cannot be easily controlled.

Table 16.2 Significant drug interactions with warfarin.

Increased anticoagulant effects (potentiation)	Reduced anticoagulant effects (inhibition)

Drugs that decrease vitamin K absorption
    Antibiotics (broad-spectrum)
    Sulphonamides
    Colestyramine
	Drugs that increase vitamin K absorption
	    Vitamin K (in food and supplements)
	    Excessive dietary fat

Drugs that inhibit cytochrome P450
    Imidazoles (ketoconazole, itraconazole, omeprazole, cimetidine, metronidazole)
    Macrolide antibiotics (erythromycin, clarithromycin)
    Antidepressants
    Ciclosporin
    Amiodarone
    Allopurinol
    Quinidine
    Disulfiram
    Ethyl alcohol (acute consumption)
	Drugs that induce cytochrome P450
	    Barbiturates
	    Phenytoin
	    Carbamazepine
	    Rifampicin
	    Griseofulvin
	    Polycyclic hydrocarbons
	    Insecticides
	    Corticosteroids
	    St. John's wort
	    Ethyl alcohol (chronic consumption)

Drugs that affect platelet function
    Aspirin
    NSAIDs
    Dipyridamole
    Clopidogrel
    Sulfinpyrazone
    Moxalactam
    Carbenicillin	

Absolute or relative overdosage of oral anticoagulants can lead to frank haemorrhage. Bleeding may occur from various sites, including the gastrointestinal tract, lung, central nervous system and skin. In these circumstances, warfarin is temporarily stopped, and the administration of fresh frozen plasma, prothrombin complex concentrate or the various coagulation factors may be necessary. In addition, phytomenadione is usually given (2.5–10 mg by slow intravenous injection) and the cause of haemorrhage should be investigated.

Fibrinolysis

Plasminogen activation

When blood coagulation occurs, the related processes of plasminogen activation and fibrinolysis are also activated. The fibrinolytic system is initiated by tissue damage and results in the conversion of plasminogen (an inactive β-globulin) to plasmin (a proteolytic enzyme). Plasmin sub-sequently breaks down fibrin to degradation products, resulting in the subsequent dissolution of the clot (Fig. 16.6). However, it is a relatively non-specific enzyme, which breaks down fibrinogen, prothrombin, factor V and factor VIII.

The main physiological activator of plasminogen is tissue-type plasminogen activator. This proteolytic enzyme is released from the endothelium of damaged blood vessels and phagocytes, or formed from proactivators in tissues by factor XIIa (activated Hageman factor). Tissue-type plasminogen activator is most effective when plasminogen is bound by fibrin, and so the formation and the action of plasmin is localised to the clot. Any circulating plasmin that is formed is immediately neutralised by antiplasmins (or plasmin inhibitors) in plasma.

Plasminogen activators are also present in many other sites and can be recovered from various secretions, where they play a physiological role in preventing fibrin deposition in ducts. Urokinase was originally identified in human urine in 1885 and later prepared from cultures

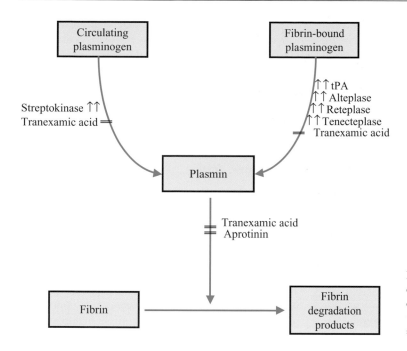

Fig. 16.6 The fibrinolytic system and the effects of fibrinolytic and antifibrinolytic drugs. tPA, tissue plasminogen activator; ↑↑, activation of the pathway is increased; ═, activation is reduced or antagonised.

of human renal cells. Several other exogenous plasminogen activators have been widely used in the treatment of venous thrombosis and pulmonary embolism and in the management of myocardial infarction.

The plasminogen activators in current clinical use are:
- streptokinase
- alteplase
- reteplase
- tenecteplase

Streptokinase

Streptokinase is a protein that was originally obtained from group C haemolytic streptococci in 1945. It activates plasminogen, forming a stable complex that results in the formation of circulating plasmin, and its half-life is approximately 40–80 minutes. Streptokinase is antigenic and its action may be partly neutralised by circulating antistreptococcal antibodies derived from previous therapy or streptococcal infections. Antibodies appear within 4–5 days of administration of streptokinase, and its use should then not be repeated for at least 12 months. Since streptokinase is antigenic, it may cause drug fever, allergic manifestations and even overt anaphylaxis. The incidence of these side effects may be reduced by the use of slow infusion rates and the administration of prophylactic steroids. Treatment may involve the use of adrenaline and both H_1- and H_2-receptor antagonists.

Streptokinase has a role in the treatment of acute myocardial infarction, deep venous thrombosis, acute pulmonary embolism and arterial thromboembolic disorders, although it is now less commonly used than other drugs. In myocardial infarction, 1,500,000 units are usually given in saline or dextrose over 60 minutes. In other conditions, 250,000 units are given over 30 minutes, followed by 100,000 units h^{-1} for 12–72 hours. Haematological monitoring, including estimations of thrombin and prothrombin times, haematocrit and platelet levels are essential during treatment. When the thrombin time has returned to a value of less than twice the normal, anticoagulants should be given in order to prevent recurrent thrombosis.

In acute myocardial infarction, streptokinase is most effective when used in patients presenting within 6 hours. It is generally considered that infarction is complete after 4–6 hours (particularly when pathological Q waves are present) and that thrombolytic therapy after this time may be of little value. Streptokinase has also been administered locally into the coronary vasculature in the treatment of myocardial infarction.

Streptokinase invariably induces systemic fibrinolysis, and the presence of free plasmin in the systemic circulation results in the consumption of various coagulation factors (mainly fibrinogen and factors V, XIII and XII). Its main adverse effects are nausea, vomiting, hypotension and bleeding. Intracerebral haemorrhage or blood loss from other sites may occur and usually necessitates the use of blood clotting factors and antifibrinolytic drugs.

Alteplase

Alteplase is a non-antigenic, single-chain, recombinant tissue plasminogen activator, which was originally derived from cultured melanoma cells. It has a much lower affinity for circulating plasminogen than for fibrin-bound plasminogen, and so it is relatively inactive in the general circulation (even at high plasma concentrations). It forms a complex with fibrin and results in the conversion of fibrin-bound plasminogen to plasmin, and so fibrinolysis affects only the thrombus.

Alteplase is rapidly cleared from the circulation by the liver and has a short half-life and brief duration of action. It is used in the treatment of myocardial infarction, pulmonary embolism and acute ischaemic stroke. In myocardial infarction, a total dose of up to 100 mg is given over 90 minutes within 6 hours of onset. A similar but more prolonged regime is given when treatment is initiated between 6 and 12 hours.

Since alteplase is non-antigenic, it does not induce the formation of antibodies or induce allergic or hypersensitivity reactions.

Reteplase

Reteplase is a similar recombinant tissue plasminogen activator, which preferentially converts fibrin-bound plasminogen to plasmin. It is less rapidly cleared from plasma than alteplase, has a longer half-life in the circulation and is non-antigenic. Reteplase is used to produce rapid thrombolysis in the treatment of myocardial infarction, and doses of 20 units are commonly given over 30 minutes.

Tenecteplase

Tenecteplase is an alternative recombinant tissue plasminogen activator which is used in the treatment of myocardial infarction. It is given as a single bolus injection, and doses of 30–50 mg are usually injected over 10 seconds.

Antifibrinolytic agents

Antifibrinolytic agents inhibit the conversion of plasminogen to plasmin or inhibit the effects of plasmin, and thus prevent or reverse the process of fibrinolysis. They have been used in the treatment of pathological states associated with excessive fibrinolytic activity and in the management of haemorrhage in haemophilic disorders. They have also been used as antidotes after overdosage of thrombolytic agents.

Antifibrinolytic agents in current clinical use are:

• tranexamic acid
• aprotinin

Tranexamic acid

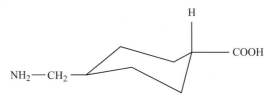

Tranexamic acid is a potent inhibitor of plasminogen activation which prevents the conversion of plasminogen to plasmin and thus inhibits fibrinolysis. In higher concentrations, it is a non-competitive inhibitor of plasmin. It can be given orally (usually 45–75 mg kg^{-1} day^{-1}) or intravenously (1.5–3 g daily in divided doses). It has been used in the prophylaxis and treatment of haemorrhage in menorrhagia and prostatic surgery, as well as during surgical procedures and dental extractions in haemophiliac patients. Tranexamic acid has also been used in the management of hereditary angioneurotic oedema and in some cases of DIC.

Aprotinin

Aprotinin is a serine proteinase inhibitor that affects many proteolytic enzymes including kallikrein (kallidinogenase), plasma kinins, trypsins and plasmin. Its activity is dependent on the inhibition of plasmin and plasmin activators, thus reducing fibrinolysis and preserving platelet function (Fig. 16.6). It has been used in the treatment of severe haemorrhage in hyperplasminaemic states, in particular those associated with excessive thrombolytic therapy or malignant disease (e.g., acute promyelocytic leukaemia). More recently, aprotinin has been successfully used to reduce blood loss during open-heart surgery and other major surgical procedures. Although concerns have been raised about its possible effects on postoperative renal function, there is no convincing evidence that this is adversely affected. Since aprotinin inhibits both trypsin and chymotrypsin, it has also been used in the treatment of acute pancreatitis. Aprotinin is antigenic and its use is usually preceded by the administration of a test dose before the drug is administered by slow intravenous infusion. It may cause localised thrombophlebitis, and severe hypersensitivity responses occur occasionally.

Other agents

Desmopressin acetate

Desmopressin acetate (DDAVP, or 1-deamino-8-D-arginine vasopressin) is a synthetic analogue of vasopressin. It has a longer duration of action than vasopressin, but has no vasoconstrictor activity. Desmopressin is mainly used in the diagnosis and treatment of diabetes insipidus. It is also used to improve haemostasis in patients with mild haemophilia or von Willebrand's disease, since it induces the release of factor VIII and factor IX from tissues and increases their concentration in the circulation. Desmopressin has also been employed to shorten the bleeding time in other conditions involving abnormal platelet function (e.g. uraemia) and has been used successfully to reduce blood loss following cardiac surgery.

Suggested reading

Anderson, J.A.M. & Saenko, E.L. (2002) Heparin resistance. *British Journal of Anaesthesia* **88**, 467–469.

Anderson, K.M., Califf, R.M., Stone, G.W., *et al.* (2001) Long-term mortality benefit with abciximab in patients undergoing percutaneous coronary intervention. *Journal of the American College of Cardiology* **37**, 2059–2065.

Aster, R.H. (1995) Heparin-induced thrombocytopenia and thrombosis. *New England Journal of Medicine* **332**, 1374–1376.

Bullingham, A. & Strunin, L. (1995) Prevention of postoperative thromboembolism. *British Journal of Anaesthesia* **75**, 622–630.

Chong, B.H. (1995) Heparin-induced thrombocytopenia. *British Journal of Haematology* **89**, 421–439.

Collins, R., Peto, R., Baigent, C. & Sleight, P. (1997) Aspirin, heparin and thrombolytic therapy in suspected acute myocardial infarction. *New England Journal of Medicine* **336**, 847–860.

Davie, E.W., Fujikawa, K. & Kisiel, W. (1991) The coagulation cascade: initiation, maintenance, and regulation. *Biochemistry* **30**, 10363–10370.

Diener, H., Cunha, L., Forbes, C., *et al.* (1996) European Stroke Prevention Study. 2. Dipyridamole and acetylsalicylic acid in the secondary prevention of stroke. *Journal of Neurological Science* **143**, 1–14.

Furie, B. & Furie, B.C. (1992) Molecular and cellular biology of blood coagulation. *New England Journal of Medicine* **326**, 800–806.

Green, C. (2003) DIC and other coagulopathies in the ICU. *Anaesthesia and Intensive Care Medicine* **4**, 147–149.

Hirsh, J. (1991) Heparin. *New England Journal of Medicine* **324**, 1565–1574.

Hirsh, J. (1991) Oral anticoagulant drugs. *New England Journal of Medicine* **324**, 1865–1873.

Hirsh, J. & Levine, M.N. (1992) Low molecular weight heparin. *Blood* **79**, 1–17.

Kaplan, K. & Francis, C. (1999) Heparin induced thrombocytopenia. *Blood Review* **13**, 1–7.

Kövesi, T. & Royston, D. (2002) Is there a bleeding problem with platelet-active drugs? *British Journal of Anaesthesia* **88**, 159–163.

Mannuccio, M. (1998) Hemostatic drugs. *New England Journal of Medicine* **333**, 245–253.

Martlew, V.J. (2000) Peri-operative management of patients with coagulation disorders. *British Journal of Anaesthesia* **85**, 446–455.

Montalescot, G., Barragan, P., Wittenberg, O., *et al.* (2001) Platelet glycoprotein IIb/IIIa inhibition with coronary stenting for acute myocardial infarction. *New England Journal of Medicine* **344**, 1895–1903.

Nichols, A.J., Ruffolo, R.R, Huffman, W.F., *et al.* (1992) Development of GPIIb/IIIa antagonists as antithrombotic drugs. *Trends in Pharmacological Sciences* **13**, 413–417.

Patrono, C. (1994) Aspirin as an antiplatelet drug. *New England Journal of Medicine* **330**, 1287–1294.

Salzman, E.W. (1992) Low-molecular-weight heparin and other new antithrombotic drugs. *New England Journal of Medicine* **326**, 1017–1019.

Schweizer, A., Höhn, L., Morel, D.R., *et al.* (2000) Aprotinin does not impair renal haemodynamics and function after cardiac surgery. *British Journal of Anaesthesia* **84**, 16–22.

Turpie, A.G., Gallus, A.S. & Hoek, J.A. (2001) A synthetic pentasaccharide for the prevention of deep-vein thrombosis after total hip replacement. *New England Journal of Medicine* **344**, 619–625.

Trivier, J.M., Caron, J., Mahieu, M., *et al.* (2001) Fatal aplastic anaemia associated with clopidogrel. *Lancet* **357**, 446.

Ware, J.A. & Heisted, D.D. (1993) Platelet-endothelium interactions. *New England Journal of Medicine* **328**, 628–635.

Weitz, J.I. & Hirsh, J. (2001) New anticoagulant drugs. *Chest* **119**, 95S–107S.

Wong, B.I., McLean, R.F., Fremes, S.E., *et al.* (2000) Aprotinin and tranexamic acid for high transfusion risk cardiac surgery. *Annals of Thoracic Surgery* **69**, 808–816.

17 Corticosteroids and Hypoglycaemic Agents

Corticosteroids

The physiological and clinical significance of the adrenal glands was first recognised by Thomas Addison approximately 150 years ago. The adrenal medulla is responsible for the synthesis and secretion of noradrenaline and adrenaline, and plays an important role in the sympathetic response to dangerous or stressful situations ('fight or flight' response). In contrast, the adrenal cortex synthesises two groups of hormones – 'mineralocorticoids' and 'glucocorticoids' – with a chemical structure based on the steroid nucleus which have different physiological effects. The mineralocorticoid hormone aldosterone is secreted by the outer cells of the adrenal cortex (the zona glomerulosa) and predominantly affects fluid and electrolyte balance. The glucocorticoid hormones – hydrocortisone (cortisol) and corticosterone – are synthesised by the inner zona fasciculata and zona reticularis, and have complex effects on carbohydrate and protein metabolism. During the past 50 years, many synthetic compounds with similar properties to hydrocortisone have been synthesised and some of these are currently used in medicine (Table 17.1). They are commonly referred to as corticosteroids (although glucocorticoids is a more precise and better term).

Hydrocortisone (cortisol)

Aldosterone

Mode of action

Glucocorticoids

Most of the pharmacological effects of glucocorticoids are dependent on their combination with intracellular steroid receptors in target cells and their subsequent effects on DNA, gene transcription and ribosomal protein synthesis. Consequently, their effects are indirect and their onset of action is relatively slow (i.e. 1–6 h).

Glucocorticoid receptors

All glucocorticoids are highly lipid-soluble and readily diffuse across cellular membranes, where they combine reversibly with glucocorticoid receptors. Two types of receptors – GRα and GRβ – are present in the cytoplasm of most cells, where they are bound in a large molecular weight complex with other proteins. Although their density is extremely variable, most cells contain between 4000 and 10,000 receptors.

Receptor activation

The activation of GRα and GRβ receptors by glucocorticoids results in conformational changes and exposes a

Table 17.1 The relative potency of some common corticosteroids

	Relative potency	Equi-effective dose (mg)
Cortisone*	0.8	12.5
Hydrocortisone*	1	10
Deflazacort	3	3
Prednisolone	4	2.5
Methylprednisolone	5	2
Triamcinolone	5	2
Betamethasone	25	0.4
Dexamethasone	25	0.4

The equi-effective anti-inflammatory doses are equivalent to the amount of hydrocortisone secreted daily by a normal adult (10–15 mg).

*Cortisone is now rarely used clinically and has been largely superseded by other corticosteroids. Both cortisone and hydrocortisone have significant mineralocorticoid activity.

DNA-binding domain. The steroid–receptor complexes then form pairs (dimers) and are transferred to the nucleus, where they are bound by specific high-affinity binding sites on DNA ('steroid responsive elements'; Fig. 17.1). The transcription of 10–100 specific target genes in the immediate vicinity of the steroid regulatory elements is either repressed or induced, resulting in changes in mRNA and ribosomal protein synthesis.

Repression of gene transcription

Repression of gene transcription is mainly mediated by inhibition of certain transcription factors, notably AP-1 (activator protein-1) and NFκB (nuclear factor κB). These factors normally activate genes concerned with the synthesis of many inflammatory mediators (Fig. 17.1). Consequently, corticosteroids decrease the synthesis of these factors by target cells, resulting in a variety of immunosuppressive and anti-inflammatory effects.

Induction of gene transcription

In contrast, the induction of gene transcription selectively increases mRNA and protein synthesis (particularly by inflammatory cells). Glucocorticoids enhance the synthesis and activity of angiotensin-converting enzyme (Chapter 14) and some endopeptidases. In addition, they induce the synthesis and intracellular translocation of a family of glycoproteins (the annexins or lipocortins). Annexin-1 inhibits phospholipase A_2 (PLA_2), which normally converts membrane phospholipids to arachidonic acid in inflammatory cells. The inhibition of PLA_2 decreases the formation of prostaglandins, leukotrienes and platelet-activating factor, and thus produces anti-inflammatory effects.

Mineralocorticoids

Aldosterone combines with steroid receptors in the distal renal tubule and the collecting ducts, and the resultant aldosterone–receptor complex then migrates to the nucleus. The modification of DNA transcription increases the number and density of Na^+ and K^+ channels in the luminal membrane and also increases the activity and expression of Na^+/K^+ ATPase in the basolateral membrane, resulting in increased reabsorption of Na^+, Cl^- and water in exchange for K^+ and H^+ elimination.

Some glucocorticoids, such as fludrocortisone, also have mineralocorticoid effects and affect electrolyte balance in the distal renal tubule. Mineralocorticoid effects are also present in glucocorticoids whose anti-inflammatory potency is relatively weak (Table 17.1) and may cause sodium retention and oedema, and thus precipitate hypertension, cardiac failure and cerebrovascular accidents in susceptible patients.

Pharmacological effects of glucocorticoids

Glucocorticoids mainly affect:
- protein and carbohydrate metabolism
- immunological competence
- inflammation

In addition, they have 'permissive' effects and their presence in body tissues may be essential for other hormones to produce their effects.

Protein and carbohydrate metabolism

Corticosteroids increase the deamination of proteins and amino acids and enhance their conversion to glucose and glycogen (gluconeogenesis). Consequently, they cause protein breakdown, reduce protein synthesis, enhance carbohydrate turnover and raise blood sugar and glycogen levels in liver and muscle. Although these actions are of little therapeutic importance, they are responsible for many of the side effects of glucocorticoids.

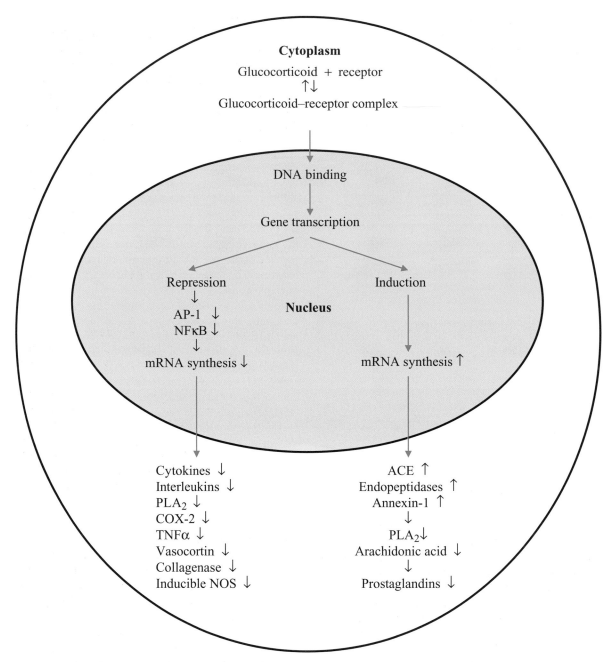

Fig. 17.1 The effects of glucocorticoids on gene transcription and the repression and induction of protein mediators of inflammation. ACE, angiotensin-converting enzyme; AP, activator protein; NF, nuclear factor; PLA$_2$, phospholipase A$_2$; COX-2, cyclooxygenase-2; TNF, tumour necrosis factor; NOS, nitric oxide synthase.

Increased protein breakdown

Increased protein breakdown causes:
- retardation of growth
- reduction in voluntary muscle mass
- thinning and ulceration of the skin and mucosae
- increased susceptibility to peptic ulceration
- striae
- osteoporosis, vertebral collapse and pathological fractures
- increased elimination of calcium, nitrogen and phosphate ions

Increased carbohydrate turnover

Increased carbohydrate turnover may cause:
- hyperglycaemia
- glycosuria
- diabetes

Immunological competence

Corticosteroids depress the activity of many cells and tissues that are concerned with immunological competence. Their chronic use causes the generalised atrophy of many lymphoid tissues such as the spleen, thymus, tonsils and lymph nodes, mainly due to a decrease in T-cell lymphocytes. After intravenous hydrocortisone, the number of circulating lymphocytes is reduced by more than 50% within 6–8 hours.

Reduced T-cell proliferation

Reduced T-cell proliferation is mainly related to the decreased synthesis of interleukin-2 (IL-2), which plays an important role in lymphocyte division and multiplication after exposure to antigens. Glucocorticoids also inhibit the synthesis and/or release of many cytokines and interleukins from T-cells, including IL-1 to IL-6, IL-8, TNF-α and TNF-δ, as well as many leucocyte and macrophage adhesion factors. Consequently, corticosteroids reduce the proliferation and the immunological competence of T lymphocytes, and this probably accounts for their effectiveness as immunosuppressant drugs after organ transplantation. Similar effects are produced in endothelial cells and macrophages.

Glucocorticoids also reduce the activity of the complement system and acute phase reactants in plasma, decrease the synthesis of IgG and IgE and inhibit the release of pharmacological mediators from mast cells and basophils.

Inflammation

All inflammatory responses are inhibited by glucocorticoids, irrespective of their cause. In acute inflammation, they decrease tissue transudation and oedema, reduce the diapedesis of neutrophils and macrophages and prevent the access of immunoglobulins to inflamed tissues. Consequently, they decrease the accumulation and activity of lymphocytes and neutrophils at sites of tissue inflammation, mainly due to the decreased synthesis and release of cytokines, interleukins and cell adhesion factors (Fig. 17.1). Most of the immunosuppressive and anti-inflammatory effects of corticosteroids in chronic inflammatory diseases are due to these changes.

Most glucocorticoids have different anti-inflammatory potencies, and cortisone and hydrocortisone are approximately 30 times less potent than betamethasone or dexamethasone (Table 17.1). This range in potency probably reflects differences in the affinity of glucocorticoids for steroid receptors.

Undesirable anti-inflammatory activity

The effects of glucocorticoids on inflammatory responses may have undesirable effects. The reduction in cellular and humoral inflammatory responses decreases resistance to infection, and may cause the reactivation of latent bacterial infections (e.g. tuberculosis), which may not be immediately apparent. Corticosteroids may also cause the reactivation of peptic ulceration, with gastrointestinal haemorrhage or perforation. Although the activity of fibroblasts and osteoblasts is decreased and bone density reduced, osteoclastic activity is increased and may lead to osteoporosis.

Permissive effects

Glucocorticoids also have indirect or permissive actions, and their presence in the body in physiological concentrations is essential in order for certain hormones (e.g. insulin, adrenaline) to produce their effects. The synthesis of adrenaline by the adrenal medulla and many of its metabolic effects, such as the synthesis of cyclic AMP by adipose tissue and subsequent lipolysis, is dependent on the presence of corticosteroids. The general pattern of fat deposition is also affected by glucocorticoids, which usually decrease adipose tissue in the limbs, but increase its deposition in the neck, supraclavicular region, trunk, shoulders and face ('buffalo hump' and 'moon face'). In the absence of glucocorticoids, blood vessels are resistant to many endogenous mediators, including adrenaline, noradrenaline and angiotensin II, since steroids promote the expression of adrenergic receptors in vascular smooth muscle. For these reasons, general anaesthesia for patients with adrenocortical insufficiency may be associated with hypotension, vascular collapse and delayed recovery (page 97).

Pharmacokinetics

Distribution

All glucocorticoids are highly lipid-soluble compounds and are absorbed in the small intestine, bound to plasma proteins and extensively metabolised by the liver. Indeed, the effects of cortisone and prednisone are dependent on their initial metabolism to hydrocortisone and prednisolone. After oral administration, the physiological steroids hydrocortisone and corticosterone are bound with high affinity by a specific plasma globulin (transcortin), which is present only in small concentrations (35 mg L^{-1}). In addition, both naturally occurring and synthetic glucocorticoids are bound by albumin.

Metabolism

After intravenous administration, hydrocortisone and aldosterone have relatively short terminal half-lives (90–120 min). They undergo extensive hepatic metabolism and are usually eliminated in urine as glucuronide or sulphate conjugates. After oral administration, the half-life of most steroids is longer due to presystemic metabolism and enterohepatic recirculation.

The pharmacokinetics of glucocorticoids may not reflect their duration of action, since there is usually a latent period after administration before their effects are apparent and some are metabolised to active derivatives. Some steroids (e.g. dexamethasone, betamethasone) may act for up to 48–72 hours.

Administration

Glucocorticoids may be administered orally or parenterally, or as local therapy to the skin, into joints or to the respiratory tract, ears or eyes.

Intravenous glucocorticoids

Intravenous steroids are most commonly used in emergency situations (e.g. shock, acute anaphylaxis, status asthmaticus). High doses can be given safely, as the risk of complications is negligible in patients on short-term therapy.

Unfortunately, intravenous steroids do not act immediately and may take up to 3–6 hours to produce their maximum effects. Hydrocortisone (100–500 mg) is normally given as the sodium succinate salt and requires reconstitution prior to injection. Although the sodium phosphate salts of hydrocortisone, betamethasone or dexamethasone can also be given intravenously, they may cause unpleasant side effects after rapid injection, particularly generalised vasodilatation and pelvic or perineal discomfort, which may be related to their hydrolysis by phosphatase enzymes.

Oral glucocorticoids

More commonly, corticosteroids are administered orally, and may be given as replacement therapy in Addison's disease, hypopituitarism or after hypophysectomy or adrenalectomy. In these conditions hydrocortisone, usually supplemented with fludrocortisone, is used. Alternatively, they may be given non-specifically for their immunosuppressive or anti-inflammatory effects and to suppress the manifestations of various diseases (Table 17.2).

Table 17.2 Conditions in which corticosteroids are used systemically in order to suppress pharmacological or pathological processes.

Active chronic hepatitis
Acute anaphylaxis
Bronchial asthma
Bronchospasm
Cerebral oedema
Crohn's disease
Exfoliative dermatitis
Haemolytic anaemia (acquired)
Malignant conditions (acute leukaemia; non-Hodgkin's lymphoma)
Nephrotic syndrome
Pemphigus
Polyarteritis nodosa
Polymyalgia rheumatica
Polymyositis
Rheumatoid arthritis
Rheumatic carditis
Systemic lupus erythematosus
Systemic sclerosis
Temporal arteritis
Thrombocytopenic purpura
Transplantation reactions
Ulcerative colitis

When oral or parenteral preparations are used, the doses required to control or suppress pathological processes may be associated with serious and unavoidable adverse effects. Indeed, some of these effects may be observed after the use of potent local preparations, particularly when used in diseases of the skin. Adverse reactions to systemic corticosteroids are often a limiting factor in their use. Although some of these reactions are due to the exaggerated pharmacological effects of steroids, others are obscure in origin (Table 17.3).

Local glucocorticoids

Local preparations of corticosteroids are used whenever possible in order to limit their systemic adverse effects. They are given by local application or administration in many conditions, including:
- diseases of the skin (eczema, lichen planus, discoid lupus erythematous and various neurodermatoses)
- diseases of the mouth (oral and perioral ulceration)
- ENT diseases (allergic rhinitis and eczematous otitis externa)
- ophthalmological conditions (allergic conjunctivitis, keratitis and uveitis)
- respiratory diseases (bronchial asthma and bronchospasm)
- intestinal conditions (ulcerative colitis and proctitis)

Suppression of pituitary–adrenal function

Undoubtedly the most serious long-term complication of corticosteroid therapy is suppression of the hypothalamic–pituitary–adrenal axis. Corticotrophin (ACTH) secretion by the anterior pituitary gland normally controls the synthesis and release of glucocorticoids by the adrenal cortex. The secretion of ACTH itself is partially controlled by a hypothalamic factor, corticotrophin releasing factor (CRF), whose release is dependent on numerous physiological and pharmacological factors, including the plasma concentrations of ACTH and hydrocortisone, as well as lipocortins, exogenous corticosteroids, opioid peptides and physical or psychological stress.

Effects of steroids on CRF and ACTH release
Corticosteroid administration suppresses CRF secretion by the hypothalamus, as well as ACTH secretion by the anterior pituitary (Fig. 17.2). Decreased secretion of ACTH reduces the physiological release of hydrocortisone and

Table 17.3 Common adverse reactions to systemic corticosteroids.

Causal effects	Reaction
Increased tissue and protein breakdown	Retardation of growth Muscle wasting Osteoporosis Vertebral collapse Fractures Avascular necrosis (femoral head) Thinning of skin, mucosae and hair Cutaneous striae Ecchymoses Subcutaneous haemorrhages Gastrointestinal bleeding Impaired wound healing
Increased carbohydrate turnover	Hyperglycaemia Glycosuria Diminished carbohydrate tolerance Diabetes mellitus
Anti-inflammatory effects	Suppression of normal immunological responses Suppression of manifestations of infection Reactivation of latent infection Peptic ulceration
Salt and water retention	Oedema Cardiac failure Hypertension Hypokalaemia
Abnormal fat deposition	Facial roundness Buffalo hump Supraclavicular fat deposition Truncal obesity
Of uncertain origin	Habituation and dependence Euphoria Psychoses Mental depression Acne Leukocytosis Cataract formation Amenorrhoea Peripheral neuropathy

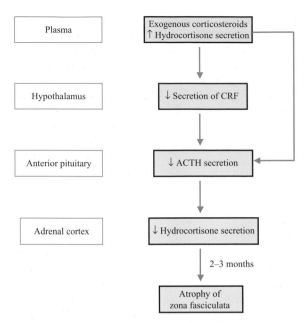

Fig. 17.2 The negative feedback control of endogenous hydrocortisone secretion by the hypothalamic–pituitary–adrenal axis. An increase in hydrocortisone secretion or exogenous corticosteroids suppresses the secretion of both corticotrophin releasing factor (CRF) by the hypothalamus and corticotrophin (ACTH) by the anterior pituitary gland.

corticosterone by the adrenal cortex to negligible levels, although the secretion of aldosterone is only slightly reduced. The functional suppression of the hypothalamic–pituitary–adrenal axis by exogenous glucocorticoids may be followed by atrophy of zona fasciculata cells, which persists for a variable time (up to 12 months) after treatment is stopped.

Response to stress

When patients are stabilised for more than 3 weeks on doses greater than the normal steroid secretion rate (10–15 mg hydrocortisone in 24 h), the sudden withdrawal of steroids is hazardous, since the hypothalamic–pituitary–adrenal axis may be suppressed and the adrenocortical response to stress may be impaired or defective. It is therefore important to slowly decrease corticosteroid dosage after chronic therapy, so that functional recovery of the axis can occur. Its physiological integrity can be tested by the morning plasma hydrocortisone concentration or the response to insulin-induced hypoglycaemia, which normally causes a prompt increase in the physiological secretion of hydrocortisone.

Modification of adrenal suppression

The suppression of the hypothalamic–pituitary–adrenal axis by systemic corticosteroid therapy can be modified by various methods, including:
- the use of as low a dose as possible, for as short a period as possible
- intermittent therapy
- the use of a single daily morning dose, in order to mimic the normal circadian rhythm of glucocorticoid secretion. The physiological secretion of hydrocortisone and corticosterone is normally maximal in the morning (8.00 a.m.) and then progressively declines to reach a nadir at 3.00 a.m.
- the use of a double dose on alternate mornings

In the past, ACTH has been used in order to limit adrenal cortical suppression and to assess adrenal function, but is no longer available in the UK. Tetracosactide (tetracosactrin) is a biologically active analogue of ACTH which is less likely to provoke hypersensitivity reactions. It is administered as a zinc phosphate complex, and its action lasts for 16–48 hours. Tetracosactide has been used to increase the secretion of endogenous steroids by the adrenal cortex and may be less likely to induce muscle atrophy, osteoporosis and retardation of growth during childhood than corticosteroids. Unfortunately, the adrenocortical response is variable and its effectiveness is limited, since it can increase the basal secretion of hydrocortisone only 5–10 times (from about 10 to 50–100 mg day^{-1}).

Corticosteroids and the metabolic response to surgery

The response to surgical stress is complex and may be influenced by the extent and nature of the surgical procedure and by drugs used during anaesthesia. One of the important metabolic responses to general anaesthesia and major surgery is an increase in the endogenous secretion rate of ACTH and hydrocortisone. The secretion rate of hydrocortisone may rise from 10–15 to 50–150 mg daily in response to operative stress and remain elevated for a variable period after surgery. Aldosterone secretion is also increased. These responses are dependent on the integrity of the hypothalamic–pituitary–adrenal axis. When patients are taking the equivalent of 10–30 mg hydrocortisone (or more) daily, the axis is partially or completely suppressed. This may persist for at least 2 months after corticosteroid therapy has been slowly reduced and stopped.

All patients on steroids, or who have recently been treated with systemic steroids, should possess a steroid card and should be aware of the possible hazards in relation to anaesthesia. In such patients, the physiological increase in hydrocortisone secretion normally associated with surgical stress may be partially obtunded or deficient, and its absence may cause severe hypotension and cardiovascular collapse during surgery. Prior to minor surgery under general anaesthesia, oral corticosteroids are usually continued until the morning of surgery and supplemented by intravenous hydrocortisone (25–50 mg) at induction. In patients undergoing more extensive surgical procedures, a similar regime is usually followed, but supplemented by parenteral hydrocortisone (50–100 mg 8-hourly) for 24 hours after moderate surgery, or 48–72 hours after major surgery. Hydrocortisone sodium succinate must also be available during surgery. During the postoperative period, the dosage of steroids is gradually reduced and progressively replaced by normal oral steroid therapy, if any. This process is usually complete by the third to fifth postoperative day. During and after bilateral adrenalectomy, a similar regime is usually followed and oral therapy (usually hydrocortisone and fludrocortisone) progressively introduced following surgery.

The use of corticosteroids during surgical procedures in patients whose steroid therapy has been stopped 3–12 months prior to surgery is less clearly defined. There is considerable evidence that the use of hydrocortisone alone on the day of surgery may provide ample protection against peripheral vascular collapse. Nevertheless, intravenous steroids should always be available during surgery.

Hypoglycaemic agents

In diabetes mellitus, there is a relative or absolute deficiency of insulin, which may be due to:
- degeneration, destruction or exhaustion of the β-cells of the islets of Langerhans
- resistance or decreased sensitivity of tissues to circulating insulin
- excessive secretion of insulin antagonists (e.g. antibodies, ACTH, corticosteroids and possibly glucagon and somatostatin)

Diabetes mellitus is usually classified as:
- insulin-dependent diabetes mellitus (IDDM, or Type I diabetes)
- non-insulin-dependent diabetes mellitus (NIDDM, or Type II diabetes)

Cause of diabetes
Current evidence suggests that Type I diabetes can be considered as a cell-mediated autoimmune disorder and that a high proportion of patients develop circulating antibodies to various structural components of β-cells. There is often a genetic predisposition to the disease, and many patients possess the HLA-DR4 histocompatibility locus. The onset of Type I diabetes is often precipitated by environmental triggering factors, such as transient viral infections. Type II diabetes is also dependent on both genetic and environmental factors, and there is often a familial tendency and a strong relationship with obesity.

Metabolic changes
In both types of diabetes, the relative or absolute deficiency of insulin results in defective carbohydrate metabolism and hyperglycaemia. The uptake of glucose by the liver and skeletal muscle is depressed and glycogen synthesis is reduced. Hyperglycaemia usually exceeds the renal threshold for glucose reabsorption (about 10 mmol L^{-1}), resulting in glycosuria, polyuria and polydipsia. Since insulin also normally promotes lipogenesis, there are also secondary effects on fat metabolism, resulting in lipolysis and the reduced uptake of triglycerides by adipose tissue. Free fatty acids in plasma are oxidised to acetyl CoA in the liver and subsequently converted to ketones (acetoacetate and β-hydroxybutyrate). The deamination of proteins and amino acids and their subsequent conversion to carbohydrate precursors (gluconeogenesis) is also increased.

Aims of treatment
The aim of the treatment of diabetes mellitus is the correction of the immediate metabolic abnormalities in carbohydrate, fat and protein metabolism, and the prevention of long-term complications, particularly retinopathy, nephropathy, neuropathy, hypercholesterolaemia and peripheral vascular damage, by the use of hypoglycaemic drugs. Current evidence suggests that most or all of these long-term complications can be prevented or avoided by the control of blood glucose within physiological limits, using individualised treatment regimes. Nevertheless, intensive treatment regimes are associated with a significantly increased risk of hypoglycaemia.

Hypoglycaemic drugs
The treatment of diabetes depends on the use of hypoglycaemic drugs, which can be divided into:
- insulin and its derivatives
- oral hypoglycaemic drugs

Insulin and its derivatives

Structure and synthesis

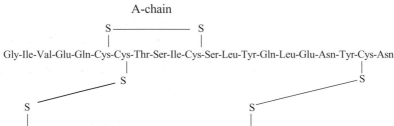

Insulin is a polypeptide with a molecular weight of approximately 5800. It contains 51 amino acid residues in two peptide chains (A and B), which are linked by two disulphide bridges. Its precursor protein (preproinsulin) is synthesised in the rough endoplasmic reticulum of the pancreatic β-cell and then partly degraded to proinsulin, in which the A and B chains are linked by a larger fragment, the connector peptide or C-peptide (Fig. 17.3). Proinsulin is then transported to the Golgi complex and converted to insulin, which is stored (with some proinsulin) in secretory granules. Consequently, when insulin is released into the circulation in response to hyperglycaemia, the C-peptide (derived from proinsulin) is also released and can be measured separately. Although the C-peptide has no known function or activity, it can be used to monitor the physiological secretion of insulin by β-cells.

Insulin secretion

The endogenous secretion of insulin is mainly dependent on the concentration of glucose in blood, although amino acids and α_2- and β_1-adrenoceptors also affect its release. An increase in the plasma concentration of glucose results in its uptake by the membrane transporter GLUT-2 in β-cells, where it is phosphorylated by glucokinase. The phosphorylation of glucose increases intracellular ATP and causes blockade of K_{ATP} channels in the β-cell membrane, resulting in depolarisation. Subsequently, voltage-dependent Ca^{2+} channels open and Ca^{2+} influx occurs, resulting in the release of insulin from β-cell granules and its secretion into the portal circulation. Insulin secretion occurs in two phases, so that an initial evanescent peak is followed by a slower, more prolonged hormonal release.

Mode of action

Insulin lowers blood sugar by activating specific insulin receptors in liver, skeletal muscle and fat. Insulin receptors consist of an extracellular (α) and an intracellular (β) domain. When the α-units are bound by insulin, the β-subunits are activated, resulting in phosphorylation of their tyrosine residues. Subsequent phosphorylation reactions increase the synthesis, activation and mobilisation of the glucose transporter GLUT-4, which migrates from the cytoplasm to the plasma membrane and increases glucose uptake. Subsequently, glucose is stored as glycogen in liver and muscle. Insulin also stimulates the synthesis of fat, and lipogenesis is increased, and so the concentration of many plasma lipids is decreased. In addition, the breakdown of proteins to carbohydrates is reduced due to inhibition of gluconeogenesis.

Metabolism

After its secretion into the portal vein, insulin has an extremely short half-life (4–6 min) and a rapid clearance (6–16 mL min^{-1} kg^{-1}). It is initially removed from the portal circulation by the liver and then metabolised by various insulin-degrading enzymes. Any insulin that enters the systemic circulation is rapidly removed by the kidney and other organs.

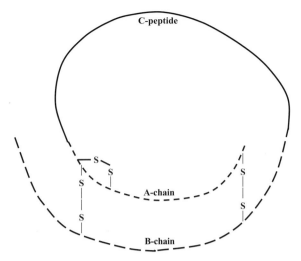

Fig. 17.3 Diagrammatic representation of the structure of proinsulin. The A-chain (- - -) and the B-chain (– – –) of insulin are connected by disulphide bridges (–S–). The C-peptide (——) is released from proinsulin when it is converted to insulin.

Animal insulins and immunological reactions

For many years, preparations of insulin used were extracted from the pancreas of pigs (porcine insulin) or cattle (bovine insulin) and purified by crystallisation. There are minor differences in the amino acid sequences of these insulins and human insulin, which differs from porcine insulin by one amino acid and from bovine insulin by three amino acids. Impure preparations of animal insulins contain proinsulin and/or C-peptide, and often cause localised or generalised insulin allergy, insulin resistance or fat atrophy (lipodystrophy). These immunological reactions can be minimised by the use of highly purified preparations of insulin, in which almost all the proinsulin and C-peptide impurities are removed by gel filtration and ion-exchange chromatography. In the UK, all insulin preparations of animal origin are now highly purified, although their use has declined significantly in recent years. Consequently, immunological reactions are now relatively uncommon.

Human insulins

During the past 25 years, human insulins have been widely used in the treatment of Type I diabetes and approximately 80–90% of patients are now stabilised on these preparations. Human insulins can be prepared by the enzymic modification of porcine insulin or synthesised by *Escherichia coli* or yeast organisms, using recombinant DNA technology. The insulin requirement of diabetic patients is usually reduced by 10–15% when bovine insulin is replaced by human insulin, although the requirements of patients stabilised on porcine insulin is usually unchanged. Hypoglycaemia may be commoner in patients stabilised on human insulin, since the hormone is commonly used in diabetic regimes that depend on the tight control of blood glucose concentrations. Some patients consider that the premonitory signs of hypoglycaemia are obtunded or blunted when animal preparations are replaced by human insulins.

Administration of insulin

Since insulin is a polypeptide, it is broken down in the gut and is given by subcutaneous injection, except in hyperglycaemic emergencies and during the perioperative period. Insulin is injected into the upper arms, thighs or abdomen, and its absorption may be affected by the site of injection and local blood flow. Consequently, absorption of insulin is increased by massage, local heat and physical exercise. It is most commonly given by portable injection devices (pen injectors) which hold the insulin in a cartridge (usually 3 mL) and deliver a metered dose. Alternatively, it can be given in conventional plastic syringes with pre-fixed or unfixed needles or reusable glass syringes with disposable needles. Although soluble insulin can be adsorbed by glass or plastic syringes, this can be avoided by the use of silicone-coated glassware.

Syringe pumps

Soluble neutral insulin or some insulin analogues can also be given by subcutaneous infusion, using a battery-operated portable syringe pump. This technique provides a continuous basal infusion of insulin, which mimics the normal secretion of endogenous insulin. The pump can be programmed to provide differential infusion rates during the day and night and to deliver supplementary bolus injections before the main meals. In spite of its disadvantages, diabetic control and the quality of life may be improved.

Monitoring

Whenever possible, insulin administration should be controlled by the frequent monitoring of blood glucose, using impregnated strips and an electronic meter. It is generally recommended that blood glucose concentrations are maintained between 4 and 7 mmol L^{-1}. Long-term diabetic control can also be assessed by the frequent measurement of the concentration of glycosylated haemoglobin (Hb_{A1c}) or fructosamine. Glycosylated haemoglobin is a covalent adduct of haemoglobin and glucose and provides an integrated measurement of hyperglycaemia over several months, since its half-life is similar to that of the erythrocyte (120 days). Concentrations of Hb_{A1c} less than 7.5% are considered to minimise the risk of vascular complications.

Insulin preparations

Soluble neutral insulin

Soluble neutral insulin is an acetate-buffered solution of insulin (pH 7.0). It is prepared from human sequence insulin or from highly purified animal insulins. After subcutaneous injection, it usually acts within 30–60 minutes and has a maximum activity between 2 and 4 hours, which lasts for up to 8 hours. Human insulin preparations may have a more rapid onset of action than animal insulins and a shorter duration of action, due to their enhanced aqueous solubility. Soluble insulin may also be given intramuscularly and intravenously, and is the most suitable preparation for diabetic emergencies and during the perioperative period. It is commonly mixed with longer-acting preparations of insulin and is widely used in many injection regimes.

Recombinant analogues of soluble insulin

- Insulin aspart
- Insulin glulisine
- Insulin lispro

Insulin aspart is a recombinant human insulin analogue in which proline (at B28) has been replaced with aspartic acid (28^B-aspartic acid-human insulin). Insulin glulisine is also a recombinant human insulin analogue, in which asparagine (at B3) is replaced by lysine and lysine (at B29) is replaced by glutamic acid (3^B-lysine-29^B-glutamic acid-human insulin). In contrast, in insulin lispro the position of two amino acid residues (proline at B28 and lysine at B29) has been reversed (28^B-lysine-29^B-proline-human insulin).

These three preparations are mainly present in solution as monomers, rather than hexamers (as with soluble insulin). Consequently, they have a faster onset of action due to their more rapid absorption, but a shorter duration of action than human soluble insulin. They control postprandial blood glucose levels when given shortly before the start of a meal and are unlikely to induce hypoglycaemic reactions. They are normally given with an intermediate- or long-acting insulin.

Isophane insulin

The duration of action of neutral insulin can be prolonged by decreasing its solubility, thus delaying its absorption after subcutaneous injection. This can be achieved by combining the hormone with various proteins (e.g. protamine) or with zinc alone in specialised conditions, as in insulin zinc suspensions.

Isophane insulin (NPH insulin) is a suspension of human or animal insulin with protamine, which slows its onset and prolongs its duration of action (Table 17.4).

Biphasic insulins

Although it can be used alone, isophane insulin is usually prepared or mixed with soluble insulin and administered as a biphasic mixture. Various proprietary preparations containing between 10 and 50% human or porcine soluble insulin are commonly used. In addition, recombinant analogues of human insulin have been complexed with protamine and used as biphasic preparations (biphasic insulin aspart and biphasic insulin lispro). Most biphasic preparations have an onset of action within 1 hour, a maximum activity between 6 and 12 hours and a duration of action of 18–24 hours (Table 17.4). Biphasic insulins are widely used in the treatment of diabetes and are commonly given subcutaneously twice daily.

Insulin zinc suspension

Insulin zinc suspension is a suspension of soluble insulin with zinc in specialised conditions, which prolongs its duration of action for 18–24 hours (and sometimes longer). It is sometimes used as a single daily subcutaneous injection in Type I diabetes. When required, it can be supplemented with soluble insulin, although not in a physical mixture.

Protamine zinc insulin

Protamine zinc insulin is a complex of bovine insulin with protamine and zinc, and has a longer duration of action than other insulins (Table 17.4). It should not be mixed with neutral soluble insulin before injection. Protamine zinc insulin is now rarely used.

Other long-acting insulins

- Insulin determir
- Insulin glargine

Table 17.4 Preparations of human and animal insulin in current use.

Type of preparation	Generic form	Name of preparation	Subcutaneous injection		
			Onset of action (h)	Maximum activity (h)	Duration of action (h)
Short acting	Soluble insulin (neutral insulin)	Actrapid (H) Velosulin (H) Humulin S (H) Insuman Rapid (H) Pork Actrapid (P) Hypurin Porcine Neutral (P) Hypurin Bovine Neutral (B)	0.5	2–4	6–8
	Insulin lispro (RHIA)	Humalog	0.2	0.5–3	3–5
	Insulin aspart (RHIA)	Novorapid	0.2	0.5–3	3–5
	Insulin glulisine (RHIA)	Apidra	0.2	0.5–3	3–5
Intermediate acting	Isophane insulin (NPH)	Insulatard (H) Humulin I (H) Insuman basal (H) Pork Insulatard (P) Hypurin Porcine Isophane (P) Hypurin Bovine Isophane (B)	2	4–12	18–24
	Biphasic isophane insulin (NPH)	Mixtard 10,20,30,40,50 (H) Humulin M3 (H) Insuman Comb 15,25,50 (H) Pork Mixtard 30 (P) Hypurin Porcine 30/70 Mix	0.5	4–12	18–24
	Biphasic insulin aspart (RHIA)	Novomix 30			
	Biphasic insulin lispro (RHIA)	Humalog Mix 25, Mix 50			
Long acting	Insulin detemir (RHIA)	Levemir			
	Insulin glargine (RHIA)	Lantus			
	Insulin zinc suspension*	Hypurin Bovine Lente (B)	3	6–15	18–24
	Protamine zinc insulin	Hypurin Bovine Protamine Zinc (B)	6	12–24	24–36

*A mixture of 30% amorphous and 70% crystalline insulin zinc suspension.

H, human sequence insulin; B, bovine highly purified insulin; P, porcine highly purified insulin; NPH, Neutral Protamine Hagedorn Insulin; RHIA, recombinant human insulin analogue.

Table 17.5 Oral hypoglycaemic agents in current use.

Drug	Proprietary preparations	Dose range (mg day^{-1})	Plasma half-life (h)	Elimination
Sulphonylureas				
Chlorpropamide	None	100–500	24–48	50% metabolised 50% excreted
Glibenclamide	Daonil Euglucon	3–15	8–12	>80% metabolised active metabolites
Gliclazide	Diamicron	40–320	9–13	>80% metabolised
Glimepiride	Amaryl	1–4	8–12	>80% metabolised
Glipizide	Glibenese Minodiab	3–40	5–9	>80% metabolised
Gliquidone	Glurenorm	15–180	3–7	>80% metabolised
Tolbutamide	None	500–2000	3–7	>95% metabolised
Meglitinides				
Neteglinide	Starlix	180–540	2–4	>80% metabolised
Repaglinide	Novonorm	1–18	2–4	>80% metabolised
Thiazolidinediones				
Pioglitazone	Actos	15–45	3–7	Active metabolites
Rosiglitazone	Avandia	4–8	4–7	Active metabolites
Other agents				
Metformin	Glucophage	500–1500	3–8	>95% excreted
Acarbose	Glucobay	50–300	4–10	>95% eliminated

These recombinant human insulin analogues form a microprecipitate in subcutaneous tissues, from which insulin is slowly absorbed. Consequently, they have a prolonged duration of action after subcutaneous injection, but do not usually cause nocturnal hypoglycaemia.

Glucagon

Glucagon is a polypeptide synthesised by the α-cells of the islets of Langerhans. It is commonly used parenterally in the emergency treatment of hypoglycaemic reactions, particularly when the administration of oral glucose is not feasible or practical.

Oral hypoglycaemic agents

Oral hypoglycaemic agents can be divided into four groups (Table 17.5):
• Sulphonylureas (and related drugs)
• Meglitinides
• Thiazolidinediones (glitazones)
• Other drugs

Sulphonylureas and related drugs

$$R_1 - \langle\bigcirc\rangle - SO_2 - NH - \overset{\overset{\displaystyle O}{\|}}{C} - NH - R_2$$

The sulphonylureas and some closely related drugs (Table 17.5) lower blood glucose by increasing insulin secretion by β-cells in the islets of Langerhans. Consequently, they may also cause degranulation and hyperplasia of functional β-cells.

Mode of action

The hypoglycaemic effects of sulphonylureas are due to the blockade of K_{ATP} channels in the cytoplasmic membrane of functional β-cells. Their competitive blockade reduces the resting potential, causing membrane depolarisation, enhanced Ca^{2+} entry and increased insulin secretion.

Some sulphonylureas may also reduce the secretion of glucagon and decrease the activity of hepatic insulinases.

Pharmacokinetics

Sulphonylureas are almost completely absorbed after oral administration. They are usually extensively metabolised in the liver, and although some of their metabolites possess hypoglycaemic activity (Table 17.5), this is not usually of clinical significance. Most sulphonylureas are highly bound to plasma proteins and have a volume of distribution similar to extracellular fluid volume (200 mL kg^{-1}) and a relatively short half-life (3–11 h). Chlorpropamide, unlike other sulphonylureas, is partly eliminated unchanged in urine and has a longer half-life (24–48 h). It may produce prolonged hypoglycaemia, particularly in elderly subjects and in patients with renal or hepatic disease.

Clinical use

Since sulphonylureas mainly act by enhancing the physiological secretion of insulin, their effects are dependent on the presence of functional β-cells. Consequently, they are mainly used in patients with Type II diabetes (i.e. maturity onset, non-insulin-dependent diabetes) who are not controlled by diet alone. Sulphonylureas are of little value in insulin-dependent diabetes, in patients with ketosis or in subjects with an insulin requirement of more than 30 units day^{-1}.

Adverse effects

All sulphonylureas tend to stimulate the appetite and may cause an increase in body weight. They may also produce gastrointestinal side effects and occasional hypersensitivity reactions (skin reactions, cholestatic jaundice and blood dyscrasias). The chronic administration of some sulphonylureas, particularly tolbutamide and chlorpropamide, is associated with alcohol intolerance, and genetically susceptible patients on these drugs may develop intense facial flushing due to vasodilatation.

Drug interactions

The hypoglycaemic effects of sulphonylureas are enhanced by some drugs and antagonised by others (Table 17.6). Some sulphonylureas (e.g. glibenclamide) produce slight diuresis, while others (e.g. chlorpropamide) can have antidiuretic effects and have been used in the treatment of diabetes insipidus.

Meglitinides

- Neteglinide
- Repaglinide

Table 17.6 Drug interactions with the sulphonylureas.

Drugs that enhance the effects of sulphonylureas	Drugs that antagonise the effects of sulphonylureas
Anticoagulants	Corticosteroids
β-Adrenergic antagonists	Diazoxide
Clofibrate	Thiazide diuretics
Fluconazole	
Miconazole	
MAOIs	
Probenecid	
Salicylates	
Sulphonamides	

Both neteglinide and repaglinide act in a similar manner to the sulphonylureas, and lower blood glucose by combining with high-affinity receptors on K$_{ATP}$ channels in islet β-cell plasma membranes. Channel blockade results in a reduction in the resting potential, depolarisation and an increase in insulin secretion. Meglitinides can compete with sulphonylureas for specific binding sites on K$_{ATP}$ channels, but have little or no effect on potassium channels in other tissues (e.g. vascular smooth muscle).

Both neteglinide and repaglinide are rapidly absorbed (within 30–60 min) and metabolised (half-life 120–240 min). Consequently, they have a short duration of action and a relatively low risk of hypoglycaemic reactions. Both drugs are used in Type II diabetes that is inadequately controlled by other measures, and may be combined with thiazolidinediones and metformin.

Thiazolidinediones (glitazones)

- Pioglitazone
- Rosiglitazone

The thiazolidinediones decrease blood glucose by reducing the resistance of peripheral tissues to insulin. Consequently, they increase insulin sensitivity, reduce glycogenolysis and impair hepatic glucose release.

Mode of action

Thiazolidinediones are bound by the nuclear receptor PPARγ (peroxisome proliferator-activated receptor gamma), which is mainly expressed in adipocytes, liver and skeletal muscle and usually forms a complex with the retinoid X receptor. They increase the binding of the complex by DNA, resulting in the transcription of genes that affect insulin sensitivity in adipose tissue and skeletal muscle. The effects of circulating insulin are enhanced, and lipogenesis and the uptake of triglycerides and unsaturated fatty acids are increased (thus reducing their plasma concentration).

Pharmacokinetics

Both pioglitazone and rosiglitazone are well absorbed after oral administration, extensively bound by plasma proteins and converted by hepatic cytochrome P450 to several active metabolites. The clearance of both drugs is reduced in hepatic impairment. Although the terminal half-lives of both drugs are relatively short (3–7 hours), their active metabolites are eliminated more slowly.

Clinical use

Thiazolidinediones have been primarily used in the treatment of Type II diabetes. They may be used alone or combined with other oral hypoglycaemic agents, such as the sulphonylureas or metformin. They usually have a relatively slow onset of action, and their maximum effects are observed only after 2–3 months. They do not cause hypoglycaemic reactions in either diabetic patients or normal subjects, unless combined with other drugs. In recent studies, rosiglitazone has been shown to impede the development of Type II diabetes in susceptible individuals.

Adverse effects

Both pioglitazone and rosiglitazone increase body weight by approximately 5%, mainly due to an increase in plasma volume and fluid retention. Ankle oedema and a mild degree of anaemia may also occur and can precipitate heart failure in susceptible individuals. Other adverse effects, including headache, fatigue and gastrointestinal disturbances, have also been reported.

Other drugs

Metformin

$$CH_3\diagdown N-C-NH-C-NH_2$$
$$CH_3\diagup$$

with NH groups double-bonded to the carbon atoms.

Metformin is a biguanide derivative that has little effect on blood glucose in normal conditions, but decreases insulin

requirements in diabetic subjects. It mainly acts by increasing the peripheral utilisation and metabolism of glucose by skeletal muscle and by reducing hepatic gluconeogenesis. It also affects fat metabolism and lowers the plasma concentration of triglycerides and LDL-cholesterol.

Metformin is extensively absorbed from the small intestine and is eliminated unchanged in urine. Although it frequently produces gastrointestinal side effects, its most serious complication is the occasional occurrence of lactic acidosis (which often has an insidious onset). Metformin may predispose patients to this condition by increasing lactate levels in blood, and its use in the elderly, in patients with renal or hepatic impairment or in alcoholic subjects may be hazardous. Nevertheless, metformin is commonly used in patients with Type II (non-insulin-dependent) diabetes who are not adequately controlled by diet and sulphonylurea drugs alone. It can be combined with other hypoglycaemic drugs (including insulin) if required.

Acarbose

Acarbose is an inhibitor of α-glucosidase, an enzyme which is present in the brush border of the small intestine and normally hydrolyses polysaccharides and disaccharides to monosaccharides. Consequently, acarbose slows the conversion of more complex sugars to monosaccharides and prevents or attenuates the normal postprandial increase in plasma glucose concentration by delaying the absorption of glucose from the small intestine.

Although acarbose is not significantly absorbed from the gut, it may cause an increase in the fermentation of unabsorbed carbohydrates. Consequently, abdominal distension, eructation and flatulence are relatively common. Hypoglycaemia should be prevented or treated with the monosaccharide dextrose (grape sugar) rather than the disaccharide sucrose (cane or beet sugar).

Acarbose is sometimes combined with other hypoglycaemic agents in the treatment of Type II diabetes.

In addition to its effects on α-glucosidase, acarbose may affect the activity of other enzyme systems that are concerned with the hydrolysis and absorption of carbohydrates.

Diabetes and general anaesthesia

Patients with diabetes are a high-risk group of surgical patients who are more likely to develop several postoperative problems, including metabolic and electrolyte abnormalities, cardiovascular sequelae, infection and delayed wound healing. Management of the disease in the perioperative period is complicated by several factors, in particular the metabolic response to stress and the effects of procedures and agents that are used during anaesthesia. The metabolic response to stress is particularly difficult to assess and varies considerably in different patients. Unfortunately, some diabetic patients may not be recognised or detected prior to surgery. The presence of glycosuria should always be excluded (or a fasting blood-glucose determined) in all patients before any operative procedure.

Surgical stress

In normal circumstances, surgical stress causes a rise in the metabolic rate, changes in carbohydrate, fat and protein metabolism, and the increased urinary elimination of nitrogen, phosphorus, potassium and calcium. The secretion of many hypothalamic, pituitary and adrenal hormones is increased. Surgical stress also affects the secretion of pancreatic hormones, and glucagon levels are increased and may be raised for several days.

Insulin secretion

Insulin secretion in non-diabetic subjects is normal or decreased during surgery, despite the presence of hyperglycaemia. It is generally accepted that the normal or reduced insulin levels are due to changes in the plasma concentration of endogenous catecholamines (mainly adrenaline). In the postoperative period, insulin secretion rises although hyperglycaemia is sustained (possibly due to enhanced gluconeogenesis). These metabolic changes are related to the extent and duration of surgery. They are slight and unimportant during minor procedures, but are enhanced during major surgery, particularly when complicated by shock or infection.

Management of diabetic patients

The management of diabetic patients during anaesthesia is aimed at the prevention of intraoperative or postoperative hypoglycaemia and the avoidance of excessive metabolic responses. Many regimes have been proposed and used for this purpose, and the management of diabetes during surgery has been a matter of some controversy. Ideally, the use of insulin should reflect the physiological changes in secretion that occur during surgical procedures in non-diabetic subjects.

Oral hypoglycaemic agents

It is generally accepted that patients who are controlled by diet alone or who are stabilised on low doses of short-acting oral antidiabetic drugs do not require additional therapy during minor surgical procedures. The morning dose should be omitted on the day of surgery. Small amounts of intravenous glucose may be required preoperatively, depending on the blood glucose concentration (which should be measured every 15 min during surgery). If persistent hyperglycaemia develops (>10 mmol L^{-1}), a glucose-insulin infusion may be required. Patients stabilised on chlorpropamide should probably be admitted to hospital several days prior to surgery and stabilised on insulin, given twice or three times daily, particularly if diabetic control is poor or major surgery is contemplated. Similarly, metformin may be stopped and changed to insulin before surgery, in order to prevent the possibility of intraoperative hypoglycaemia and lactic acidosis. The aim of these procedures is to ensure that diabetic patients are well controlled, normoglycaemic, non-ketotic and have adequate glycogen reserves prior to surgery.

Glucose–insulin–potassium infusion during surgery

In the past, several different regimes have been used for the administration of insulin and the control of blood glucose levels during surgery and the perioperative period. One common method involved the administration of half the daily insulin requirements on the morning of surgery, followed by the infusion of sufficient dextrose to maintain normoglycaemia (or slight hyperglycaemia). It is now recognised, particularly when patients are undergoing major surgical procedures, that these regimes are less satisfactory than methods based on the intravenous infusion of soluble insulin and the frequent monitoring of its effects on blood glucose. In diabetic patients stabilised on insulin who are undergoing major surgical procedures, infusions of glucose, insulin and potassium salts are now widely used during the perioperative period. One common regime is based on the administration of dextrose (10%) containing potassium chloride (20 mmol L^{-1}) and soluble insulin (20 units L^{-1}) at the rate of 100 mL h^{-1} on the day of surgery. The method depends on the frequent monitoring of serum potassium and blood glucose (at 60-min intervals) in order to regulate the dosage of insulin. If the blood glucose is 10–15 mmol L^{-1}, 30 units L^{-1} should be added; if the blood glucose is more than 15 mmol L^{-1}, 40 units L^{-1} should be added, while if the blood glucose is less than 5 mmol L^{-1}, 10 units L^{-1} should be used. This regime can be modified if hyperglycaemia is more marked or if fluid restriction is necessary due to cardiac failure. Blood glucose concentrations should be measured at 30–60-minute intervals. Although there is no danger of patients receiving insulin alone, some may be absorbed by glass or by plastic. Alternatively, dextrose (5%, with KCl approximately 10 mmol L^{-1}) and insulin can be separately infused, with the rate of insulin infusion (usually 2–4 units h^{-1}) controlled by frequent blood glucose determinations. The added KCl should be regulated to maintain plasma concentrations within normal limits (3.5–5.0 mmol L^{-1}). In many centres, separate infusions of dextrose and insulin are now commonly employed during surgery.

Postoperative management

In the postoperative period, there is commonly an increased insulin requirement, particularly if infection or other complications occur, and a moderate degree of hyperglycaemia is not unusual. Consequently, frequent monitoring of blood glucose may be needed to prevent the development of decompensation or ketosis. Infusion of fluids containing glucose, insulin and potassium salts may be continued for several days, while normal feeding is gradually established. As soon as the patient can take food or fluids orally, normal antidiabetic drug therapy can be resumed and the intravenous regime can be terminated. Insulin requirements may be 10–20% more than usual, particularly if the patient is unwell. Some patients may relapse and become persistently hyperglycaemic or may require additional soluble insulin or even reversion to an intravenous regime. Emergency surgery (particularly in the uncontrolled or ketotic diabetic patient) presents particular problems, and it is generally accepted that ketosis and abnormal fluid balance must be controlled before anaesthesia is induced.

Monitoring during surgery

It should be emphasised that the optimum control of diabetic patients during surgery depends on the frequent measurement of blood glucose (and potassium) concentrations. Blood glucose can be rapidly determined on the ward or in theatre by semiquantitative methods (i.e. glucose testing strips with an electronic glucose meter) which provide a relatively accurate assessment of the metabolic state. The determination of urinary glucose during the perioperative period may be extremely misleading and does not reflect blood glucose concentrations.

Drug interactions

Although some inhalational agents (ether and cyclopropane) can cause hyperglycaemia, most agents in current use, including nitrous oxide, all fluorinated agents, thiopental, propofol, opioid analgesics and all muscle relaxants, have little or no effect on blood glucose. Nevertheless, other drugs that may be used in the perioperative period, including ketamine, diazoxide, adrenaline, β-adrenoceptor antagonists and corticosteroids, may significantly modify blood glucose levels.

β-Adrenoceptor antagonists are particularly hazardous, since they may induce and potentiate hypoglycaemia but obscure all its peripheral clinical signs.

Increased secretion of endogenous adrenaline may cause marked hyperglycaemia in the nervous and excitable patient. Similarly, hypoxia and hypercarbia increase adrenaline secretion, and may cause a considerable rise in blood glucose concentration.

Suggested reading

Alberti, K.G.M.M. & Thomas, D.J.B. (1979) The management of diabetes during surgery. *British Journal of Anaesthesia* **51**, 693–710.

Barnes, P.J. & Adcock, I. (1993) Anti-inflammatory actions of steroids: molecular mechanisms. *Trends in Pharmacological Sciences* **14**, 436–441.

Barnett, A.H. & Owens, D.R. (1997) Insulin analogues. *Lancet* **349**, 47–51.

Best, L. (2002) Pharmacological control of blood sugar. *Anaesthesia and Intensive Care Medicine* **3**, 346–348.

Bolli, G.B. & Owens, D.R. (2000) Insulin glargine. *Lancet* **356**, 443–445.

Cheatham, B. & Kahn, C.R. (1995) Insulin action and the insulin signaling network. *Endocrinological Reviews* **16**, 117–142.

Christiansen, C.L., Schurizek, B.A., Malling, B., *et al.* (1988) Insulin treatment of the insulin-dependent diabetic patient undergoing minor surgery – continuous intravenous infusion compared with subcutaneous administration. *Anaesthesia* **43**, 533–537.

Chrousos, G.P. (1995) The hypothalamic–pituitary–adrenal axis and immune-mediated inflammation. *New England Journal of Medicine* **332**, 1351–1362.

Dornhorst, A. (2001) Insulinotropic meglitinide analogues. *Lancet* **358**, 1709–1716.

Dunnet, J.M., Holman, R.R., Turner, R.C., *et al.* (1988) Diabetes mellitus and anaesthesia – a survey of the peri-operative management of the patient with diabetes mellitus. *Anaesthesia* **43**, 538–542.

Flower, R.J. (1988) Lipocortin and the mechanism of action of the glucocorticoids. *British Journal of Pharmacology* **94**, 987–1015.

Fonseca, V., Rosenstock, J., Patwardhan, R., *et al.* (2000) Effect of metformin and rosiglitazone combination therapy in patients with Type 2 diabetes mellitus: a randomized controlled trial. *Journal of the American Medical Association* **283**, 1695–1702.

Funder, J.W. (1997) Glucocorticoid and mineralocorticoid receptors, biology and clinical relevance. *Annual Review of Medicine* **48**, 231–240.

Gill, G.V. & Alberti, K.G.M.M. (1989) Surgery and diabetes. *Hospital Update* **5**, 327–336.

Heald, A. (2002) Adrenocortical hormones. *Anaesthesia and Intensive Care Medicine* **3**, 327–330.

Kahn, C.R. (1994) Banting Lecture. Insulin action, diabetogenes, and the cause of type II diabetes. *Diabetes* **43**, 1066–1084.

Marx, J. (1995) How the glucocorticoids suppress immunity. *Science* **270**, 232–233.

McAnulty, G.R. (2000) Anaesthetic management of patients with diabetes mellitus. *British Journal of Anaesthesia* **85**, 80–90.

Owens, D.R., Zinman, B. & Bolli, G.B. (2001) Insulin today and beyond. *Lancet* **358**, 739–746.

Philipson, L.H. & Steiner, D.F. (1995) Pas de deux or more: the sulfonylurea receptor and K^+ channels. *Science* **268**, 372–373.

Porter, A.L. & McCrirrick, A. (2002) Anaesthetic management of the diabetic patient. *Anaesthesia and Intensive Care Medicine* **3**, 316–319.

Ramirez, V.D. (1996) How do steroids act? *Lancet* **347**, 630–631.

Saltiel, A.R. & Pessin, J.E. (2002) Insulin signaling pathways in space and time. *Trends in Cell Biology* **12**, 65–70.

Scherpereel, P.A. (2001) Perioperative care of the diabetic patient. *European Journal of Anaesthesia* **18**, 227–294.

Tan, G. (2002) The pancreas. *Anaesthesia and Intensive Care Medicine* **3**, 330–333.

White, M.F. & Kahn, C.R. (1994) The insulin signaling system. *Journal of Biological Chemistry* **269**, 1–4.

Wilckens, T. (1995) Glucocorticoids and immune function, physiological relevance and pathogenic potential of hormonal dysfunction. *Trends in Pharmacological Sciences* **16**, 193–197.

Glossary

The glossary contains most of the common abbreviations used in the book. The mathematical symbols used in Chapters 2 and 3 are defined separately. Common chemical symbols (e.g. H^+, K^+, Na^+ and Ca^{2+}) have not been included.

Units of length, mass, volume and time

m	metre
mm	millimetre
μm	micrometre (micron)
nm	nanometre
kg	kilogram
g	gram
mg	milligram
μg	microgram
ng	nanogram
L	litre
mL	millilitre
μL	microlitre
h	hour
min	minute
s	second
ms	millisecond
μs	microsecond

Other abbreviations

ACE	angiotensin converting enzyme
AChE	acetylcholinesterase
ACTH	adrenocorticotrophic hormone
ADH	antidiuretic hormone
AHG	anti-haemophilic globulin
ADP	adenosine diphosphate
AMP	adenosine monophosphate
AMPA	α-amino-3-hydroxy-5-methyl-4-isoxazole proprionic acid
ATP	adenosine triphosphate
ANP	atrial natriuretic peptide
APD	action potential duration
APTT	activated partial thromboplastin time
ATP	adenosine triphosphate
AT	angiotensin
AV	atrioventricular
BChE	butyrocholinesterase (plasma cholinesterase)
cAMP	cyclic adenosine monophosphate
CCK	cholecystokinin
cGMP	cyclic guanosine monophosphate
CGRP	calcitonin gene-related peptide
ChE	cholinesterase
CNS	central nervous system
COMT	catechol-O-methyltransferase
COX	cyclooxygenase
CRF	corticotrophin releasing factor
CSF	cerebrospinal fluid
CTZ	chemoreceptor trigger zone
CVS	cardiovascular system
CYP	isoforms of the cytochrome P450 enzyme system
δ-ALA	delta-aminolaevulinic acid
Da	Dalton (unit of molecular weight)
DDAVP	desmopressin acetate
DIC	disseminated intravascular coagulation
EC	excitation–contraction
ECF	extracellular fluid
ECG	electrocardiogram
ED_{50}	median effective dose
EDRF	endothelial-derived relaxant factor (nitric oxide)
EEG	electroencephalogram
EMLA	eutectic mixture of local anaesthetics
ENT	ear, nose and throat
EPP	endplate potential
ET	endothelin
FRC	functional residual capacity
GABA	γ-aminobutyric acid
GH	growth hormone

GMP	guanosine monophosphate
GTP	guanosine triphosphate
GTN	glyceryl trinitrate (nitroglycerine)
G6PD	glucose-6-phosphate dehydrogenase
^{3}H	tritium labelled
HMWK	high molecular weight kininogen
HSP	heat shock protein
5-HT	5-hydroxytryptamine
Hz	hertz (a frequency of 1 stimulus per second)
ICP	intracranial pressure
IgE	immunoglobulin E
IgG	immunoglobulin G
i.m.	intramuscular
INR	international normalized ratio
IPPV	intermittent positive pressure ventilation
IP$_3$	inositol trisphosphate
ISA	intrinsic sympathomimetic activity
i.u.	international unit
i.v.	intravenous
IVRA	intravenous regional analgesia
kDa	kiloDaltons (units of molecular weight)
kPa	kilopascals (1 kilopascal = 7.5 mm Hg)
LD$_{50}$	median lethal dose
LMWH	low molecular weight heparin
MAC	minimum alveolar concentration
MAO	monoamine oxidase
MAOI	monoamine oxidase inhibitors
MAP	muscle action potential
MEPP	miniature endplate potential
MHPG	3-methoxy-4-hydroxy-phenylethylene-glycol
MSH	melanocyte stimulating hormone
mV	millivolt
MW	molecular weight
NADPH	reduced nicotinamide adenine dinucleotide phosphate
NANC	non-adrenergic non-cholinergic
NGF	nerve growth factor
NK	neurokinin
NMDA	N-methyl-D-aspartate
NO	nitric oxide
NOS	nitric oxide synthase
NRM	nucleus raphe magnus
NSAID	non-steroidal anti-inflammatory drug
NTS	nucleus tractus solitarius
P$_{CO_2}$	carbon dioxide tension
P$_{ACO_2}$	alveolar carbon dioxide tension
Pa$_{CO_2}$	arterial carbon dioxide tension
PABA	para-aminobenzoic acid
PAF	platelet activating factor

pH	$-\log_{10}[H^+]$
pKa	$-\log_{10}[K]$ (dissociation exponent)
PAG	periaqueductal grey matter
PG	prostaglandin
PGI$_2$	prostacyclin
PLA$_2$	phospholipase A$_2$
p.p.m.	parts per million
PDE	phosphodiesterase
PRA	plasma renin activity
PT	prothrombin time
REM	rapid eye movement
RNA	ribonucleic acid
SA	sinoatrial
s.c.	subcutaneous
SLE	systemic lupus erythematosus
SNP	sodium nitroprusside
sp.gr	specific gravity
$t_{1/2}$	half-life
t.d.s.	thrice daily
THF	tetrahydrofolate
TNF	tumour necrosis factor
tPA	tissue type plasminogen activator
TX	thromboxane
TXA$_2$	thromboxane A$_2$
UDP	uridine diphosphate
v/v	volume for volume
VMA	vanillylmandelic acid (3-methoxy-4-hydroxy-mandelic acid)

Greek letters

α	alpha
β	beta
γ	gamma
δ	delta
ε	epsilon
κ	kappa
λ	lambda
μ	mu
ν	nu
π	pi
ρ	rho
σ	sigma

Symbols

$\approx$	approximately equals
$\propto$	is proportional to
∞	infinity

Index